cytology and microscopic anatomy

The National Veterinary Medical Series for Independent Study

cytology and microscopic anatomy

H.-Dieter Dellmann, Docteur-Vétérinaire, Habil.

Clarence Hartley Covault Distinguished Professor
Department of Veterinary Anatomy
Iowa State University
College of Veterinary Medicine
Ames, Iowa

Jeanine R. Carithers, Ph.D.

Professor Emeritus
Department of Veterinary Anatomy
Iowa State University
College of Veterinary Medicine
Ames, Iowa

SANS TACHE

Williams & Wilkins

BALTIMORE • PHILADELPHIA • HONG KONG
LONDON • MUNICH • SYDNEY • TOKYO

A WAVERLY COMPANY
1996

Williams
& Wilkins

Acquisitions Editor: Elizabeth A. Nieginski
Development Editors: Melanie Cann, Lynne Stockton
Managing Editor: Amy G. Dinkel
Copy Editor: Stephen Jensen
Production Coordinator: Peter J. Carley
Illustrator: Birck Cox
Editorial Coordinator: Beth Goldner

The publisher gratefully acknowledges the Professional Examination Service (PES) for providing information about the format and content of the National Board Examination (NBE) for Veterinary Medical Licensing.

Williams & Wilkins
Suite 5025
Rose Tree Corporate Center
Building Two
1400 N. Providence Road
Media, PA 19063 USA

Printed in the United States of America

Library of Congress Cataloging-in-Publication Data
Dellmann, Horst-Dieter.
Cytology and microscopic anatomy / H.-Dieter Dellmann, Jeanine R. Carithers.
p. cm. — (The National veterinary medicine series for independent study)
Includes index.
ISBN 0-683-01467-6
1. Veterinary histology—Outlines, syllabi, etc. 2. Veterinary histology—Examinations, questions, etc. 3. Veterinary cytology—Outlines, syllabi, etc. 4. Veterinary cytology—Examinations, questions, etc. I. Carithers, Jeanine R. II. Title. III. Series.
SF757.3.D437 1995
636.089'1018'076—dc20 95-14964
CIP

96 97 98
10 9 8 7 6 5 4 3 2 1

Contents

Preface

This book is designed to provide a succinct overview of histology for students in veterinary medicine. It covers essential information to be reviewed in preparation for National Board Examinations. The first four chapters cover cytology. They are followed by six chapters devoted to the basic tissues, and by twelve chapters dealing with the microscopic anatomy of organs or organ systems. The outline format permits fast retrieval of facts, and the information and explanations are concise to facilitate and enhance the reviewing process. Each chapter is followed by multiple-choice study questions with answers and explanations for immediate feedback, and a comprehensive examination concludes the book. We hope that this book fulfills the purpose for which it was designed, and we encourage constructive criticism from students and other readers.

H.-Dieter Dellmann
Jeanine R. Carithers

Acknowledgments

We thank the College of Veterinary Medicine at Iowa State University, and especially the Department of Veterinary Anatomy, for encouraging us to accept the invitation to write this book and for providing the academic and physical environment in which the writing could be accomplished. Mr. Randy DenAdel's skillful assistance in the photolaboratory is gratefully acknowledged. We appreciate the excellent editorial input provided by Melanie Cann, and we thank the anonymous reviewers for their comments and helpful suggestions.

Chapter 1

The Nucleus and Organelles of Protein Synthesis

I. NUCLEUS.

NUCLEUS. All eukaryotic cells have a nucleus. In exceptional cell types (e.g., mammalian red blood cells), the nucleus may be lost after the cell matures. Certain cell types (e.g., skeletal muscle cells) normally have more than one nucleus.

A. Fine structure and function (Figure 1-1). The nucleus is a restricted region containing the cell's genetic material, deoxyribonucleic acid (DNA). Its contents, collectively called **nucleoplasm,** are separated from the rest of the cell, which is called the **cytoplasm,** by a double-layered membranous envelope.

1. **Nucleoplasm.** The nucleoplasm contains **chromatin** and the **nucleolus.**
   - a. **Chromatin** consists of **DNA** and **protein**. Proteins in chromatin modulate the transcription of DNA.
     - (1) **DNA contains genetic information.**
     - (2) **DNA directs protein synthesis,** thus regulating the cell's activities.
       - (a) **Transcription of DNA is the first step in protein synthesis.** During transcription, DNA is used as a template (pattern) for synthesis of **ribonucleic acid (RNA)** molecules.
         - (i) **Euchromatin** contains DNA that is being transcribed; it is uncoiled (i.e., extended) to facilitate access by enzymes involved in RNA synthesis and nucleotides, which are the building blocks of RNA. Because the euchromatin is extended, the regions it occupies are electron lucent (Figure 1-2A; see Figure 1-1).
         - (ii) **Heterochromatin** contains DNA that is not involved in transcription. This chromatin is condensed; therefore, it appears as electron-dense regions in the nucleus. In females, the second X chromosome remains coiled during interphase; this **sex chromatin** (or **Barr body**) has a characteristic location in each cell type and can be seen as a nuclear appendage in some neutrophils (see Figure 8-8D).
         - (iii) Chromatin shifts back and forth between heterochromatic and euchromatic forms whenever the amount or variety of proteins synthesized by the cell is altered.
       - (b) **Replication** of DNA occurs before cell division. During replication, an exact copy of each DNA molecule is formed using the original DNA as a template.
         - (i) After replication, each DNA molecule becomes very tightly wound into a darkly staining **chromosome** during prophase of mitosis.
         - (ii) During cell division, chromosomes containing identical DNA molecules pass to each of the daughter cells.
   - b. The **nucleolus,** a distinct spheroidal structure comprising thick cords of electron-dense fibrils and granules interspersed with electron-lucent regions (see Figure 1-1), is the site of ribosomal RNA (rRNA) production. The electron-dense regions contain rRNA and protein, and the electron-lucent regions contain portions of DNA called **nucleolar organizers** that encode rRNA.
     - (1) The rRNA combines with protein from the cytoplasm before leaving the nucleus via nuclear pores (see I A 2 a) to form ribosomes in the cytoplasm.
     - (2) When cells increase their level of protein synthesis, their nucleoli increase in size and may increase in number. Conversely, nucleoli become smaller and fewer when protein synthesis declines.
   - c. **Water** and a variety of **soluble molecules** surround the chromatin and nucleolar material.

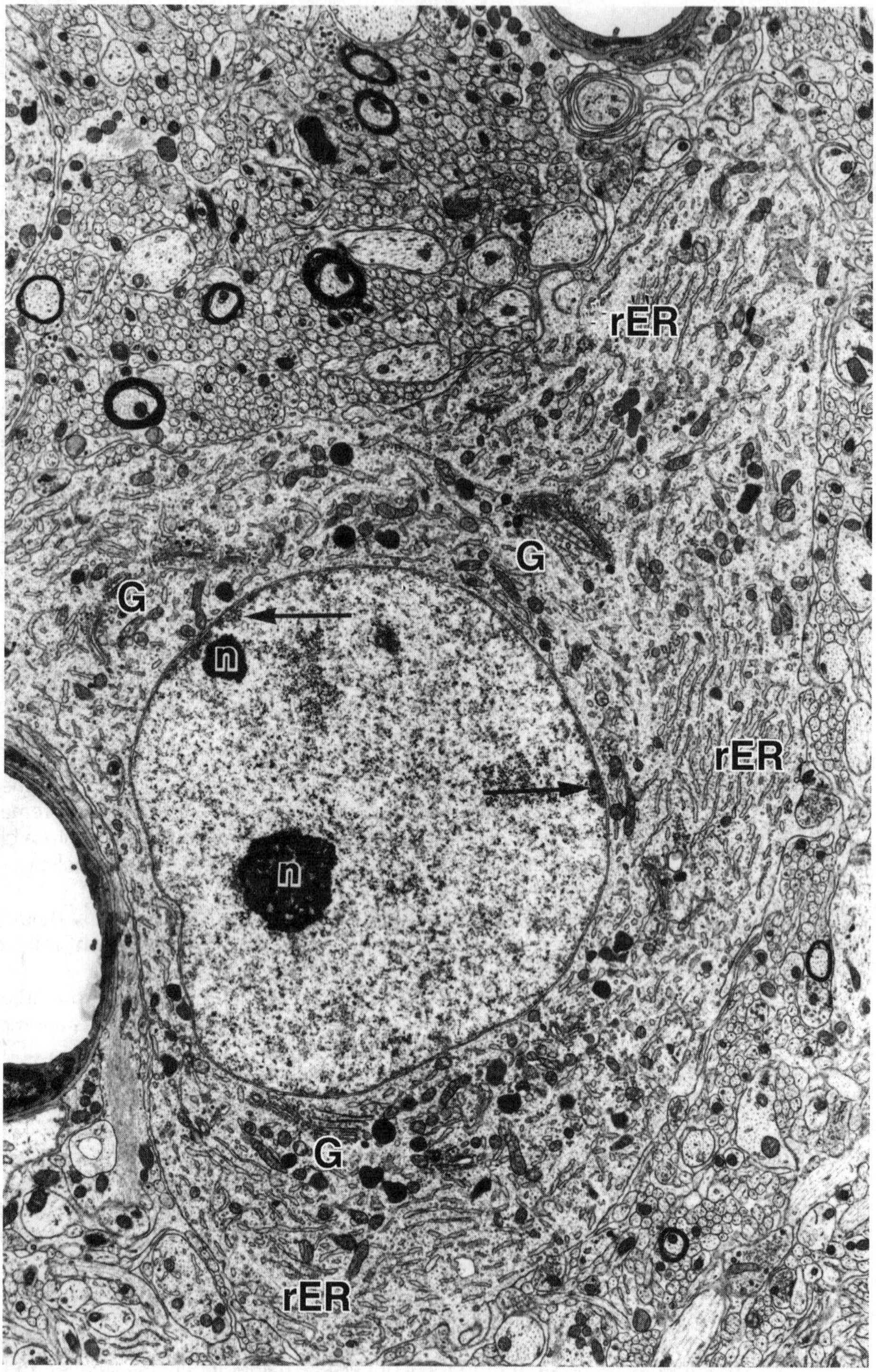

Figure 1-1. Electron micrograph of a nerve cell with a large nucleus that contains two nucleoli (*n*). Areas occupied by euchromatin appear light because euchromatin is uncoiled (i.e., extended) for ease of ribonucleic acid (RNA) transcription. A small amount of inactive heterochromatin, which appears dark because it is condensed, lies adjacent to the nuclear envelope (*arrows*). Components of the Golgi complex (*G*) lie on all sides of the nucleus, and several peripheral accumulations of rough endoplasmic reticulum (*rER*) are present.

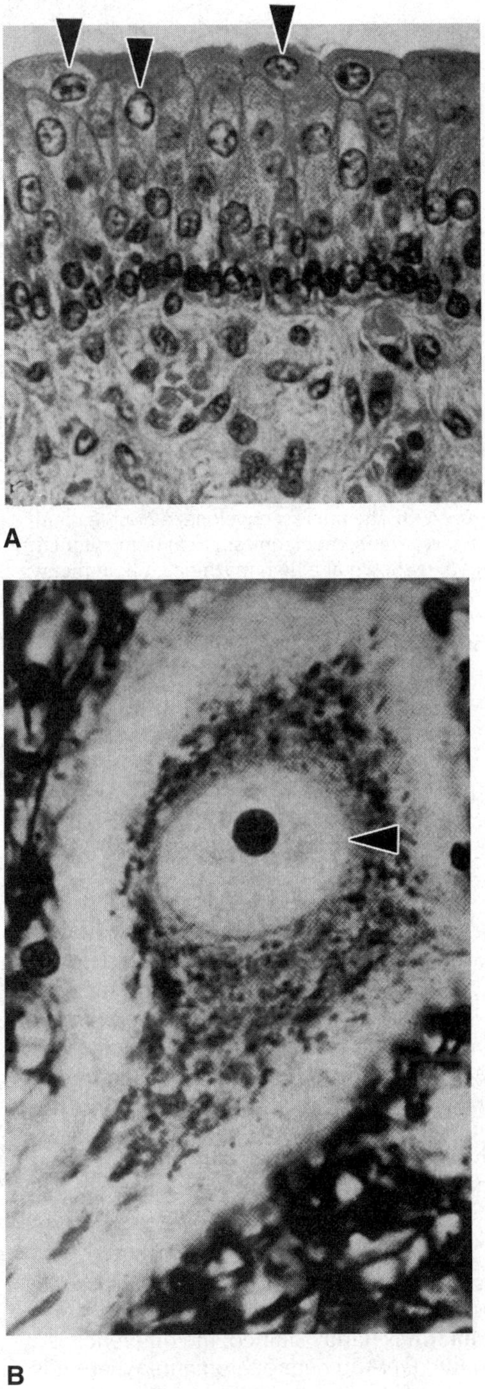

Figure 1-2. Light micrographs of cells sectioned through their nuclei (*arrows*). (*A*) Patterns of light euchromatin and darkly stained heterochromatin are noticeable in these nuclei. Hematoxylin–eosin. (*B*) A nerve cell active in protein synthesis. Its large nucleus appears pale because most of its chromatin is active euchromatin. The large nucleolus is densely stained. The pale chromatin and distinct nucleolus are both signs of active protein synthesis. Cresyl violet–Luxol fast blue. (Reprinted from Dellmann H-D: *Textbook of Veterinary Histology,* 4th ed. Baltimore, Williams & Wilkins, 1993, pp 3, 22.)

2. **Nuclear envelope.** The nuclear envelope separates the nucleus from the cytoplasm (Figure 1-3).
   a. It **consists of two membranes,** which are fused at many points to form **nuclear pores**. The pores permit restricted movement of molecules between the cytoplasm and nucleoplasm.
   b. The outer membrane can be continuous with membranes of the **rough endoplasmic reticulum (rER),** in which case the space enclosed by the two membranes (perinuclear cisterna) communicates directly with the rER cisternae.

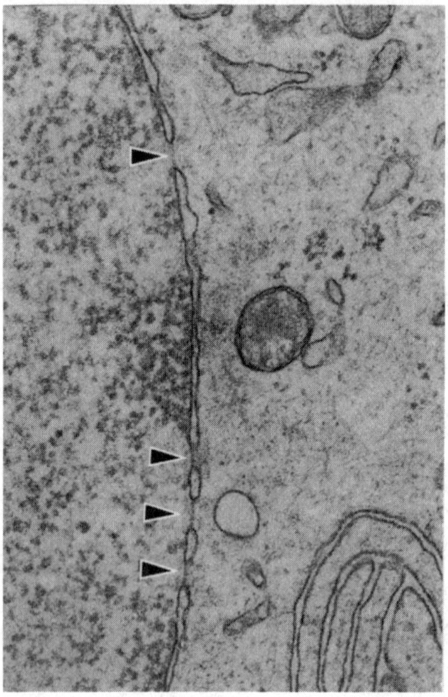

Figure 1-3. The nuclear envelope, a double membrane separating nucleoplasm (*left*) from cytoplasm (*right*), is shown at a high magnification. In many spots the two membranes fuse to form nuclear pores (*arrows*). Nuclear pores permit selective passage of materials between the nucleoplasm and the cytoplasm.

c. The nuclear envelope disappears during cell division and is reformed from the rER after mitosis.

B. Light-microscope appearance (see Figure 1-2)

1. Most stains that are used to reveal histologic structure depend on the formation of electrostatic linkages between the acidic and basic components of the staining mixture and the tissue.
   a. Tissue elements that bind more readily with basic dyes are said to be **basophilic;** those that stain with acidic dyes are termed **acidophilic**.
   b. The intensity of coloration is directly related to the concentration of anionic or cationic sites in the structure being stained.
   c. The most commonly used staining mixture is **hematoxylin and eosin (H&E)**.
      (1) **Hematoxylin** acts like a **basic dye;** therefore, it stains chromatin and other acidic structures (e.g., ribosomes, glycosaminoglycans) **blue**.
      (2) **Eosin,** which is an **acidic dye,** stains most other components of the cytoplasm and intercellular material **red or pink**.
2. The nucleus, due to the pronounced basophilia of the DNA in its chromatin, is usually a striking feature of a cell at the light-microscope level.
   a. **Euchromatin** is pale, whereas **heterochromatin** is darkly stained; the difference is due to the greater concentration of basophilic DNA in heterochromatin, where it is condensed, than in euchromatin, where it is extended.
      (1) The ratio of euchromatin to heterochromatin is a good indication of how active a cell is: More active cells have more euchromatin; therefore, their nuclei are larger and lighter (see Figure 1-2B).
      (2) Even in very euchromatic nuclei, such as those in active secretory cells and large neurons, the periphery of the nucleus is marked by a thin layer of heterochromatin.

b. **Nucleoli** are the most darkly stained structures in cells processed with standard stains, because of their highly concentrated basophilic RNA. They are most prominent in cells that are actively synthesizing proteins (e.g., secretory cells, neurons, and malignant neoplasms).
c. The **nuclear envelope** and its pores are well below the limit of resolution with the light microscope; however, the location of the membranes is usually marked by a layer of basophilic heterochromatin that coats the inner membrane of the nuclear envelope between pores.

II. ORGANELLES OF PROTEIN SYNTHESIS.

Protein synthesis is programmed by nuclear DNA, but it is completed in the cytoplasm.

A. RNA molecules

1. **Three types of RNA molecules** pass through nuclear pores to enter the cytoplasm, where they collaborate to produce peptides and proteins.
   a. **Messenger RNA (mRNA)** encodes the amino acid sequence to be produced. The portion encoding one amino acid is called a codon. For each type of protein synthesized in a cell, mRNA with a specific codon sequence is produced.
   b. **Ribosomal RNA (rRNA).** Ribosomes, which contain RNA, activate successive codons on the mRNA molecule. All ribosomes in a cell are similar; they are not specific for a certain type of mRNA or amino acid.
   c. **Transfer RNA (tRNA).** Each molecule of tRNA, also called soluble RNA (sRNA), can form a complex with only one type of amino acid. The tRNA then recognizes a corresponding activated codon and aligns its amino acid to be incorporated into the forming peptide chain.

2. **Translation.** The process in which a specific protein is synthesized using the coded message transcribed from DNA onto a molecule of mRNA is called translation.

B. Ribosomes

1. **Formation** (see Figure 1-4). Ribosomes are cytoplasmic granules approximately 11 nm in diameter.
   a. In the cytoplasm, ribosomal subunits from the nucleolus combine to form ribosomes when they interact with a molecule of mRNA.
   b. Each ribosome has a small subunit that binds to mRNA at the "start codon," and a large subunit that helps form the peptide bond and holds the growing peptide chain. Part of the recognition site for tRNA is present on each subunit.
   c. Numerous ribosomes, each creating a separate peptide chain, become associated with each mRNA molecule. Such a group of ribosomes is called a **polyribosome,** often shortened to **polysome** (Figure 1-4, *inset*).

2. **Distribution.** Some ribosomes are free within the cytoplasm; others are attached by their large subunits to membranes of the endoplasmic reticulum (ER).

3. **Function.** Ribosomes are the engines of protein synthesis; the total number of ribosomes in a cell is directly related to the rate of protein synthesis.
   a. **Free (unattached) ribosomes** synthesize protein for use within the cytoplasm.
   b. **Ribosomes attached to the ER** synthesize proteins for secretion, lysosomal enzymes, and proteins for new membranes.

4. **Light-microscope appearance**
   a. Individual ribosomes and polysomes are far below the limits of resolution with the light microscope.
   b. Cells containing large numbers of free ribosomes (e.g., neurons, rubriblasts, and rapidly growing cells, including malignant neoplasms) are basophilic, because of the nucleic acid (the RNA) in the ribosomes.

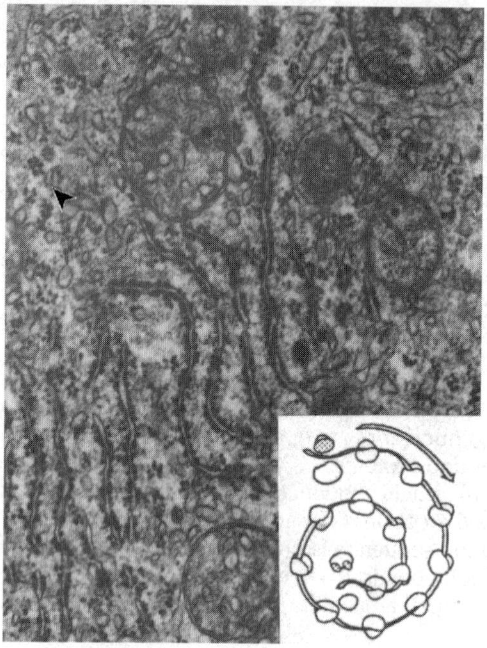

Figure 1-4. Electron micrograph of rough endoplasmic reticulum (rER). In addition to polysomes on the rER, this cell contains many free polysomes (*arrow*). (Reprinted with permission from Dellmann H-D: *Textbook of Veterinary Histology,* 4th ed. Baltimore, Williams & Wilkins, 1993, p 3.) The *inset* shows how a polysome comprises a series of ribosomes attached to a molecule of messenger ribonucleic acid (mRNA).

c. Large fluctuations in the number of ribosomes can be detected at the light-microscope level as changes in cytoplasmic basophilia.

C. Rough endoplasmic reticulum (rER)

1. **Structure and distribution** (see Figures 1-1 and 1-4)
   - **a.** The rER (so called because ribosomes attached to its outer surface give it a rough appearance) is usually in the form of flattened cisternae, often joined by tubules.
   - **b.** In cells with very abundant rER, the cisternae are packed like lamellae (i.e., stacks of parallel cisternae). These are typically concentrated in the part of the cell that is nearest to the surface where amino acids and other nutrients enter the cell from nearby blood vessels (Figure 1-5).
2. **Functions.** The rER synthesizes proteins for secretion and lysosomal enzymes; it also synthesizes proteins, carbohydrates, and lipids for membranes.
   - **a. Protein synthesis** (Figure 1-6). The two large classes of proteins produced in the rER are secretory products, which are exported, and lysosomal enzymes, which remain in the cell. Both are packaged in membranes that are also produced by the rER.
     - **(1)** Each mRNA molecule for proteins that are destined to enter the lumen of the rER encodes a **signal peptide sequence** at the beginning of the new peptide chain. This signal peptide sequence binds to a cytoplasmic signal recognition protein, which interacts with a receptor in the rER membrane, and the ribosome becomes attached to the ER membrane.
     - **(2)** Proteins synthesized by attached ribosomes enter the cisternal cavity as they are formed; there they are isolated from other cytoplasmic components and undergo further processing (see Figure 1-6).
       - **(a)** The signal sequence is usually removed.
       - **(b)** Disulfide bonds form, establishing secondary and tertiary conformations.
       - **(c)** Oligosaccharides are added to most proteins.
   - **b. Membrane synthesis.** Membranes for all parts of the cell are also synthesized by the rER; therefore, some rER is typically present even in cells that do not secrete proteins.
     - **(1)** The protein components of membranes are produced by the attached ribosomes.
     - **(2)** The lipid and carbohydrate components are synthesized by enzymes that are integral parts of the ER membrane itself.

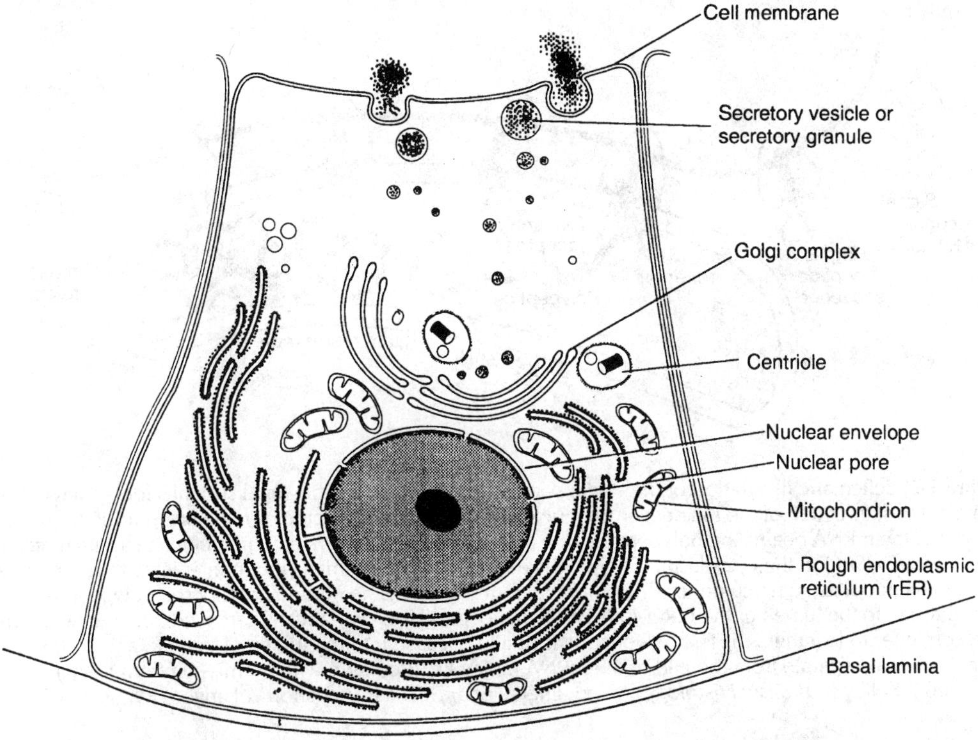

Figure 1-5. Schematic drawing of the organization of organelles in a polarized secretory cell. Rough endoplasmic reticulum (rER) is concentrated in the basal cytoplasm, near the bottom of the drawing. This part of the cell is closest to the underlying capillaries, the source of the amino acids that will be used in protein synthesis. The many mitochondria in this region provide a ready source of energy. The Golgi complex is above the nucleus, where its immature face receives transfer vesicles from the subjacent rER and its mature face gives rise to secretory vesicles that occupy the apical cytoplasm. Secretory products are released by exocytosis (i.e., by fusion of the secretory vesicle with the apical plasma membrane and opening of its lumen to the extracellular space), as shown at the top of the drawing. (Adapted with permission from Dellmann H-D: *Textbook of Veterinary Histology,* 4th ed. Baltimore, Williams & Wilkins, 1993, p 2.)

3. Light-microscope appearance

a. Individual cisternae of rER are too small for resolution with the light microscope.

b. The membrane of rER has no staining affinity, but the attached ribosomes are intensely basophilic. Therefore, concentrations of rER are visible, and examples in some cell types are so characteristic that they have been named.

(1) Clumps of basophilic rER and free ribosomes in nerve cells are called Nissl bodies or Nissl substance (see Figure 1-2B).

(2) Stacks of basophilic rER in gland cells are called ergastoplasm.

c. The amount of rER in a cell is directly related to the rate of synthesis of lysosomal enzymes and protein for export. Therefore, a cell's secretory activity may be estimated by its basophilia.

D. Golgi complex

1. Structure and distribution (Figure 1-7)

a. The Golgi complex is composed of 3–15 parallel cisternae and associated vesicles.

b. The **cisternae** of the Golgi complex are usually represented as they appear in polarized cells, where they form a compact stack at the apical pole of the nucleus (see

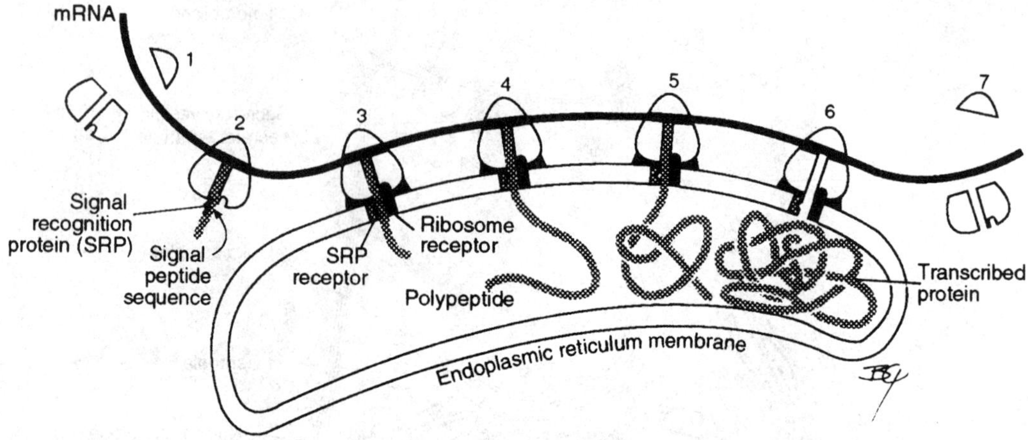

Figure 1-6. Schematic illustration of the signal peptide hypothesis. (*1*) Ribosomal subunits form a new ribosome at the start codon of the messenger ribonucleic acid (*mRNA*) molecule. (*2*) The first portion (signal codon) of the mRNA begins the polypeptide with a signal peptide sequence, which binds to a signal recognition protein (SRP) in the cytoplasm. (*3*) The SRP and the large ribosomal subunit interact with receptors in the rough endoplasmic reticulum (rER) membrane, forming a transmembrane pore for the polypeptide to pass through to the lumen of the rER. (*4, 5*) The signal peptide is enzymatically removed, and the polypeptide continues to lengthen. (*6*) The polypeptide is finally released into the lumen of the rER, and (*7*) the ribosomal subunits separate from the end of the mRNA molecule. (Redrawn with permission from Junqueira LC, Carneiro J, Kelley RO: *Basic Histology,* 7th ed. Englewood Cliffs, NJ, Appleton & Lange, 1992, p 119.)

Figure 1-5). However, the overall shape of the stacks of cisternae is variable in unpolarized cells; for example, they form a widespread network in endocrine and nerve cells (see Figure 1-1).

(1) The convex surface of the cisternae nearer the nucleus (proximal) is called the forming, or *cis,* face.

(2) The concave surface facing the plasma membrane (distal) is called the mature, or *trans,* face.

c. Small **transfer vesicles** are most numerous near the forming face and edges of the cisternal stack. They bud off ribosome-free areas of the rER and carry proteins to the Golgi complex, where they fuse with the forming face (see Figure 1-7).

d. Secretory vesicles and **condensing vacuoles** (see II D 2 b) form at the mature face.

(1) Secretory vesicles move directly to the cell membrane.

(2) Condensing vacuoles, which are not released immediately, give rise to **secretory granules**.

2. Functions

a. Newly synthesized proteins from the rER are transferred to the Golgi complex for final processing and packaging.

(1) Processing takes place while the proteins move toward the mature face of the Golgi complex.

(a) Unnecessary segments of the peptide chain are removed.

(b) Carbohydrates are synthesized in the Golgi complex and added to some glycoproteins; other carbohydrates are removed.

(c) Lipids are synthesized or imported from smooth endoplasmic reticulum (sER) and complexed with proteins.

(d) Water is removed, conserving it for the cell and concentrating the secretory material.

(2) Acid hydrolases, enzymes destined for lysosomes, are segregated from the secretory products that will be released from the cell.

b. Completed products leave the mature face of the Golgi complex.

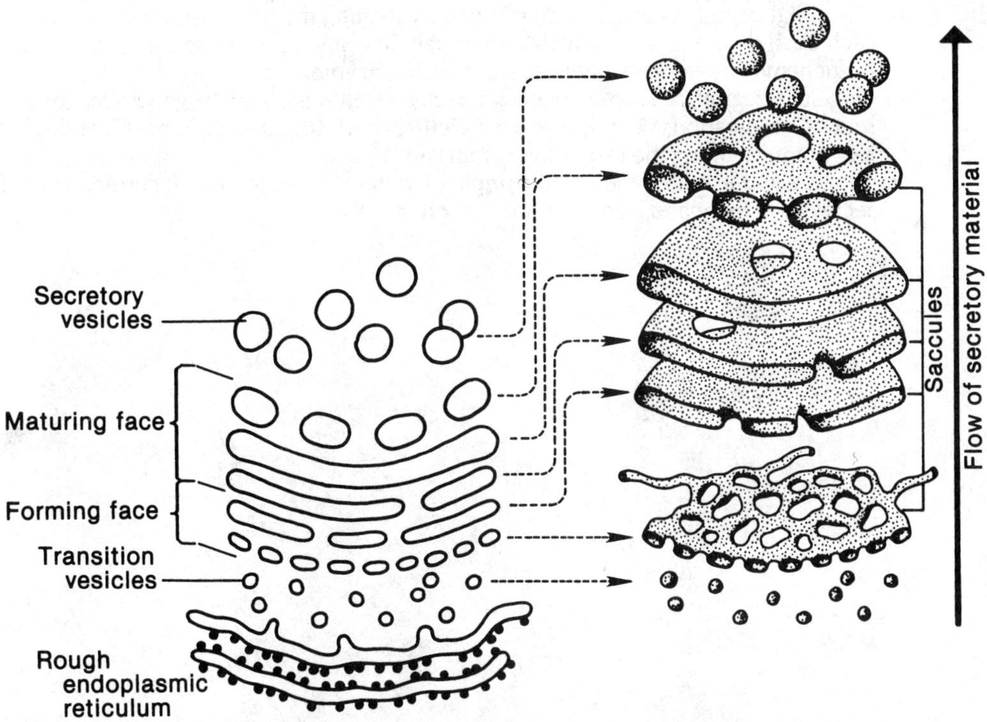

Figure 1-7. Diagram of the secretory pathway through the rough endoplasmic reticulum (rER) and Golgi complex. (Reprinted from Thorpe NO: *Cell Biology.* New York, John Wiley, 1984, p 360.)

(1) In cells that secrete constantly (i.e., **constitutive secretion**), small secretory vesicles carry their products directly to the cell membrane.
   (a) **Exocytosis** (release) begins with fusion of the secretory vesicle and the cell membrane.
   (b) The fused portion of the membrane immediately breaks down, opening the lumen of the vesicle and releasing its contents to the exterior of the cell (see Figure 1-5).
   (c) The addition of new membrane to the cell surface during exocytosis is balanced by internalization of membrane to be degraded or recycled.

(2) In cells that store secretory products to be released in response to some stimulus (i.e., **regulated secretion**), secretory products are packaged in **condensing vacuoles,** where further concentration leads to formation of **secretory granules** (those containing digestive enzymes are called **zymogen granules**). Secretory granules can accumulate in large numbers.

(3) Vesicles containing lysosomal enzymes (transport vesicles) move into the cytoplasm to fuse with endolysosomes containing material to be digested.

c. Membranes are also processed in the Golgi complex.
   (1) Membranes that will enclose secretory material become altered so that they can fuse with the plasma membrane.
   (2) A glycocalyx is added to future cell membrane.
   (3) Membranes in certain regions of the Golgi complex are prepared to enclose lysosomal enzymes.

3. Light-microscope appearance

a. The size of the Golgi complex is usually within the limit of resolution of the light microscope, but it does not stain with routine histologic stains.

b. The Golgi complex can be demonstrated by treating the tissue with heavy metals such as silver or osmium, which accumulate in cisternae at the forming face, or by histochemically demonstrating characteristic enzymes.
c. The Golgi region can sometimes be detected as an unstained "negative image" in routine preparations of cells that have well-stained structures such as rER and secretory granules filling the rest of the cytoplasm.
d. The size and extent of the Golgi complex are directly related to the current level of secretory activity and lysosome production in the cell.

STUDY QUESTIONS

DIRECTIONS: Each of the numbered items or incomplete statements in this section is followed by answers or completions of the statement. Select the **one** numbered answer or completion that is **best** in each case.

1. Chromatin can exist in any of several forms. Which group of terms refers to forms of chromatin?

(1) Heterochromatin, euchromatin, and ergastoplasm
(2) Heterochromatin, euchromatin, and chromosomes
(3) Chromosomes and basophilic bodies
(4) Heterochromatin, euchromatin, and ribosomes
(5) Ribosomes, chromosomes, and ergastoplasm

2. Transcription differs from replication in that:

(1) deoxyribonucleic acid (DNA) is not involved in transcription.
(2) DNA is involved only in transcription.
(3) transcription occurs primarily in the cytoplasm.
(4) transcription is ribonucleic acid (RNA) synthesis, and replication is DNA synthesis.
(5) transcription is protein synthesis, and replication is DNA synthesis.

3. Translation is defined as a process in which:

(1) messenger RNA (mRNA) is produced from a deoxyribonucleic acid (DNA) template.
(2) the genetic information of the cell is copied before mitosis.
(3) mRNA, transfer RNA (tRNA), and ribosomal RNA (rRNA) are involved in synthesizing protein.
(4) ribosomes are produced in the nucleolus.
(5) euchromatin is converted to heterochromatin.

4. Which of the following is a change that is visible at the light-microscope level in a cell that is increasing its secretory activity?

(1) An increase in the ratio of euchromatin to heterochromatin
(2) A decrease in the size and number of nucleoli
(3) An increase in cytoplasmic acidophilia
(4) An increase in the size and complexity of the Golgi complex
(5) An increase in the number of transfer vesicles from the rough endoplasmic reticulum (rER)

5. All of the following are characteristics of nucleoli *except*:

(1) they are a site of ribonucleic acid (RNA) production.
(2) they are composed primarily of RNA and protein.
(3) there may be several in one nucleus.
(4) they are composed of heterochromatin.
(5) they are larger in active cells than they are in inactive cells.

6. The nuclear envelope can *best* be described as:

(1) a single membrane that separates nucleoplasm from cytoplasm.
(2) a structure formed by the Golgi complex.
(3) an organelle that is visible using the light microscope.
(4) a membrane separating the nucleolus from the rest of the nucleoplasm.
(5) a pair of membranes enclosing a cisternal cavity that may open into that of the rough endoplasmic reticulum (rER).

7. Ribosomes and polysomes can be *best* described as:

(1) free in the cytoplasmic matrix when they are engaged in making proteins for intracellular use.
(2) unable to make proteins that will remain in the cell when they are attached to the rough endoplasmic reticulum (rER).
(3) acidophilic in very large accumulations.
(4) gradually decreasing in number when a cell increases its level of secretory activity.
(5) synthesized by nuclear heterochromatin.

8. What is the main function of the rough endoplasmic reticulum (rER) in secretory cells?

(1) Synthesis of carbohydrates
(2) Synthesis of fats
(3) Synthesis of proteins for intracellular use
(4) Complexing fats and carbohydrates with proteins for export
(5) Synthesis of proteins for export

9. All of the following statements regarding the rough endoplasmic reticulum (rER) are true *except*:

(1) it is the source of membranes for other parts of the cell.
(2) its membranes appear rough in electron micrographs because of attached ribosomes.
(3) in cells with large accumulations of rER, it is concentrated in the part of the cell nearest to the source of nutrients.
(4) large accumulations are visible with the light microscope as basophilic regions.
(5) it is present only in cells that secrete proteins.

10. The Golgi complex is the site of all of the following activities *except*:

(1) synthesis and addition of carbohydrates to glycoproteins.
(2) attachment of lipids to proteins to form lipoproteins.
(3) release of the transfer vesicles that carry secretory products to condensing vacuoles.
(4) separation of lysosomal enzymes from secretory products.
(5) addition of glycocalyx to future cell membranes.

DIRECTIONS: Each group of items in this section consists of numbered options followed by a set of numbered items. For each item, select the **one** numbered option that is most closely associated with it. Each numbered option may be selected once, more than once, or not at all.

Questions 11–15

Match each descriptive phrase with the associated structure.

(1) Nucleolus
(2) Nuclear envelope
(3) Euchromatin
(4) Heterochromatin
(5) Nucleoplasm

11. Material enclosed by the nuclear envelope

12. Site of ribosome production

13. Structure with attached ribosomes on its outer surface

14. An indication of an active cell when it predominates

15. Condensed chromatin not currently being transcribed

Questions 16–20

Match each descriptive phrase with the associated structure.

(1) Free ribosome
(2) Attached ribosome
(3) Polysome
(4) Rough endoplasmic reticulum (rER)
(5) Golgi complex

16. Has a role in conservation of cellular water

17. Directly responsible for synthesis of proteins for extracellular use

18. A membrane system that sequesters newly formed proteins

19. A cluster of granules associated with a messenger ribonucleic acid (mRNA) molecule

20. Abundant in cells that produce large amounts of protein for intracellular use

ANSWERS AND EXPLANATIONS

1. The answer is 2 *[I A 1 a (2) (a) (i)–(ii), (b) (i)].* Heterochromatin, euchromatin, and chromosomes are all terms that refer to forms of chromatin. Heterochromatin and euchromatin are present in the nuclei of nondividing (interphase) cells, and chromosomes are in dividing cells. Heterochromatin is condensed chromatin that is not currently involved in transcription, whereas euchromatin is extended (uncoiled) chromatin that is undergoing transcription. Chromosomes are formed by separation and condensation of the chromatin containing each individual deoxyribonucleic acid (DNA) molecule. Ergastoplasm is an accumulation of rough endoplasmic reticulum (rER) in a secretory cell. Ribosomes are ribonucleoprotein granules involved in cytoplasmic protein synthesis.

2. The answer is 4 *[I A 1 a (2) (a)].* Deoxyribonucleic acid (DNA) is used as a template for both transcription and replication, but in the former ribonucleic acid (RNA) is synthesized, whereas in the latter DNA is formed. Transcription of messenger RNA (mRNA) is the first step in protein synthesis (i.e., the first step in translation); replication of DNA precedes cell division. Both processes occur in the nucleus.

3. The answer is 3 *[II A].* Each of the three types of ribonucleic acid (RNA) plays an essential role in translation, or protein synthesis. Messenger RNA (mRNA) encodes the new protein by means of a series of sites that recognize and interact only with specific ribosomal RNA (rRNA) molecules. The transfer RNA (tRNA) molecules each carry a specific amino acid to be inserted in the growing peptide chain, and rRNA activates successive sites on the mRNA so that its interaction with tRNA can occur. The synthesis of mRNA from deoxyribonucleic acid (DNA) is called transcription, and genetic information is copied before mitosis in the process called replication. Protein synthesis occurs only in the cytoplasm. No special name is attached to the condensation and dispersion of chromatin when euchromatin is converted to heterochromatin and back to euchromatin.

4. The answer is 1 *[I A 1 a, B 2 a (1)].* An increase in the ratio of euchromatin to heterochromatin is visible at the light-microscope level in a cell that is increasing its secretory activity. Because protein synthesis begins with the production of messenger RNA (mRNA), chromatin containing the deoxyribonucleic acid (DNA) that encodes the necessary ribonucleic acid (RNA) is converted from condensed heterochromatin to extended euchromatin when the cell increases its protein secretory activity. Nucleoli increase in size (and sometimes in number) to provide the additional ribosomes needed. The increased RNA (primarily ribosomal) in the cytoplasm makes it more basophilic. The number of transfer vesicles and the size and complexity of the Golgi complex do increase, but these changes are not visible at the light-microscope level.

5. The answer is 4 *[I A 1 b].* Nucleoli are not composed of heterochromatin; they consist primarily of protein and ribonucleic acid (RNA) that is produced in them. Because nucleoli increase in size and, in certain cells, also in number when protein synthesis increases, they are good indicators of the synthetic activity of a cell.

6. The answer is 5 *[I A 2].* The nuclear envelope is reformed after cell division by the rough endoplasmic reticulum (rER), and its outer membrane and lumen sometimes retain continuity with that organelle. The double-layered nuclear envelope and its pores are below the resolving power of the light microscope, although a layer of peripheral heterochromatin that lies along the inner membrane marks its position between the nucleoplasm and the cytoplasm.

7. The answer is 1 *[II B 3 a].* Proteins made in association with free polysomes are used within the cell. Ribosomes of the rough endoplasmic reticulum (rER) make membrane proteins and lysosomal enzymes that will remain in the cell as well as proteins for export. The nucleolus produces more and more ribosomes when the cell increases its secretory activity. The nucleic acid in ribosomes causes increased cytoplasmic basophilia when the ribosomes become sufficiently numerous in active secretory cells.

8. The answer is 5 *[II C 2].* Although it is true that certain proteins that are produced by attached ribosomes (membrane proteins and lysosomal enzymes) do remain in the cell, the main function of the rough endoplasmic reticulum (rER) in secretory cells is synthesis of proteins for export. Synthesis of fats and carbohydrates is primarily associated with the Golgi complex, where they may be complexed with proteins from the rER in the process of forming a final secretory product.

9. The answer is 5 *[II C 2 b]*. Because membranes for other organelles are formed by the rough endoplasmic reticulum (rER), small amounts of rER are found in cells that do not secrete proteins. In cells with abundant rER, the rER is typically concentrated in the part of the cell that is nearest to its nutrient supply. Because the ribosomes that are attached to the rER are intensely basophilic, large accumulations of rER are visible with the light microscope. The attached ribosomes give the rER a rough appearance under the electron microscope.

10. The answer is 3 *[II D 1 c]*. Transfer vesicles pinch off of the rough endoplasmic reticulum (rER) to carry newly formed proteins to the cisternae of the Golgi complex. Condensing vacuoles form directly from cisternae at the mature face of the Golgi complex. Synthesis of carbohydrates and complexing of carbohydrates and lipids with proteins take place in the Golgi complex. Enzymes that are destined for lysosomes (i.e., acid hydrolases) are separated in the Golgi complex from the secretory products that will be released from the cell. The Golgi complex also adds glycocalyx to membranes that are destined to become cell membranes.

11–15. The answers are: 11-5 *[I A]*, **12-1** *[I A 1 b]*, **13-2** *[I A 2]*, **14-3** *[I B 2 a (1)]*, **15-4** *[I A 1 a (2) (a) (ii)]*. Nucleoplasm is the material enclosed by the nuclear envelope, which is a double membrane with ribosomes on its outer (cytoplasmic) surface. Included in the nucleoplasm are euchromatin, where ribonucleic acid (RNA) is transcribed; heterochromatin, the condensed chromatin not currently active in RNA production; and the nucleolus, the site of ribosomal RNA (rRNA) production. A high ratio of euchromatin to heterochromatin and a large nucleolus are signs of secretory activity.

16–20. The answers are: 16-5 *[II D 2 a (1) (d)]*, **17-4** *[II C 2]*, **18-4** *[II C 2 a (2)]*, **19-3** *[II B 1 c]*, **20-1** *[II B 3]*. Ribosomes that become attached to the same messenger ribonucleic acid (mRNA) molecule constitute a polysome. Cells that produce large amounts of protein for use in the cytoplasmic matrix have many free ribosomes. In contrast, ribosomes that synthesize proteins for export (or for lysosomes or membranes) are attached to membranes of the rough endoplasmic reticulum (rER). The membranes of this organelle sequester newly formed proteins that are lysosomal enzymes or are appropriate for export, but that might interfere with the normal activity of the cell if they were free in the cytoplasm. Packaged proteins are then transferred to the Golgi complex, where, among other processing steps, excess water is removed and conserved for the cell.

Chapter 2

Other Membranous Organelles

I. LYSOSOMES (Figure 2-1)

A. Structure

1. **Lysosomes** are **membranous vesicles,** usually 0.2–0.4 μm in diameter, that contain many different **hydrolytic enzymes** for intracellular digestion.
   a. **Major enzyme groups** include esterases, glycosidases, and peptidases, all with maximal activity at the acid pH maintained in the lysosomes.
   b. Lysosomes may also contain a variety of **other structures and materials undergoing digestion** (Figure 2-1; see I B 2).
2. **Multivesicular bodies** (see Figure 2-4) are small vesicles that contain smaller vesicles. They are present in most cell types and are most numerous in cells with many lysosomes. They fuse with lysosomes and endocytic vesicles and function as lysosomes; they cannot be distinguished from other lysosomes light microscopically.

B. Formation (Figure 2-2)

1. **Transport vesicles** released from the Golgi complex contain acid hydrolases that are segregated from the rest of the cell by the bounding membrane. These transport vesicles **fuse with endolysosomes,** which contain material to be digested, **to form lysosomes**.
2. The material being digested in lysosomes may be derived from three sources:
   a. **Cytoplasmic elements**
      (1) Organelles or excess secretory granules may be surrounded by membranes derived from the endoplasmic reticulum (ER), forming structures called **autophagosomes**.

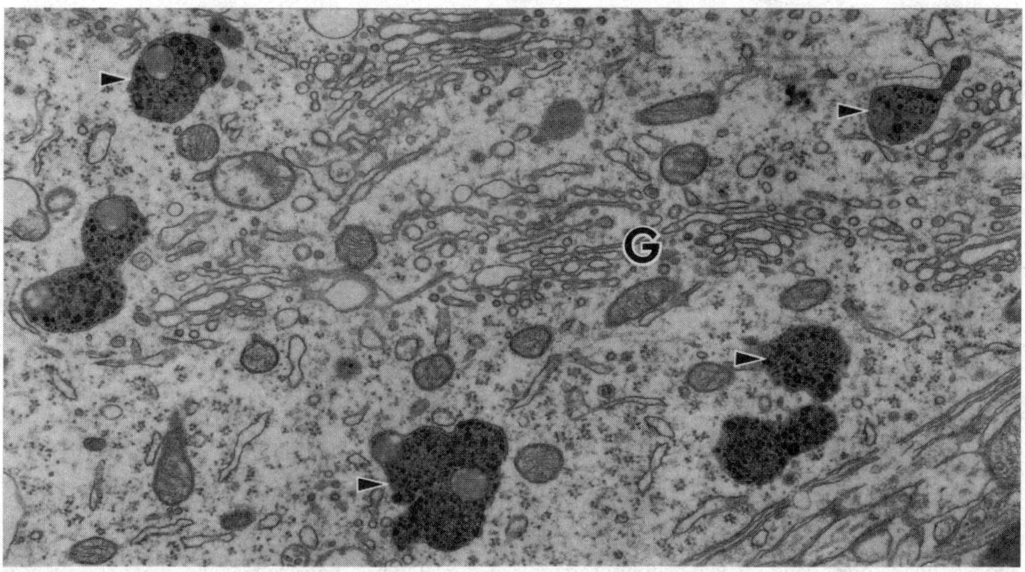

Figure 2-1. Electron micrograph of a phagocytic cell, showing several lysosomes with varied contents (*arrows*). The section also passes through the cisternae of the Golgi complex (*G*).

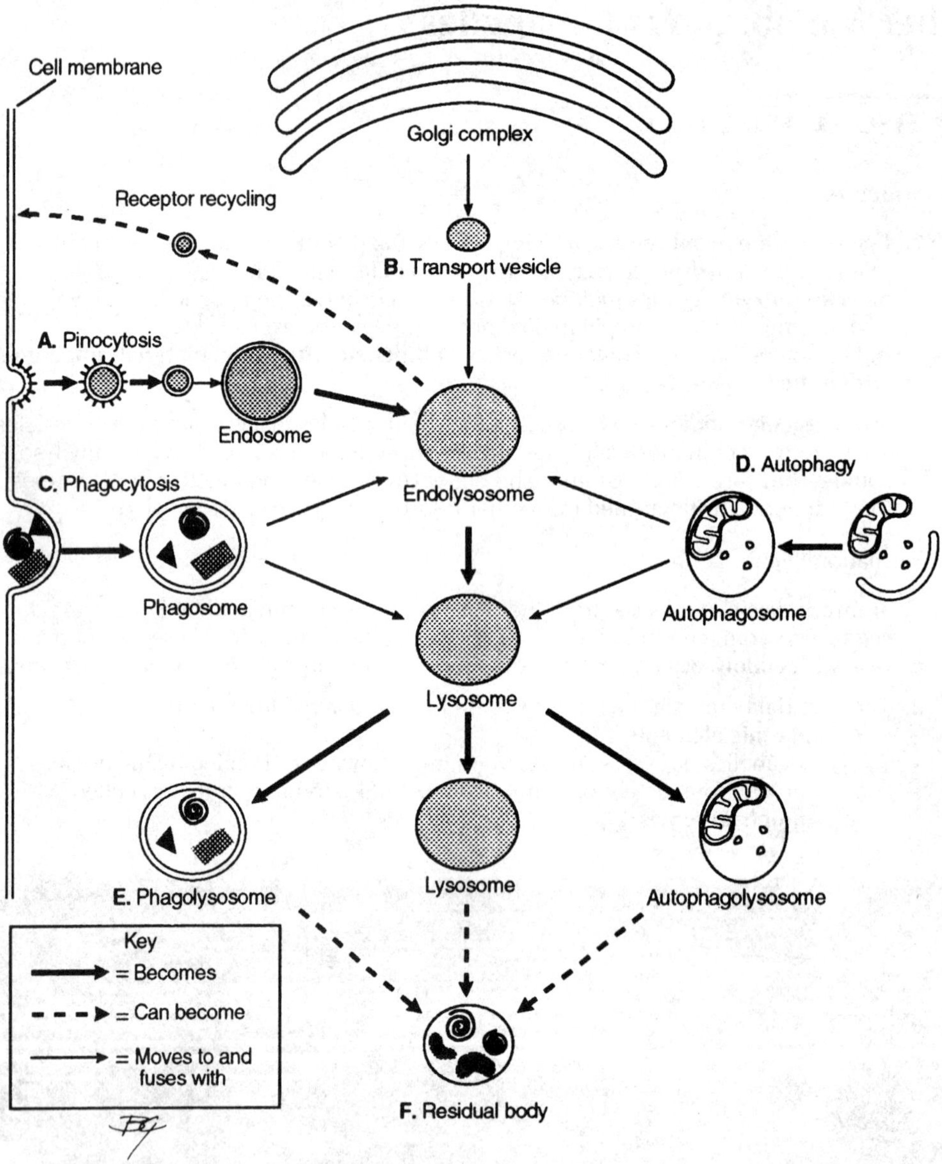

Figure 2-2. Schematic diagram of the formation of different types of lysosomes. (*A*) Vesicles formed by pinocytosis lose their bristle-like coating of clathrin and fuse with endosomes, the organelles responsible for sorting incoming material. Endosomes become endolysosomes; the acidic environment of the endolysosome permits dissociation of certain components, such as membrane receptors, for recycling. (*B*) Transport vesicles carry lysosomal enzymes from the mature face of the Golgi complex to endolysosomes to form mature lysosomes. (*C*) Phagocytosis (heterophagy) produces phagosomes, which contain extracellular material. (*D*) Autophagy produces autophagosomes, which contain cytoplasmic components. (*E*) Phagosomes and autophagosomes can fuse with endolysosomes or with mature lysosomes to become phagolysosomes or autophagolysosomes, respectively. Digested molecules pass through the lysosomal membrane to the cytosol (i.e., the cytoplasmic matrix) to be used for cell processes. (*F*) Undigestible materials accumulate within the lysosome, which becomes a residual body when its enzymes are exhausted.

(2) An autophagosome may fuse with a mature lysosome or with an endolysosome to form an **autophagolysosome**.

b. **Pinocytic vesicles. Pinocytosis** is the **cellular ingestion of fluids** (see also Chapter 4 III A 2).

(1) Pinocytic vesicles fuse with **endosomes** initially and then become endolysosomes.

(2) Transport vesicles carrying newly synthesized hydrolytic enzymes from the Golgi complex fuse with endolysosomes, and digestion is initiated.

(3) Additional changes in the bounding membrane produce mature lysosomes.

c. **Phagosomes (heterophagosomes). Phagocytosis** is the **cellular ingestion of particulate matter** (see also Chapter 4 III A 1).

(1) Phagosomes are formed only in cells that are specialized to take up macromolecules or microorganisms by regulated endocytosis.

(2) Fusion of phagosomes with lysosomes or endolysosomes produces **phagolysosomes** (heterolysosomes).

C. **Fate.** If the lysosome contains undigestible material, it becomes a **residual body** when its enzymes are exhausted (see Figure 2-2).

D. **Functions.** Lysosomes contain scores of different acid hydrolases that, collectively, are able to **break down** all of the major constituents of the cell. The relative abundance of specific enzymes varies depending on the function of the cell. Lysosomes in neutrophils, for example, are especially well adapted to destroy bacteria, and lysosomes in thyroid cells assist in the release of thyroid hormone.

1. **Autophagy** refers to digestion of all or parts of **the cell itself**. This process permits recycling of raw materials from cellular components that are deteriorating, that are superfluous as a result of reorganization of the cell, or that can be spared to maintain the cell during starvation.

2. **Crinophagy** is a special type of autophagy that involves the degradation of excess hormone-containing secretory granules.

3. **Heterophagy** is the digestion of material from outside the cell.

a. Lysosomes in phagocytic cells derived from white blood cells inactivate potentially harmful foreign invaders, including bacteria. Some of the most dangerous microorganisms are those that have evolved a defense against lysosomal digestion (e.g., an enzyme-resistant waxy coat).

b. Although most frequently associated with defense, heterophagy can also conserve useful molecules (e.g., as when reabsorbed protein in the kidney is broken down for reuse of its components).

E. **Clinical significance**

1. **Tissue damage.** Release of lysosomal enzymes from white blood cells contributes to tissue damage at the site of inflammation, although the damage is minimal because the pH of the tissue is significantly above the optimum pH for lysosomal enzyme activity.

2. **Particle diseases.** Lysosomes are particularly susceptible to exogenous substances, including drugs, toxins, and particles, because the lysosomes fuse with vesicles containing extracellular materials brought into the cell via endocytosis. Particle diseases result when cells phagocytose certain undigestible substances, such as silica dust or asbestos.

a. These particles damage the lysosomal and cell membranes, causing leakage of lysosomal enzymes.

b. Released enzymes kill the cell, releasing more destructive enzymes, as well as the offending particles, into the surrounding tissue.

c. Other cells phagocytose the particles, and the cycle is repeated.

3. **Storage diseases.** In storage diseases, a certain substrate is not completely digested by the lysosomes because of a congenital lack of a necessary enzyme or activator protein.
   a. The substrate accumulates until it interferes with cell function.
   b. Long-lived cells are particularly susceptible; storage diseases (e.g., gangliosidoses, globoid cell leukodystrophy) most often involve the nervous system.

4. **Infection.** A congenital lack of lysosomal enzymes that are necessary for bactericidal or fungicidal action, or failure of the Golgi complex to package the enzymes properly, results in susceptibility to severe infections.

F. Light-microscope appearance

1. Most lysosomes are too small to be seen easily with the light microscope, but in some phagocytic cell types they may be large and noticeable. Examples of lysosomes that can be seen with the light microscope include azurophilic granules in monocytes and other white blood cells, specific granules in eosinophils, and many phagolysosomes in actively phagocytic cells.

2. The fine structure of lysosomes is highly variable because it depends on the contents of the lysosome. Therefore, **positive identification** at both light- and electron-microscope levels **requires histochemical or cytochemical identification of hydrolytic enzymes**. The presence of acid phosphatase is commonly used to histochemically identify lysosomes.

3. **Residual bodies** are often easily identifiable by their accumulations of **lipofuscin,** a yellow-brown lipid called "wear and tear pigment." Lipofuscin granules are most numerous in long-lived cells (e.g., muscle and nerve cells).

II. PEROXISOMES (MICROBODIES)

A. Fine structure

1. Peroxisomes are **small vesicles that contain oxidative enzymes,** including **peroxidase** and **catalase**. All components of peroxisomes are taken up from the cytosol.

2. Their **size and fine structure** are quite variable, depending on the species and the cell type. Peroxisomes appear to have granular contents, and in most mammalian species they contain a crystalloid core composed of urate oxidase.

B. Distribution

1. Peroxisomes are present in almost all cells, but are **largest** and **most numerous in** the **liver** and **kidney**.

2. Peroxisomes increase in number by **growth** and **fission**.

C. Functions

1. **Peroxide (H_2O_2) formation.** Peroxisomes form peroxide by removing hydrogen from specific substrates and combining it with molecular oxygen.
   a. **Catalase uses the peroxide to oxidize other substrates.**
   b. The **energy** from these metabolic oxidations is **dissipated as heat if it is not used directly for metabolic processes**. In contrast, mitochondria use energy from oxidation to produce chemical energy in the form of adenosine triphosphate (ATP).

2. **Fatty acid oxidation** and **gluconeogenesis**
   a. **Fatty acid oxidation** by peroxisomes in the **liver generates energy**.
   b. **Gluconeogenesis** occurs in peroxisomes when **amino acids** and **fatty acids** are **converted to carbohydrates**.

3. **Bactericidal action.** Peroxide in phagocytic cells has bactericidal potency.
4. **Detoxification.** Certain toxic molecules are detoxified by oxidative reactions in peroxisomes. For example, alcohol dehydrogenases in peroxisomes can degrade alcohol.

D. Light-microscope appearance

1. Most peroxisomes are just above the limit of resolution with the light microscope.
2. Specific enzymes in peroxisomes can be demonstrated with special stains.

III. SMOOTH ENDOPLASMIC RETICULUM (sER) (Figure 2-3)

A. Formation, structure, and distribution

1. In a number of cell types, rough endoplasmic reticulum (rER) gives rise to a specialized membrane that is free of ribosomes. These membranes comprise the smooth-surfaced sER, a system of anastomosing tubules (and sometimes cisternae and vesicles, depending on the cell type).
2. Generally, cells that develop sER are involved in lipid metabolism or are specialized to regulate movements of certain ions (e.g., calcium, chloride).

B. Functions. The functions of sER vary widely among cell types.

1. **Lipid synthesis.** The sER is responsible for lipid synthesis in liver cells, cells that produce steroid hormones, and intestinal absorptive cells.
   a. **Steroids** are lipids synthesized by the sER. Cholesterol is produced in the liver, whereas androgens, estrogens, progesterone, and adrenal steroids are produced by endocrine cells in the gonads and the adrenal cortex, respectively.
   b. **Intestinal absorptive cells** absorb monoglycerides and fatty acids that have been broken down from triglycerides in the intestinal lumen. These building blocks are transported to the sER where triglycerides are reconstituted before being released to the extracellular space.

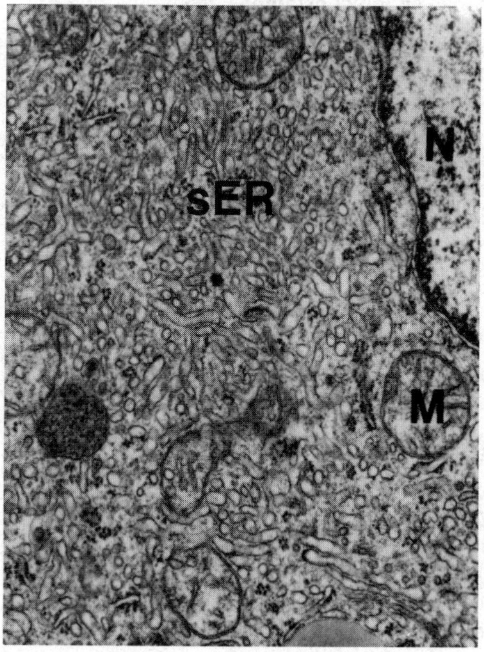

Figure 2-3. Electron micrograph of a portion of the cytoplasm in a cell with abundant smooth endoplasmic reticulum (*sER*). A portion of the nucleus (*N*) is shown at the *upper right,* and a mitochondrion (*M*) is indicated. (Reprinted with permission from Dellmann H-D: *Textbook of Veterinary Histology,* 4th ed. Baltimore, Williams & Wilkins, 1993, p 4.)

2. **Metabolism of lipid-soluble substances.** The sER in liver cells metabolizes lipid-soluble substances.
   a. Exposure to barbiturates or other lipid-soluble substances, including carcinogens, opiates, insecticides, and alcohol, causes proliferation of the sER in liver cells. The hypertrophy of the sER increases the number of its integral enzymes, which accelerates metabolization of all lipid-soluble substances and can reduce the effectiveness of a given dose of other drugs given concurrently.
   b. Some substances, such as carbon tetrachloride, are converted to a toxic form by the sER.
3. **Regulation of ion concentration.** In some cells, sER regulates cytoplasmic concentrations of ions.
   a. sER sequesters and releases calcium ions in muscle cells, thereby regulating contraction and relaxation.
   b. sER sequesters chloride ions in the cells that produce hydrochloric acid in the stomach.
4. **Glycogen metabolism.** sER is involved in glycogen metabolism in liver cells. Glycogen is the storage form of carbohydrates.

C. Light-microscope appearance

1. Individual components of sER are too small for the resolving power of the light microscope.
2. Because sER has no ribosomes, it is not basophilic and the acidophilia of its membranes cannot be distinguished from that of other cytoplasmic components. Therefore, even in large, dense accumulations, its presence can be determined only with the electron microscope.

IV. MITOCHONDRIA

A. Structure and distribution

1. Mitochondria range from spherical or ovoid to very elongated, thread-like shapes. They can divide and fuse, and they move and change shape constantly.
2. They are formed of **two membranes,** one within the other (Figures 2-4 and 2-5).
   a. The **outer membrane** is a cytoplasmic vesicle that resembles other cytoplasmic vesicles.
   b. The **inner membrane** parallels the outer membrane except where it projects into the center in shelf-like folds called **cristae** (see Figure 2-4). In cells that produce steroids, the folds are replaced by tubular or vesicular formations (see Figure 2-5).
      (1) The inner membrane differs from other membranes in the cell in that its **inner surface** is covered with tiny granules that contain enzymes **involved in ATP production**.
      (2) The **mitochondrial matrix** occupies the space within the inner membrane. Small **matrix granules** are composed primarily of calcium phosphate.
3. Mitochondria are proportional in size and number to the energy requirements of the cell and are concentrated in the parts of the cell that require the most energy.
   a. They are very abundant in the striated ducts of salivary glands and certain kidney tubules near the basal membrane, where they provide energy for pumping ions across the large plasma membrane.
   b. They are aligned along the contractile apparatus in skeletal muscle cells.
   c. They are most numerous near the rER in secretory cells.

B. Source.
Mitochondria are believed to have evolved from aerobic bacteria that established synergistic relationships with anaerobic true cells.

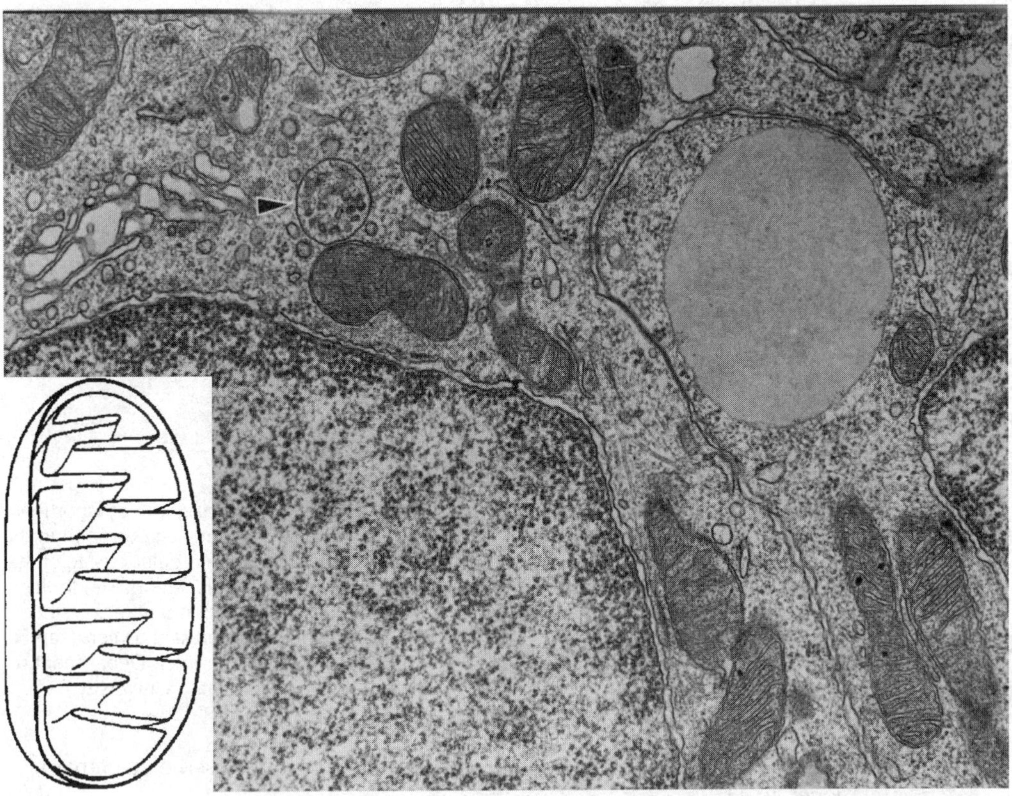

Figure 2-4. Electron micrograph of several mitochondria. A portion of the nucleus is at the *lower left,* a multivesicular body is indicated by the *arrow,* and a lipid droplet appears as a homogeneous, gray circular area at the right. The *inset* is a cutaway view of a mitochondrion showing the inner and outer membranes.

1. Although mitochondria depend on the cell for most of their proteins, they contain DNA and ribosomes of the types found in bacteria and they produce some of their own proteins.
2. Unlike other organelles, which are synthesized under the control of nuclear DNA from both parents, mitochondria are inherited only from the maternal parent. **All mitochondria** in an individual are **derived from mitochondria in the ovum**.

C. Functions

1. **Cellular respiration.** Mitochondria are the organelles of cellular respiration. These "powerhouses" of the cell oxidize nutrients (burn fuel) to produce ATP (a high-energy compound) and heat.
   - **a.** Substrates derived from nutrients are metabolized in the mitochondrial matrix to produce acetyl coenzyme A, which is then processed by enzymes of the tricarboxylic acid (TCA) cycle. Hydrogen atoms released by this series of oxidations pass to the inner membrane.
   - **b.** Enzymes integral to the inner membrane are organized into functional units that act as chemical mass production lines.
     - **(1)** Hydrogen atoms from the matrix are transported along a series of enzymes called the respiratory chain.
     - **(2)** The reactions of the respiratory chain are coupled with **oxidative phosphorylation** reactions, in which adenosine diphosphate (ADP) is converted to ATP.

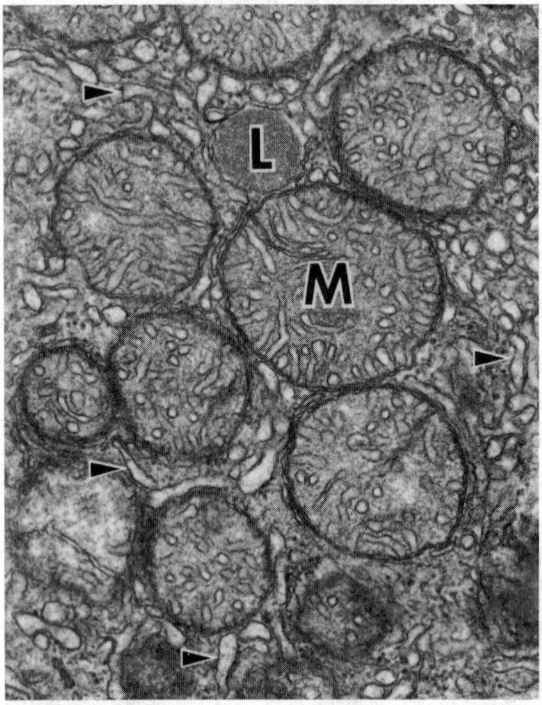

Figure 2-5. Electron micrograph of a portion of the cytoplasm of a steroid-secreting cell in the corpus luteum. Note the tubular cristae of the mitochondria (*M*). Tubular smooth endoplasmic reticulum (sER) is abundant (*arrows*). A lipid droplet (*L*) is also present. (Micrograph courtesy of Dr. M. H. Stromer, Department of Animal Science, Iowa State University.)

Therefore, the energy released during electron transport is used efficiently to generate ATP.

c. ATP passes to the cytosol (cytoplasmic matrix) to be used as a source of metabolic energy that can power other reactions.

2. Steroid biosynthesis. In steroid-producing cells, mitochondria assist in steroid biosynthesis.

3. Calcium concentration. Matrix granules that concentrate calcium phosphate are believed to help maintain a characteristically low level of calcium in the cytosol.

D. Light-microscope appearance

1. The average-sized mitochondrion is within the limits of resolution of the light microscope, and mitochondria are often observed in living cells using phase microscopy.
2. Mitochondrial membranes are **stained by iron hematoxylin** and can be demonstrated by special stains for oxidative enzymes.
3. In cells where they are fairly large and their image is not confused by the staining reaction of neighboring structures, mitochondria may be clearly visible in routine preparations. They are especially well demonstrated in the striated ducts of salivary glands and in certain tubules in the kidney.

STUDY QUESTIONS

DIRECTIONS: Each of the numbered items or incomplete statements in this section is followed by answers or completions of the statement. Select the **one** numbered answer or completion that is **best** in each case.

1. Lysosomes typically arise from which one of the following?

(1) Synergistic organisms that have entered eukaryotic cells
(2) Fission of mitochondria
(3) Phagocytosis
(4) The rough endoplasmic reticulum (rER) and the Golgi complex
(5) Endosomes that have exhausted their supply of hydrolytic enzymes

2. Which one of the following correctly describes endosomes or lysosomes?

(1) Endosomes contain hydrolytic enzymes and the contents of pinocytic vesicles with which they have fused.
(2) Multivesicular bodies are endosomes that have not yet been supplied with hydrolytic enzymes.
(3) The contents of lysosomes are the same in all cell types for a given species.
(4) Autophagolysosomes can be involved in cellular reorganization.

3. Which of the following statements *best* describes a lysosomal function?

(1) Heterophagy occurs when a lysosome fuses with a secretory granule.
(2) Heterophagy is important in defense responses.
(3) Crinophagy is a special type of autophagy that breaks down cellular components after cell death.
(4) Autophagy is the intracellular digestion that occurs in transport vesicles.
(5) Autophagy enables cells to break down phagocytosed molecules for reuse in the body.

4. At the light-microscope level, individual lysosomes:

(1) have a characteristic yellow-brown color.
(2) are usually large enough to detect easily.
(3) can be identified with certainty only in phagocytic cells.
(4) can be identified with certainty only by histochemical tests for the presence of hydrolytic enzymes.
(5) are uniform in size and appearance within a given cell type.

5. The functions of peroxisomes (microbodies) are:

(1) similar to those of mitochondria, in that they produce energy in the form of adenosine triphosphate (ATP).
(2) unlike those of lysosomes, in that they contain no known enzymes.
(3) related to their ability to oxidize certain organic compounds.
(4) limited by their inability to degrade peroxidase.
(5) related to protein synthesis.

6. The structure and distribution of peroxisomes:

(1) are remarkably consistent across cell types and species.
(2) are consistent across species, but their distribution is limited to liver and kidney cells.
(3) usually permit them to be detected with the light microscope with appropriate staining reactions.
(4) depend on the structure and distribution of materials in the vesicles with which they have fused.
(5) are visible only at the fine structural level.

7. Smooth endoplasmic reticulum (sER) is associated with which one of the following functions?

(1) Protein synthesis
(2) Lipid metabolism
(3) Packaging of secretory material for export
(4) Formation of lysosomes
(5) Energy production

8. Which one of the following statements *best* describes the smooth endoplasmic reticulum (sER)?

(1) It usually consists of an anastomosing system of smooth-surfaced tubules.
(2) When it is abundant, its presence is easily detected at the light-microscope level due to its basophilia.
(3) It is derived from the Golgi complex.
(4) It is present to some degree in almost all cells.
(5) It is most abundant in protein-secreting cells.

9. Which one of the following statements is true regarding functions of the smooth endoplasmic reticulum (sER)?

(1) It generates energy or heat in the liver by oxidizing fatty acids.
(2) It produces hydrolytic enzymes in white blood cells that will become tissue phagocytes.
(3) It inactivates hydrochloric acid absorbed by cells lining the stomach.
(4) It breaks down lipids (fats) absorbed by intestinal lining cells into components that are soluble in the blood.
(5) It regulates contraction of muscle cells by sequestering and releasing calcium ions.

10. Which of the following statements *best* describes the origin of mitochondria?

(1) They are believed to be derived originally from anaerobic bacteria.
(2) Their proteins are programmed by nuclear DNA and they are produced by the rough endoplasmic reticulum (rER) and the Golgi complex.
(3) Approximately half of the mitochondria in an individual arise from mitochondria contributed by the spermatozoon during fertilization.
(4) All of the mitochondria in an individual are derived from maternal mitochondria in the ovum.
(5) Mitochondrial enzymes are programmed by nuclear DNA.

11. Mitochondrial components are responsible for specific biochemical processes, including which one of the following?

(1) Metabolism of substrates derived from food to produce acetyl coenzyme A in the mitochondrial matrix
(2) Production of acetyl coenzyme A in the compartment between the inner and outer membranes
(3) Processing of acetyl coenzyme A by the enzymes of the tricarboxylic acid (TCA) cycle in the compartment between the inner and outer membranes
(4) Respiration and adenosine triphosphate (ATP) production on the inner membrane
(5) Production and storage of ATP in the mitochondrial matrix

12. Mitochondria are *best* described by which one of the following statements?

(1) They are formed of two membranous sacs, one within the other.
(2) They are formed by a single cytoplasmic membrane that is folded in on itself to resemble a layered structure.
(3) They can be seen with the light microscope only by using special stains to demonstrate their enzymes.
(4) They are most numerous in parts of the cell where little other activity is taking place.
(5) They occupy fixed positions in the cell.

13. All of the following statements regarding smooth endoplasmic reticulum (sER) in the liver are true *except:*

(1) it can be responsible for drug interactions that alter the effectiveness of a given dose of medicine.
(2) it is involved in the metabolism of glycogen.
(3) it decreases in amount after exposure to lipid-soluble drugs.
(4) it helps synthesize steroids, notably cholesterol.
(5) it can convert harmless substances to toxic compounds.

14. All of the following statements regarding the roles of lysosomes in disease processes are true *except*:

(1) lysosomes in certain white blood cells contain enzymes that can inactivate pathogenic bacteria.
(2) inability to fight certain fungal diseases can result from the congenital absence of a specific lysosomal enzyme.
(3) storage diseases result from the congenital absence of a specific lysosomal enzyme.
(4) particle diseases involve exposure of the same undigestible particles to lysosomes in a series of phagocytic cells.
(5) release of lysosomal contents from white blood cells contributes to wound healing.

ANSWERS AND EXPLANATIONS

1. The answer is 4 *[I B]*. Lysosomal enzymes and membranes are produced by the rough endoplasmic reticulum (rER) and the Golgi complex. Mitochondria are believed to be derived from aerobic microorganisms that established synergistic relationships with anaerobic eukaryotic cells. They can replicate by fission. Phagocytosis produces phagosomes, which fuse with lysosomes or endolysosomes. Exhausted lysosomes are called residual bodies.

2. The answer is 4 *[I D 1; Figure 2-2]*. Autophagolysosomes are important elements in cellular reorganization. They can, for example, digest portions of the cell's machinery that are no longer needed when the cell's level of activity decreases and use the components for protein synthesis. Autophagolysosomes can also convert portions of the cell to raw materials for survival during periods of starvation. Endosomes fuse with pinocytic vesicles, but they do not contain hydrolytic enzymes. Multivesicular bodies contain hydrolytic enzymes and function as lysosomes. The enzymatic contents of lysosomes are specific for each cell type. Lysosomes in white blood cells, for example, are supplied with enzymes that destroy bacteria or that can digest most other phagocytosed materials.

3. The answer is 2 *[I D 3]*. Heterophagy, which is digestion of material from outside the cell (i.e., phagocytosed material), occurs primarily in defense responses of white blood cells. Fusion of a lysosome or endolysosome with secretory granules is a feature of crinophagy, a special category of autophagy that purges hormone-producing cells of "stale" stored hormones. Autophagy occurs in lysosomes that have been formed by fusion of a lysosome or endolysosome with an autophagic vesicle.

4. The answer is 4 *[I F 1–3]*. The best way of identifying a structure as a lysosome at either the light-microscope or fine structural level is by identifying the hydrolytic enzymes it contains, because the size and appearance (including color) are highly variable, depending on the great variety of possible vesicles with which the lysosome may fuse. In most cells, the largest lysosomes are just at or below the resolving power of the light microscope, so they are difficult to detect. Active phagocytes are notable exceptions; they often contain very large phagolysosomes. Residual bodies, which are membrane-bounded accumulations of undigestible material that no longer contain enzymes, often contain lipofuscin, which imparts a golden-brown hue.

5. The answer is 3 *[II C]*. The peroxidase in peroxisomes can promote (catalyze) oxidation of some organic compounds. The energy that is produced by these oxidative reactions, however, is not used to generate adenosine triphosphate (ATP), as it is in mitochondria; if it is not used directly to power some reaction, it generates heat, thus contributing to maintenance of body temperature. Peroxidases in liver cells generate energy by oxidizing fatty acids, and in phagocytic cells peroxidases are produced for their antibacterial action. Peroxidase is but one of the enzymes in peroxisomes. Among their other important enzymes are catalase, which promotes decomposition of hydrogen peroxide, and alcohol dehydrogenase, which degrades alcohol. Peroxisomes are not involved in protein synthesis.

6. The answer is 3 *[II D]*. Most peroxisomes are just large enough for resolution with the light microscope, when special stains are used to identify their specific enzymes. Their size and appearance are quite variable, depending on species and cell type. Their contents usually appear granular, but may be amorphous or appear crystalline. Although they are larger and far more numerous in certain cells in the liver and kidneys, peroxisomes are present in almost all cells.

7. The answer is 2 *[III B 1–2]*. Smooth endoplasmic reticulum (sER) in liver cells plays an important role in synthesizing lipids and metabolizing lipid-soluble substances. In cells that secrete steroid hormones, sER is involved in lipid synthesis; in intestinal absorptive cells, it is responsible for reconstituting triglycerides (fats) from absorbed monoglycerides and fatty acids. Because no ribosomes are attached to sER membranes, no synthesis of lysosomal enzymes or other proteins can occur. The Golgi complex, which is also formed of smooth-surfaced membranes, is the organelle that packages secretory material for export from the cell and forms lysosomal enzymes. Mitochondria are the major producers of energy, supplemented by peroxisomes in some cells.

8. The answer is 1 *[III A 1].* The smooth endoplasmic reticulum (sER) usually comprises anastomosing smooth-surfaced tubules only, although cisternae and vesicles are present in some cells. In a number of cell types, the rough endoplasmic reticulum (rER) gives rise to a specialized membrane without ribosomes [the smooth endoplasmic reticulum (sER)]. sER cannot be detected at the light-microscope level because, lacking ribosomes, it has no staining affinity for basic stains, and its staining with acid stains is similar to that of most cytoplasmic components. This organelle exists only in certain cells, generally those that are involved in lipid metabolism or that regulate movements of certain ions. It is not characteristic of protein-secreting cells; in those cells, rER is abundant.

9. The answer is 5 *[III B 3 a].* Smooth endoplasmic reticulum (sER) is arranged around and between the contractile elements in skeletal muscle cells, where it initiates contraction by releasing calcium ions and then causes relaxation by taking the calcium up again. Peroxisomes are the organelles that can produce energy to power biochemical reactions or be released as heat in the liver. Rough endoplasmic reticulum (rER) is responsible for producing lysosomal enzymes in all cells, including white blood cells. The lining cells of the stomach do not contain sER. sER in certain glandular cells of the stomach helps produce hydrochloric acid by sequestering chloride ions, and its role in intestinal lining cells is to reassemble triglycerides from fatty acids and monoglycerides that have been absorbed from the intestinal lumen.

10. The answer is 4 *[IV B 2].* Only the sperm head, which contains no mitochondria, enters the oocyte during fertilization; therefore, all mitochondria form by division of maternal mitochondria present in the ovum. Mitochondria are believed to be derived from aerobic microorganisms that established synergistic relationships with anaerobic eukaryotic cells. It is their ability to use oxygen to produce energy that makes them essential components of mammalian cells. Although mitochondria depend on the cell's nucleus for most nuclear functions, and their outer membrane is a typical cytoplasmic membrane, they contain DNA and produce some of their own protein.

11. The answer is 4 *[IV C 1 b].* Enzymes responsible for oxidative phosphorylation [i.e., enzymes of the respiratory chain and adenosine triphosphate (ATP) production] are precisely arranged in the inner membrane. Acetyl coenzyme A is produced in the mitochondrial matrix from products of digestion (primarily fatty acids and pyruvate) that enter mitochondria from the cytoplasmic matrix. Enzymes of the tricarboxylic acid (TCA) cycle are located in the mitochondrial matrix, which is enclosed within the space formed by the inner membrane. ATP leaves the inner membrane (where it is produced) to pass through the outer membrane to the cytosol, where it provides power for many different cellular processes.

12. The answer is 1 *[IV A 2].* Mitochondria are formed of an outer membrane that is simply a cytoplasmic vesicle and an inner membrane that is different from all other membranes in the cell. The inner membrane is folded, forming shelf-like cristae that project into the mitochondrial matrix enclosed by the inner membrane. Most mitochondria are large enough to be demonstrated with the light microscope, and the larger ones may be visible in routine preparations. They can also be demonstrated by special stains. Mitochondria are constantly moving about in the cytoplasm, but most are concentrated in the most active regions of the cell, where there is the greatest demand for the energy they provide.

13. The answer is 3 *[III B 2 a].* Exposure to lipid-soluble drugs, including alcohol, causes proliferation of the smooth endoplasmic reticulum (sER) in liver cells. This provides more capacity for metabolizing and inactivating the drugs, and it also accelerates the processing of all other lipid-soluble substances, which is why the sER is involved in the mechanisms of many drug interactions. In liver cells, the sER is also involved in the metabolism of glycogen and the synthesis of cholesterol, a steroid. Some substances (e.g., carbon tetrachloride) are converted to a toxic form by the sER.

14. The answer is 5 *[I E 1]*. The release of lysosomal enzymes by white blood cells that migrate to wounds and sites of inflammation contributes to tissue damage in these areas. White blood cells enter the tissue to fight infection. Certain ones become phagocytic cells that are specially equipped to destroy most infectious agents. A congenital lack of enzymes with fungicidal or bactericidal action in an animal's white blood cells can render the animal incapable of destroying infectious fungi or of fighting bacteria. Storage diseases result from the congenital absence of a specific lysosomal enzyme, leading to the accumulation of an undigested compound that then interferes with cell function. Particle diseases result when cells phagocytose an undigestible substance (e.g., silica dust), which damages the lysosomal and cell membranes. The cell dies, releasing its contents into the surrounding tissue, where the offensive particles are once again phagocytosed by new cells in an endless cycle.

Chapter 3

Cytoskeletal Elements and the Cytoplasmic Matrix

I. CYTOSKELETAL ELEMENTS.

Three types of **filamentous structures—microfilaments, intermediate filaments,** and **microtubules**—are classified as cytoskeletal elements. Cytoskeletal elements are responsible for **cellular movement** and provide support for the cell.

A. Microfilaments (F-actin, actin filaments)

1. **Structure**
   a. **Microfilaments** are the **thinnest** cytoplasmic filaments (**6–8 nm in diameter**).
   b. These **filamentous polymers** are composed of actin, a globular protein (i.e., G-actin). In most cells, only about half of the actin is found as F-actin; the remainder is depolymerized.

2. **Distribution**
   a. In **muscle cells,** microfilaments (which combine with the proteins tropomyosin, troponin, and α-actinin to form **thin filaments**) are arranged in **linear arrays**. These arrays are highly ordered in skeletal and cardiac muscle (see Figure 10-5).
   b. In most **other cells,** microfilaments are **concentrated near the cell membrane.** For example, in **surface epithelial cells,** microfilaments combine with other types of filaments to form a **terminal web in the apical cytoplasm** (see Figure 4-7A).

3. **Function.** Microfilaments are **contractile**.
   a. In **muscle cells,** thin filaments interact with thick (i.e., myosin) filaments to produce **cellular contraction**. Myosin is a dimeric protein; thick filaments comprise many overlapping myosin dimers.
   b. In **other cells,** microfilaments cause **movement of the cell membrane**.
      (1) Microfilaments are necessary for separation of daughter cells after cell division, ameboid movements, extension of processes, contraction of microvilli, and endocytosis.
      (2) These movements may also involve interaction with myosin; however, in nonmuscle cells, myosin may not polymerize to form thick filaments, or its filamentous form may be transitory.

4. **Light-microscope appearance.** Individual microfilaments are too slender to be visible light microscopically.
   a. **Pronounced acidophilia** marks sites **where microfilaments are abundant,** such as the **brush border** (i.e., a layer of microvilli on the apical surface of intestinal absorptive cells).
   b. The orderly, interdigitating arrangement of thin and thick filaments **in skeletal and cardiac muscle cells** produces **cross-striations** that are visible light microscopically (see Figure 10-4).

B. Intermediate filaments

1. **Structure**
   a. Intermediate filaments measure **7–11 nm in diameter,** which means that they are thicker than microfilaments and thinner than thick filaments and microtubules.
   b. Intermediate filaments are composed of filamentous proteins. They are **chemically heterogenous** (i.e., they are composed of different proteins in different cell types).

2. **Function.** All intermediate filaments are **flexible** and **exhibit tensile strength**. They **support cells** and **maintain their shape**.
   a. **Keratin filaments (tonofilaments)** are strong filaments that **protect surface epithelial cells from shearing forces** and **limit the permeability of the epithelium**.

(1) They are attached by dense plaques to the cell membrane, and are most numerous at cell junctions, especially desmosomes (see Chapter 4 II A 2 b; Figures 4-4 and 4-7A).

(2) Keratin filaments in different cell types differ chemically and have different physical properties. For example, skin cells produce soft keratin, but cells in hair follicles and claw beds produce hard keratin.

b. Desmin filaments are abundant in **muscle cells,** where they **hold the thick and thin filaments in place** and **anchor them to the cell membrane**.

c. Vimentin filaments are located in **cells derived from the mesenchyme,** including many cells in the developmental stages. They **hold the nucleus in place** and **may define organelle-free nuclear–cytoplasmic channels** adjacent to nuclear pores.

d. Neurofilaments (Figure 3-1) and **glial fibrillary acidic protein (GFAP)** are found in **neurons** and **astrocytes,** respectively. They help to **support the asymmetric shapes and extensive processes** that are characteristic of these cell types.

e. Spectrin filaments are found in **red blood cells**. They **protect the erythrocyte from shearing forces** that are encountered as the cell circulates. In addition, spectrin filaments **support the asymmetric shape of the cell**.

3. Light-microscope appearance

a. Like the other cytoskeletal elements, **individual intermediate filaments** are **too small to be seen** with the light microscope.

b. Bundles of intermediate filaments, such as the **tonofibrils** that support cells in the epidermis of the skin and the **neurofibrils** that maintain the long cytoplasmic processes of nerve cells, **are visible** light microscopically.

C. Microtubules

1. Structure

a. Microtubules are slender (**25 nm in diameter**), unbranched, hollow filaments. They **vary in length** and may be as long as several hundred μm (Figure 3-2).

b. Formation. Microtubules are formed of **tubulin,** a dumbbell-shaped dimer consisting of the globular proteins **α-tubulin** and **β-tubulin**.

(1) **Polymerization.** Tubulin subunits polymerize in a tight helix to form microtubules (Figure 3-3A).

(a) Polymerization is initiated at **microtubule-organizing centers** (e.g., in the **cytocentrum,** a gelated region of the cytoplasm that generally excludes other organelles, and in other locations throughout the cytoplasm).

(b) Polymerization (and depolymerization) takes place at the ends of the microtubules in response to **cellular regulatory signals**. Although the ratio of tubulin subunits in tubules to those dissolved in the cytosol may remain constant, individual microtubules are constantly growing or shrinking.

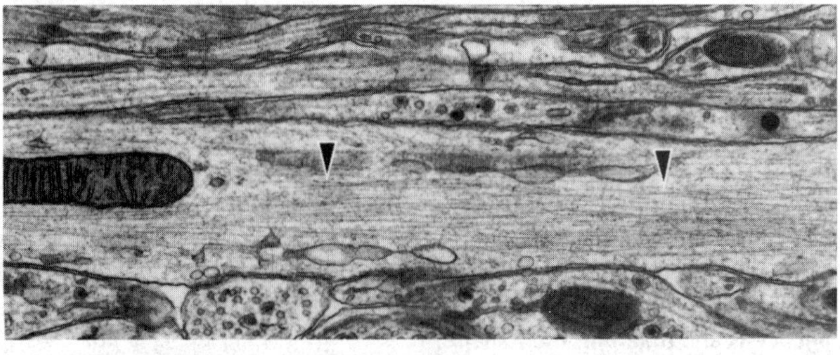

Figure 3-1. Intermediate filaments, indicated by the *arrows,* form the cytoskeletal core of this nerve cell (neuron) process. Intermediate filaments in neurons are called neurofilaments.

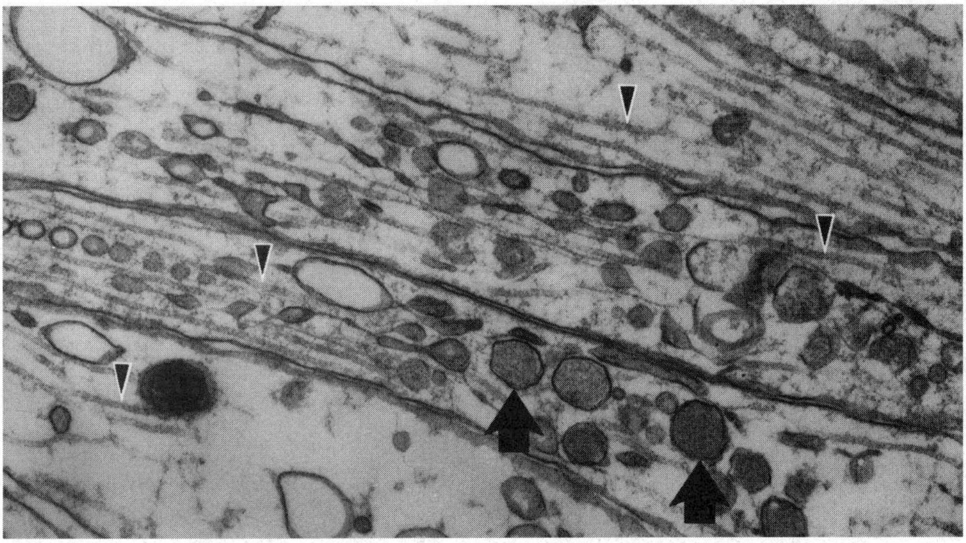

Figure 3-2. In axonal processes, such as this one from a neurosecretory neuron, microtubules (indicated by the *small arrowheads*) have a dual function. They provide semirigid support for the elongated cell process and also aid in movements of substances to and from the axonal terminal. Secretory granules, indicated by the *large arrows,* are en route along the microtubules to their point of release at the axon terminal.

(2) **Depolymerization.** Several drugs, including colchicine and the antineoplastic agent vincristine, cause depolymerization of microtubules, thereby halting the functions that depend on these structures.

2. **Distribution.** Microtubules may be distributed individually in the cytoplasm or organized into bundles, as in the extended processes of nerve cells (see Figure 3-2).
   a. The **mitotic apparatus (spindle)** is formed of microtubules. Some microtubules radiate from the poles, some join the poles, and others join chromosomes to the poles.
   b. **Centrioles.** Each centriole is a short cylinder that is composed of nine sets of three microtubules (Figure 3-4; see Figure 3-3B).
      (1) **Distribution**
         (a) Centrioles occur in **pairs,** with one centriole oriented perpendicularly to the other. Most cells have one pair of centrioles, but multinucleated cells may have many pairs.
         (b) Centrioles usually lie near the **center of the cell**. They are often located near the mature face of the Golgi complex in the cytocentrum.
      (2) **Functions**
         (a) Centrioles act as **poles during cell division**.
            (i) Before cell division occurs, a new centriole is assembled at one end of each existing centriole so that a pair of centrioles is provided for each daughter cell.
            (ii) The two centrioles, each with its newly formed daughter centriole, move to opposite ends of the cell, where they **organize the assembly of the mitotic apparatus** and form the **poles** toward which the chromosomes move.
         (b) Centrioles **organize the formation of basal bodies, which anchor cilia** and **flagella** in the cytoplasm. In addition, centrioles can act as basal bodies themselves.

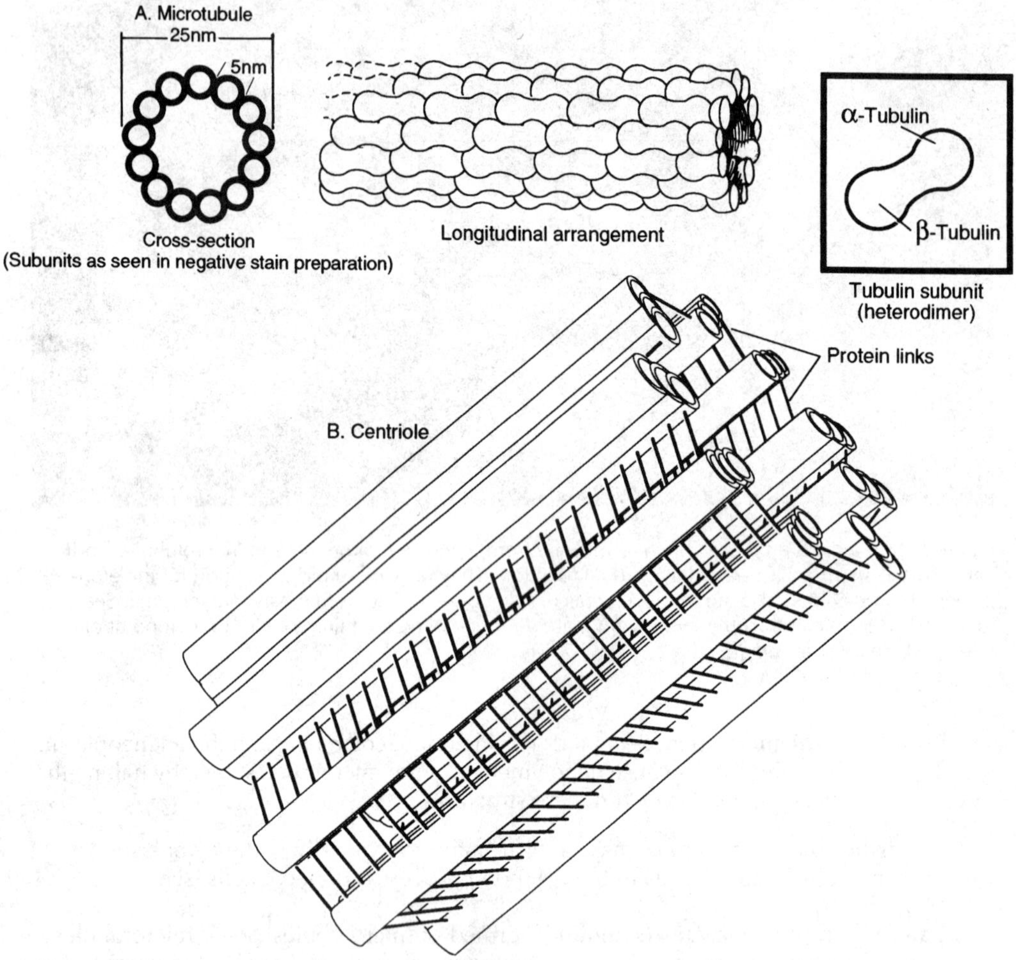

Figure 3-3. Microtubule and centriole formation. (*A*) Microtubules are formed by polymerization of tubulin subunits in a spiral with thirteen subunits per turn. This substructure is visible in electron-microscope preparations. (*B*) Centrioles are formed by nine triplets of microtubules that are arranged like vanes in a pinwheel. Some subunits are shared between adjacent microtubules within the triplets. (Adapted with permission from Junqueira LC, Carneiro J, Kelley RO: *Basic Histology,* 7th ed. Englewood Cliffs, NJ, Appleton & Lange, 1992, p 46.)

c. **Basal bodies, cilia,** and **flagella** (see Chapter 4 II B; Figure 4-6) also contain microtubules. The microtubules in centrioles, basal bodies, cilia, and flagella are quite stable compared with the highly labile microtubules in other parts of the cell.

3. **Functions**
   a. **Organization of cellular components**
      (1) Microtubules determine the position of the rough endoplasmic reticulum (rER) and the Golgi complex.
      (2) They influence the distribution of intermediate filaments. In some cases (e.g., during separation of daughter cells after cell division), they determine the distribution of actin filaments.
      (3) They are essential for the formation of cytoplasmic processes in some cell types, such as neurons.

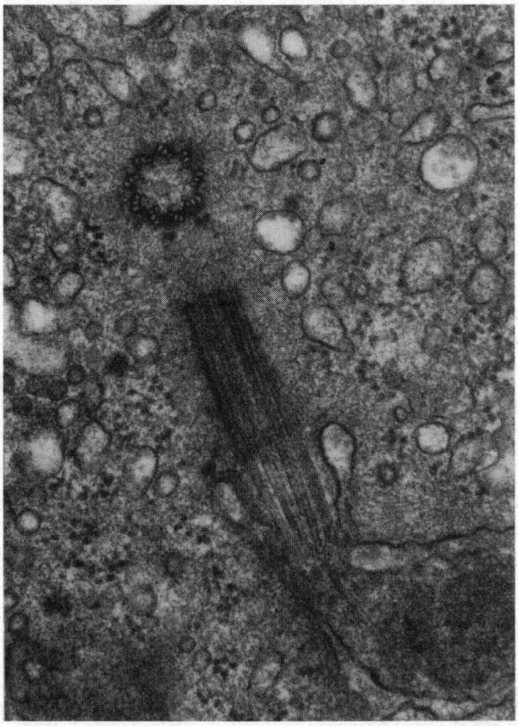

Figure 3-4. Electron micrograph showing a pair of centrioles in a neuron. One centriole, at the *upper left,* is seen in cross-section. The other, which is cut along its longitudinal axis, has assumed the role of basal body by organizing the formation of a small cilium (*lower right*).

b. Cytoskeletal support. Microtubules are **major skeletal elements** in asymmetric cells.

(1) The helical substructure of microtubules makes them **semirigid**. Without microtubules, expenditure of energy would be necessary to maintain irregular cellular shapes.

(2) Microtubules help to **support nerve cell processes** that can exceed 1 m in length. In addition, they help to **maintain the flattened discoid shape of red blood cells** and **platelets**.

c. Intracellular movement systems

(1) Microtubules **direct the movement of certain organelles and other cytoplasmic components** along defined routes. They are essential for the following processes:

(a) Movement of **transfer vesicles** from the rER to the immature face of the Golgi complex

(b) Movement of **secretory vesicles and granules** to the plasma membrane during secretion

(c) Movement of **endocytotic vesicles** into the cell

(d) Movement of **transcytotic vesicles** across the cell from one surface to another

(e) Movement of materials to and from the cell body via the nerve cell processes (i.e., retrograde and anterograde transport, respectively), in a process known as **axonal transport**

(f) Movement of **pigment granules** between the cell body and processes in melanocytes to produce changes in skin color

(2) Microtubules in the mitotic apparatus **move chromosomes to the poles of the daughter cells during karyokinesis** (i.e., nuclear division).

4. Light-microscope appearance

a. Individual microtubules are below the limit of resolution with the light microscope.

b. Centrioles. Iron hematoxylin is commonly used to demonstrate centrioles, although a number of other dyes may be used as well. Centrioles appear as **minute rods** within the cytocentrum.

II. CYTOPLASMIC INCLUSIONS

A. Definition. Inclusions were originally defined as structures that do not participate in cellular metabolism. Many are transitory cytoplasmic deposits. However, many inclusions are now known to play metabolic roles.

B. Types of inclusions. The following structures are traditionally classified as inclusions:

1. **Storage forms of foodstuffs** (e.g., fat, carbohydrates) include **lipid droplets** (see Figure 2-4) and **glycogen deposits.**
   a. Stored foodstuffs provide a **constant source of energy for the cell.**
   b. The lipid droplets that are stored in fat cells **provide energy for the entire body between feedings.**
2. **Residual bodies** (see Figure 2-2), which store unmetabolized residues of incomplete lysosomal digestion, may accumulate for the life of the cell. Long-lived, nondividing cells, such as neurons and cardiac muscle cells, accumulate a golden-brown pigment known as **lipofuscin** in their residual bodies.
3. **Pigments** are characteristic of some cells.
   a. **Melanin** is a pigment with a brownish-black form and a reddish-yellow form. It protects the nuclei of skin cells from ultraviolet radiation and provides color for the skin and hair. This coloring helps to camouflage animals from predators.
   b. **Hemoglobin** is a red, iron-containing pigment that transports oxygen and carbon dioxide in red blood cells.
   c. **Hemosiderin,** which contains iron, and **bilirubin,** which does not, are yellowish-brown pigments that are produced by hemoglobin degradation.
      (1) Iron conserved in hemosiderin is reused to make hemoglobin in new red blood cells.
      (2) Bilirubin plays a role in digestion and absorption. It is secreted in the bile.
4. **Secretory granules** (see Figure 3-2), which are eventually released from the cell, and **phagosomes** (see Figure 2-2), which fuse with endosomes or lysosomes, are often classified as inclusions.
5. **Crystals** are present in some cell types. For example, insulin-secreting cells in the pancreas of some species contain insulin crystals. Although the exact composition and function of these crystals have not been determined, most are believed to be proteinaceous.

C. Light-microscope appearance

1. When viewed light microscopically after routine histologic procedures, both **lipid droplets** and **glycogen deposits** appear as empty areas.
   a. **Lipid droplets** have **distinct, smooth outlines.**
   b. **Glycogen deposits** have irregular and indistinct outlines.
2. **Pigment** color is independent of the stain used: Lipofuscin is yellowish-brown, and melanin is brownish-black.

III. CYTOPLASMIC MATRIX (HYALOPLASM, CYTOSOL)

A. Location and composition. The **cytoplasmic matrix** occupies the intracellular space between organelles and inclusions. It contains water and soluble molecules, including molecular building blocks of the organelles and cytoskeletal elements, enzymes, and other factors involved in metabolic reactions. Researchers disagree regarding the extent to which the matrix is a homogeneous sol (i.e., a colloidal fluid), versus a combination of solvated regions and structured, semirigid gelated regions.

1. **Sol.** The **endoplasm,** which surrounds the organelles, is a sol. **Cytoplasmic streaming** moves organelles and solutes around rapidly in the endoplasmic matrix.

2. **Gel**
   a. The **cytocentrum,** which is the spherical region surrounding the centrioles, is a gel.
   b. The **ectoplasm,** which is the peripheral cytoplasm, contains no membranous organelles, but may contain many filaments. The ectoplasmic matrix is usually gelated but **can undergo rapid sol–gel transformation,** especially in ameboid cells.

B. Functions

1. The cytoplasmic matrix **permits diffusion of soluble materials** to various parts of the cell and is itself the **site of many metabolic reactions**.
2. **Gelated regions limit the movement of organelles.**

C. Light-microscope appearance. The cytoplasmic matrix is featureless light microscopically.

STUDY QUESTIONS

DIRECTIONS: Each of the numbered items or incomplete statements in this section is followed by answers or completions of the statement. Select the **one** numbered answer or completion that is **best** in each case.

1. Would it be justifiable to call microtubules and the other cytoplasmic filaments the "musculoskeletal system" of the cell? Explain.

(1) Yes, because microtubules and the other filaments are all contractile and provide rigidity or tensile strength to the cell.
(2) Yes, because microtubules and the other filaments provide rigidity to the cytoplasm, and intermediate filaments effect movement of the plasma membrane.
(3) Yes, because functionally, microtubules correspond to bone and cartilage, intermediate filaments correspond to tendons and ligaments, and microfilaments correspond to muscle.
(4) No, because each type of filament has only a support function or a contractile function, not both.
(5) No, because microtubules and cytoplasmic filaments have only cytoskeletal function.

2. Which one of the following statements *best* describes microfilaments in nonmuscle cells?

(1) Microfilaments are composed of tubulin subunits.
(2) Microfilaments in nonmuscle cells do not contain actin.
(3) Microfilaments are fairly uniformly distributed in the endoplasmic cytosol.
(4) Most microfilaments are located near the cell membrane.
(5) Microfilaments form the contractile core of cilia and flagella.

3. Which one of the following is a major function of microfilaments?

(1) Separation of daughter cells after cell division
(2) Beating of cilia
(3) Movement of chromosomes to the poles during cell division
(4) Support of the asymmetric shapes of nerve cell processes
(5) Attachment of thick filaments to the cell membrane

4. Which one of the following statements *best* describes intermediate filaments?

(1) Although all intermediate filaments have the same molecular character, they are given different names in different cells.
(2) Keratin filaments are abundant in muscle cells, where they support and attach contractile filaments.
(3) Intercellular junctions are supported primarily by vimentin filaments.
(4) Bundles of tonofilaments, called tonofibrils, can be seen light microscopically.
(5) Spectrin filaments are characteristic of surface epithelial cells.

5. Which one of the following statements *best* describes the structure of microtubules?

(1) Their helical substructure makes them semirigid.
(2) They are tubular polymers composed of actin.
(3) They contain both actin and myosin.
(4) They rarely form bundles or associate with other microtubules.
(5) Their value as cytoskeletal elements is enhanced by their permanence.

6. Which one of the following cytoplasmic inclusions is a storage form for nutrients?

(1) Melanin
(2) Bilirubin
(3) Glycogen
(4) Hemosiderin
(5) Residual bodies

7. One of the functions of microtubules is:

(1) forming the contractile core of microvilli.
(2) providing flexibility to cell processes.
(3) anchoring intercellular junctions.
(4) preventing movement of organelles into the ectoplasm.
(5) transporting materials back and forth between the cell body and processes of certain cell types.

8. Which one of the following statements about the structure and distribution of centrioles is true?

(1) Centrioles are composed of nine spirally arranged microtubules.
(2) Centrioles usually lie between the nucleus and the Golgi complex.
(3) Just before cell division occurs, a cell contains at least four centrioles.
(4) Centrioles lie adjacent to the cytocentrum, an amorphous gelated region that surrounds the centrioles and the nucleus.
(5) After cell division, each daughter cell contains a single centriole.

9. Hyaloplasm and cytosol refer to:

(1) the gelated region underlying the cell membrane.
(2) the endoplasmic reticulum (ER).
(3) all of the protein-secreting organelles.
(4) the material that occupies the regions between organelles.
(5) all cytoskeletal elements.

10. Which one of the following inclusions resembles an empty area with an indistinct, irregular surface in routine light-microscope preparations?

(1) Glycogen
(2) Lipid
(3) Phagosomes
(4) Residual bodies
(5) Pigment granules

11. Which one of the following statements *best* describes the cytoplasmic matrix?

(1) The endoplasmic matrix is a semirigid gel.
(2) Streaming movements of the endoplasmic matrix move organelles around rapidly.
(3) Metabolically important molecules diffuse through the cytoplasmic matrix, but metabolic reactions occur only in or on the membranous surfaces of organelles.
(4) The ectoplasmic matrix is a gelated region that contains few organelles or cytoskeletal elements.
(5) Sol–gel transformation of the ectoplasmic matrix is rare, and is limited to cells that are well supported by attachments to adjacent structures.

12. All of the following functions would be affected by depolymerization of microtubules *except*:

(1) secretion.
(2) contraction of muscle cells.
(3) mitosis.
(4) ciliary action.
(5) maintenance of the shape of cell processes.

ANSWERS AND EXPLANATIONS

1. The answer is 3. *[I A 3, B 2, C 3 b]*. The microtubules and other cytoplasmic filaments could be considered the "musculoskeletal system" of the cell. Microtubules are semirigid structures that provide mechanical support to the cell and its processes in the way that bone and cartilage do for the vertebrate body. The intermediate filaments correspond to the strong fibrous attachments of the tendons and ligaments, in that they provide tensile strength and support to the cell and its processes. Microfilaments are contractile proteins in muscle cells as well as other cell types. Intermediate filaments are not contractile and are not directly involved in cellular movements. Microtubules and microfilaments have roles in both cellular support and movement.

2. The answer is 4 *[I A 2 b]*. Because microfilaments are involved in plasmalemmal movements in nonmuscle cells, most are located near the cell membrane. Microfilaments in all cells are formed by the polymerization of globular actin molecules (G-actin) to form long filaments (F-actin). The contractile internal core of cilia and flagella is formed by microtubules.

3. The answer is 1 *[I A 3 b (1)]*. Microfilaments are involved in movement of the cell membrane, such as takes place during separation of the daughter cells after cell division, ameboid movements, and endocytosis. Beating of cilia is accomplished by interactions between microtubules in their core. Chromosome movement during mitosis also depends on microtubules, which form the mitotic apparatus (spindle). Although microfilaments aid in the formation of cytoplasmic processes, it is the semirigid character of microtubules that provides long-term support for permanent asymmetric processes, such as those of nerve cells, without the expenditure of energy. Thick filaments are not attached directly to the plasma membrane. Actin filaments are anchored to the cell membrane by intermediate filaments.

4. The answer is 4 *[I B 3 b]*. Tonofibrils are bundles of tonofilaments that are large enough to be seen light microscopically. Tonofilaments, which are composed of keratin, are especially important in epithelial cells, where they anchor intercellular junctions, thereby maintaining the integrity of surfaces that are exposed to frictional or shearing forces. Although all intermediate filaments are similar in size and function cytoskeletally, their constituent proteins differ according to cell type. Contractile filaments in muscle cells are supported by and attached to the cell membrane by desmin filaments. Vimentin is most abundant near the nucleus in cells that are derived from the mesenchyme. Spectrin filaments form a reinforcing layer under the plasma membrane of red blood cells.

5. The answer is 1 *[I C 3 b (1)]*. Microtubules are formed when tubulin subunits polymerize in a tight, semirigid helix. They do not contain actin or myosin. Although microtubules may be distributed singly in the cytoplasm, they commonly form sheets or bundles, or even combine to form other cytoplasmic structures, such as centrioles and cilia. Microtubules in centrioles, cilia, and flagella are relatively stable, but most are highly labile, forming and dissolving readily as needed.

6. The answer is 3 *[II B 1]*. Glycogen deposits, which are the storage form of carbohydrates, and lipid droplets, which are the storage form of fats, are the most common nutrient-containing cytoplasmic inclusions. Melanin is a pigment, as are bilirubin, which does not contain iron, and hemosiderin, which does. Residual bodies contain materials that the cell cannot metabolize.

7. The answer is 5 *[I C 3 c (1) (e)]*. The role of microtubules in transporting materials between the cell body and cell processes has been extensively studied in nerve cells. In neurons, microtubules are essential for the movement of membranes and other essential materials into processes called axons, which lack protein-synthesizing capability, and for the return of chemical messages from the axon ending to the cell body. Microfilaments form the contractile core of microvilli. Microtubules provide rigidity, not flexibility, to cell processes. Intermediate filaments provide tensile strength without loss of flexibility, and also anchor intercellular junctions. Organelles are limited to the endoplasmic cytosol by the physical character of the cytoplasmic matrix, which is usually gelated in the ectoplasm.

8. The answer is 3 *[I C 2 b]*. Centrioles are always found in pairs, and just before cell division occurs, a new centriole forms in association with each member of the original pair, making a total of four centrioles. Multinucleated cells may have many pairs of centrioles, typically one pair for each nucleus. Centrioles are composed of 27 microtubules that are arranged in nine groups of three. They usually lie near the mature face of the Golgi complex, which is the side opposite the nucleus, within a gelated region called the cytocentrum. The cytocentrum contains no other structures. In a good light-microscope preparation, the centrioles can be seen as small rods in the cytocentrum.

9. The answer is 4 *[III A]*. Hyaloplasm and cytosol are synonyms for the cytoplasmic matrix, which occupies the regions between organelles and other formed cytoplasmic elements. The ectoplasm, a gelated region underlying the cell membrane, is part of the cytoplasmic matrix. The endoplasmic reticulum (ER), like all other cytoplasmic organelles, lies within and is surrounded by the cytoplasmic matrix.

10. The answer is 1 *[II C 1 b]*. Glycogen, which is extracted, or is not stained by routine techniques, comprises scattered aggregations of submicroscopic granules in the cytoplasm. Therefore, deposits of glycogen have an irregular surface. Lipid droplets, which also appear as empty areas in routine preparations, have a well-defined outline. Phagosomes and residual bodies are preserved and well stained in most sections, and pigment granules are visible even in unstained preparations.

11. The answer is 2 *[III A 1]*. Cytoplasmic streaming moves organelles around the endoplasm and is important for distributing solutes around the cell. Cytoplasmic streaming is possible because the endoplasmic matrix is a sol, not a semirigid gel. Streaming carries molecules to and from organelles, and also facilitates the molecular encounters that are necessary for the many reactions that occur in the matrix. Few organelles penetrate the gelated ectoplasm, but many cytoskeletal elements are located there. Actin is particularly abundant in this region, which is near the cell membrane. Sol–gel transformation of the ectoplasm can occur rapidly. It is especially important in motile cells that are undergoing ameboid motion.

12. The answer is 2 *[I A 3 a, C 3]*. Muscle contraction is accomplished by the interaction of thin filaments, which contain microfilaments, and myosin. Secretion, mitosis, ciliary action, and maintenance of the shape of cell processes depend on microtubules. Microtubules move transfer vesicles from the rough endoplasmic reticulum (rER) to the Golgi complex and secretory granules from the Golgi complex to the cell membrane during secretion. They also form the mitotic apparatus that moves chromosomes to the poles during mitosis. Microtubules form the motile cores of cilia and flagella, and also maintain the shape of permanent cell processes.

Chapter 4

Cellular Membranes and Adaptations of the Cell Surface

I. CELLULAR MEMBRANES

A. Description.

Membranes surround the cell and divide it into compartments.

1. A **cell membrane (plasma membrane, plasmalemma)** surrounds the cell, forming a semipermeable barrier between the cytoplasm and the extracellular environment.
2. **Intracellular membranes** separate the nucleus from the cytoplasm. They also separate the interiors of organelles and most inclusions from the cytosol (i.e., the cytoplasmic matrix between the organelles and cytoskeletal components).

B. Composition.

All cellular membranes comprise a **lipid bilayer** and **associated proteins** (Figure 4-1).

1. The **lipid bilayer** is a double layer of lipid molecules that forms the boundary.
   a. **Phospholipids, cholesterol,** and **glycolipids** make up the lipid bilayer.
   b. Each lipid molecule has two **nonpolar (hydrophobic) tails,** which are directed into the membrane interior, and a **polar (hydrophilic) head** that faces one surface or the other.
2. **Proteins** are the major membrane component by weight. They lie within and upon the lipid bilayer (see Figure 4-1).
   a. **Integral (intrinsic) membrane proteins** have a nonpolar portion that lies within the lipid bilayer.

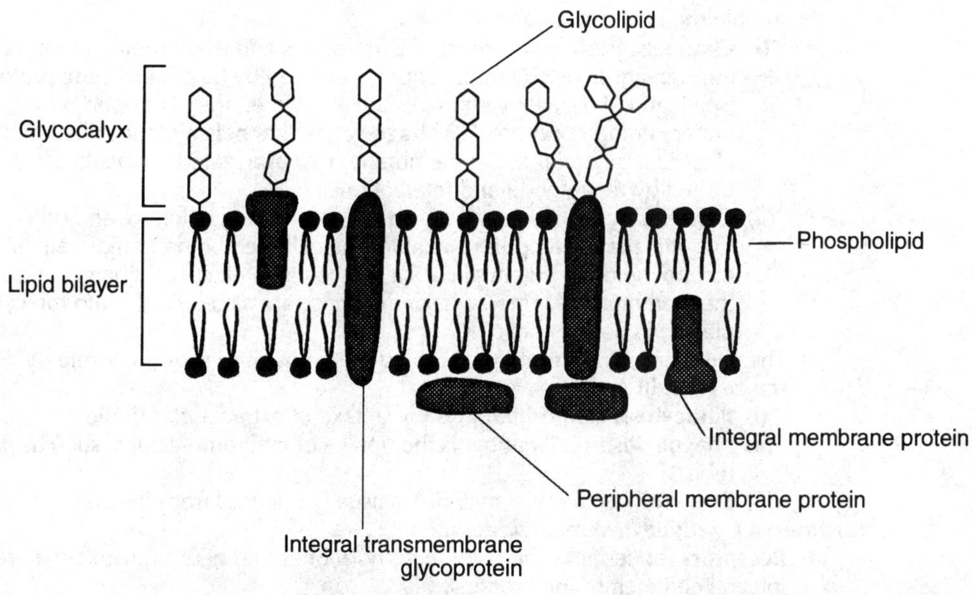

Figure 4-1. Schematic drawing of the cell membrane. The intracellular (cytosol-facing) surface is toward the bottom, and the extracellular face is toward the top. Collectively, the surface oligosaccharides constitute the glycocalyx. (Reprinted with permission from Dellmann H-D: *Textbook of Veterinary Histology,* 4th ed. Baltimore, Williams & Wilkins, 1993, p 2.)

(1) Some integral membrane proteins, called **transmembrane proteins,** extend all the way through the membrane so that polar portions are exposed on both membrane surfaces. Other integral membrane proteins are exposed only to one membrane surface or the other (see Figure 4-1).

(2) Many integral protein molecules are able to drift about in the plane of the membrane. However, certain transmembrane integral proteins attach to elements adjacent to the membrane. Integrin is a transmembrane protein that attaches to both cytoskeletal proteins and extracellular molecules.

b. **Peripheral (extrinsic) membrane proteins** lie outside the lipid bilayer because they lack a nonpolar region that can extend into the bilayer. They are held by weak electrostatic forces to the surface.

C. Types of cellular membranes

1. **Cell membranes** (see Figure 4-1)

a. **Composition.** Like all cellular membranes, the cell membrane comprises a lipid bilayer with integral and extrinsic proteins. In addition, **oligosaccharides** (small carbohydrates) form a layer called the **glycocalyx** on the extracellular surface of the cell membrane.

(1) **Glycoproteins.** Many oligosaccharides are attached to integral or extrinsic membrane proteins, forming glycoproteins. Most membrane proteins are actually glycoproteins.

(2) **Glycolipids.** Other oligosaccharides are attached to lipids in the outer layer, forming glycolipids.

b. **Functions.** Cell membrane functions are depicted in Figure 4-2.

(1) **Selective barrier.** The cell membrane determines which substances enter or leave the cell, thereby controlling the composition of the cytoplasm.

(a) The **lipid bilayer** is a **semipermeable barrier.**

(i) It is relatively **impermeable to most water-soluble molecules;** however, **lipid-soluble substances readily diffuse** through the lipid bilayer.

(ii) Water passes freely because the molecules are very small and electrically neutral.

(b) Proteins in the cell membrane form **channels** and act as **carriers** for water-soluble molecules and ions.

(i) **Channels. Passive transport** of certain ions and small molecules occurs through aqueous channels, or pores, formed by transmembrane proteins (see Figure 4-1). Many channels are **gated** (i.e., they are open only under certain conditions). **Voltage-gated channels** are controlled by the electrical potential of the membrane; **receptor-gated channels** are controlled by receptor–ligand interactions.

(ii) **Carriers. Active transport** of sodium, potassium, calcium, and other ions via enzymatic pumps enables the cell membrane to maintain an electrochemical potential (i.e., a difference in electrical charge) across the membrane. Amino acids and glucose are also brought into the cytoplasm via active transport.

(c) The cell membrane's motility and plasticity allow it to take up or release substances (see III A–B).

(i) **Pinocytosis** (cell drinking) is the uptake of extracellular liquids.

(ii) **Phagocytosis** (cell eating) is the uptake of macromolecules, such as proteins.

(iii) **Exocytosis** is the way material is usually released from the cell.

(2) **Interface with environmental factors**

(a) **Receptors** for certain molecules (e.g., hormones and neurotransmitters) are integral cell membrane proteins.

(i) **Receptor-mediated functions** include hormone actions, antigen recognition, phagocytosis, and neurotransmission.

(ii) **Receptor abnormalities** can profoundly affect cellular function. Many diseases involve receptor abnormalities.

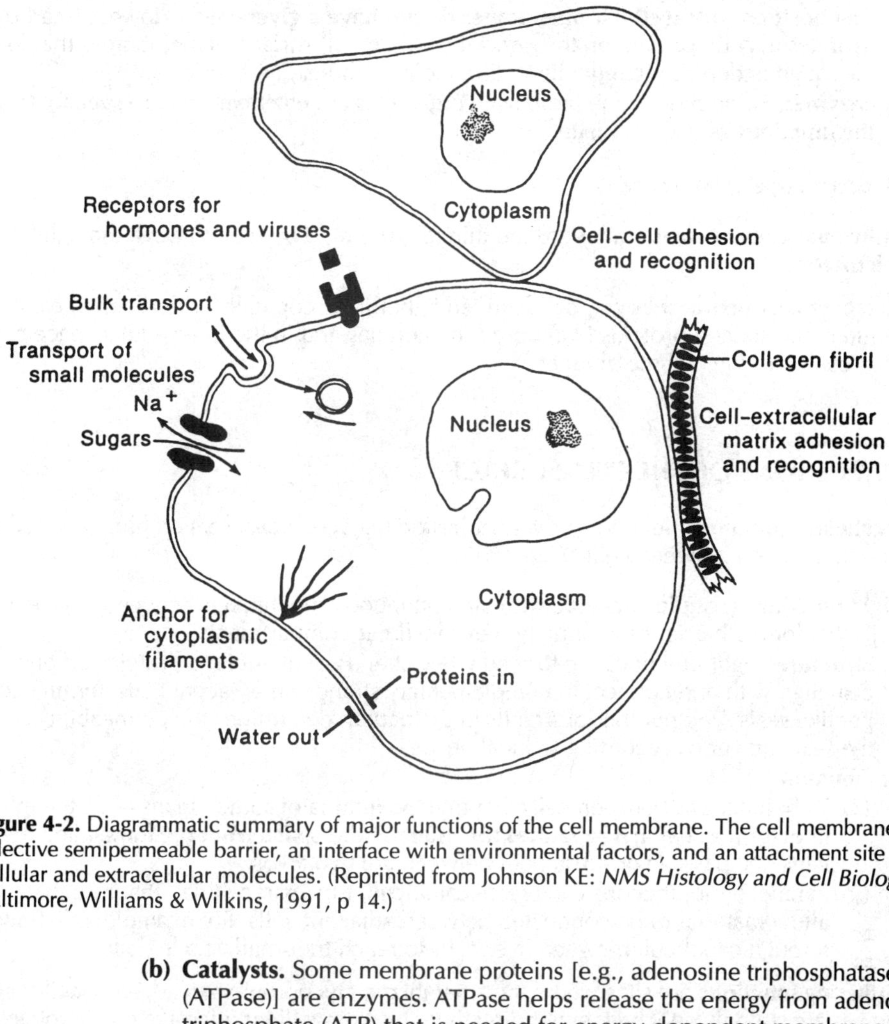

Figure 4-2. Diagrammatic summary of major functions of the cell membrane. The cell membrane acts as a selective semipermeable barrier, an interface with environmental factors, and an attachment site for intracellular and extracellular molecules. (Reprinted from Johnson KE: *NMS Histology and Cell Biology,* 2nd ed. Baltimore, Williams & Wilkins, 1991, p 14.)

- **(b) Catalysts.** Some membrane proteins [e.g., adenosine triphosphatase (ATPase)] are enzymes. ATPase helps release the energy from adenosine triphosphate (ATP) that is needed for energy-dependent membrane functions (e.g., active transport).
- **(c) Junctions.** Integral cell membrane proteins called cell adhesion molecules (CAMs) can form specialized junctions between cells or between cells and extracellular components (see also II A 1–3).
- **(d) Intercellular recognition.** Oligosaccharides in the glycocalyx probably serve as surface recognition factors.
  - **(i) Contact inhibition,** which regulates the degree to which normal cells grow and divide, involves recognition of specific surface factors.
  - **(ii) Immune responses** are based on recognition of "nonself" versus "self" surface factors.
  - **(iii) Morphogenesis** (i.e., the formation of the various tissues, organs, and body parts) depends on identification of neighboring cells during development.

(3) Fortification. Extrinsic membrane proteins may strengthen the membrane or hold other membrane proteins in position. Microfilaments and intermediate filament proteins (e.g., spectrin) can be extrinsic membrane proteins.

2. Intracellular membranes. Intracellular membranes resemble cell membranes, with the following exceptions:

a. Size. Intracellular membranes are **slightly thinner** than cell membranes.

b. **Composition. Intracellular membranes do not have a glycocalyx.** However, carbohydrates may be present on the noncytosol (luminal) surface of membranes that form the rough endoplasmic reticulum (rER), Golgi complex, and vesicles.

c. **Enzymes.** Some membrane proteins in organelles are enzymes that are **specific to the functions of the organelle**.

D. Light-microscope appearance

1. **Individual cellular membranes** are too thin (8–10 nm) to be seen through the light microscope.

2. **Adjacent cell membranes** can be identified light microscopically when seen in cross-section. The stained proteins in apposed membranes and in the intercellular space mark the position of the cell membranes.

II. ADAPTATIONS OF THE CELL SURFACE

A. Intercellular junctions.

Junctions provide adhesion between cells, seal off lumina, or allow for communication between cells (Figure 4-3).

1. **Tight junctions (zonulae occludentes)** are continuous attachments between adjacent cells that form a barrier separating two extracellular compartments.
   a. **Structure.** Tight junctions are formed when strands of membrane proteins on one cell align with and connect to complementary strands on adjacent cells, forming zipper-like seals. The number of strands in the pattern determines the permeability of the seal and varies according to local needs.
   b. **Function**
      (1) Tight junctions between cells that line the lumina of some organs (e.g., the intestine) form a seal that **separates the intercellular space from the lumen** and prevents the passage of substances between the two areas.
      (2) Parallel tight junctions can create **canaliculi,** tiny extracellular channels that allow material to be conducted between adjacent cells. For example, bile flows through canaliculi between liver cells to reach the smallest bile ducts.

2. **Adhering junctions** are sites where transmembrane glycoproteins in adjacent cell membranes are strongly attached, either directly or by extracellular adhesive glycoproteins (e.g., fibronectin). They are supported at the cytoplasmic membrane surface by attachments to intracellular cytoskeletal elements.
   a. A **zonula adherens (intermediate junction, belt desmosome)** is a type of adhering junction that joins adjacent cells around their entire perimeter. A zonula adherens usually parallels and supports a zonula occludens (see Figure 4-3).
      (1) **Structure.** Intercellular adhesive glycoproteins bond to integrins (see I B 2 a) in the closely apposed cell membranes.
      (2) **Function**
         (a) Contractile microfilaments are attached to the cytoplasmic surface of integrins in the cell membrane by proteins in the junctional region.
         (b) Zonulae adherentes prevent adjacent cells from pulling away from each other when microvilli and terminal webs in the apical cytoplasm contract. These junctions are especially well developed where the surface layer is exposed to frictional or shearing forces.
   b. A **desmosome (macula adherens, spot desmosome)** is a circular adhering junction. Desmosomes are located at discrete spots along the surface of the cell (Figure 4-4; see Figure 4-3).
      (1) **Structure**
         (a) **Extracellular surface.** A **dense plaque,** believed to be the interwoven filamentous portions of transmembrane linker glycoproteins that attach the two cells, exists between the apposed cell membranes.

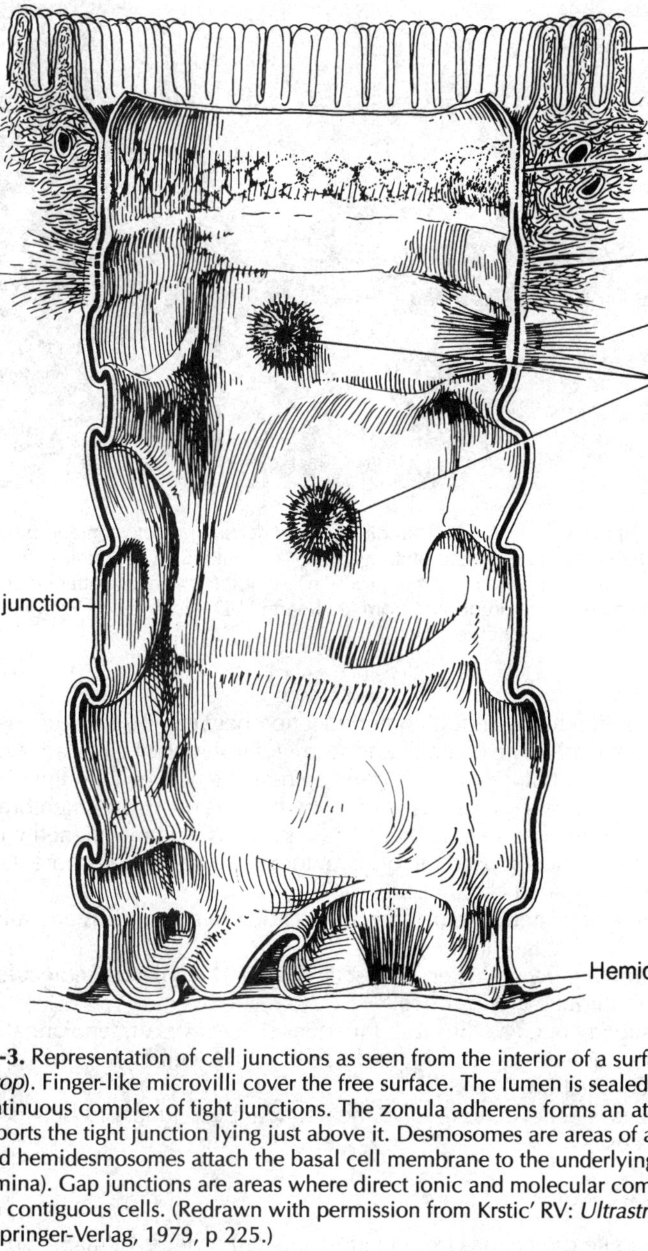

Figure 4-3. Representation of cell junctions as seen from the interior of a surface cell lining the intestinal lumen (*top*). Finger-like microvilli cover the free surface. The lumen is sealed from the intercellular spaces by a continuous complex of tight junctions. The zonula adherens forms an attachment band that parallels and supports the tight junction lying just above it. Desmosomes are areas of attachment between adjacent cells, and hemidesmosomes attach the basal cell membrane to the underlying extracellular material (i.e., the basal lamina). Gap junctions are areas where direct ionic and molecular communication is possible between contiguous cells. (Redrawn with permission from Krstic' RV: *Ultrastructure of the Mammalian Cell.* Berlin, Springer-Verlag, 1979, p 225.)

(b) Cytoplasmic surface. Dense plaques that contain intracellular attachment proteins are located on the cytoplasmic side of the junctional cell membrane. The attachment proteins join the cytoplasmic ends of the transmembrane linker molecules to cytoplasmic tonofilaments.

(2) Function. Desmosomes hold adjacent cells (i.e., groups or layers of cells) together.

(a) Desmosomes are most numerous in the surface layer of the skin and other surface layers that are subjected to shearing forces, but they are also present between cells in many different tissues.

(b) Hemidesmosomes resemble desmosomes and attach surface cells to underlying extracellular material rather than to other cells [see Chapter 5 II C 2 a (1) (b)].

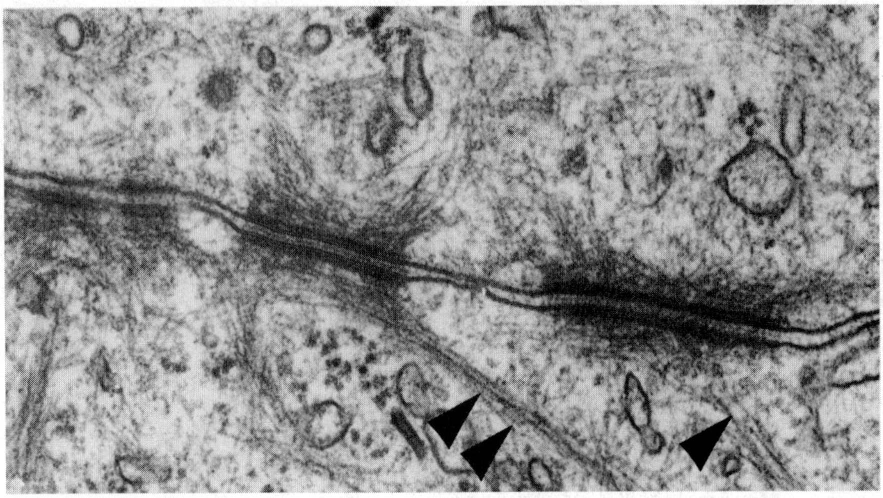

Figure 4-4. Electron micrograph of two desmosomes. The intermediate dense line between and parallel to the adjacent cell membranes is believed to be formed by transmembrane linking glycoproteins. Tonofilaments (*arrowheads*), a type of intermediate filament, can be seen inserting into the dense attachment plaque on the cytoplasmic surface of the membrane. (Reprinted from Dellmann H-D: *Textbook of Veterinary Histology,* 4th ed. Baltimore, Williams & Wilkins, 1993, p 13.)

3. **Gap (communicating) junctions** permit communication between cells (Figure 4-5). The region of apposition may be large or small and is irregular in outline. The apposing cell membranes are very close, but a narrow (3 nm) gap remains between the lipid bilayers.
   a. **Structure.** Tubular channels (pores) are formed by clusters of six transmembrane proteins that project into the intercellular gap. These proteins become aligned with corresponding proteins in the apposed membrane, forming a continuous pore. Gap junctions contain many such channels.
   b. **Functions.** Gap junctions **permit rapid communication between cells** and allow certain groups of cells to act as a unit.
      (1) **Metabolic coupling** occurs when nutrients, ions, and regulatory molecules are rapidly spread through groups of cells.
      (2) **Electrical coupling** occurs when gap junctions pass waves of depolarization between cells, such as nerve and muscle cells, whose cell membranes are specialized for conduction.
      (3) **Morphogenesis** is believed to involve the abundant gap junctions between embryonic cells.

B. Cilia and flagella

1. Cilia are hair-like, motile projections from the free (apical) surfaces of many types of cells (Figure 4-6). Many cell types have a single cilium, and certain cells (e.g., those lining the air-conducting passages of the respiratory system) have several hundred cilia.
   a. **Structure**
      (1) Each cilium projects from a **basal body** (see Figure 4-6A) that is anchored in the apical cytoplasm by a filamentous rootlet. The structure of basal bodies is identical to that of centrioles (see Chapter 3 I C 2 b).
      (2) The **axoneme** (i.e., the motile apparatus in the shaft) comprises arrays of **microtubules** and their complex interconnections. These microtubules are arranged in a characteristic cylindrical pattern (see Figure 4-6B).
         (a) **Nine peripheral doublets** (i.e., nine pairs of microtubules) grow into the cilium from each triplet in the basal body. The doublets slide relative to each other to cause ciliary movement.

A

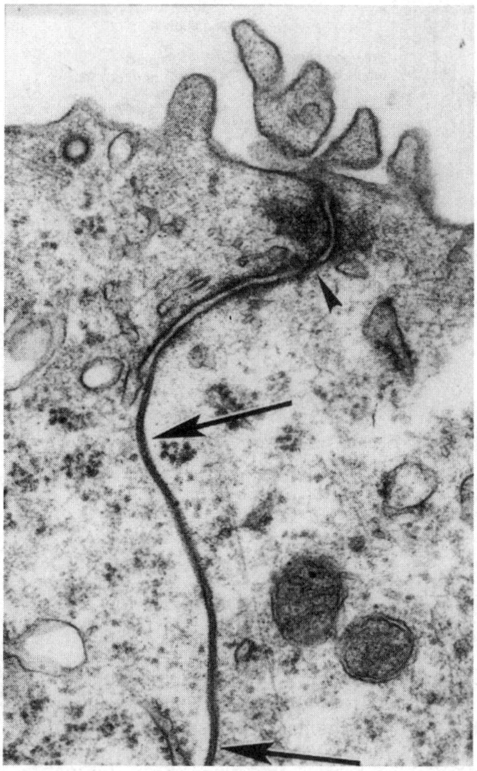

B

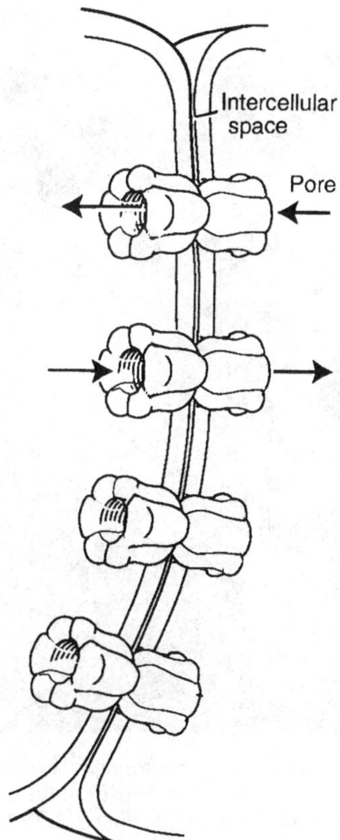

Figure 4-5. Gap junctions. (*A*) Electron micrograph showing a gap junction (*arrows*) between two ependymal cells. A zonula adherens (*arrowhead*) is also visible. Reprinted from Dellmann H-D: *Textbook of Veterinary Histology,* 4th ed. Baltimore, Williams & Wilkins, 1993, p 13.) (*B*) Schematic representation of a portion of a gap junction, demonstrating how clusters of transmembrane proteins are arranged and aligned with those in the neighboring cell to form a continuous channel through which ions and small molecules can pass (*arrows*).

- **(i) Dynein,** a protein with ATPase activity, forms short arms on each peripheral doublet.
- **(ii)** Dynein hydrolyzes ATP to release energy that is used to slide the doublets relative to each other.

(b) Two central singlet microtubules are in the middle of the cylinder.

b. Functions

(1) Movement of extracellular material. Microtubules in the shaft of the cilium generate a **rigid action stroke** and a **flexible recovery stroke**.

(a) Mechanism. A **mucociliary apparatus,** found in certain mucous membranes, is formed by richly ciliated cells and mucous cells or glands.

- **(i)** Coordinated strokes of hundreds of cilia resemble waves that keep a surface sheet of mucus constantly moving.
- **(ii)** The sticky surface of the mucous layer adheres to particles or cells that touch it and carries them along in the desired direction.
- **(iii)** The deeper layers of mucus are less viscous, minimizing resistance to the recovery strokes of the cilia.

(b) Applications

- **(i)** In the **respiratory system,** the mucociliary apparatus removes particulate matter.
- **(ii)** In parts of the **reproductive system,** the mucociliary apparatus transports secretions as well as the oocyte.

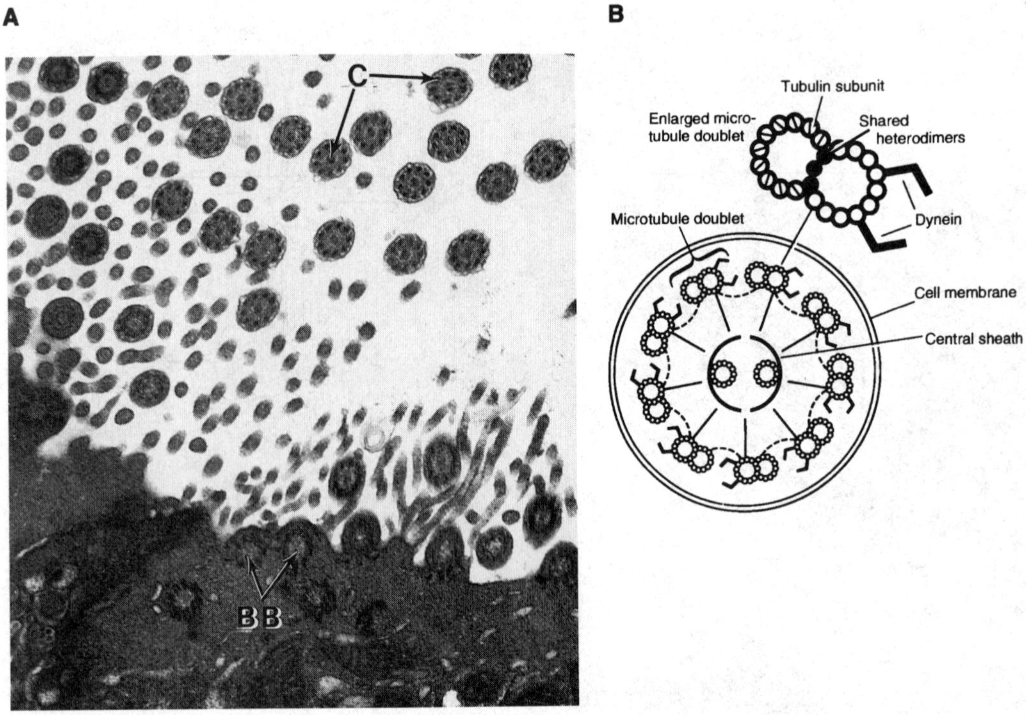

Figure 4-6. Cilia. (*A*) Electron micrograph showing cilia (*C*) on cells lining the lumen of the trachea. Each cilium is anchored by a basal body (*BB*) in the cytoplasm. (Reprinted from Johnson KE: *NMS Histology and Cell Biology,* 2nd ed. Baltimore, Williams & Wilkins, 1991, p 47.) (*B*) Schematic representation of a cross-section through the shaft of a cilium to show its microtubular substructure (i.e., the axoneme). The dynein arms on each doublet have adenosine triphosphatase (ATPase) activity; they are involved in the sliding of doublets relative to each other during ciliary movement. (Redrawn with permission from Junqueira LC, Carneiro J, Kelley RO: *Basic Histology,* 7th ed. Englewood Cliffs, NJ, Appleton & Lange, 1992, p 46.)

(2) **Sensory receptors.** Some cilia are modified to serve a sensory function. They function as:
   (a) Photoreceptors in the eye
   (b) Chemoreceptors in the nose (olfactory epithelium)
   (c) Sensory portions of hair cells in the ear

2. **Flagella** are longer than cilia and are present only on spermatozoa in mammals.
   a. **Structure.** Each flagellum has the same microtubular core as cilia, plus additional structures. The single flagellum arises from one of the cell's two centrioles, which serves as its basal body.
   b. **Function.** Flagella are instrumental to cell locomotion.

3. **Light-microscope appearance**
   a. **Individual cilia** and **flagella** are usually about 200 nm in diameter and 10 μm in length (longer, in the case of flagella). At high magnification, they are slender projections from the free surface.
   b. **Basal bodies** can also be detected if the specimen is well prepared.

C. **Microvilli** are very fine, finger-like projections from the free surface of many cells.

1. **Structure** (Figure 4-7A)
   a. Each microvillus is covered by a cell membrane with a surface **glycocalyx**.

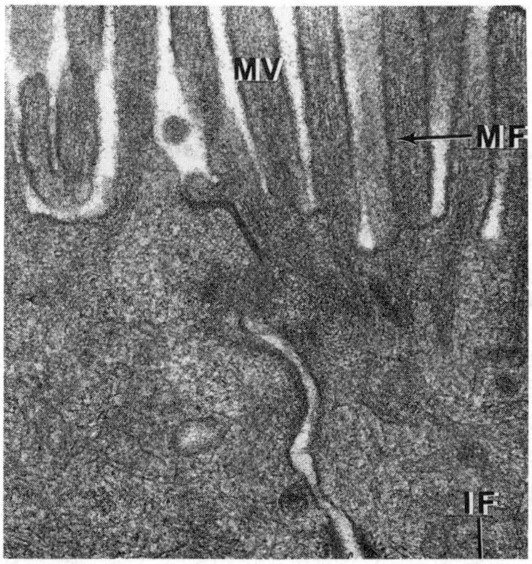

A

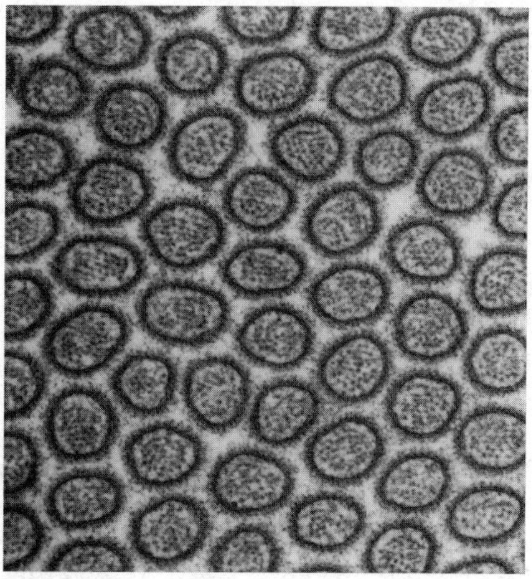
B

Figure 4-7. Microvilli. (*A*) Longitudinal sections through microvilli (*MV*) reveal that the bundles of microfilaments (*MF*) that form the cores of microvilli insert into the terminal web. (Reprinted from Johnson KE: *NMS Histology and Cell Biology,* 2nd ed. Baltimore, Williams & Wilkins, 1991, p 49.) (*B*) Cross-sections through microvilli that have been sectioned in a plane parallel to the cell surface. Notice that each microvillus has a core of microfilaments and a "fuzzy" surface, the glycocalyx. (Reprinted from Dellmann H-D: *Textbook of Veterinary Histology,* 4th ed. Baltimore, Williams & Wilkins, 1993, p 3.)

b. Each microvillus contains a **core of 20–30 microfilaments** (see Figure 4-7B). The microfilaments are attached at one end to the inner surface of the cell membrane at the tip of the microvillus, and their other end is enmeshed in the terminal web in the apical cytoplasm.

2. Function. Microvilli tremendously **increase the surface area available for absorption**. Cells that are specialized for absorption (e.g., those lining the intestine) have large numbers of microvilli arranged in orderly arrays.

a. The actin contained in the cores of microvilli enables them to contract, pumping absorbed molecules toward the cell body.

b. The glycocalyx is very well developed on microvilli in the intestinal lining to facilitate the uptake of substances.

3. Light-microscope appearance

a. Individual microvilli, with diameters of only about 80 nm, cannot be seen through the light microscope.

b. Brush (striated) borders. Where microvilli combine to form a layer of closely spaced projections (e.g., on intestinal absorptive cells), striations perpendicular to the surface can be detected at higher magnifications. In brush borders, large amounts of stain are absorbed by the actin, which is acidophilic, and the glycoproteins in the glycocalyx.

c. In the **epididymis,** microvilli are very long and branched. Clumps of these microvilli are easily seen and may be mistaken for cilia.

III. TRANSIENT ADAPTATIONS OF THE CELL SURFACE

A. Endocytosis is the general term for any process used by the cell to bring in material from its surroundings (see Figure 2-2).

1. **Phagocytosis**
   a. **Process.** Phagocytosis is a **regulated** (i.e., receptor-mediated) **process** by which the cell ingests particles or large molecules.
      (1) **Binding.** Receptors on the cell surface bind to the particle to be phagocytosed.
      (2) **Enclosure.** Cytoplasmic processes gradually envelop the particle by progressive binding of additional receptors in the cell membrane to the particle surface.
      (3) **Separation.** The portion of the membrane surrounding the particle separates from the rest of the cell membrane and is released into the cytoplasm. The new membrane-bounded vesicle is called a **phagosome** or **phagocytic vesicle**.
      (4) **Digestion.** After phagocytosis, the phagosome fuses with a **lysosome,** which digests the material with its hydrolytic enzymes (see Chapter 2 I A–B).
   b. **Significance.** Phagocytosis is not important in most vertebrate cells; however, many white blood cells are actively phagocytic.

2. **Pinocytosis**
   a. **Process.** Pinocytosis is a **constitutive process** (i.e., it is continuous and unregulated) by which the cell ingests fluids. Like phagocytosis, it occurs by invagination and separation of a vesicle, but unlike phagocytosis, the vesicles that are ingested are very small (Figure 4-8).
   b. **Types.** Both nonselective and selective pinocytosis occur.
      (1) **Nonselective pinocytosis** is the **random** ingestion of extracellular fluid.
      (2) **Selective pinocytosis** is **mediated by receptors**.
         (a) **Ligands.** Macromolecules or small particles that bind to specific surface receptors are called ligands. Examples of ligands include **regulatory molecules** and **essential cellular components**. For example, iron bound to the ligand transferrin is concentrated through selective pinocytosis in developing red blood cells for hemoglobin synthesis.
            (i) Ligands can be transported into a cell against a concentration gradient.
            (ii) After pinocytosis, ligands may be processed in several different ways.

Fusion. Pinocytic vesicles fuse with endosomes, which become endolysosomes. An acidic environment permits dissociation of the receptor before the endolysosome becomes a lysosome. The receptor is returned to the cell membrane and reused.

Degradation. Both ligand and receptor may be degraded.

Recycling. Both the ligand and its receptor may be recycled to the cell membrane. For example, the iron-carrying protein ligand transferrin gives up its iron to the cell and is subsequently recycled along with its receptor.

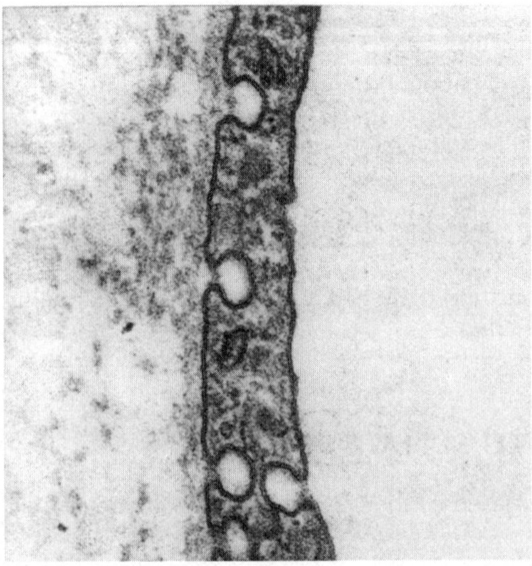

Figure 4-8. Electron micrograph showing pinocytic vesicles in an endothelial cell lining the lumen of a capillary. The trilaminar appearance characteristic of the cell membrane in electron micrographs is also well displayed. The cell membrane, like most cellular membranes, comprises parallel dense lines with a lighter central region when seen in cross-section. (Reprinted from Dellmann H-D: *Textbook of Veterinary Histology,* 4th ed. Baltimore, Williams & Wilkins, 1993, p 6.)

Transcytosis. Some ligands are carried across the cell and released into a different extracellular compartment by exocytosis. Transcytosis occurs across placental cells and the endothelial cells lining some blood vessels.

c. **Clathrin** is a fibrous protein that helps membranes curve into vesicles by forming a basket-like array on the cytoplasmic membrane surface. Selective pinocytosis generally occurs where clathrin is associated with the cell membrane.
   (1) Sites of pinocytic uptake are called **coated pits,** because clathrin looks like a fuzzy layer in electron micrographs. The vesicles they give rise to have the fuzzy layer on the outer surface and are called **coated vesicles**.
   (2) Clathrin separates from the membrane before the vesicle fuses with an endosome.

B. **Exocytosis** is the release of the contents of vesicles or granules from a cell. Like endocytosis, it has constitutive and regulated forms (see Chapter 1 II D 2 b).

1. **Fusion.** A cytoplasmic vesicle membrane fuses with the cell membrane.
   a. The contents of **secretory vesicles** are released continuously by **constitutive exocytosis**.
   b. The contents of **secretory granules** are stored until the cell is stimulated to release them by **regulated exocytosis**.
2. **Discharge.** A pore to the exterior immediately forms at the point of fusion, and the contents of the vesicle are discharged from the cell.
3. **Recycling.** The membrane is retrieved by endocytosis and recycled.

STUDY QUESTIONS

DIRECTIONS: Each of the numbered items or incomplete statements in this section is followed by answers or completions of the statement. Select the **one** numbered answer or completion that is **best** in each case.

1. Which one of the following statements correctly describes the structure of *all* cellular membranes?

(1) One surface is covered with a glycocalyx.
(2) Integral membrane proteins have a nonpolar region that lies within the lipid bilayer.
(3) Integral membrane proteins are fixed in specific sites by attachment to adjacent structures, but peripheral (extrinsic) proteins can drift to different areas of the membrane.
(4) Peripheral membrane proteins do not have a polar region that can attach them to the membrane.
(5) Nonpolar ends of lipid molecules face both surfaces of the membrane.

2. Which one of the following statements regarding the cell membrane's role in controlling the composition of the cytoplasm is true?

(1) The lipid bilayer is impermeable to water.
(2) Integral membrane proteins are the main barrier in the semipermeable membrane.
(3) Transmembrane proteins permit the passive passage of certain ions and small molecules.
(4) Amino acids and glucose enter the cell through protein channels.
(5) Active transport of ions maintains electrical neutrality across the membrane.

3. An important function of certain membrane oligosaccharides is believed to be:

(1) acting as receptors for hormones and neurotransmitters.
(2) forming intercellular junctions to separate extracellular compartments.
(3) acting as surface recognition factors.
(4) forming intercellular junctions for communication between adjacent cells.
(5) releasing energy to power certain membrane functions.

4. Desmosomes are characterized by:

(1) integral membrane proteins, which are apposed in adjacent cell membranes.
(2) intercellular filamentous material, which attaches the apposing cell membranes to each other.
(3) contractile microfilaments, which are attached to the cytoplasmic surface of the junction.
(4) their limited distribution in surface tissues.
(5) their proximity to tight junctions.

5. Beating of cilia involves:

(1) a rigid action stroke and a flexible recovery stroke.
(2) interaction between microtubules and microfilaments in the core of the shaft.
(3) interaction between microfilaments in the shaft and myosin in the basal bodies.
(4) release of energy from adenosine triphosphate (ATP) stored in the dynein arms of the peripheral microtubules.
(5) rapid polymerization and depolymerization of microtubules in the core of the shaft.

6. Which one of the following statements *best* describes motile cellular processes?

(1) Flagella are generally shorter and less numerous than cilia, which they otherwise resemble.
(2) The energy for ciliary movement comes from anaerobic glycolysis.
(3) Cilia are often present on surface cells, but are very rare on other cell types.
(4) Individual cilia are too slender to detect with a light microscope.
(5) A centriole serves as the basal body for the flagellum of a spermatozoon tail.

7. Microvilli are *best* characterized structurally by:

(1) their lack of internal structure.
(2) their lack of affinity for routine histologic stains.
(3) their surface glycocalyx and microfilamentous core.
(4) their typical location on the basal surface of absorptive cells.
(5) their typical location on the apical surface of secretory cells.

8. Phagocytosis is *best* described as:

(1) a regulated endocytic process.
(2) a constitutive reaction of a cell to any particulate matter it touches.
(3) a means for imbibing large amounts of liquids quickly.
(4) a process common to most vertebrate cells.
(5) a lysosomal process.

9. Which one of the following statements *best* characterizes events that occur during selective pinocytosis?

(1) Receptors from the cell membrane are destroyed by lysosomal digestion.
(2) Receptor–ligand interactions occur at the cell membrane.
(3) Ligands in the extracellular fluid are adsorbed by clathrin on the outer surface of the cell membrane.
(4) Clathrin is destroyed by lysosomal digestion.
(5) Specific substances can be selected for uptake but cannot be moved into the cell against a concentration gradient.

10. Intracellular membranes resemble cell membranes, *except* they:

(1) have different enzymes as integral membrane proteins.
(2) are slightly thicker.
(3) do not have oligosaccharides associated with their surface.
(4) do not have transmembrane proteins.
(5) are the same on both surfaces.

11. All of the following occur during exocytosis *except*:

(1) constitutive release of secretory granules.
(2) constitutive release of secretory vesicles.
(3) recycling of cellular membranes.
(4) fusion of a cytoplasmic membrane with the cell membrane.
(5) loss of material from the cell.

DIRECTIONS: Each group of items in this section consists of numbered options followed by a set of numbered items. For each item, select the **one** numbered option that is most closely associated with it. Each numbered option may be selected once, more than once, or not at all.

Questions 12–14

Match each type of intercellular junction with the function it performs.

(1) Present only in surface layers, where it prevents layers of surface cells from being disrupted by shearing forces
(2) Transfers waves of depolarization from cell to cell
(3) Permits direct chemical communication between the cytoplasmic matrices of adjacent cells
(4) Forms spots of tight attachment between neighboring cells
(5) Forms impermeable barriers between extracellular compartments

12. Tight junction

13. Desmosome

14. Zonula adherens

ANSWERS AND EXPLANATIONS

1. The answer is 2 *[I B 2 a].* Only nonpolar regions of proteins can lie within the lipid bilayer. Although the cell membrane has a glycocalyx, which is formed in the rough endoplasmic reticulum (rER) and Golgi complex, many intracellular membranes have no associated oligosaccharides. Some integral membrane proteins appear to be attached to anchoring structures, but many drift freely within the plane of the membrane. Peripheral (extrinsic) membrane proteins do have polar regions; however, they lack nonpolar regions that can insert in the lipid bilayer. Therefore, peripheral membrane proteins are held only by weak electrostatic forces to the surface. The nonpolar ends of lipid molecules are in the core of the lipid bilayer; their polar ends are exposed.

2. The answer is 3 *[I C 1 b (1) (b) (i)].* Transmembrane proteins form aqueous channels or pores through which certain ions and small molecules can pass freely. The lipid bilayer is freely permeable to water, although it is quite impermeable to most water-soluble molecules. The lipid bilayer constitutes the main barrier in the semipermeable membrane. Amino acids and glucose enter the cell with the help of protein carriers. Active transport mechanisms for sodium, potassium, and calcium ions enable the cell to maintain an electrochemical potential across the membrane.

3. The answer is 3 *[I C 1 b (2) (d)].* Oligosaccharides are believed to be the surface recognition factors involved in such important processes as contact inhibition, appropriate immune responses, and morphogenesis. The receptors that recognize surface factors as well as other substances, such as hormones, neurotransmitters, and immune substances, are proteins. Integral membrane proteins are responsible for forming intercellular junctions. Tight junctions separate extracellular regions (such as an organ lumen from the interstitial space) and gap junctions allow intercellular communication between adjacent cells. Enzymes [e.g., adenosine triphosphatase (ATPase), which releases energy from high-energy compounds] are also proteins.

4. The answer is 1 *[II A 2 b (1)].* Transmembrane linker glycoproteins on adjacent cell membranes interact to attach the cells together at desmosomes. The cytoplasmic end of these proteins is attached to the cytoskeletal tonofilaments via a prominent intercellular, dense plaque adjacent to the cell membrane. Intercellular filamentous material bonds the apposed membranes of zonulae adherentes (intermediate junctions, belt desmosomes), the other type of adhering junction. Apposition of integral membrane proteins in adjacent cell membranes also occurs in both tight junctions, where the proteins form a continuous barrier, and gap junctions, where the proteins form channels joining the cytoplasmic matrix of the two cells. Microfilaments are attached to zonulae adherentes, where they are involved in contraction of the terminal web and nearby microvilli, but they are not associated with desmosomes. Desmosomes are most numerous in surface tissues, but they are present in other types of tissue as well. Zonulae adherentes are typically parallel to tight junctions, which they support. Desmosomes, however, can occur anywhere two cells are juxtaposed.

5. The answer is 1 *[II B 1 b (1)].* Microtubules in the shafts of cilia generate a rigid action stroke and a flexible recovery stroke that enable cilia to perform one of their primary functions, transport. The rigid action stroke is determined by the orientation of the two central singlet microtubules, and the flexible recovery stroke prepares the cilium for the next cycle. Microfilaments are not present in the shaft of the cilia, and myosin is not a component of basal bodies. Adenosine triphosphatase (ATPase) is stored in dynein, not adenosine triphosphate (ATP). Beating of cilia uses energy from ATP, which is released by the ATPase activity of the dynein arms of the peripheral doublets. Although microtubules that are free in the cytoplasm form and dissolve readily, microtubules that are organized to form cilia, flagella, and centrioles are quite stable.

6. The answer is 5 *[II B 2 b].* One of the two centrioles in the spermatozoon serves as the basal body for its flagellum. In other cell types, centrioles organize the formation of basal bodies. Flagella are longer than cilia. The energy for ciliary movement is released through an oxidative, not an anaerobic, process. Adenosine triphosphatase (ATPase) in the dynein arms acts on adenosine triphosphate (ATP) to release energy. Individual cilia can be detected at higher magnifications with a light microscope, and basal bodies can also be detected in good preparations. Although cilia are most numerous on surface cells, most (possibly all) cells have one small cilium.

7. The answer is 3 *[II C 1]*. The glycocalyx, which covers all cell membranes, is especially well developed on certain microvilli (e.g., those on cells of the intestinal lining). Their internal structure consists of a core of 20–30 microfilaments. Both the glycocalyx and the actin in the microfilamentous core are acidophilic; therefore, an intensely stained border marks cells with numerous microvilli. Most microvilli are on the apical (free) surface of absorptive cells.

8. The answer is 1 *[III A 1 a]*. Phagocytosis is a regulated, not constitutive, process that occurs only when it is triggered by interaction of an extracellular object or substance with surface receptors on the phagocytic cell. Endocytosis includes all processes that bring material into cells; phagocytosis, which is endocytosis of solids, not liquids, is an endocytic process. Phagocytosis is a process common to one-celled animals, where it serves a nutritive function. In vertebrates, phagocytosis is a specialized activity of certain cells, primarily white blood cells of the defense system. It is not until after phagocytosis is completed that phagosomes fuse with lysosomes, where their contents are digested.

9. The answer is 2 *[III A 2 b (2)]*. Selectivity is achieved by interactions of cell membrane surface receptors with specific molecules called ligands. Some receptors are eventually destroyed by fusion of pinocytic vesicles with endosomes and then lysosomes, but many are released from endosomes to be recycled to the cell membrane. Clathrin is a fibrous protein on the cytoplasmic, not outer, surface of the cell membrane. It helps membranes curve into vesicles and then is released from the membrane before fusion of the pinocytic vesicle with other cytoplasmic vesicles. A major advantage of selective pinocytosis is that it enables cells to take in regulatory molecules, essential cellular components, and other specific substances against a concentration gradient. For example, selective pinocytosis is responsible for the high concentration of iron found in developing red blood cells.

10. The answer is 1 *[I C 2]*. The enzymes in each membrane are specific for the functions performed by that organelle or inclusion. Intracellular membranes are slightly thinner than cell membranes. They often have oligosaccharides associated with their luminal surface, especially in the rough endoplasmic reticulum (rER) and Golgi complex, where the cell membrane originates. Transmembrane proteins are found in all types of membranes. Different populations of both lipids and proteins can be found on the two surfaces of all membranes. In the rER, for example, the enzymes for lipid synthesis are on the cytosol surface, and those that synthesize oligosaccharides are on the luminal surface.

11. The answer is 1 *[III B 1 b]*. Secretory granules are stored in the cytoplasm until some signal causes their release; that is, they are released by regulated exocytosis. Secretory vesicles are released automatically, by constitutive exocytosis, as soon as they are formed. The cellular membrane is retrieved by endocytosis and recycled. A cytoplasmic vesicle membrane fuses with the cell membrane, and the material is expelled from the cell through a pore to the exterior.

12–14. The answers are: 12-5 *[II A 1]*, **13-4** *[II A 2 b]*, **14-1** *[II A 2 a]*. Tight junctions separate extracellular compartments. Some tight junctions prevent the contents of an organ with a lumen (e.g., the intestine) from entering the intercellular spaces. Others define a channel (canaliculus) between adjacent secretory cells leading to a duct.

Desmosomes can be compared with snaps, because they mechanically attach adjacent cells to each other at specific spots. They are most numerous in surface layers, but are also present in many other locations.

Zonulae adherentes (intermediate junctions, belt desmosomes) form continuous bands that mechanically attach adjacent surface cells to each other near their free border. They are especially well developed where the surface layer is exposed to frictional or shearing forces.

Chapter 5
Epithelium

I. INTRODUCTION

A. Definitions

1. **Cytology** is the study of cells.
2. **Histology** is the microscopic study of tissues, which comprise groups of structurally similar cells. The billions of cells present in a single animal are arranged into tissues.
3. **Organology** is the study of organs, which are formed by the integration of several tissues to perform specific functions.

B. Four basic tissues

1. **Epithelium** covers and lines all body surfaces except joint cavities and the rostral (anterior) surface of the iris. Epithelium also forms the secretory portions of glands.
2. **Connective tissue** (see Chapters 6, 7, and 8) is specialized for support, protection, or energy storage.
   a. Intercellular material is a major component of most connective tissues.
   b. Connective tissue underlies all epithelium.
   c. Examples of specialized connective tissues include bone, cartilage, fat, and blood.
3. **Muscle** (see Chapter 10) contains cells that are specialized for contraction.
   a. **Skeletal** muscle moves body parts.
   b. **Cardiac (heart)** and **smooth muscle** change the shapes of organs.
4. **Nervous tissue** (see Chapter 9) contains cells that are specialized for conduction. Nervous tissue forms the brain, spinal cord, autonomic ganglia, and nerves.

C. Embryologic origins of tissues

1. Tissues are derived embryologically from **three primary germ layers: ectoderm, mesoderm,** and **entoderm (endoderm)**.
   a. **Ectoderm** is the **outer germ layer**.
   b. **Mesoderm** is the **middle germ layer**.
   c. **Entoderm** is the **inner germ layer**.
2. **Epithelium** is derived from all three germ layers.
   a. **Ectoderm** forms the **epidermis** (the epithelial surface of the skin) and structures derived from epidermis.
   b. **Mesoderm**
      (1) Mesoderm forms **mesothelium,** which is the lining of closed body cavities (peritoneal, pleural, and pericardial).
      (2) Mesoderm forms **endothelium,** which lines the cardiovascular system.
   c. **Entoderm** forms the lining of the gastrointestinal tract and all its diverticula.
3. **Other basic tissues**
   a. Most **connective tissue** and **muscle tissue** are derived from **mesoderm**.
   b. **Nervous tissue** is derived from **ectoderm**.

D. **Membranes** comprise epithelium and its underlying connective tissue.

1. **Mucous membranes** are coated by mucus from surface epithelial cells or glands that open onto the surface. Mucous membranes, also called **wet membranes,** line organ systems that communicate with the exterior of the body.
2. **Serous membranes** line closed body cavities; therefore, their epithelial component is mesothelium. They are lubricated by a watery fluid that is produced passively as a transudate from the blood.
3. **Skin (integument)** is another example of a membrane.

II. CHARACTERISTICS OF EPITHELIA

A. **Arrangement.** Epithelial cells lie close together with little intercellular material. The cells in an epithelial sheet are usually similar in structure.

B. **Polarization.** Epithelial cells are **polarized** with respect to the underlying connective tissue and the free surface. All substances that enter or leave the body must pass through an epithelial layer; therefore, the organelles and cytoskeletal elements are oriented relative to those movements (Figure 5-1).

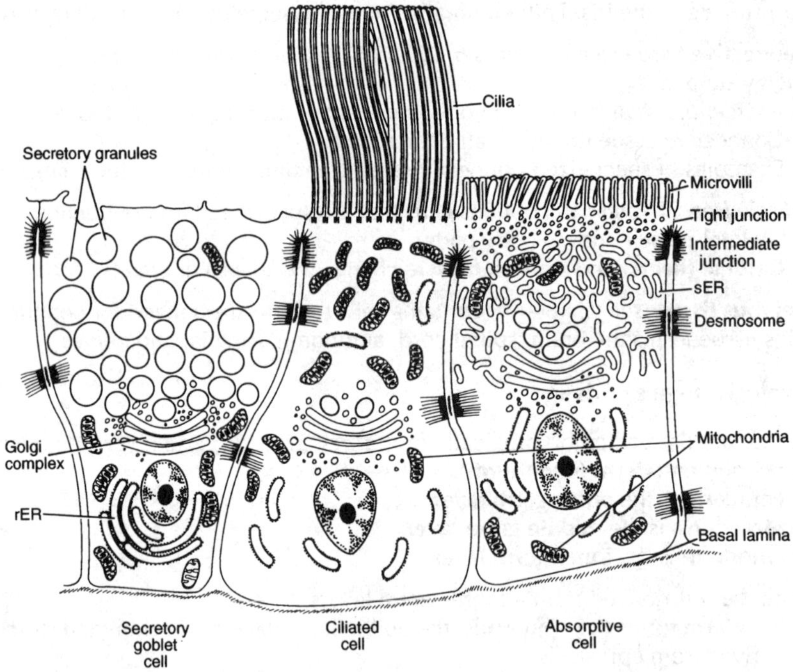

Figure 5-1. This schematic representation of three cells in a hypothetical simple columnar epithelium shows a secretory goblet cell, a ciliated cell, and an absorptive cell with microvilli. Intermediate and tight junctions, seen as terminal bars light microscopically, join all the cells at the apical ends of their lateral cell membranes. A basal lamina is indicated beneath the basal cell membranes. Some rough endoplasmic reticulum (*rER*), mitochondria, and a supranuclear Golgi complex are present in all cells. In the secretory cell, a larger amount of rER is concentrated in the basal cytoplasm, and stored secretory granules have accumulated in the apical cytoplasm. In the ciliated cell, many mitochondria occupy the apical cytoplasm near the basal bodies of the cilia. The free surface of the absorptive cell is covered with microvilli, and abundant smooth endoplasmic reticulum (*sER*) is in the apical cytoplasm for processing of absorbed substances.

1. **Basal cytoplasm**
   a. Cytoplasmic structures located in the basal cytoplasm are close to the entry point of nutrients and substrates arriving from capillaries in the underlying connective tissue.
   b. The **nucleus,** most of the **rough endoplasmic reticulum (rER),** and many **mitochondria** are located in the basal cytoplasm.
2. **Apical cytoplasm**
   a. The **Golgi complex** typically lies near the apical pole of the nucleus, with its mature face toward the surface.
   b. In cells that undergo regulated secretion, **secretory granules** await the signal for exocytosis in the cell apex, near their point of release.
   c. In absorptive cells, **organelles that modify substances absorbed through the free surface** [e.g., the smooth endoplasmic reticulum (sER), which processes absorbed lipids in the small intestine] are concentrated in the apical cytoplasm.
   d. In ciliated cells, many **mitochondria** occupy the apical cytoplasm. Adenosine triphosphate (ATP) produced by mitochondria is needed to power ciliary action.

C. Surface characteristics

1. **Apical free surface**
   a. **Cell membrane.** The composition of the cell membrane of the apical free surface differs from that of the basolateral surfaces. For example, the apical cell membrane may contain proteins that transport a certain molecule into the cytoplasm, whereas the basolateral membrane contains proteins that transport the same molecule out of the cell. In addition, glycoproteins and glycolipids are usually more numerous in the apical membrane.
   b. **Modifications.** Specializations of the apical free surface are common in surface epithelia.
      (1) **Microvilli** (see also Chapter 4 II C) cover the free surface of absorptive cells.
      (2) **Cilia** (see also Chapter 4 II B). Ciliated cells are present in many mucous membranes (see Figure 14-1). For example:
         (a) In the upper respiratory system, cilia continuously move a sticky sheet of mucus and captured foreign particles toward the pharynx.
         (b) In the uterine tubes, cilia help move released oocytes and fertilized ova toward the uterus.
         (c) Cilia on many sensory epithelial cells are modified to play a role in sensory perception; in this capacity, they are no longer motile.
      (3) **Keratin** (see Chapter 20 II A 6). Keratinization (cornification) strengthens the surface layers of stratified squamous epithelia in locations that are exposed to friction and shearing forces (e.g., the epidermis of the skin is keratinized stratified squamous epithelium). Keratinization is accomplished by replacing all other intracellular components with keratin.
   c. **Adhesiveness.** The free surface is not adhesive.
      (1) Because the apical surface of epithelium is **not sticky,** substances that come into contact with the surface do not adhere; therefore, even very narrow epithelium-lined lumina do not become occluded.
      (2) In many areas, a **well-developed glycocalyx** contributes to the nonadhesive surface by electrostatically repelling negatively charged particles and other cells. The glycocalyx is especially thick in the small intestine.
2. **Basal surface.** The **basement membrane** is a continuous amorphous layer that lies beneath the epithelium, separating the epithelium from the adjacent connective tissue (see Figure 5-2). Exceptions include the endothelium of capillaries, in which the basement membrane may be discontinuous, and the lymphatic capillaries, which lack a basement membrane.
   a. **Structure of the basement membrane**
      (1) The **basal lamina** is an amorphous layer that is always present as a continuous sheet that parallels the basal cell membrane of the epithelium.

(a) The basal lamina, which is seen only with the electron microscope, is **produced by the epithelial cells.**

(b) **Hemidesmosomes** attach the basal cells of the epidermis to the underlying basal lamina.

(2) A **reticular lamina** is a fibrous layer that is often present. It is produced by the adjacent connective tissue.

b. **Composition of the basement membrane**

(1) **Type IV collagen,** which is highly glycosylated (i.e., linked to many carbohydrate groups), forms highly cross-linked elastic networks instead of fibrils. Type IV collagen is unique to basal laminae.

(2) **Laminin,** a glycoprotein, has binding sites for the basal cell membrane and for type IV collagen.

(3) **Proteoglycans** (e.g., heparan sulfate) are also present; these substances are known to mediate cell–substrate adhesion.

(4) **Fibrillar collagen** forms the reticular lamina when this layer is present.

c. **Functions of the basement membrane**

(1) The basement membrane provides **support** and an **attachment site for the epithelial layer.**

(2) The basal lamina **separates the epithelium from the underlying connective tissue** and **limits the movement of macromolecules between the two tissues.** Muscle cells and nervous tissue are also separated from connective tissue by a basal lamina.

(a) In glomeruli of the **kidney,** the basement membrane is very thick and acts as an **ultrafiltration barrier,** preventing the loss of large proteins from the blood [see Chapter 15 II B 1 a (3)].

(b) The thick basement membrane of the **trachea** inhibits bacterial invasion.

(c) **Loss of a continuous basement membrane** is characteristic of many invasive tumors and is considered **evidence of metastasis** of cancer cells.

d. **Light-microscope appearance of the basement membrane.** Stains reveal the basement membrane when it is thick enough to be detected light microscopically. Most commonly used is the **periodic acid–Schiff (PAS) reaction,** which demonstrates the carbohydrate-rich macromolecules of the basement membrane.

3. **Lateral surfaces.** Intercellular junctions (see also Chapter 4 II A) are numerous.

a. **Tight junctions** and **zonulae adherentes** are unique to epithelia. They appear under the light microscope as **terminal bars** (Figure 5-2C&E) between the apices of adjacent cells in some epithelia.

(1) **Tight junctions** prevent the translocation of membrane proteins between the apical and basolateral compartments of the cell membrane. In epithelia that line lumina, tight junctions form a seal that separates the lumen from the intercellular space.

(2) **Zonulae adherentes** are adhesive junctions that hold the cells together.

b. **Gap junctions** may also be present, allowing communication between cells within an epithelial layer.

c. **Desmosomes** are most numerous and best developed in epithelia that are subject to shearing forces.

D. **Cytoskeletal elements** (see also Chapter 3 I A–B). **Microfilaments** and **tonofibrils** (bundles of intermediate filaments) are often abundant in surface epithelia. All epithelia contain **keratin tonofilaments,** which are unique to epithelia.

E. **Vascularity.** Epithelia are **avascular.**

1. They are **supplied by diffusion** from blood vessels and lymphatics in the underlying connective tissue.

2. **Lymphocytes** from the blood are commonly seen migrating through the epithelial lining of certain organ systems that communicate with the external environment, such as the digestive tract.

F. **Innervation.** Most surface epithelia are not innervated. Exceptions include the cornea, the epidermis of the skin, the gustatory (taste) regions in the digestive system, the olfactory epithelium in the respiratory system, and the inner ear.

III. CLASSIFICATION OF EPITHELIA

A. Epithelia are classified according to the **number of cell layers** and the **shape of the cells.**

1. **Number of cell layers**
   a. **Simple epithelia** are a single cell layer thick. All cells extend from the basal lamina to the free surface (see Figure 5-2A–C).
   b. **Stratified epithelia** have two or more layers of cells (see Figure 5-2D).
   c. **Pseudostratified epithelia** appear to be stratified, because the cells are not all the same height and because their nuclei lie at different levels. All cells in a pseudostratified epithelium lie on the basal lamina, but some of the cells do not reach the free surface (see Figure 5-2E).

2. **Shape of the cells.** (Stratified epithelia are classified according to the shape of the cells in the surface layer.)
   a. **Squamous cells** are flat (see Figure 5-2A).
      (1) **Simple squamous epithelia** (e.g., **mesothelium, endothelium**) are characteristic of surfaces through which metabolites or gases must move rapidly.
      (2) **Stratified squamous epithelium** is by far the most common type of stratified epithelium (see Figure 5-2D). Examples include the surface layer of the skin and the lining of the cranial and caudalmost portions of the digestive system.
   b. **Cuboidal cells** are approximately as high as they are wide (see Figure 5-2B).
      (1) They may be specialized for absorption or secretion.
      (2) **Simple cuboidal epithelium.** Examples include the lining of many tubules in the kidneys and many small ducts.
   c. **Columnar cells** are taller than they are wide (see Figure 5-2C).
      (1) **Simple columnar epithelium.** Examples include the lining of the digestive tract from the esophagealgastric junction to the anus, and the lining of parts of the respiratory and female reproductive systems.
      (2) **Pseudostratified columnar epithelium.** Examples include the characteristic linings of most of the upper airways and parts of the male reproductive tract.

B. **Special types of epithelium**

1. **Transitional epithelium** is a pseudostratified epithelium (see Figure 5-2F) that lines most of the urinary tract. The shapes of cells in transitional epithelium change when the organs they line are distended.

2. **Cytogenic (seminiferous) epithelium** is a stratified epithelium that lines the seminiferous tubules of the testes. It comprises supportive cells and developing male germ cells.

IV. GLANDULAR EPITHELIA

A. **Cellular components of glands**

1. **Glandular epithelial cells** are **specialized for secretion** (i.e., the synthesis and release of some product). Cells of other tissue types may also be secretory (e.g., connective tissue cells secrete intercellular materials; nerve cells secrete neurotransmitters).

2. **Myoepithelial cells** are contractile cells with long, slender processes that form basket-like assemblies around the secretory units of some glands.

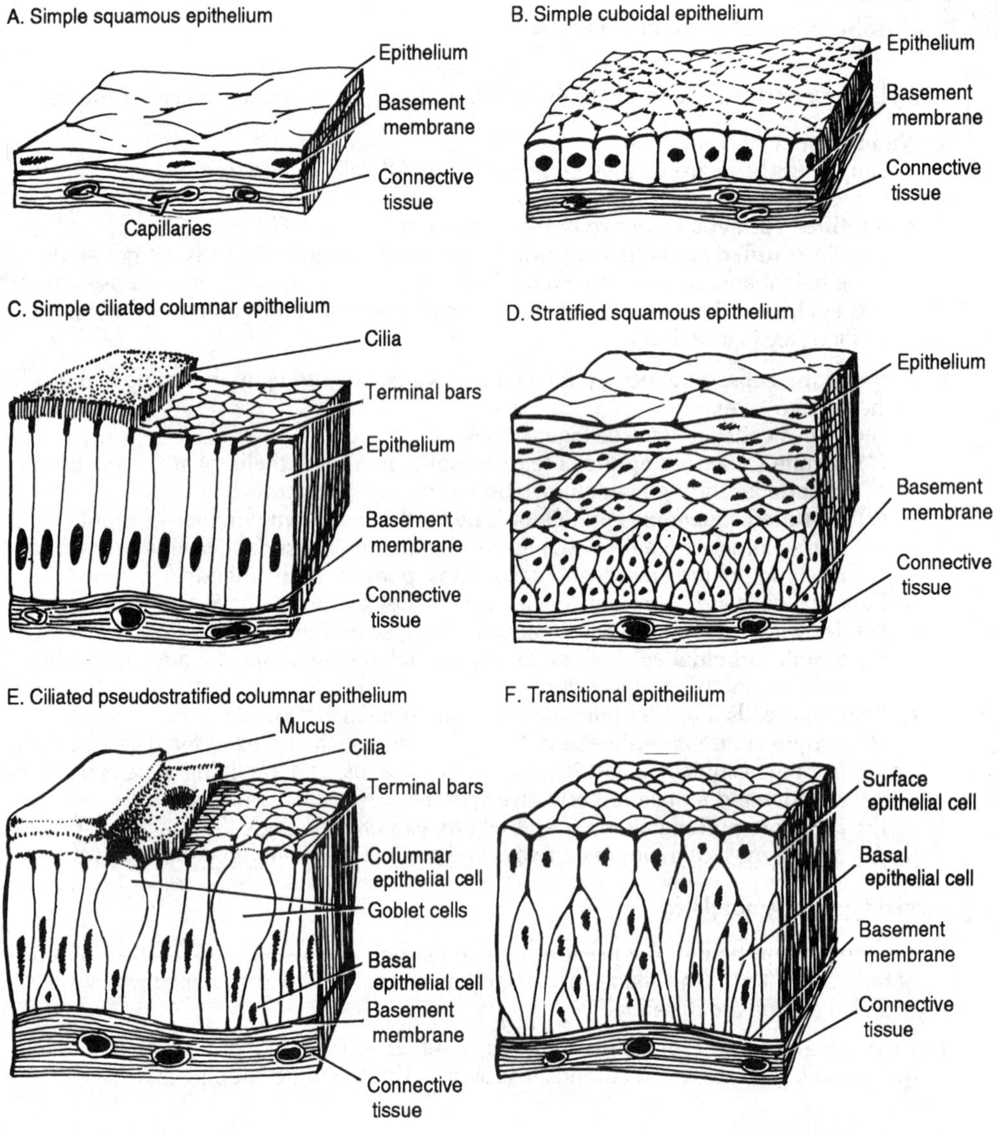

Figure 5-2. Schematic drawings of the most common types of surface epithelia with the basement membrane and connective tissue on which they lie. (*A*) Simple squamous epithelium. (*B*) Simple cuboidal epithelium. (*C*) Ciliated simple columnar epithelium. Notice that the tight and intermediate junctions, which appear as terminal bars in longitudinal sections through the cells, form a continuous seal and attachment between the apices of the cells. (*D*) Stratified squamous epithelium. The cells above the basal layer have no contact with the basement membrane. (*E*) Ciliated pseudostratified epithelium with goblet cells. The mucus secreted by goblet cells forms a continuous layer on the surface. Ciliary movement moves the mucus along in a sheet. (*F*) Transitional epithelium. Although this epithelium appears to be stratified light microscopically, each cell has a process that extends to the basement membrane. When the epithelium is distended, it appears to have only two or three cell layers. (Modified and redrawn with permission from Junqueira LC, Carneiro J, Kelley RO: *Basic Histology,* 7th ed. Englewood Cliffs, NJ, Appleton & Lange, 1992, pp 76–77.)

a. Although myoepithelial cells resemble smooth muscle cells because they contain actin and contract in response to nervous or humoral stimuli, they are true epithelial cells.

b. **Contraction** of myoepithelial cells **helps expel secretory products. Milk let-down** results from contraction of myoepithelial cells in the mammary gland.

B. General structure of glands

1. **Parenchyma and stroma**

a. **Parenchyma** is the specific (characteristic) functional part of an organ. In glands, the parenchyma is the secretory epithelium.

b. **Stroma** is the supportive part of an organ, typically formed by connective tissue, as it is in large glands. Blood vessels and nerves are distributed to all parts of the gland through the stroma.

(1) **Reticular fibers** are delicate connective tissue elements that support the smallest (microscopic) lobules and individual secretory units of glands.

(2) **Septa** are sheets of connective tissue that divide the large glands into lobes and lobules.

(3) The **capsule** is a layer of connective tissue that surrounds the entire gland.

2. Glands are **classified anatomically** based on the shape of their secretory units and the complexity of their duct system.

a. **Secretory units**

(1) **Tubular secretory units** are **elongated** (Figure 5-3A–D & H).

(a) Examples of **simple tubular glands** are found in the intestines.

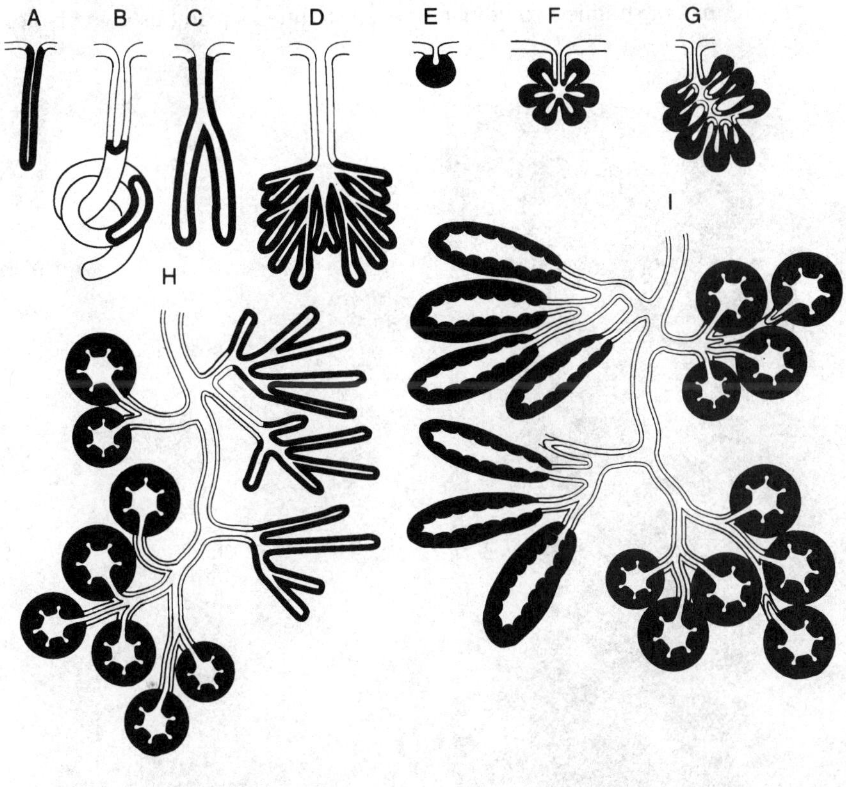

Figure 5-3. Schematic drawing of different forms of exocrine glands. (*A*) Simple tubular; (*B*) Simple coiled tubular; (*C, D*) Simple branched tubular; (*E*) Simple acinar; (*F, G*) Simple branched acinar; (*H*) Compound tubuloacinar on the *left,* compound tubular on the *right;* (*I*) Compound acinar. Secretory portions are *black;* excretory ducts are *double lines.* (Redrawn and modified with permission from Fawcett DW: *A Textbook of Histology,* 11th ed. London, Chapman & Hall, 1985, pp 94–95.)

(b) Examples of **branched tubular glands** are found in the stomach (see Figure 5-3C&D).

(c) Examples of **coiled tubular glands** include sweat glands (Figure 5-4).

(2) **Acinar secretory units** are **spherical** or **flask-shaped**. Sebaceous glands are examples of simple branched acinar glands.

(3) **Tubuloacinar secretory units** comprise a **secretory tubule and a cluster of acini** that open into the tubule (see Figure 5-3H).

(a) Submucosal glands in the small intestines are examples of simple tubuloacinar glands.

(b) Most large glands, including the major salivary glands and the pancreas, are compound tubuloacinar glands.

b. **Duct system.** Glands that release their secretions to the body surface (i.e., **exocrine glands**) often do so through a duct or a system of ducts.

(1) **Simple glands** lack a duct or have a **single, unbranched excretory duct** (see Figure 5-3A–G). Simple glands that have several secretory units are called **simple branched glands** (see Figure 5-3C, D, F, & G).

(2) **Compound glands** have a **branching duct system** that drains many secretory units (see Figure 5-3H&I). Most compound glands are large enough to be named (e.g., parotid gland, pancreas).

(a) **Branching excretory ducts,** which are **merely conductive** and not secretory, drain the secretory product (see Figure 5-3H&I). The smallest ducts are lined by simple cuboidal epithelium; the epithelium typically increases in thickness in proportion to the size of the duct. Depending on the size and location of the gland, the lining may be simple columnar, pseudostratified columnar, or stratified columnar, or even stratified squamous in the largest ducts.

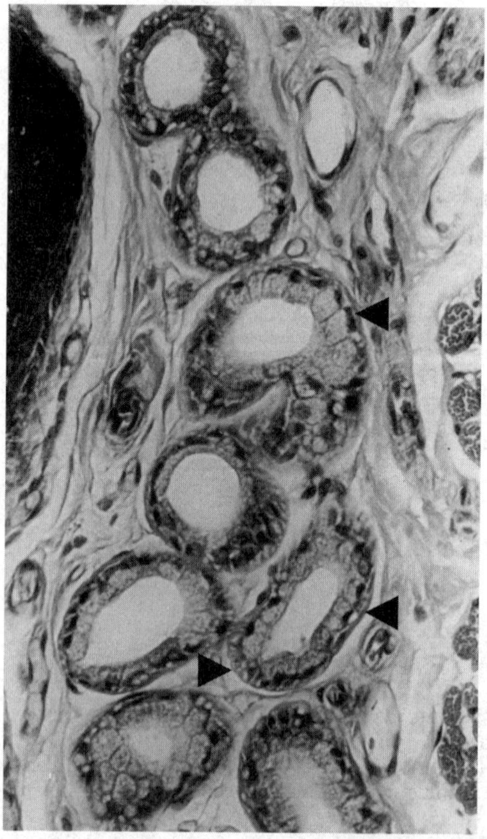

Figure 5-4. Light micrograph of a simple coiled tubular gland. Myoepithelial cell processes (*arrows*) surround the tubule.

(i) **Intralobular ducts** drain portions of lobules and are located within the lobules, where they are surrounded by secretory units.
(ii) **Interlobular ducts** (Figure 5-5) drain entire lobules and are located in the connective tissue septa between lobules.
(iii) **Lobar ducts** drain the lobes.
(iv) The **main duct** drains the entire gland.

(b) **Smaller ducts,** some of which **contribute to the secretory product,** are also present in certain glands.
(i) **Intercalated ducts** (Figure 5-6) join secretory acini with secretory ducts. They are most easily seen in the pancreas.
(ii) **Secretory ducts** occur in some glands; they contribute to the secretory product of the gland.
(iii) **Striated ducts** (see Figure 5-6), which are prominent in major salivary glands, contribute to the electrolyte and water content of the secretory product. Their basal striations result from parallel arrays of mitochondria lying in parallel folds of basal cell membrane. The mitochondria provide energy for active transport of ions across the basal membrane.

C. **Other classifications of glands.** Glands may be classified according to where their product is released, the number of secretory cells, the method (or mode) of secretion, and the secretory product.

1. **Where the product is released**
   a. **Exocrine glands** release their product to a body surface directly or by way of a duct.
   b. **Endocrine glands** (see Chapter 19) release their product to the intercellular spaces, where the product is carried away by the blood.

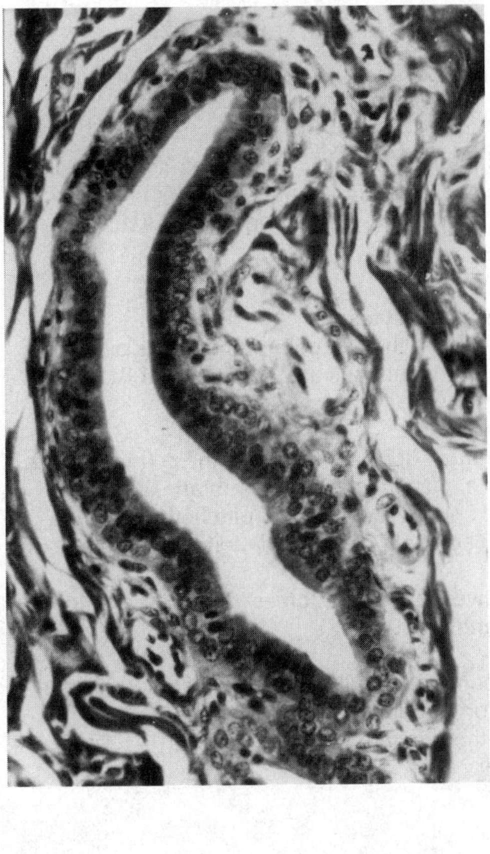

Figure 5-5. Interlobular duct in a salivary gland. The duct is lined by stratified columnar epithelium and surrounded by connective tissue of the septum.

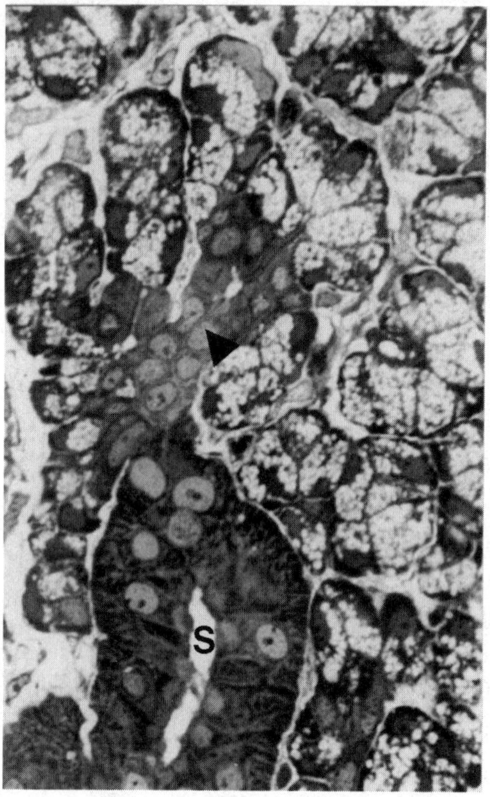

Figure 5-6. Intercalated duct (*arrow*) leading from secretory acinus to striated duct (*S*) in a salivary gland. Mitochondria are visible in the basal portions of the cells lining the striated duct.

2. **Number of secretory cells**
   a. **Unicellular**
      (1) **Goblet cells,** which exhibit regulated secretion of mucin, are unicellular glands.
      (2) **Isolated endocrine cells** are also present in many epithelia.
   b. **Multicellular.** Most glands are multicellular glands. In avians, some multicellular glands are intraepithelial, but in mammals, multicellular glands expand into the connective tissue. In the case of endocrine glands, the connection to the surface no longer exists.

3. **Method of secretion**
   a. **Merocrine glands** secrete their products by **exocytosis.**
      (1) The secretory vesicle or granule fuses with the cell membrane and is expelled without loss of any other cellular components (see also Chapter 4 III B).
      (2) Most secretory products are released by exocytosis.
   b. **Apocrine glands**
      (1) In apocrine glands, the **secretory granule** does not fuse with the cell membrane. Instead, it **evaginates the free surface,** pushing the cell membrane and a thin layer of cytoplasm in front of it. The entire **evagination is pinched off,** and the secretory product and its surrounding cytoplasm and cell membrane are released from the cell.
      (2) Apocrine secretion occurs in most **sweat glands** of domestic animals and in the **release of lipids from mammary gland cells.**
   c. **Holocrine glands**
      (1) In holocrine glands, **entire cells** become filled with secretory material, disintegrate, and are released as the secretory product.
      (2) **Sebaceous glands,** the oil glands of the skin, are holocrine glands.

4. Secretory product. Glands that open onto a mucous membrane may be classified as mucous, serous, or mixed mucoserous.

a. Mucous glands

(1) **Mucous cells** secrete **mucin,** which combines with water outside the cell to form **mucus,** a **viscous** substance that **contains** many **acidic glycoproteins.**

(2) **Light-microscope appearance.** Mucous cells usually look "empty" in routine preparations because the rER and small heterochromatic (dark-staining) nucleus are pushed to the basal cytoplasm by the unstained mucin droplets in the apical cytoplasm (Figure 5-7).

b. Serous glands

(1) **Serous cells** secrete a watery product that is rich in proteins and neutral glycoproteins.

(2) **Light-microscope appearance**

(a) The nucleus of a serous cell is more euchromatic (light-staining) and more centrally located than that of a mucous cell, and the cytoplasm is often distinctly basophilic because of abundant rER (see Figure 5-7).

(b) In the serous cells of the pancreas, stored zymogen granules make the apical cytoplasm acidophilic.

c. Mixed mucoserous glands

(1) Mucous cells and serous cells may be in separate secretory units or they may coexist in the same secretory unit (see Figure 5-7).

(2) When both cell types are combined in the same secretory unit, the serous cells are typically pushed to the periphery, where they form crescent-shaped serous **demilunes** (see Figure 5-7).

(3) The secretory products of the serous cells reach the lumen by passing through tiny **canaliculi** between mucous cells.

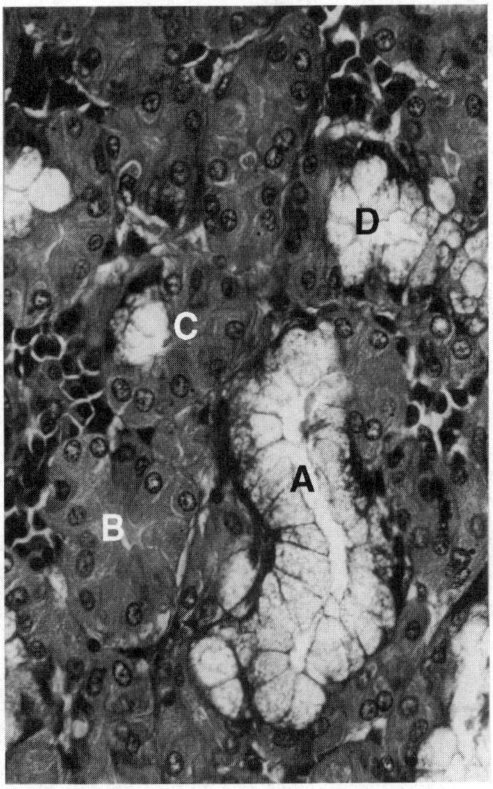

Figure 5-7. Tubular and acinar secretory units in a mixed mucoserous salivary gland. A tubular mucous secretory unit (*A*) is surrounded by serous acini (*B*) and several mixed mucoserous acini. In one of the mixed acini, serous and mucous cells are side by side in the acinus (*C*); in another, mucous cells form the acinus (*D*), with a demilune of serous cells.

V. REGENERATION OF EPITHELIA

A. **Repair and renewal mechanisms** are well developed in epithelia because the surface location of epithelia exposes them to stress and damage.

1. **Stem cells.** A self-renewing population of stem cells in the basal epithelium is responsible for cell renewal.
   a. **Renewal rates** vary from a few days in some epithelia to years in others. Cells are replaced continually in the epidermis of the skin and the lining of the digestive tract and less frequently in other areas.
   b. Division of a stem cell is believed to produce one cell that remains a relatively undifferentiated stem cell and another that gives rise to one or more mature cells typical of that epithelium.
2. **Ameboid movement.** Although normally nonmotile, epithelial cells may exhibit ameboid movement to **cover surface wounds**.

B. **Pathology.** Most **malignant tumors** are of epithelial origin (carcinomas). Malignancies are characterized by failure of the mechanisms that normally control and limit cell proliferation and spreading.

STUDY QUESTIONS

DIRECTIONS: Each of the numbered items or incomplete statements in this section is followed by answers or by completions of the statement. Select the **one** numbered answer or completion that is **best** in each case.

1. Which of the following is a basic tissue?

(1) Epidermis
(2) Blood
(3) Connective tissue
(4) Brain
(5) Smooth muscle

2. Mesoderm is the embryonic germ layer that gives rise to:

(1) the epidermis of the skin.
(2) the glands and hair follicles associated with the skin.
(3) nervous tissue.
(4) the lining of the cardiovascular system.
(5) the lining of the digestive system.

3. Which of the following statements *best* describes epithelial tissue?

(1) A wide variety of cell types is usually present.
(2) It is derived from ectoderm and mesoderm.
(3) The free surface adheres readily to particles and other cell types.
(4) There is little intercellular material.
(5) The basal cell surface and connective tissue abut.

4. Which of the following statements describes the usual pattern of epithelial cell polarization?

(1) The rough endoplasmic reticulum (rER) and Golgi complex are located in the basal cytoplasm near the source of nutrients.
(2) Mitochondria are concentrated in the basal cytoplasm of ciliated cells.
(3) The apical free surface of absorptive cells has many cilia.
(4) The rER and many mitochondria are concentrated in the basal cytoplasm of secretory cells.
(5) The basal lamina covers the basal and lateral cell membranes but is absent on the free surface.

5. Which one of the following statements regarding intercellular junctions in epithelia is true?

(1) Tight junctions and zonulae adherentes are found only in epithelia.
(2) Tight junctions provide for adhesion between the apical regions of cells.
(3) Tight junctions allow communication between adjacent cells.
(4) Zonulae adherentes prevent apical membrane proteins from mixing with basolateral membrane proteins.
(5) Hemidesmosomes are components of junctional complexes.

6. Surface epithelia are classified as:

(1) simple if all cells touch the basement membrane.
(2) pseudostratified if the nuclei are at different levels.
(3) stratified if the cells are flat.
(4) columnar if the cells are taller than they are wide.
(5) transitional if the cells in the superficial layer are a different shape than the basal cells.

7. Which one of the following statements *best* describes secretion?

(1) Secretion is unique to epithelium.
(2) Secretion refers to both synthesis and release of a cellular product.
(3) Secretion is release of a synthesized product without loss of cytoplasmic elements.
(4) Secretion in compound glands occurs in cells lining the secretory units and excretory ducts.
(5) Secretion is a function of the stroma of a gland.

8. Glands are classified anatomically as:

(1) simple if they secrete mucin.
(2) compound if they have multiple secretory units.
(3) compound if they are drained by a branching system of excretory ducts.
(4) tubuloacinar if they have an unbranched excretory duct.
(5) acinar if they have elongated secretory units.

9. The duct system of a compound gland may include:

(1) striated ducts, so named because they have a striated apical border of microvilli to reabsorb water from the secretory product.
(2) intercalated ducts that drain into secretory ducts.
(3) interlobular ducts that are surrounded by secretory units within the lobules.
(4) a lobar duct that drains each lobule.
(5) either excretory ducts, or secretory ducts and striated ducts.

10. Which one of the following statements is true regarding glands that open onto a mucous membrane?

(1) The products of mucous glands are rich in proteins and neutral glycoproteins.
(2) Mucous demilunes are characteristic of mixed mucoserous glands.
(3) The products of mucous cells are released through tiny canaliculi.
(4) The secretory product of serous glands is viscous and sticky.
(5) Serous glands appear more basophilic than mucous glands in routine preparations.

11. Which of the following statements regarding glands is true?

(1) The parenchyma of a compound gland includes the capsule, septa, and reticular fibers that support individual lobules and secretory units.
(2) Glands are classified anatomically according to the shape of the secretory cells.
(3) Holocrine secretion occurs in most glands.
(4) Contraction of myoepithelial cells in the mammary glands is responsible for milk let-down.
(5) Myoepithelial cells are smooth muscle cells that are closely associated with secretory units of glands.

12. Which one of the following statements is true of histologic membranes?

(1) Mucus-secreting cells are characteristic of the surface epithelium of mucous membranes.
(2) Serous membranes are lubricated by the products of serous glands that open onto their surface.
(3) Histologic membranes comprise an epithelium and its underlying connective tissue.
(4) Membranes are lubricated by either mucous or serous fluids.
(5) "Wet membrane" is another term for serous membrane.

Questions 13–15

Refer to the micrograph.

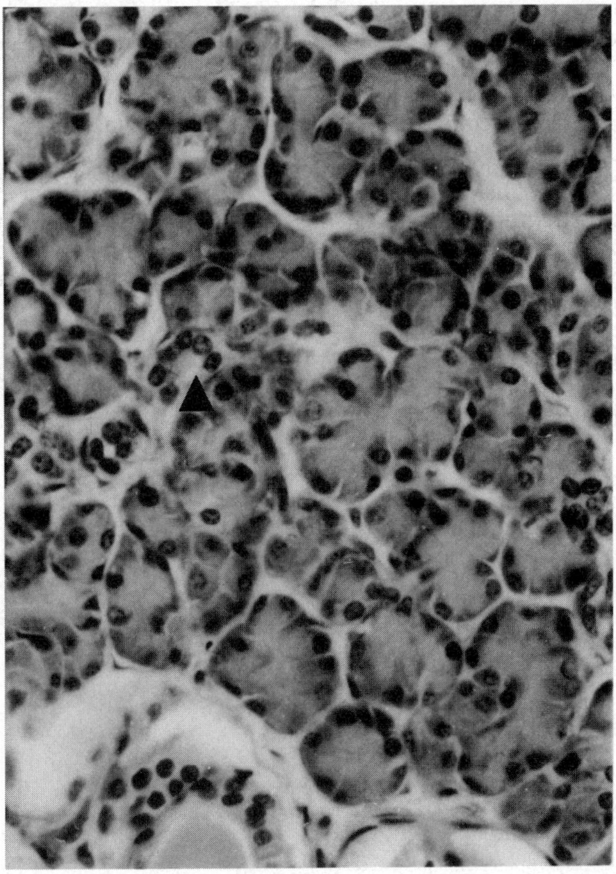

13. Identify the structure indicated by the arrow.

(1) A tubular secretory unit
(2) An acinar secretory unit
(3) A serous demilune
(4) An intercalated duct
(5) An interlobular duct

14. According to secretory product, what type of gland is illustrated?

(1) Mucous
(2) Serous
(3) Mixed mucoserous

15. According to method of secretion, what type of gland is illustrated?

(1) Merocrine
(2) Apocrine
(3) Holocrine

DIRECTIONS: Each of the numbered items or incomplete statements in this section is negatively phrased, as indicated by an italicized word such as *not, least,* or *except*. Select the **one** numbered answer or completion that is **best** in each case.

16. All of the following are true statements regarding epithelial polarity *except:*

(1) all substances that enter or leave the body must pass through an epithelial layer.
(2) brush or striated borders are characteristic surface specializations of absorptive cells.
(3) the composition of the apical cell membrane differs from that of the basolateral cell membrane.
(4) hemidesmosomes are associated only with the basal cell membrane.
(5) in cells with regulated secretion, secretory granules accumulate in the basal cytoplasm.

17. All of the following are functions of the basement membrane *except:*

(1) supporting the epithelial layer.
(2) separating epithelium from underlying muscle, nervous, or connective tissue.
(3) acting as an ultrafiltration barrier.
(4) inhibiting bacterial invasion through a wet membrane.
(5) attaching the epithelial layer to the underlying tissue.

ANSWERS AND EXPLANATIONS

1. The answer is 3 *[I B]*. Connective tissue is one of the four basic tissues. The other basic tissues are epithelium, muscle, and nervous tissue. Together the basic tissues comprise all the specific types of tissue in the body. Epidermis is a type of epithelium. Blood is a type of connective tissue. The brain is one of the structures composed of nervous tissue. Smooth muscle is one of the three types of muscle.

2. The answer is 4 *[I C 2 b (2)]*. Mesoderm gives rise to endothelium, the epithelial lining of the heart, blood vessels, and lymph vessels. The epidermis and its associated glands and hair follicles arise from ectoderm, as does nervous tissue. The lining of the digestive tract develops from entoderm.

3. The answer is 4 *[II A]*. Epithelial cells are very close together with very little intercellular matrix. In fact, their cellularity makes most epithelial layers stand out when viewed with the light microscope. Although some epithelia have several cell types (e.g., columnar ciliated cells and columnar secretory cells), the cells are usually similar in structure. Epithelium is derived from all three germ layers: ectoderm, mesoderm, and entoderm. The nonadhesiveness of the free surface is an essential characteristic of epithelia. It prevents the epithelial surface from adhering to adjacent surfaces and allows small epithelium-lined lumina to remain open. All epithelia lie on connective tissue, but the basal cell surface is separated from the connective tissue by a basement membrane.

4. The answer is 4 *[II B 1 b]*. In secretory cells, most of the rough endoplasmic reticulum (rER) and many mitochondria as well as the cell nucleus occupy the basal portion of the cell. Therefore, the substrates that have diffused from capillaries in the underlying connective tissue and have been absorbed through the basal cell membrane immediately encounter the synthetic machinery of the cell. The products of synthesis in the rER are passed to the Golgi complex at the apical pole of the nucleus as they move toward their point of exocytosis through the apical cell membrane. In ciliated cells, mitochondria are concentrated in the apical cytoplasm, which is where the adenosine triphosphate (ATP) they produce is used as chemical energy for ciliary action. The surface area of absorptive cells is increased by the presence of microvilli. The basal lamina, a component of the basement membrane that closely parallels the basal surface of the epithelium, does not extend along the lateral cell membranes.

5. The answer is 1 *[II C 3 a]*. Tight junctions and zonulae adherentes are present only in epithelia. The tight junctions form a seal between cells that separates the lumen from the intercellular tissue space and also prevents inappropriate mixing of apical and basolateral membrane proteins. Because tight junctions are not strongly adhesive, zonulae adherentes, strong adhesive junctions adjacent to the tight junctions, support the tight junctions. The other components of the junctional complex are desmosomes, the attachment plaques joining adjacent lateral cell membranes. Hemidesmosomes are present only on the basal cell surface of certain epithelial cells, where they attach the epithelium to the basement membrane.

6. The answer is 4 *[III A 2 c]*. Columnar cells are taller than they are wide. Stratified columnar epithelium, which is relatively rare, has columnar cells in the surface layer. To be classified as simple, all cells must both touch the basement membrane and reach the free surface. All cells also lie on the basement membrane in pseudostratified epithelia, but not all reach the free surface. Although the cell nuclei lie at different levels in pseudostratified epithelia (because of the varying cell heights), this is not a criterion for classification. Stratified epithelia refers to those with more than one layer of cells; epithelia with flat cells are classified as squamous. Cells in the superficial layer of most stratified epithelia are a different shape than the basal cells. Transitional epithelium is a special type of pseudostratified epithelium that lines most of the urinary tract; its cells change shape when the lumen of the organ is distended.

7. The answer is 2 *[IV A 1]*. The process of secretion includes both synthesis and release of a cellular product. Although the secretory cells of glands are epithelial, secretion also occurs in many cell types in which it is not the primary function (e.g., nerve cells). Cytoplasmic elements and portions of the cell membrane or even the entire cell are lost during apocrine and holocrine secretion. Excretory ducts are defined as ducts that merely carry the secretory product without contributing to it. The portion of a gland that is secretory is called the parenchyma; the stroma is the supportive tissue.

8. The answer is 3 *[IV B 2 b (2)]*. The presence of a branching system of excretory ducts is the characteristic feature of a compound gland. Secretion of mucus occurs in glands ranging from the simplest unicellular glands (goblet cells) to large compound glands. Simple branched glands, as well as compound glands, have multiple secretory units. A gland is defined as tubuloacinar if it has a secretory duct draining a cluster of acini. Most compound glands are tubuloacinar glands. Acinar glands have spherical or flask-shaped secretory units. If glands have elongated secretory units, they are classified as tubular.

9. The answer is 2 *[IV B 2 b (2) (b) (i)]*. Intercalated ducts, which are the smallest ducts, join the acini and secretory ducts; their beginning is surrounded by the secretory acinus in some glands. Striated ducts are so named because the elongated mitochondria aligned in parallel folds of the basal cell membranes have a striated appearance. They regulate the water and electrolyte content of the secretory product. Intralobular, not interlobular, ducts lie within the lobules. Interlobular ducts, which drain each lobule, are in connective tissue septa between lobules. Lobar ducts are present only in glands large enough to have several lobes, which they drain. Excretory ducts are always present in compound glands; secretory ducts, striated ducts, or both, may also be present.

10. The answer is 5 *[IV C 4 b (2)]*. Because they contain more rough endoplasmic reticulum (rER) and their nuclei are larger and more centrally located, serous glands appear more basophilic than mucous glands in routine preparations. Mucin, the product of mucous glands, contains many acidic glycoproteins; proteins and neutral glycoproteins are characteristic of serous secretions. In mixed mucoserous glands, the serous cells are pushed to a peripheral location in the secretory units by the bulging mucous cells, forming crescent-shaped serous demilunes. The products of the displaced serous cells reach the lumen through narrow canaliculi between the mucous cells. Mucin, secreted directly into the lumen by mucous cells, combines with water outside the cell to form viscous, sticky mucus.

11. The answer is 4 *[IV A 2 b]*. Myoepithelial cells wrap long, slender processes around secretory units of certain glands, including mammary glands, and their contraction helps expel secretory products. In mammary glands, this response to nervous or humoral stimuli is called milk let-down. Myoepithelial cells are true epithelial cells. They lie beneath the secretory cells, extending their processes between the secretory cells and the basement membrane. The parenchyma of any organ is the portion that performs the major functions of the organ. In glands, the parenchyma is the secretory epithelium. Glands are classified anatomically according to the shape of the secretory units and the complexity of the excretory duct system. Holocrine secretion, in which the entire cell disintegrates and becomes part of the secretory product, occurs only in sebaceous glands in domestic animals.

12. The answer is 3 *[I D]*. A membrane is formed by an epithelium and its underlying connective tissue. Mucous membranes are coated by mucus that may come from surface cells or from deeper glands that open onto the surface. Serous membranes are lubricated by a watery transudate from the blood; they have no relationship to serous glands. Not all membranes are serous or mucous membranes. Skin, for example, is a membrane that is lubricated by sebaceous glands. Mucous membranes are often called wet membranes.

13–15. The answers are: 13-4 *[Figure 5-6]* **14-2** *[Figure 5-7]*, **15-1** *[IV C 3]*. This intercalated duct can be recognized by its lining of epithelial cells that are much smaller than cells in the surrounding secretory units and the fact that it is closely surrounded by secretory units, which would not be true for an interlobular duct.

All the secretory cells are fairly darkly stained and have round or oval nuclei, which are characteristics of serous cells.

Apocrine glands and holocrine glands all are associated with the skin. All other glands are merocrine. Serous glands, such as the one shown here, are associated only with mucous membranes.

16. The answer is 5 *[II B 2 b]*. Secretory granules accumulate in the apical cytoplasm between the mature face of the Golgi complex and the apical cell membrane, through which they will be released. Because epithelia cover or line all body surfaces, all substances must pass through an epithelium to enter or leave the body. Brush borders are formed by a layer of parallel uniform microvilli that amplify the apical surface area of absorptive cells. The composition of the apical cell membrane differs from that of the remaining cell membrane because it is adapted to fulfill the functions of the free surface rather than to face other cells. In certain locations in the body, the apical cell membrane may actually transport the same material inward that is transported outward by the basolateral membrane. Hemidesmosomes attach certain epithelia to the underlying basal lamina; hence, they are associated only with the basal cell membrane.

17. The answer is 2 *[II C 2]*. The basement membrane separates epithelium from connective tissue only; muscle and nervous tissue do not underlie epithelium. The basement membrane acts as a support and provides a basis of attachment for the epithelium. In addition, it serves as an important barrier (e.g., it prevents the loss of large molecules from the blood in kidney glomeruli and prevents invasion by bacteria in the trachea).

Chapter 6

Connective Tissue

I. INTRODUCTION

A. Structure

1. **Cells** and **extracellular material** comprise connective tissue. Extracellular material is characteristically present in relatively large amounts in connective tissue and, in some cases, is the major functional element.
2. Connective tissues form a continuous layer, or **continuum,** that is separated from the other basic tissues by basal laminae.

B. Functions.

Functions. Some forms of connective tissue are highly specialized [e.g., bone and cartilage (see Chapter 7), blood (see Chapter 8)]. Connective tissue functions include:

1. **Support.** Connective tissues surround and support the other basic tissues and form the stroma of most organs.
2. **Transportation.** The blood carries cells, solutes, and gases, and the ground substance of connective tissue (see II A) permits diffusion of nutrients and waste to and from cells.
3. **Energy source.** Connective tissues store energy and release it on signal as chemical energy or heat energy.
4. **Storage.** Connective tissues store water and electrolytes. The main electrolyte in loose connective tissue is sodium. Bone is involved in calcium balance.
5. **Inflammation and tissue repair** (see II C 2)

C. Development of connective tissue (Figure 6-1)

1. **Mesoderm** gives rise to **mesenchyme,** the embryonic connective tissue.
2. **Mesenchyme** condenses and differentiates to form specific structures, such as **bone, cartilage, ligaments, fat, blood cells,** and **blood vessels. Loose connective tissue** is formed from the remaining mesenchyme.

II. STRUCTURE OF CONNECTIVE TISSUE.

The structural components of connective tissue are ground substance, fibers, and cells.

A. Ground substance

Ground substance, which is amorphous and colorless, occupies the space between cells and fibers.

1. **Composition.** Ground substance has two main constituents, glycosaminoglycans and structural glycoproteins.
   a. **Glycosaminoglycans** are linear polysaccharides.
      (1) **Hyaluronic acid** is the most abundant and the least viscous of the glycosaminoglycans.
         (a) Hyaluronic acid is **not sulfated.**
         (b) It **does not bind covalently** to proteins.

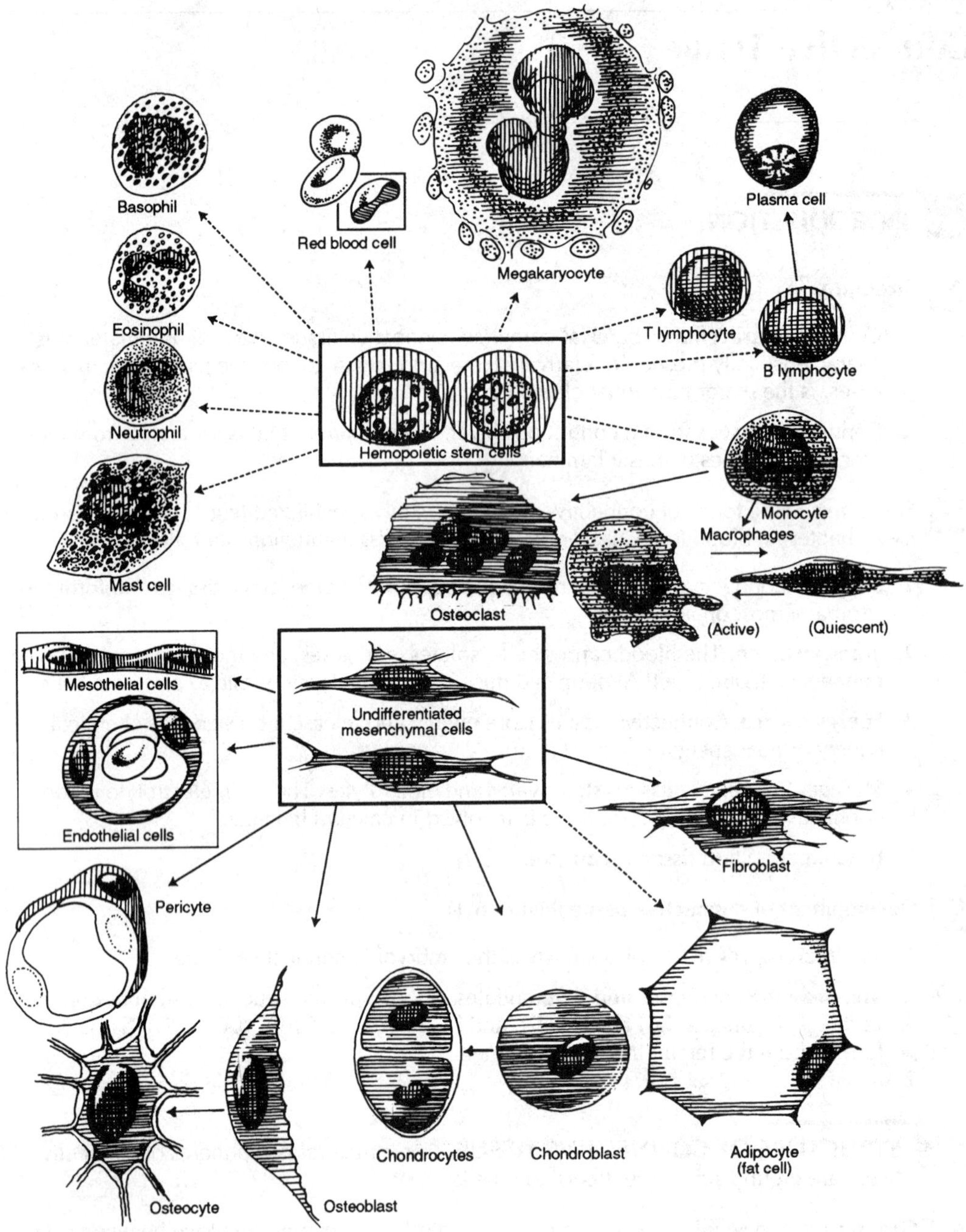

Figure 6-1. Simplified representation of connective tissue cell derivations from embryonic mesenchyme cells. (Endothelium and mesothelium, shown in the *box at left,* are epithelial derivatives of mesenchyme.) *Dotted lines* indicate lineages where intermediate cell types have not been illustrated. Vascular smooth muscle cells (not illustrated) also retain important mesenchymal capabilities. The cells are not drawn to scale; adipocytes, megakaryocytes, and osteoclasts are often much larger than illustrated. (Redrawn with permission from Junqueira LC, Carneiro J, Kelley RO: *Basic Histology,* 7th ed. Englewood Cliffs, NJ, Appleton & Lange, 1992, p 119.)

(2) **Sulfated glycosaminoglycans** bind covalently with a protein core, forming a proteoglycan molecule.

(a) **Structure. Proteoglycans** are macromolecules comprising a protein core to which many unbranched glycosaminoglycans are bound.

(i) Proteoglycans are similar in shape to a **bottle brush,** with the protein as the stem and the glycosaminoglycans as the radiating bristles.

(ii) The glycosaminoglycans in proteoglycans usually have a negative charge, which makes them intensely **hydrophilic.**

Layers of **solvation water** surround each proteoglycan as a result of this hydrophilia.

The **volume of each molecule is** greatly **increased when** fully **hydrated.**

(iii) A **molecular net** forms when the negatively charged carbohydrates on proteoglycans bind to collagen.

(b) **Types.** There are four major types of sulfated glycosaminoglycans:

(i) **Dermatan sulfate** occurs mainly in tissues that are rich in collagen type I (e.g., tendons, ligaments, fibrocartilage, and dermis).

(ii) **Chondroitin sulfate** occurs mainly in types of cartilage that are rich in collagen type II (e.g., hyaline cartilage, elastic cartilage).

(iii) **Heparan sulfate** occurs mainly in reticular fibers, which contain collagen type III, and in basement membranes.

(iv) **Keratan sulfate** occurs mainly in bone, cartilage, and the cornea.

(3) **Distribution**

(a) The ratio of sulfated glycosaminoglycans to hyaluronic acid is greater in firmer tissues than in softer ones.

(b) In cartilage, proteoglycans bind to hyaluronic acid chains, forming large, rigid molecular aggregates.

b. **Structural glycoproteins** are composed of a protein with attached carbohydrates.

(1) **Structure.** Unlike proteoglycans, the protein usually predominates and the carbohydrates are often branched.

(2) **Function.** Glycoproteins help attach cells to each other and to their extracellular substrate. Important glycoproteins include fibronectin and laminin.

(a) **Fibronectin** is able to bind with cells, glycosaminoglycans, and collagen. It is produced by some epithelial cells as well as by fibroblasts (see II C 1 c).

(b) **Laminin** helps attach epithelial cells to the basal laminae.

c. **Tissue fluid** is the small amount of **unbound water** in the connective tissue.

(1) Tissue fluid contains **ions** and **small plasma proteins** that have leaked out of the capillaries.

(2) **Edema** is abnormal accumulation of tissue fluid.

2. **Functions**

a. **Diffusion.** The ground substance is a medium for diffusion of nutrients and wastes to and from cells.

b. **Storage.** Hydration layers on the proteoglycans are important storage sites for water and electrolytes.

c. **Protection.** Viscous ground substance is an impediment to movement of bacteria and other foreign material. Some of the most invasive bacteria are those that secrete hyaluronidase, which breaks down hyaluronic acid and other glycosaminoglycans.

3. **Light-microscope appearance.** Under the light microscope, the ground substance appears to be unstained because it is so dilute; therefore, the areas it occupies appear empty.

B. Fibers. There are three types of protein fibers in connective tissue: collagen fibers, reticular fibers, and elastic fibers.

1. **Collagen fibers** are the most abundant of the fibers.

a. **Classification.** There are several different types of collagen, the best known of which are collagen types I through IV. All are glycosylated, but the carbohydrate content differs among types.
   (1) **Collagen type I,** the most abundant type, **forms collagen fibers**.
      (a) Type I is present in **fibrous structures** (e.g., tendons, organ capsules, dermis).
      (b) Type I provides tensile strength in **bone**.
   (2) **Collagen type II forms thin fibrils.**
      (a) Fibrils are visible only under the electron microscope.
      (b) Most collagen type II is found in **cartilage**.
   (3) **Collagen type III forms fibrils or thin fibers.**
      (a) Type III is the main component of **reticular fibers**.
      (b) Type III can copolymerize with other collagen types, usually collagen type I.
   (4) **Collagen type IV does not form fibrils or fibers.**
      (a) If type IV polymerizes, it is as a **lattice** that can be deformed.
      (b) Type IV is located in **basal laminae**.

b. **Formation of collagen fibrils and fibers**
   (1) **Components**
      (a) **Procollagens,** which are soluble, are secreted by the cell. The type of procollagen produced depends on the location of the tissue in the body.
      (b) **Tropocollagen** is formed outside the cell by enzymatic removal of portions of the procollagen peptides.
         (i) **Collagen fibrils** are formed by polymerization of overlapping parallel tropocollagen subunits. The type of procollagen determines the strength of the cross-linkages between tropocollagen molecules and, therefore, the strength of the collagen fibril.
         (ii) **Collagen fibers,** visible under the light microscope, are formed spontaneously by aggregation of fibrils in collagen types I and III.
   (2) **Abnormalities.** A series of enzymes, cofactors, and other extracellular substances are involved in collagen fiber formation from procollagen secretion on. Because so many factors are involved, collagen synthesis is susceptible to disruption at many points.
      (a) **Faulty enzymes** or **disease processes** may cause collagen abnormalities.
      (b) **Sclerosis** is a condition caused by **excessive** accumulation of **collagen**.

c. **Light-microscope appearance**
   (1) Collagen is acidophilic.
   (2) It stains blue or green with common trichrome stains.

d. **Physical properties.** Collagen is:
   (1) **Inelastic**
   (2) **Strong,** with a tensile strength greater for its mass than steel
   (3) **Flexible**
   (4) **Birefringent**
   (5) **Unstable.** Boiling or acid treatment denatures collagen, producing **gelatin**. These treatments are used to tenderize tough cuts of meat.

e. **Functions.** Collagen is the most abundant protein in the body, constituting almost one third of the body's dry weight.
   (1) Collagen fibers form tendons, ligaments, capsules of organs, and dermis.
   (2) Collagen provides the tensile strength of bone and cartilage.

2. **Reticular fibers** are very thin strands.
   a. **Structure.** Reticular fibers are composed of loosely packed thin fibrils of type III collagen, with a carbohydrate-rich surface coating of glycoproteins and proteoglycans.
   b. **Light-microscope appearance.** Reticular fibers are not stained by routine methods but can be demonstrated with the periodic acid–Schiff (PAS) reaction or with silver stains.
   c. **Functions**
      (1) **Support.** Delicate networks of reticular fibers support the smallest subunits of tissues and organs. Reticular fibers are particularly numerous in:
         (a) **Blood-forming tissues** (e.g., bone marrow, lymphatic organs), where they are produced by reticular cells

(b) **Smooth muscle,** where they are produced by smooth muscle cells
(c) **Basement membranes,** where they form the reticular layer
(2) **Tissue integrity.** Deficiency of collagen type III can lead to arterial and intestinal ruptures.

3. **Elastic fibers**
a. **Formation of elastic fibers**
(1) **Components**
(a) **Proelastin** is secreted from the cell.
(b) **Elastin** is produced by polymerization of proelastin. Elastin is a three-dimensional reticulum that can be deformed and then recover its shape.
(2) Elastin is deposited among thin glycoprotein-containing microfibrils, which are resistant to tension. Elastin exists in fibers as well as in laminae (sheets). Elastic laminae are characteristic of the walls of some blood vessels.
b. **Light-microscope appearance**
(1) Elastic fibers are **acidophilic.**
(2) They appear bright because they are **refractile** (i.e., capable of deflecting light).
(3) Elastic fibers are larger than individual collagen fibers, and, unlike collagen fibers, they are branched.
c. **Physical properties**
(1) **Deformability.** Elastic fibers can be stretched to 50% longer than their original length.
(2) **Elasticity.** Elastic fibers return to their original dimensions following deformation without the expenditure of energy. The elastic properties of a specific structure are determined by the proportions of elastin and microfibrils.
(3) **Limited tensile strength.** The tensile strength of elastic fibers is limited; therefore, they are always supported by a network of collagen fibers.
(4) **Stability.** Elastic fibers are resistant to boiling, acid, and alkali extraction.
d. **Functions**
(1) **Shape retention.** Elastic fibers are most numerous in structures subjected to frequent deformation, such as skin and the lungs, where they return the structures to their original form.
(2) **Maintenance of blood flow.** Elastic fibers and laminae in arteries act as auxiliary pumps; elastic recoil propels the blood between pulses. Smooth muscle cells in blood vessels produce these elastic fibers and laminae.
(3) **Support.** Elastic fibers in the nuchal ligament help support the head in grazing animals.

C. **Cells** (see Figure 6-1)

1. **Resident cells.** Cells that are normally present in connective tissue are called resident cells. Most arise from mesenchyme, although some are immigrants from the blood and are derived from hemopoietic stem cells.
a. **Mesenchymal cells** are undifferentiated embryonic connective tissue cells. Their long, slender processes form a loose network in mesenchyme.
b. **Pericytes** are spindle-shaped or branched cells that lie on the surface of capillaries and venules. They are a reserve population of relatively undifferentiated connective tissue cells that may differentiate into other connective tissue cell types or into smooth muscle.
c. **Fibroblasts** are the characteristic cell type of connective tissue.
(1) **Structure.** Fibroblasts are usually spindle-shaped but may have multiple processes (stellate). Their shape is determined by their extracellular substrate.
(2) **Light-microscope appearance**
(a) **Inactive cells.** In quiescent fibroblasts (i.e., **fibrocytes**), the cytoplasm is acidophilic; therefore, it blends with the extracellular components, and only the heterochromatic (darkly staining) nucleus is visible.
(b) **Active cells.** During growth and wound healing, when secretory activity is stimulated, the cells are enlarged, have more processes, and the cytoplasm is basophilic. Fibroblasts may become migratory during wound healing.

(3) **Function.** Fibroblasts secrete the extracellular components of connective tissue (i.e., the ground substance and the three types of connective tissue fibers).

d. **Reticular cells** are similar in appearance to fibroblasts, but they are present only in reticular connective tissue. They produce reticular fibers.

e. **Adipocytes** (fat cells) are specialized to synthesize and store lipid.

(1) **White adipose cells**

(a) **Structure**

(i) White adipose cells contain a single large lipid droplet (i.e., they are **unilocular**) formed by fusion of smaller droplets during development.

(ii) Lipid displaces the heterochromatic nucleus and the cytoplasm to the periphery of the cell. Cross-sections through these cells in routine preparations resemble a **signet ring,** with the nucleus as the signet and the cytoplasm as the ring surrounding the unstained lipid droplet (see Figure 6-8A).

(b) **Functions**

(i) **Energy storage and production.** Most white adipose cells metabolize their lipid stores to produce **chemical energy** when the animal's diet does not meet its energy needs (see III F).

(ii) **Support and cushioning.** Cells in certain locations, such as the digital pad and around the kidneys, provide structural support and cushioning. These cells do not respond to metabolic signals.

(2) **Brown adipose cells**

(a) **Structure.** Brown adipose cells contain several lipid droplets (i.e., they are **multilocular**) and many large mitochondria.

(b) **Function.** Brown adipose cells metabolize their lipid stores to produce **heat.**

f. **Mast cells** are derived from hemopoietic stem cells.

(1) **Structure.** Mast cells are **ovoid** (egg-shaped) or **angular** cells that are most frequently located in the loose connective tissue near small blood vessels. The cytoplasm of mast cells is **granular**. The granules are of different sizes within a single cell.

(2) **Composition of granules.** Granule contents may include:

(a) **Heparin,** which is an anticoagulant. Heparin also stimulates endothelial cell motility, promoting angiogenesis.

(b) **Histamine,** which dilates small blood vessels and increases their permeability

(i) Histamine produces **edema** of the surrounding tissue and increases white blood cell **diapedesis** (i.e., the migration of blood cells through the walls of capillaries and venules into the tissue).

(ii) Histamine also causes **contraction of smooth muscle in** the walls of **small airways.**

(c) **Chemotactic mediators,** which attract white blood cells [e.g., eosinophil chemotactic factor of anaphylaxis (ECF-A), which attracts eosinophils].

(d) **Arachidonic acid,** which promotes the production of substances that cause dilation of small blood vessels

(e) **Leukotrienes,** which cause smooth muscle to contract

(3) **Light-microscope appearance**

(a) **Achromatic (nonstaining).** In most species, the granules are unstained in routine preparations.

(b) **Metachromatic.** The granules stain metachromatically with appropriate stains. For example, after staining with toluidine blue, the mast cell granules look purple but the other cellular components are the same color as the dye (i.e., blue).

(4) **Functions.** Mast cells are classified as **paracrine** cells because the contents of their granules act on nearby cells. Specific granules contain mediators of inflammation and immediate hypersensitivity.

(a) **Inflammation.** Degranulation of mast cells helps initiate the inflammation reaction.

(b) **Immediate hypersensitivity.** Mast cells are important mediators of immediate hypersensitivity, the allergic reaction that occurs within minutes after the second exposure to an antigen.

(i) When an animal is first exposed to an antigen, cells of its immune system produce a class of specific antibodies called **immunoglobulin E (IgE)**.
(ii) The IgE molecules become concentrated on the surface of mast cells (and basophils in the blood).
(iii) If the same antigen re-enters the body, it binds with the IgE molecules on the mast cells, which triggers exocytosis of the specific granules.
(iv) Massive degranulation can cause **anaphylactic shock**.

g. Macrophages (histiocytes)

(1) **Origin.** Macrophages are derived from hemopoietic stem cells. Their immediate source is white blood cells called **monocytes**.

(2) **Structure.** Macrophages vary widely in appearance, depending on the function they are performing and the tissue in which they are located.
(a) They are **irregular** in outline, with an **eccentric nucleus**.
(b) When they become actively phagocytic, they increase in size, extend pseudopodia, and become more irregular in shape.
(c) Active cells have an extensive Golgi complex and many lysosomes. They acquire cytoplasmic vacuoles and granules.

(3) **Distribution.** Most of the macrophage life span is spent in loose connective tissue or reticular connective tissue, where they live for several months. The **mononuclear phagocyte system (MPS)** is composed of macrophages throughout the body. In certain regions, macrophages have been given special names, such as:
(a) **Kupffer cells** in the liver
(b) **Alveolar macrophages (dust cells),** which can remove particles from the lungs both nonselectively and by receptor-mediated phagocytosis
(c) **Osteoclasts** in bone
(d) **Microglia** in the central nervous system (CNS)

(4) **Functions**
(a) **Phagocytosis** [see also Chapter 8 II B 3 b (1)]. The phagocytic activity of macrophages is important for:
(i) Digestion of microorganisms and foreign particles
(ii) Removal of cellular debris after an inflammation reaction has occurred
(iii) Removal of aged and abnormal red blood cells
(b) **Secretion.** Macrophages secrete many cytokines, substances that are involved in immunologic responses, defense, and healing, such as:
(i) Interleukins (substances that affect other white blood cells)
(ii) Pyrogens (fever-inducing substances)
(iii) Growth factors

2. **Immigrant cells** are hemopoietic stem cell-derived white blood cells that have entered the connective tissue by diapedesis. White blood cells in connective tissue are called **free cells** because they are motile. Immigrant cells usually enter the tissue during an inflammation reaction (Figure 6-2); however, some of these cells are present normally in certain locations, notably the lamina propria (i.e., the connective tissue component of mucous membranes) of the intestine. Once in the tissue, they do not return to the blood.

a. Basophils are so called because they contain basophilic granules.

(1) **Comparison with mast cells.** Basophil granules are similar (identical in many species) to those of mast cells. Basophils resemble mast cells functionally, but they arise from different stem cells.

(2) **Functions**
(a) **Inflammation.** Basophils enter injured tissue, where their degranulation promotes the inflammation reaction (see also Chapter 8 II B 6 b).
(b) **Allergy.** Basophils are the source of blood histamine during allergic reactions.

b. Neutrophils [phagocytes, microphages, polymorphonuclear leukocytes (PMNLs)]

(1) **Structure**
(a) **Lysosomes** and specific granules are present in neutrophils; however, they are usually not visible in routine preparations in most domestic animals.
(b) **Nuclei** are multilobulated and heterochromatic.

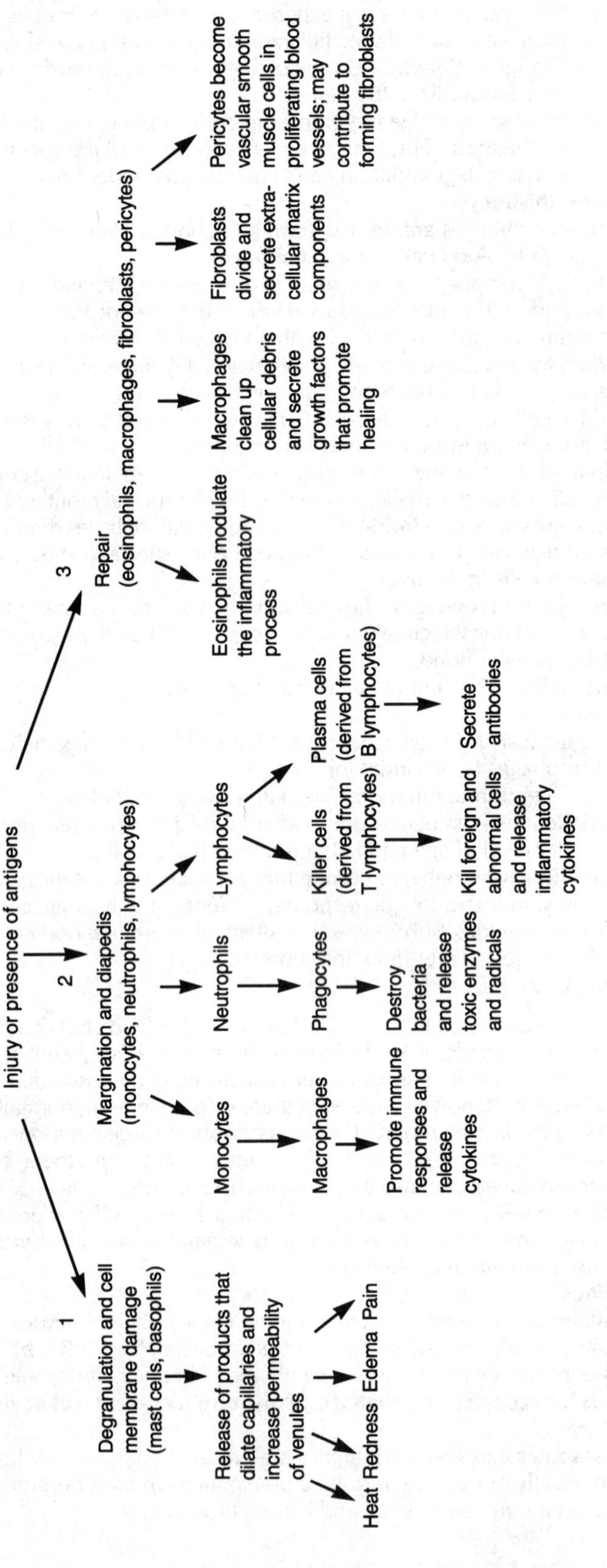

Figure 6-2. Role of connective tissue resident and immigrant cells in inflammation and tissue repair.

(2) **Functions.** Neutrophils are the **first line of defense** against pathogenic bacteria; products of the immune system and chemicals released by bacteria quickly attract large numbers of neutrophils to the injured tissue (see also Chapter 8 II B 4 b).

(a) **Antibacterial activity.** Neutrophils have two types of granules, which contain both enzyme and nonenzyme proteins with antibacterial activity.

(b) **Phagocytosis.** Neutrophils phagocytose microorganisms and small particles.

(3) **Pus** is formed by accumulations of dead neutrophils, bacteria, and partially digested material. Neutrophils are sometimes called pus cells.

c. **Eosinophils** contain eosinophilic granules.

(1) **Structure.** Eosinophils usually have a **bilobed nucleus**. Specialized lysosomes are the specific granules of eosinophils.

(2) **Functions.** Eosinophils increase in number in the tissue during allergic reactions and in parasitic and other types of disease.

(a) **Phagocytosis.** Eosinophils phagocytose antigen–antibody complexes and certain parasites; however, they are not actively phagocytic toward other particles.

(b) **Hydrolysis.** Eosinophils release enzymes that break down important chemical mediators of allergic reactions, including histamine.

d. **Lymphocytes**

(1) **Structure.** Lymphocytes contain a small amount of slightly basophilic cytoplasm and a relatively large heterochromatic nucleus.

(2) **Distribution.** Lymphocytes are present in **chronically inflamed tissue**. They are also present normally in the lamina propria of the digestive tract and, to a lesser extent, the respiratory and female reproductive tracts.

(3) **Functions.** There are many different types of lymphocytes, but they cannot be distinguished structurally. The two main classes are T lymphocytes and B lymphocytes.

(a) **T lymphocytes** initiate **cell-mediated immune responses**. They can be very long-lived.

(b) **B lymphocytes** are responsible for **humoral immunity**. When stimulated by an antigen, B lymphocytes secrete antibodies and give rise to clones of plasma cells.

e. **Plasma cells**

(1) **Structure**

(a) Plasma cells have an **eccentric nucleus** with a characteristic **clumped heterochromatin pattern,** described as resembling a **wagon wheel** or a **clock face**.

(b) An abundance of **free polysomes** (multiple units of ribosomes) give the cytoplasm a basophilic appearance.

(c) Near the nucleus, the pale-staining Golgi complex is often visible against the dark cytoplasm.

(2) **Distribution.** Like the B lymphocytes from which they arise, plasma cells are present in chronically inflamed tissue and in the mucous membranes of certain organ systems.

(3) **Function.** Plasma cells produce immunoglobulins (antibodies) for 10–20 days, after which time the cells die.

III. TYPES OF CONNECTIVE TISSUES

A. Embryonic connective tissues

1. **Mesenchyme** is composed of mesenchymal cells and amorphous material. A few fibers may also be present.

2. **Mucous connective tissue** is primarily ground substance with a few fibers and fibroblasts. It is present in the umbilical cord and hypodermis and persists in isolated locations, including the pulp of developing teeth and the comb of poultry.

B. **Loose connective tissue** (Figure 6-3)

1. **Structure**
   a. **Ground substance.** Loose connective tissue contains a large amount of ground substance that is especially rich in **hyaluronic acid** and is, therefore, quite **viscous**. Because areas containing ground substance look like empty spaces (areolae) microscopically, loose connective tissue is often called areolar tissue.
   b. **Fibers.** Loose connective tissue contains relatively **few fibers;** however, all three types of fibers may be present. Their relative abundance varies in different locations in the body.
   c. **Cells. Fibroblasts** and **macrophages** are the most abundant cells. All types of immigrant cells may be present and are especially numerous in the lamina propria of mucous membranes.
   d. **Blood supply.** Loose connective tissue is **very vascular**.
2. **Distribution**
   a. Loose connective tissue fills spaces between other structures and supports epithelia.
   b. The **subcutis** (subcutaneous tissue), the **lamina propria,** and the **tela submucosa** are loose connective tissues.
3. **Functions**
   a. **Movement.** Loose connective tissue is flexible, permitting limited movement between adjacent structures or layers.
   b. **Storage.** Abundant ground substance makes loose connective tissue an important storage site for water and electrolytes.

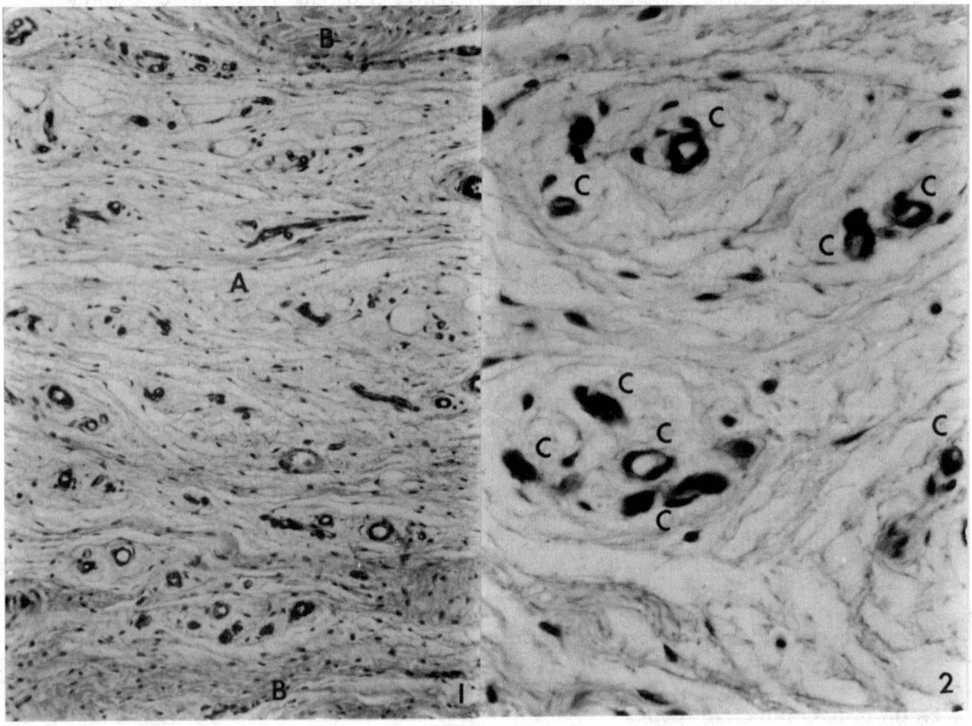

Figure 6-3. Loose connective tissue. (*1*) At low magnification, the loose connective tissue occupying most of the field (*A*) can be compared with dense irregular connective tissue near the bottom of the field (*B*). (*2*) At higher magnification, capillaries (*C*) and loosely arranged fibers are shown. (Reprinted with permission from Dellmann H-D: *Textbook of Veterinary Histology,* 4th ed. Baltimore, Williams & Wilkins, 1993, p 34.)

C. Dense connective tissue appears white on gross examination. It is classified as dense irregular or dense regular connective tissue, depending on the organization of its fibers.

1. **Dense irregular connective tissue** (Figure 6-4)
   a. **Structure.** Dense irregular connective tissue consists mostly of **bundles of collagen fibers running in many different directions**. **Fibroblasts** are the predominant cell type present.
   b. **Distribution.** Dense irregular connective tissue is found in most organ capsules, under mucocutaneous membranes, and in the dermis.
   c. **Functions.** Because of the random arrangement of its fibers, dense irregular connective tissue resists stress in several directions. Therefore, it **supports and protects the organs and skin**.
2. **Dense regular connective tissue** (Figure 6-5)
   a. **Structure.** Dense regular connective tissue consists mostly of bundles of **parallel collagen fibers**. In the cornea, fibers in different layers run at right angles. **Fibroblasts** are the only cell type present.
   b. **Distribution.** Dense regular connective tissue forms tendons, aponeuroses (muscle terminations and attachments), ligaments, and the cornea.
   c. **Functions**
      (1) Dense regular connective tissue resists stress along the linear axis of the fibers, providing the musculoskeletal system with strong attachments that flex but do not change in length.
      (2) In the cornea, its regular arrangement provides both strength and transparency.

D. Dense elastic tissue (Figure 6-6) appears yellow on gross examination.

1. **Structure.** Dense elastic tissue consists of **large parallel elastic fibers,** each surrounded by a supportive network of much **smaller collagen fibers** that prevent the elastic fibers from being overstretched. **Fibroblasts** are the only cells present.

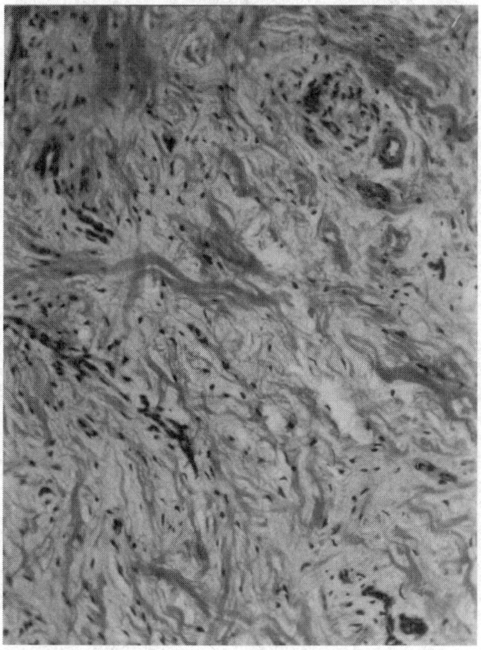

Figure 6-4. Dense irregular connective tissue. Randomly arranged bundles of collagen fibers and dark nuclei of fibroblasts are shown. (Reprinted with permission from Dellmann H-D: *Textbook of Veterinary Histology,* 4th ed. Baltimore, Williams & Wilkins, 1993, p 31.)

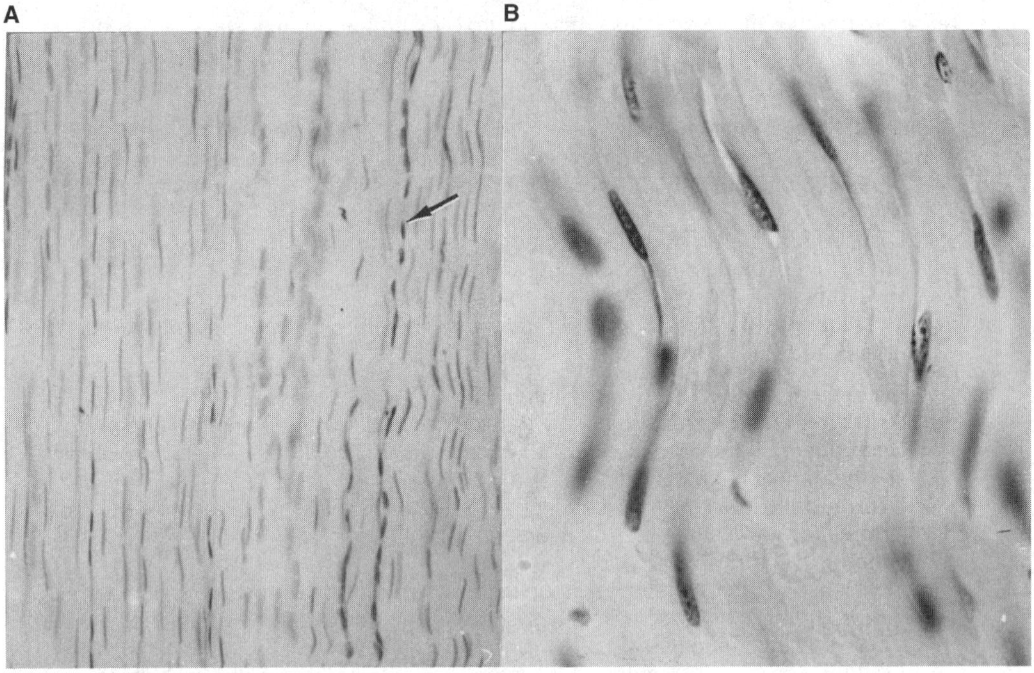

Figure 6-5. Dense regular connective tissue. (*A*) Low magnification. (*B*) High magnification. Fibroblasts (*arrow*) can be seen between the parallel bundles of collagen fibers. (Reprinted with permission from Dellmann H-D: *Textbook of Veterinary Histology,* 4th ed. Baltimore, Williams & Wilkins, 1993, p 37.)

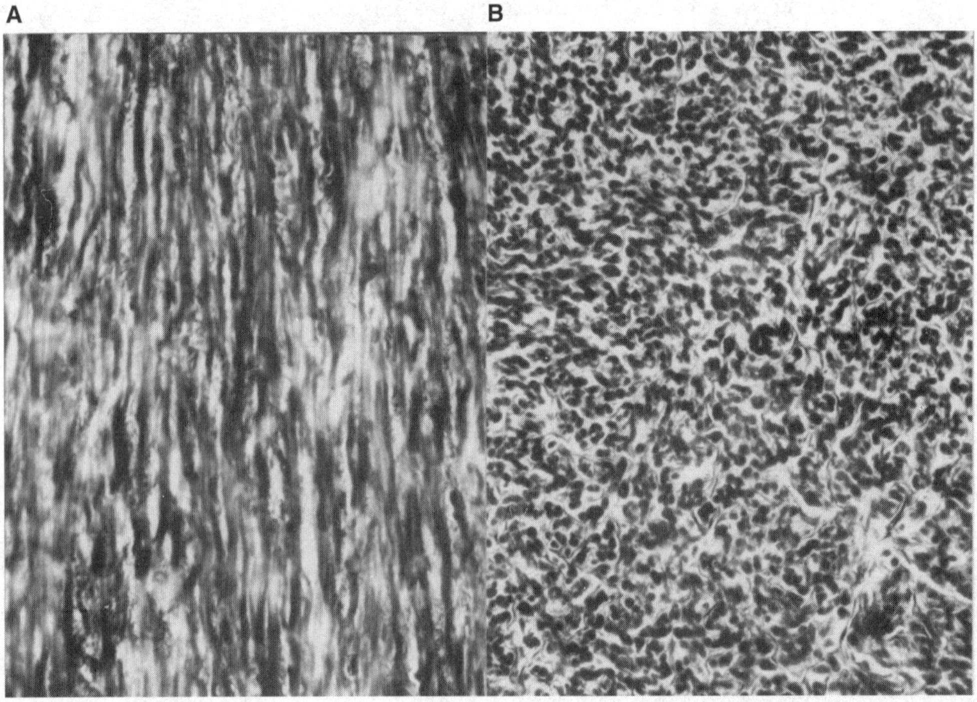

Figure 6-6. Elastic tissue in (*A*) longitudinal section and (*B*) cross-section. The large elastic fibers are surrounded by a network of collagen fibers.

2. **Distribution.** Dense elastic tissue forms the **nuchal ligament** and certain other ligaments of the vertebral column. Large arteries also contain elastic tissue (see Chapter 11).
3. **Functions.** The linear orientation of elastic elements in ligaments helps maintain the alignment of the vertebral column. Elastic recoil helps raise the head of grazing animals.

E. **Reticular tissue** (Figure 6-7)

1. **Structure.** Reticular tissue is a special type of loose connective tissue composed of **reticular cells** and **reticular fibers**.
   - **a.** The spindle-shaped or stellate cells form an open three-dimensional network, or reticulum.
   - **b.** Reticular fibers lie along the surfaces of reticular cells and are ensheathed by cytoplasmic processes of these cells. Reticular fibers support the reticulum.
   - **c.** Reticular tissue is always continuous with dense irregular connective tissue.
2. **Distribution.** Reticular tissue is the supportive element of all blood-forming tissues.
3. **Functions.** Reticular tissue forms the **stroma** of all the blood-forming tissues. It provides a supportive framework with large open spaces for the immigrant cells in bone marrow and lymphoid organs.

F. **Adipose tissues** are specialized to synthesize and store fats. They are highly cellular and are richly vascularized and innervated.

1. **White adipose tissue** (Figure 6-8A) is usually white on gross examination, but it is yellow in older animals of some species. Functions of adipose tissue include:
   - **a. Energy storage and production.** White adipose tissue is a reservoir of **chemical energy** that provides a continuous source of energy although feeding is intermittent.
     - **(1) Secretion.** Adipose cells secrete enzymes that enter the adjacent capillaries where they release fatty acids from triglycerides in chylomicrons and lipoproteins in the blood.
     - **(2) Absorption and storage.** The fatty acids are absorbed by the surrounding adipose cells, where triglycerides are reconstituted and stored. Adipose cells also synthesize triglycerides from other metabolic substrates (e.g., glucose).
     - **(3) Oxidation.** When energy is needed, the stored fat is oxidized to produce adenosine triphosphate (ATP). The rate of oxidation is highly responsive to nervous and hormonal stimuli.
   - **b. Structural support and cushioning**
   - **c. Insulation**
2. **Brown adipose tissue** (see Figure 6-8B) is brown in the fresh state because its cells contain many large mitochondria.

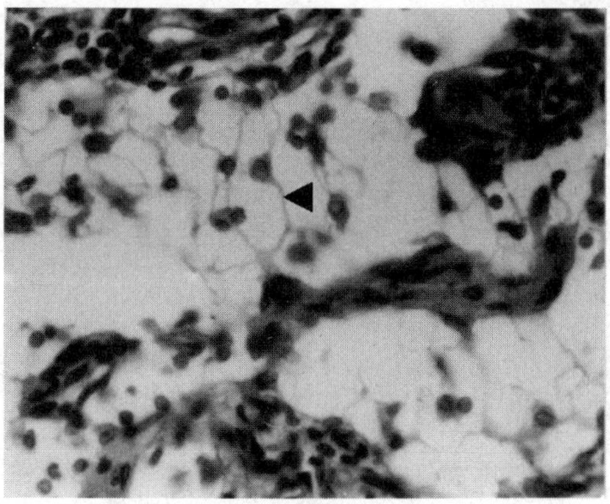

Figure 6-7. Reticular connective tissue. The long, slender processes of reticular cells (*arrow*) are connected to form a three-dimensional network. The reticular fibers are not stained. (Reprinted with permission from Dellmann H-D: *Textbook of Veterinary Histology,* 4th ed. Baltimore, Williams & Wilkins, 1993, p 38.)

A B

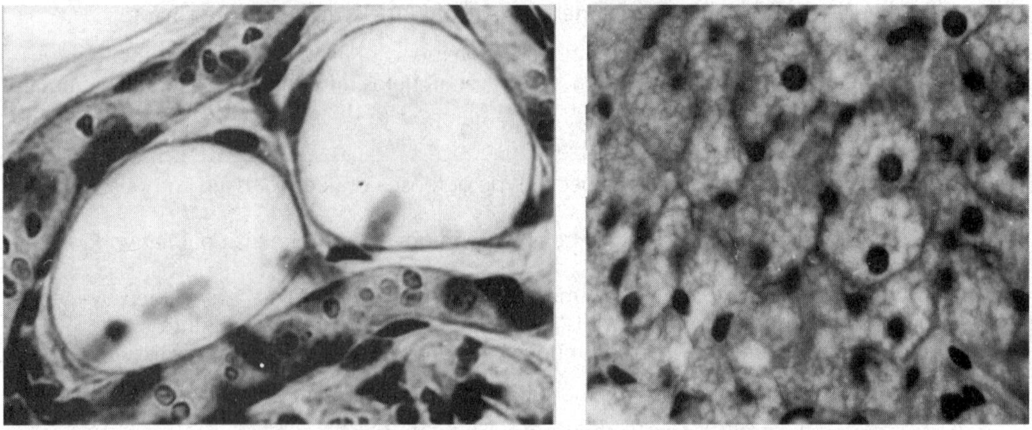

Figure 6-8. (*A*) Two white adipose cells surrounded by capillaries. Each adipose cell contains one large lipid droplet. (*B*) Brown adipose tissue. Each cell contains numerous small lipid droplets. (Reprinted with permission from Dellmann H-D: *Textbook of Veterinary Histology,* 4th ed. Baltimore, Williams & Wilkins, 1993, pp 38, 39.)

a. **Distribution.** Brown adipose tissue is limited to certain areas in the body, including the **axilla, mediastinum, perirenal fat,** and **mesenteries**. The largest accumulation is usually in the **interscapular region** (i.e., between the shoulder blades).

b. **Function.** Brown adipose tissue is a reservoir of **heat energy**.

   (1) Its mitochondria can oxidize lipids to produce heat instead of ATP.

   (2) Nervous stimulation activates brown adipose tissue on exposure to cold temperatures to **warm the blood** and **raise body temperature**.

      (a) Brown adipose tissue is especially well developed in **hibernating animals,** where it raises the body temperature on arousal from hibernation.

      (b) It is also important for maintaining body temperature in **infant animals**.

STUDY QUESTIONS

DIRECTIONS: Each of the numbered items or incomplete statements in this section is followed by answers or by completions of the statement. Select the **one** numbered answer or completion that is **best** in each case.

1. Which one of the following statements *best* describes the development of connective tissue?

(1) Connective tissue is the only type of tissue that forms from mesenchyme.
(2) Mesenchyme gives rise to mesoderm, the embryonic connective tissue.
(3) Mesenchyme remaining after other structures are formed becomes loose (areolar) connective tissue.
(4) Connective tissue arises from all three primary germ layers.
(5) The different types of connective tissue become separated by other types of tissue during development.

2. Which one of the following statements is true of the glycosaminoglycans of the ground substance?

(1) Hyaluronic acid binds covalently to collagen fibers and other proteins.
(2) Hyaluronic acid is the most viscous of the glycosaminoglycans.
(3) Solvation water is bound to positively charged glycosaminoglycans.
(4) Sulfated glycosaminoglycans bind covalently with protein to form macromolecules that are shaped like bottle brushes.
(5) Dermatan sulfate occurs mainly with reticular fibers.

3. Which one of the following statements regarding structural glycoproteins is true?

(1) They are primarily carbohydrates.
(2) They attach cells to each other.
(3) Keratan sulfate and chondroitin sulfate are important glycoproteins.
(4) They contain polymerized hyaluronic acid.
(5) They are produced only by connective tissue cells.

4. Which of the following is an important function of the ground substance?

(1) It is a storage site for electrolytes.
(2) It permits free diffusion of macromolecules to and from cells.
(3) It contains hyaluronidase, which inhibits bacterial migration through the tissue.
(4) It keeps the surfaces of connective tissue fibers from becoming attached to other tissue elements.
(5) It forms a continuous layer that separates connective tissue from other types of tissue.

5. Which one of the following statements regarding collagen is true?

(1) Collagen is a structural proteoglycan.
(2) The distribution of collagen is limited to tough, semirigid structures.
(3) Collagen type IV does not form fibrils or fibers.
(4) Collagen type III is the most abundant type of collagen.
(5) Collagen type I forms reticular fibers.

6. Which of the following occurs in the formation of collagen fibers?

(1) Insoluble procollagen is formed immediately after its precursor molecule is secreted.
(2) Tropocollagen assembles to form fibrils outside the cell.
(3) Diversity is achieved by differences in the way the common precursor molecule is arranged in tropocollagen.
(4) Once procollagen is present in sufficient concentration, the remaining steps in fibrillogenesis occur spontaneously.
(5) Collagen fibrils and fibers are visible under the light microscope.

7. Which of the following is a characteristic of collagen?

(1) It exhibits basophilia.
(2) It has elastic properties.
(3) It resists treatment with acids.
(4) It has greater tensile strength than steel.
(5) It becomes tougher when it is boiled.

8. Which of the following is a characteristic of elastic fibers?

(1) They are synthesized only by connective tissue cells.
(2) They are intensely basophilic.
(3) They are denatured by boiling or treatment with acids or alkalis.
(4) They are surrounded by a network of collagen fibers.
(5) They are thinner than collagen fibers.

9. Which one of the following statements regarding connective tissue cells is true?

(1) Quiescent fibroblasts lack the capacity to become motile.
(2) Fibroblasts are intensely acidophilic during growth and wound healing.
(3) Reticular cells produce collagen fibers and reticular fibers.
(4) Mesenchymal cells are the characteristic cell type of loose and dense connective tissues.
(5) Pericytes are considered a reserve population of relatively undifferentiated cells.

10. Plasma cells and certain B lymphocytes share which one of the following characteristics?

(1) Antibody secretion
(2) Nonspecific phagocytosis
(3) Receptor-mediated phagocytosis
(4) Secretion of substances that cause contraction of smooth muscle in small airways
(5) Long life in the connective tissue

11. White and brown adipose tissues share which one of the following characteristics?

(1) They convert an intermittent feeding pattern to a constant source of chemical energy.
(2) Their cells resemble signet rings because of the single large lipid droplet in the center.
(3) Their mitochondria oxidize lipids to produce heat.
(4) They consist primarily of extracellular materials.
(5) They are highly responsive to nervous stimuli.

12. Which one of the following occurs during an inflammation reaction?

(1) Eosinophils secrete substances that initiate the inflammation response.
(2) Basophils migrate into the injured tissue and differentiate into mast cells.
(3) Pericytes cause vasodilation of capillaries, leading to edema in the surrounding tissue.
(4) Macrophages phagocytose bacteria and tissue debris and secrete growth factors.
(5) B lymphocytes that are stimulated by antigens become killer cells.

DIRECTIONS: Each of the numbered items or incomplete statements in this section is negatively phrased, as indicated by an italicized word such as *not, least,* or *except*. Select the **one** numbered answer or completion that is **best** in each case.

13. All of the following cells are members of the mononuclear phagocyte system (MPS) *except:*

(1) Kupffer cells in the liver.
(2) histiocytes in loose connective tissue.
(3) microglia in the central nervous system (CNS).
(4) osteoclasts in the bone.
(5) pericytes in the cardiovascular system.

14. All of the following structures are composed of dense regular connective tissue *except:*

(1) tendons.
(2) organ capsules.
(3) ligaments.
(4) aponeuroses.
(5) the cornea of the eye.

DIRECTIONS: The group of items in this section consists of numbered options followed by a set of numbered items. For each item, select the **one** numbered option that is most closely associated with it. Each numbered option may be selected once, more than once, or not at all.

Questions 15–17

Match each characteristic with the cell it describes.

(1) Mast cell
(2) Neutrophil
(3) Macrophage
(4) Eosinophil

15. Contains two types of antibacterial lysosomes

16. Releases enzymes that hydrolyze histamine

17. Releases substances that initiate the inflammation reaction

Questions 18–22

Match each characteristic with the connective tissue it describes.

(1) Loose connective tissue
(2) Dense irregular connective tissue
(3) Reticular connective tissue
(4) Dense regular connective tissue

18. Forms the lamina propria of most mucous membranes

19. Forms the dermis

20. Characteristic of blood-forming organs

21. Able to resist deformation and tearing in all directions

22. Consists primarily of ground substance that is rich in hyaluronic acid and contains fibers of all types

ANSWERS AND EXPLANATIONS

1. The answer is 3 *[I C 2]*. Mesenchyme condenses and differentiates to form specific structures, and what remains between those structures becomes loose connective tissue. Among the structures that form from mesenchyme are blood vessels, including the smooth muscle in their walls. Mesenchyme, the embryonic connective tissue, arises from mesoderm, the middle layer of the three primary germ layers. All connective tissues remain in contact as a continuum through the body.

2. The answer is 4 *[II A 1 a (2) (a)]*. Proteoglycans are macromolecules formed by a linear central core of protein (corresponding to the stem of a bottle brush) and glycosaminoglycans that radiate from the core like bristles. Hyaluronic acid does not bind to proteins, and it is the least viscous of the glycosaminoglycans. Most glycosaminoglycans in proteoglycans have a negative charge, which makes them strongly hydrophilic and causes them to become surrounded by layers of solvation water. Dermatan sulfate is so named because it is abundant in the dermis, where it is associated with thick collagen fibers. It is also abundant in tendons, ligaments, fibrocartilage, and other tissues that contain many thick collagen fibers. The sulfated glycosaminoglycan that occurs with reticular fibers is heparan sulfate.

3. The answer is 2 *[II A 1 b (2)]*. Glycoproteins help attach cells to each other and also to their extracellular substrate. They are primarily proteins. Keratan sulfate and chondroitin sulfate are not glycoproteins; they are sulfated glycosaminoglycans. Hyaluronic acid is also a glycosaminoglycan, and it does not bind with proteins. Structural glycoproteins, such as fibronectin and laminin, can be produced by some epithelial cells as well as by connective tissue cells.

4. The answer is 1 *[II A 2 b]*. The hydrophilic proteoglycans in the ground substance interact electrostatically with water and cations, creating a storage site for water and electrolytes. Sodium is the most abundant cation present. Although the ground substance permits water, ions, and small molecules to pass to and from cells, it limits the movement of macromolecules and microorganisms. Hyaluronidase is secreted by some very invasive bacteria. It breaks down hyaluronic acid, thereby decreasing the viscosity of the ground substance and permitting the microorganism to migrate through it. The ground substance contains molecules that attach connective tissue fibers to other elements of the connective tissue and that attach other types of tissue to the connective tissue. Separation between tissue types is maintained, however, by the basal laminae produced by other tissues where they are apposed to the connective tissue.

5. The answer is 3 *[II B 1 a (4)]*. Collagen type IV, which is characteristic of the basal lamina, does not form fibrils or fibers. Collagen is a glycoprotein, not a proteoglycan. It is very widely distributed in structures ranging from delicate, pliable basement membranes to bone. It is, in fact, the most abundant protein in the body, constituting almost one-third of its dry weight. Collagen type I is the most abundant type; it forms the bulk of the tough, fibrous tendons, ligaments, and organ capsules. Collagen type III is characteristic of reticular fibers.

6. The answer is 2 *[II B 1 b]*. After tropocollagen is formed from procollagen outside the cell, it assembles to form fibrils, which combine to form fibers. Procollagens are the soluble precursor molecules that are secreted by the cell. Differences among the several types of procollagen are responsible for the diversity among collagens in different structures. To proceed correctly, the steps in collagen synthesis require a series of interactions with other molecules, including enzymes and cofactors. Collagen fibrils are visible under the electron microscope, but only collagen fibers are large enough to be seen under the light microscope.

7. The answer is 4 *[II B 1 d (2)]*. For its weight, collagen has greater tensile strength than steel. It is acidophilic. It is inelastic, a property that is related to its supportive and protective functions. It is denatured by either acid treatment or boiling, yielding gelatin. Cooking tough cuts of meat with vinegar or acidic vegetables and moist heat exploit these properties of collagen.

8. The answer is 4 *[II B 3 c (3)]*. Elastic fibers have limited tensile strength; therefore, they are always surrounded by a network of supportive collagen fibers. Elastic fibers (and elastic laminae) are synthesized by the smooth muscle cells in certain blood vessels, not only by connective tissue cells. They are acidophilic. Unlike collagen, elastic fibers are resistant to boiling, acid, and alkali extraction. They are usually thicker than collagen fibers.

9. The answer is 5 *[II C 1 b]*. Pericytes, so called because they lie on the surface of capillaries and venules, are considered a reserve population of cells that can differentiate into other connective tissue cell types. Quiescent fibroblasts (also called fibrocytes) have the ability to become active again and may become migratory during wound healing. When their synthetic activity is stimulated, their cytoplasm is very basophilic because of the abundance of rough endoplasmic reticulum (rER) and free polysomes. Reticular cells produce reticular fibers, but not collagen fibers. Mesenchymal cells are embryonic connective tissue cells; fibroblasts are the characteristic cell type of loose and dense connective tissues.

10. The answer is 1 *[II C 2 d (3) (b), e (3)]*. When stimulated by an antigen, B lymphocytes begin to secrete antibodies, even as they are dividing to produce a clone of cells that will differentiate into plasma cells, which are specialized to secrete antibodies. Neither cell type is phagocytic, nor do they secrete vasoactive substances. Some B lymphocytes are long-lived; but once a cell has differentiated into a plasma cell, it lives only another 10–20 days.

11. The answer is 5 *[III F 1 a (3), 2 b (2)]*. Both white and brown adipose tissues are highly responsive to nervous stimuli; however, the trigger for stimulating white adipose tissue is the body's need for food energy, and the trigger for stimulating brown adipose tissue is cold temperatures. Even in starving animals, brown adipose cells do not lose their lipid stores. White adipose cells resemble signet rings, but brown adipose cells are multilocular. Heat is a by-product of oxidation in all cells (in fact, mitochondria are responsible for the body heat), but only in brown adipose tissue is heat production a primary function. Both types of adipose tissue are highly cellular (i.e., they contain very little extracellular material).

12. The answer is 4 *[II C 1 g (4); Figure 6-2]*. In the early stages after an injury, macrophages help neutrophil-derived microphages engulf and destroy bacteria. Later, macrophages clean up the tissue to prepare it for repair by phagocytosing cellular debris. They also promote repair by secreting growth factors. Basophils and mast cells, not eosinophils or pericytes, secrete substances that initiate the inflammation response, including capillary vasodilation and edema. Basophils and mast cells are very similar in their staining reactions, contents, and function; however, they arise from two different stem cell types, and basophils do not become mast cells. B lymphocytes give rise to antibody-secreting plasma cells; it is T lymphocytes that become killer cells.

13. The answer is 5 *[II C 1 b, g (3)]*. Pericytes are relatively undifferentiated cells that can differentiate into other types of connective tissue, but not into macrophages. Kupffer cells, histiocytes, microglia, and osteoclasts are all monocyte-derived members of the mononuclear phagocyte system (MPS).

14. The answer is 2 *[III C 1 b]*. Organ capsules are composed of dense irregular connective tissue, whereas tendons, ligaments, aponeuroses, and the cornea are all composed of dense regular connective tissue. The parallel arrangement of collagen fibers in tendons is very regular; the arrangement in the cornea, where different layers of fibers are at right angles to each other, is less regular.

15–17. The answers are: 15-2 *[II C 2 b (2) (a)]*, **16-4** *[II C 2 c (2) (b)]*, **17-1** *[II C 1 f (4)]*. Neutrophils, which are the first line of defense against pathogenic bacteria, have two types of granules that contain both enzyme and nonenzyme proteins with antibacterial activity.

Eosinophils release enzymes that hydrolyze histamine. In addition, eosinophils release other chemicals that are involved in allergic reactions.

Degranulation of mast cells releases substances that initiate the inflammation reaction. In most domestic species, mast cell granules are unstained with routine methods but can be demonstrated with metachromatic stains. Heparin, an anticoagulant found in mast cell granules, also stimulates the growth of new blood vessels. Other granule contents, notably histamine, cause contraction of smooth muscle in the small airways. Massive degranulation of mast cells and basophils can cause anaphylactic shock. Mast cell degranulation is a regulated event that occurs on the second exposure to a given antigen.

18–22. The answers are: 18-1 *[III B 2 b]*, **19-2** *[III C 1 b]*, **20-3** *[III E 2]*, **21-2** *[III C 1 c]*, **22-1** *[III B 1 a, b]*. Loose connective tissue, which consists primarily of ground substance that is rich in hyaluronic acid and contains fibers of all types, forms the lamina propria of most mucous membranes.

Dense irregular connective tissue, which forms the dermis, is best able to resist mechanical stress in all directions because it consists primarily of collagen fibers (which have greater tensile strength for their mass than steel) running in all directions. Dense regular connective tissue, formed by bundles of parallel collagen fibers, resists stress in the axis of the fibers but is subject to lateral deformation.

Reticular connective tissue, which does not contain collagen or elastic fibers, is characteristic of blood-forming organs, including both the bone marrow and lymph organs. It is a loose connective tissue that is designed to accommodate many immigrant cells, the developing blood cells.

Chapter 7

Cartilage and Bone

I. INTRODUCTION.

INTRODUCTION. Cartilage and bone are supportive connective tissues. The extracellular matrix, which is formed and maintained by the cells, is specialized to provide this support.

II. CARTILAGE

A. Basic structure

1. **Cells**
   a. **Chondrocytes** are the cells of cartilage.
      (1) **Structure.** Chondrocytes are round or oval. Active chondrocytes contain abundant rough endoplasmic reticulum (rER) and have a well-developed Golgi complex.
      (2) **Function.** Chondrocytes secrete the proteins and glycosaminoglycans that form and maintain the extracellular matrix.
   b. Chondrocytes are contained in **lacunae,** which are cavities within the extracellular matrix (Figure 7-1).
2. **Matrix.** The extracellular matrix, called the chondromatrix, comprises fibrils and fibers embedded in an amorphous ground substance that is rich in glycosaminoglycans and proteoglycans.
3. **Vascularity.** Cartilage is avascular. Nutrients and wastes diffuse into and out of the cells through solvation water (i.e., water bound to matrix components). The thickness of cartilage is, therefore, limited.
4. **Covering. Perichondrium** is the dense irregular connective tissue that encapsulates most cartilage (see Figures 7-1 & 7-3).
   a. The **outer fibrous layer** consists of dense connective tissue.
   b. The **inner cambium layer** contains chondrogenic cells that are capable of becoming **chondroblasts** (cartilage-producing cells).

B. Embryologic origin

1. **Mesenchyme** cells differentiate into **chondroblasts,** forming **protochondral tissue** in **chondrification centers.**
2. **Chondroblasts** retract their processes and begin to secrete amorphous ground substance and procollagen.
3. **Chondrocytes,** the resultant cells, are surrounded by **chondromatrix** and occupy **lacunae.**

C. Growth and repair

1. **Interstitial growth**
   a. **Process**
      (1) **Mitotic division of chondrocytes** gives rise to isogenous groups of two to eight cells.

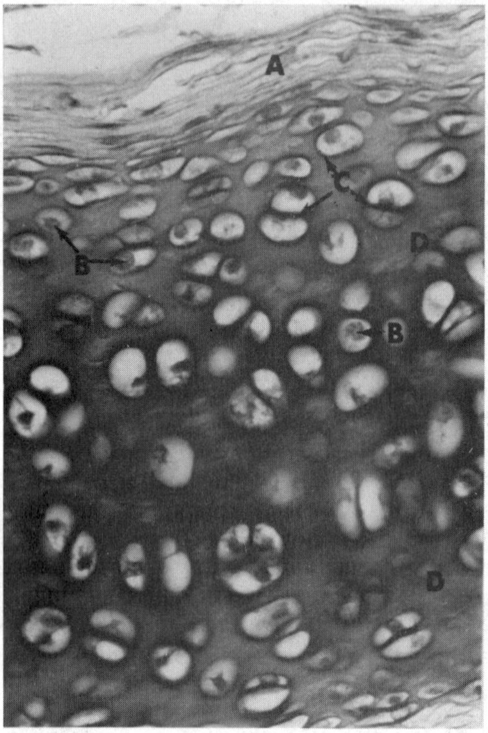

Figure 7-1. Hyaline cartilage. The perichondrium (*A*) that surrounds the cartilage mass is dense irregular connective tissue. Chondrocytes (*B*) occupy lacunae in the matrix. The chondrocytes are flattened near the perichondrium and become more spherical in the deeper portions of the tissue. The more darkly stained rim around the lacunae (*C*) results from a greater concentration of ground substance in those regions. The homogeneous cartilage matrix appears gray. (Reprinted with permission from Dellmann H-D: *Textbook of Veterinary Histology,* 4th ed. Baltimore, Williams & Wilkins, 1993, p 40.)

(2) The cells secrete matrix components, expanding the cartilage from within and separating the cells within each isogenous group.

b. Applications

(1) Interstitial growth is important in **physeal (growth) plates,** where it is responsible for elongation of long bones.

(2) Interstitial growth is also used to continually replace worn cartilage at **synovial surfaces**.

(3) Interstitial growth occurs only in **recently formed cartilage,** which is still somewhat pliant.

2. Appositional growth

a. Process

(1) Chondrogenic cells in the cambium layer of the perichondrium differentiate into chondroblasts.

(2) Secretion of matrix components by these cells increases the thickness of the cartilage.

b. Applications

(1) Appositional growth **increases the girth of the cartilage**.

(2) Most **repair** is by appositional growth.

3. Repair is **limited,** especially in the adult cartilage, where the ability to undergo interstitial growth is greatly reduced. Large deficits are usually replaced by dense connective tissue or fibrocartilage (see II D 3).

D. Classification. Three types of cartilage are distinguished according to the types of fibers they contain.

1. Hyaline cartilage is the most abundant type of cartilage. Its thin fibrils are mostly collagen type II. Hyaline cartilage is so named because of its glassy appearance in the fresh state (see Figure 7-1).

a. **Structure**

(1) **Chondrocytes**

(a) The chondrocytes of hyaline cartilage are **flattened or elliptical near the surface** of the cartilage and gradually become **spherical deeper in the tissue** (see Figure 7-1).

(b) **Isogenous groups** of chondrocytes are formed by mitosis of chondrocytes.

(2) **Amorphous ground substance**

(a) **Chondromucoproteins,** which are the proteoglycans of cartilage, contain chondroitin 4-sulfate, chondroitin 6-sulfate, and keratan sulfate.

(b) **Chondronectin** is a glycoprotein that helps attach chondrocytes to collagen in the matrix.

(c) **Hyaluronic acid** is present in small amounts.

(d) **Water** is abundant. It accounts for 75% of the total weight. Most water is bound electrostatically (solvation water) to glycosaminoglycans.

(3) **Fibers**

(a) **Collagen type II,** which forms **thin fibrils,** is the major fibrous element of hyaline cartilage.

(b) The collagen fibrils cannot be distinguished under the light microscope because they are small and their refractive index is similar to that of the ground substance that surrounds them.

(4) **Perichondrium** covers all hyaline cartilage except that forming articular surfaces in joints.

b. **Physical properties.** Hyaline cartilage is:

(1) **Rigid.** The matrix is rigid because of many cross-links between proteoglycans, hyaluronic acid, and collagen (Figure 7-2).

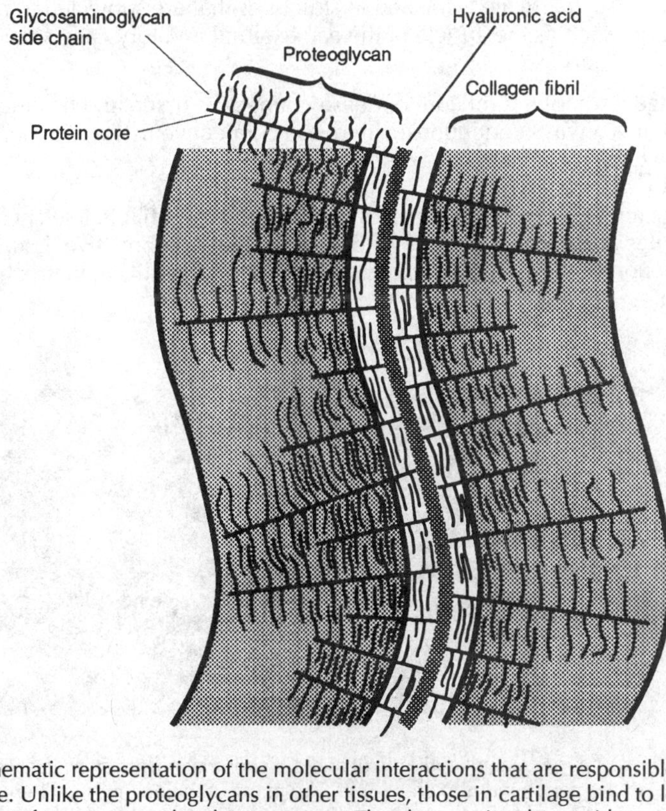

Figure 7-2. Schematic representation of the molecular interactions that are responsible for the rigidity of hyaline cartilage. Unlike the proteoglycans in other tissues, those in cartilage bind to long polymers of hyaluronic acid to form macromolecular aggregates. The glycosaminoglycan side arms of the proteoglycans have a net negative charge that causes them to bind electrostatically to collagen. Layers of solvation water are also bound to the glycosaminoglycans and contribute to the volume and rigidity of the tissue.

(a) As in other types of connective tissue, the shape of the proteoglycan molecule resembles a bottle brush in form, with a central protein core and projecting glycosaminoglycans that look like bristles.
(b) One end of the protein core binds to a long hyaluronic acid polymer in the ground substance. Up to 200 proteoglycans may be attached to the same hyaluronic acid molecule. In contrast, proteoglycans of loose and dense fibrous connective tissues do not bind to hyaluronic acid.
(c) The glycosaminoglycan side chains of the proteoglycan bind to collagen fibrils electrostatically, as they do in loose and dense connective tissues.

(2) **Resilient.** The high water content of the matrix allows the cartilage to act as a shock absorber, which is especially important in articular cartilages.

c. **Functions**

(1) **Support.** Hyaline cartilage provides resilient support for structures, including:
(a) The walls of the larger respiratory airways
(b) The nictitating membrane (i.e., the third eyelid)
(c) The attachment sites of the ventral ends of the ribs to the sternum
(d) The articular surfaces

(2) **Friction reduction.** The articular cartilages provide smooth sliding surfaces for movement at the joints.

(3) **Embryologic skeleton.** Hyaline cartilage forms a temporary skeleton in the embryo.

(4) **Growth.** Lengthening of long bones is possible because of interstitial growth of hyaline cartilage in the physeal plate.

2. **Elastic cartilage (Figure 7-3)**

a. **Structure.** Elastic cartilage has the same structure as hyaline cartilage, except that it contains many **branching elastic fibers** in addition to **collagen type II**.

b. **Function.** Elastic cartilage is located in structures that are subjected to mechanical deformation, such as the auricle of the ear, external auditory canals, auditory tubes, epiglottis, and larynx.

3. **Fibrocartilage** resembles a mixture of dense connective tissue and hyaline cartilage (Figure 7-4). It is always continuous with dense connective tissue and merges with adjacent hyaline cartilage, ligaments, tendons, or bone.

a. **Structure**

(1) Fibrocartilage consists of **bundles of collagen type I fibers** interspersed with **spicules of cartilage**. It forms when cells in dense connective tissue differentiate into chondroblasts and secrete a small amount of cartilage matrix between the collagen fibers.

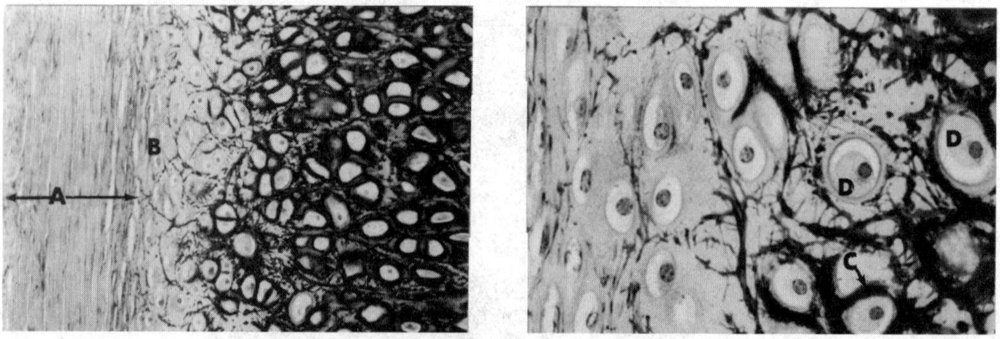

Figure 7-3. Elastic cartilage at a low magnification (*left*) and a higher magnification (*right*). The fibrous layer (*A*) and cellular layer (*B*) of the perichondrium are visible. The many branching elastic fibers have been blackened (*C*). Chondrocytes (*D*) nearly fill the lacunae. (Reprinted with permission from Dellmann H-D: *Textbook of Veterinary Histology*, 4th ed. Baltimore, Williams & Wilkins, 1993, p 41.)

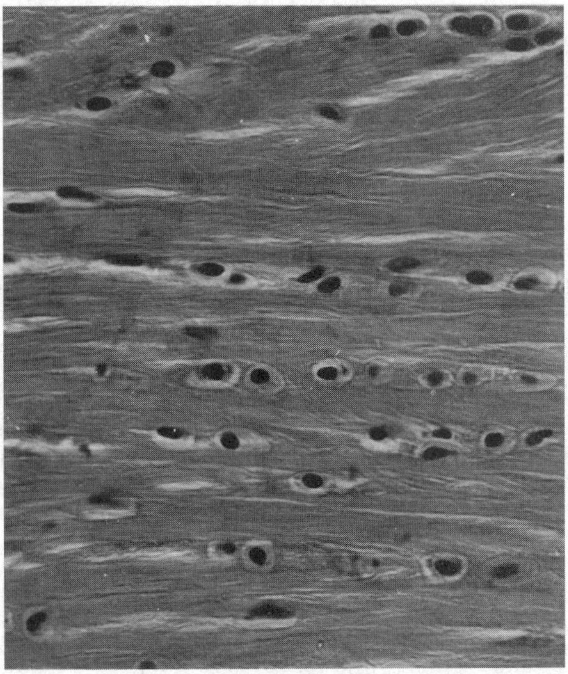

Figure 7-4. Fibrocartilage. Spherical chondrocytes lie between thick bundles of collagen fibers. As is often the case, the sparse chondromatrix cannot be distinguished. (Reprinted with permission from Dellmann H-D: *Textbook of Veterinary Histology,* 4th ed. Baltimore, Williams & Wilkins, 1993, p 42.)

(2) Each cartilage spicule may contain one cell, or a long row of spherical or ovoid cells. The matrix is often difficult or impossible to see using a light microscope.

(3) **No perichondrium** is present.

b. **Function.** Fibrocartilage is associated with the **skeletal system** in sites where rigid support with great tensile strength is needed (e.g., intervertebral discs, menisci, attachment sites of tendons and ligaments to bone).

III. BONE.

Bone is a tissue in which the matrix is mineralized, giving it rigidity. Bones are organs in which bone is the primary tissue.

A. Functions

1. **Support.** Bones support and protect soft tissues and organs.
2. **Leverage.** Bones are the rigid components of leveraged movement systems. They increase the forces produced by muscular contraction.
3. **Storage.** Bone tissue is a storage site for certain ions.

   a. **Calcium** levels in the blood are precisely regulated. Blood calcium is continuously interchanged with bone calcium.

   (1) **Parathormone** (parathyroid hormone) increases blood calcium levels by stimulating the breakdown of bone matrix by both osteoclasts and osteocytes. Osteocytic osteolysis affects only a thin layer of matrix adjacent to the osteocyte, but its cumulative effect is physiologically important.

   (2) **Calcitonin** is a hormone that inhibits osteoclasts and, therefore, decreases blood calcium levels.

(3) Calcium ions also pass back and forth continuously between interstitial tissue and hydroxyapatite crystals in the most recently formed (and less mineralized) lamellae (i.e., layers of bone).

b. The storage and release of **phosphate** and other ions by the bone are also regulated.

B. Basic structure

1. Cells

a. **Osteoblasts synthesize the organic matrix** of bone and **promote mineralization** (Figure 7-5).

(1) **Structure.** Osteoblasts, which are **cuboidal to columnar,** lie in a **single layer** on bone surfaces that are growing. **Cytoplasmic processes** are attached by **gap junctions** to processes of neighboring osteoblasts and processes of osteocytes (see III B 1 b) in adjacent bone.

(2) Osteoblasts have very **basophilic cytoplasm** (see Figure 7-5) because of their well-developed rER. They are **polarized** with their secretory surface facing the bone.

b. **Osteocytes,** which **maintain the bone matrix,** are osteoblasts that have surrounded their cell body and processes with bone matrix (see Figures 7-5 & 7-6).

(1) Osteocytes lie in **lacunae** in the bone matrix. In mature bone, they are located at the junctions of adjacent **lamellae**.

(2) Narrow matrix channels called **canaliculi** (see Figure 7-6) run between adjacent lacunae, both within a lamella and between adjacent lamellae. Lacunae nearest to the surface have canaliculi that go to the surface.

(a) The canaliculi house the long, slender osteocyte processes, which are connected by **gap junctions** to processes of adjacent osteocytes and osteoblasts **(surface cells).**

(b) Because bone matrix is impermeable, osteocyte processes and gap junctions in the canalicular system are responsible for exchange of metabolites between osteocytes and blood. Some exchange also occurs through the small amount of ground substance between the processes and walls of the canaliculi.

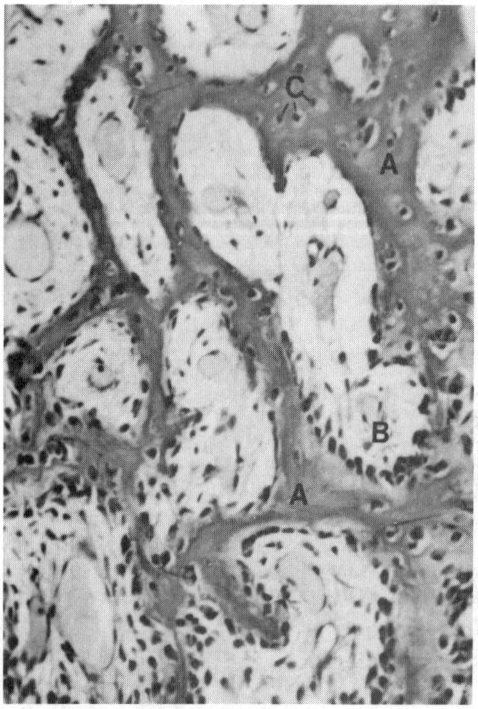

Figure 7-5. Cells of bone tissue. The surface of the bone (*A*) is covered by darkly stained osteoblasts (*B*). Osteocytes (*C*) are surrounded by bone. Blood vessels are present in the lightly stained mesenchyme. (Reprinted with permission from Dellmann H-D: *Textbook of Veterinary Histology,* 4th ed. Baltimore, Williams & Wilkins, 1993, p 46.)

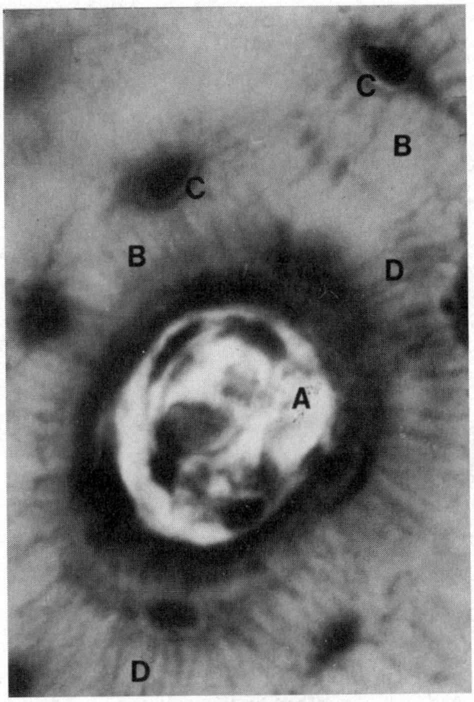

Figure 7-6. Central canal (*A*) of an osteum surrounded by lamellae of bone (*B*). Osteocytes (*C*) occupy lacunae between lamellae. The lacunae are joined to each other and to the central canal by canaliculi, which appear as radiating streaks in this preparation (*D*). (Reprinted with permission from Dellmann H-D: *Textbook of Veterinary Histology,* 4th ed. Baltimore, Williams & Wilkins, 1993, p 43.)

c. **Osteoclasts** secrete enzymes and acid that **break down the bone matrix,** and they phagocytose the resulting debris (Figure 7-7).
   (1) **Structure.** Osteoclasts, which are found on bony surfaces, are **giant multinucleated cells** derived by fusion of monocytes; therefore, they are members of the mononuclear phagocyte system (MPS).
   (2) Active osteoclasts contain many **lysosomes** and, facing the bone, they have a highly folded irregular surface called the **ruffled border** (see Figure 7-7).

2. **Matrix.** The matrix of bone has both organic and inorganic components, each contributing about half of the dry weight.
   a. **Organic matrix**
      (1) **Components**
         (a) **Collagen type I** is the primary organic component of the matrix.
         (b) A small amount of **ground substance** is also present.
      (2) **Function.** The organic matrix provides **tensile strength**. If it is removed, the remaining bone is easily crumbled.
   b. **Inorganic matrix**
      (1) **Components**
         (a) **Calcium** and **phosphorus,** mostly in the form of plate-shaped crystals of **hydroxyapatite,** are the primary inorganic components of the matrix.
         (b) Other ions, including **bicarbonate, citrate, magnesium, potassium,** and **sodium** are also present.
      (2) **Functions**
         (a) **Ion exchange.** A hydration layer of water and ions surrounding the hydroxyapatite crystals is the medium for exchange of ions between bone matrix and blood.
         (b) **Strength.** The inorganic matrix enables bone to resist **compressive stress**.

3. **Vascularity.** Bone is richly vascularized (Figure 7-8A).

4. **Covering. Periosteum** is the dense connective tissue that covers bone, except where it is covered by articular cartilage.
   a. The **outer fibrous layer** of periosteum is dense irregular connective tissue.

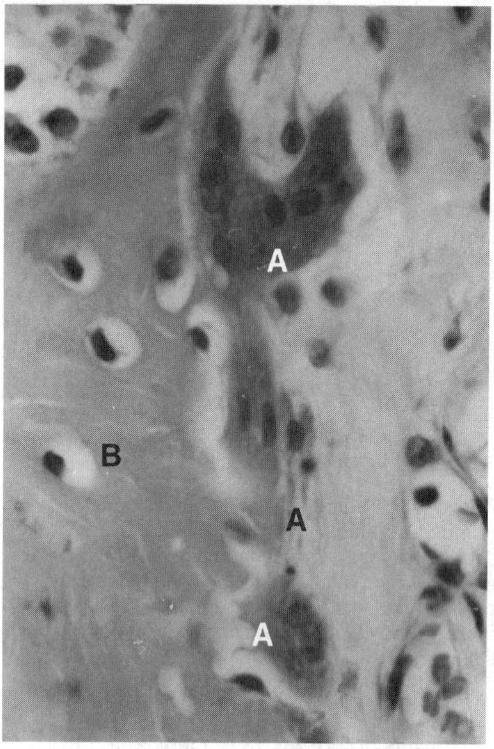

Figure 7-7. Several osteoclasts (*A*) lie in erosion lacunae on the surface of a spicule of bone (*B*). Several nuclei are visible in the osteoclast at the top of the field. The osteoclast's frothy-appearing peripheral cytoplasm is the ruffled border.

b. The **inner cambium layer** of periosteum contains **osteogenic (osteoprogenitor) cells** that are capable of differentiating into osteoblasts or chondroblasts.
c. **Nerve endings** in the periosteum are responsible for much of the pain associated with injury to a bone.

5. **Lining. Endosteum** lines all the interior surfaces, including marrow spaces and vascular canals. The endosteum, which contains osteogenic cells, meets the cambium layer of the periosteum at the external openings of the vascular canals that perforate the bone, forming a continuous layer of osteogenic cells.

6. **Bone marrow,** which contains blood-forming tissue and fat-storing cells, occupies cavities within bone.
   a. **Red bone marrow** contains a large proportion of developing blood cells.
   b. **Yellow bone marrow** contains predominantly fat-storing cells.

C. Organization

1. **Compact bone** (see Figure 7-8B)
   a. **Histologic structure.** The matrix and osteocytes of compact bone are arranged in well-defined lamellar patterns.
      (1) **Osteons** (see Figure 7-8) contain four to twenty concentrically arranged lamellae surrounding a central (osteonal) canal (see Figure 7-6). Central canals and their osteons often branch.
         (a) **Capillaries** in the central canal supply osteocytes. These capillaries arise from vessels, housed in **perforating canals,** that penetrate the bone (see Figure 7-8A). Capillaries also arise from the small anastomosing branches of the vessels that run from osteon to osteon in **communicating canals**.
         (b) **Collagen fibers** within each lamella have a helical arrangement that is at different angles in adjacent lamellae.

A

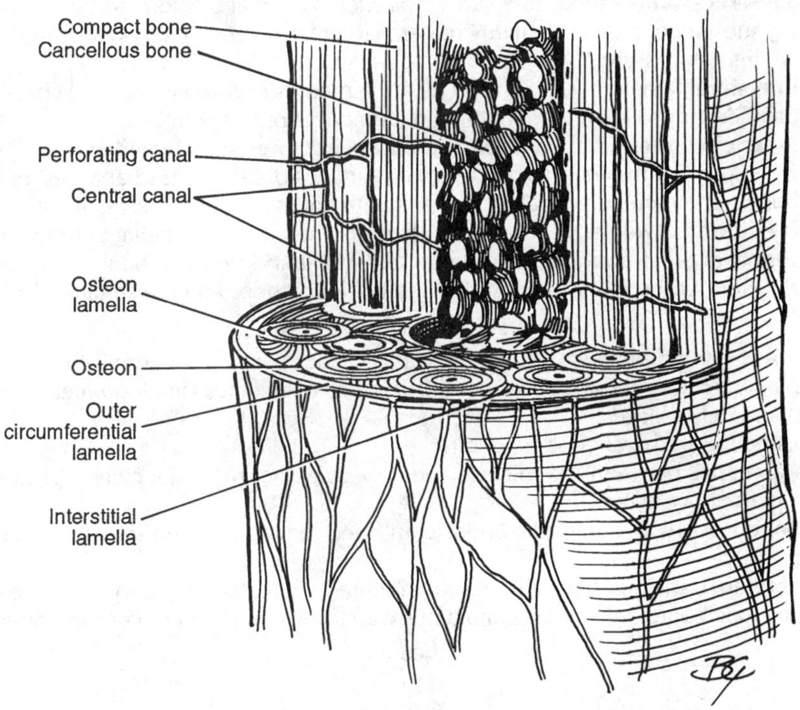

B

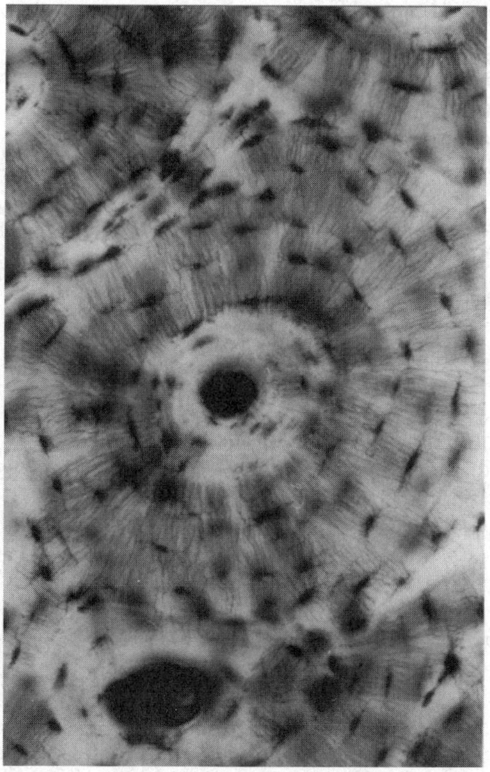

Figure 7-8. (*A*) Schematic drawing of a portion of an adult bone. Common lamellar patterns illustrated in the compact bone are osteons, outer circumferential lamellae, and interstitial lamellae. The central canals of the osteon are represented in longitudinal section along the longitudinal cut surface. They communicate with perforating canals that carry vascular branches from blood vessels in the periosteum (visible on the *left*). (Redrawn with permission from Dellmann H-D: *Textbook of Veterinary Histology,* 4th ed. Baltimore, Williams & Wilkins, 1993, p 44.) (*B*) Ground compact bone. This bone has been dried and then mechanically ground to a thin layer. This process does not preserve bone cells. One complete cross-section through an osteon is surrounded by portions of other osteons. Between the osteons are interstitial lamellae, which are remnants of older osteons that have been partially destroyed during remodeling.

(c) A **reversal (cement) line** surrounds each osteon and is formed by cementing substance, a layer of highly mineralized matrix. This line is visible under the light microscope.

(2) **Interstitial lamellae** (see Figure 7-8) are remnants of osteons that have been partially destroyed during remodeling of compact bone (see III D 2).

(3) **Inner circumferential lamellae** and **outer circumferential lamellae** (see Figure 7-8A) parallel the internal and external surfaces of the shafts (diaphyses) of long bones. They are adjacent to the endosteum and periosteum, respectively.

(4) **Plexiform networks** are formed by sheets of intersecting lamellae. These and a variety of other arrangements are present in flat and irregular bones.

b. Distribution. Compact bone forms the shaft of long bones and the surface of all adult bones.

2. Cancellous (spongy) bone is contiguous with compact bone (see Figure 7-8A).

a. Histologic structure. Cancellous bone is a lattice of spicules (small pointed projections) and trabeculae.

(1) **Lamellae** are parallel or concentric.

(2) **Capillaries** between the spicules and trabeculae nourish osteocytes. Vascular canals are very rare.

(3) **Bone marrow** occupies the endosteum-lined spaces between spicules and trabeculae.

b. Distribution. Cancellous bone is present in some irregular and flat bones and the ends of some long bones, where it is contiguous with the surface layer of compact bone.

D. Classification

1. Primary (woven, immature, new) bone is the first type of bone to be formed during development or repair.

a. Its **lacunae** and **collagen fibers** are **randomly arranged**.

b. Its matrix contains less mineral than that of mature bone.

c. Its gross organization **resembles cancellous bone.**

2. Secondary (lamellar, mature) bone replaces almost all primary bone in the adult. It is produced only by remodeling of primary bone (see III F).

a. Lacunae are arranged in layers in an **orderly** fashion.

b. The **collagen fibers** are **parallel** within a lamella and their orientation is approximately perpendicular in adjacent lamellae. This organization provides great tensile strength.

c. Secondary bone contains a much **higher concentration of inorganic matrix** than does primary bone, making the bone more rigid.

d. Most secondary bone is compact, but in some areas (e.g., the epiphyses of long bones) it may be cancellous.

E. Osteogenesis.

Bone can form directly in mesenchyme, or it may replace a temporary cartilage skeleton.

1. Intramembranous osteogenesis is direct formation of primary bone in mesenchyme or osteogenic connective tissue. It is responsible for development of most of the flat bones of the skull, the mandible, and for all appositional growth and repair.

a. Mesenchymal condensation. Mesenchymal tissue condenses (i.e., becomes more cellular) in primary ossification centers (areas where bone will begin to form).

(1) **Osteogenic cells** form from mesenchymal cells, retaining their processes and attachments to adjacent cells.

(2) **Several primary ossification centers** form for each bone.

b. Osteoblasts. Multiple groups of osteogenic cells within each ossification center differentiate to become osteoblasts.

(1) **Osteoid.** Osteoblasts secrete ground substance and collagen first. This organic matrix, in which the collagen fibers are randomly oriented, is called osteoid.

(2) **Matrix granules** that contain alkaline phosphatase and calcium phosphate are then released.

(a) **Alkaline phosphatase** permits precipitation of the mineral salts.

(b) **Calcium phosphate** is deposited on collagen fibrils.

(3) **Spicules.** The osteoblasts become surrounded by mineralized matrix, forming spicules of primary bone (Figure 7-9).

(4) **Blood vessels** grow into the areas between spicules.

c. **Growth.** Spicules continue to grow and eventually fuse to form a spongy structure with blood vessels in the interstices (see Figure 7-5). Mesenchyme remaining between the bone and blood vessels gives rise to bone marrow.

d. **Expansion.** The mesenchyme adjacent to the primary ossification centers continues to condense and differentiate into osteoblasts, adding bone to the surface by **appositional growth**.

e. **Fusion.** All primary ossification centers for a given bone eventually fuse.

2. **Endochondral osteogenesis** is a process in which primary bone formation is integrated with removal of a temporary hyaline cartilage skeleton. It occurs in the development of the weight-bearing short and long bones, where temporary support is needed early in development.

a. **Removal of cartilage** begins in primary ossification centers within the cartilage.

(1) Chondrocytes hypertrophy (Figure 7-10), which enlarges their lacunae, leaving only thin septa and spicules of matrix.

(2) The septa and spicules that are not destroyed become calcified, which increases their ability to withstand compression.

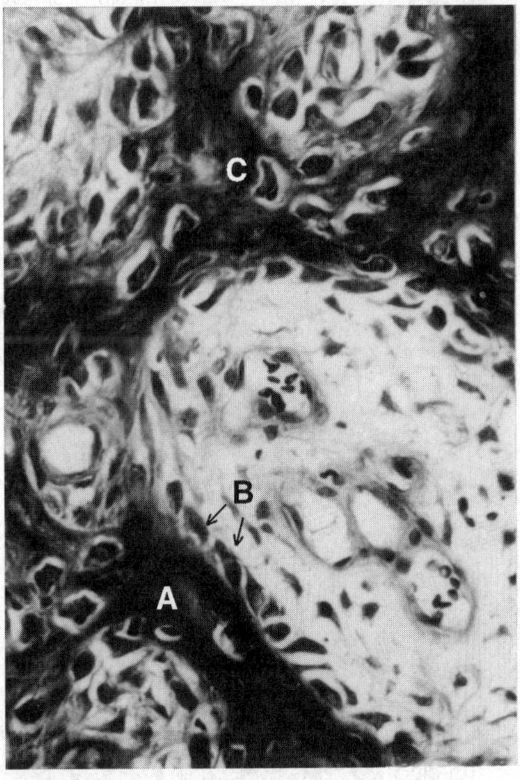

Figure 7-9. Bone being formed by intramembranous osteogenesis. Bone spicule (*A*) is formed by osteoblasts (*B*), which lie on the surface of the bone. The intense cytoplasmic basophilia of the active osteoblasts is evident. Collagen fibers are visible in the matrix (*C*) of this primary bone.

A

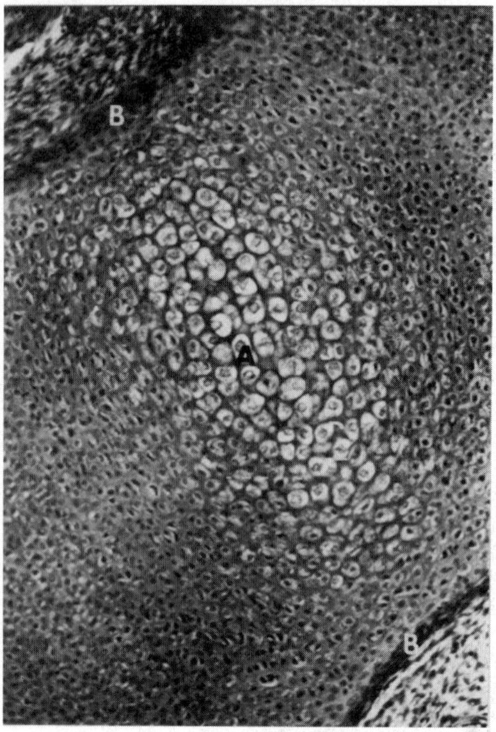

Figure 7-10. Endochondral osteogenesis. (*A*) Cartilage model of a long bone in which the primary center of ossification is beginning to form. Hypertrophied chondrocytes (*A*) have reduced the matrix to thin partitions. The bony collar will form in the perichondrium (*B*) surrounding this region. (*B*) Schematic drawing of the formation of bone on septa of calcified cartilage. A layer of osteoblasts is separated from the cartilage by newly formed bone. A capillary, which carried osteoprogenitor cells into the tissue, is also shown. (Reprinted and redrawn with permission from Dellmann H-D: *Textbook of Veterinary Histology,* 4th ed. Baltimore, Williams & Wilkins, 1993, pp 47, 50.)

B

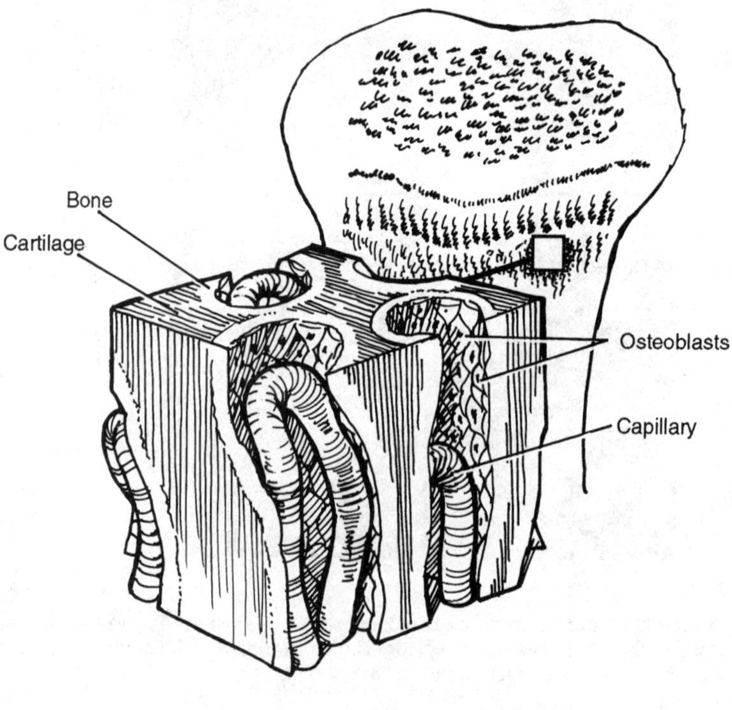

(3) The lacunae fuse and the chondrocytes suddenly die (i.e., programmed death takes place), leaving open channels in the calcified matrix.

b. Formation of bone takes place on the surface of the calcified cartilage matrix (see Figure 7-10).

(1) Capillary loops grow into the channels created by the death of chondrocytes.

(2) Osteoprogenitor cells are carried into the channels on capillaries. They move to the surface of the calcified cartilage matrix, where they form a layer of osteoblasts (see Figure 7-10).

(3) Bone matrix is formed on the surface of the calcified cartilage matrix by secretion of osteoid and matrix granules (see III C 1 b).

(4) More bone is added by additional osteoblasts, which differentiate from osteoprogenitor cells.

3. Formation of a long bone. Both intramembranous and endochondral osteogenesis are involved in the formation of the long bones of the extremities.

a. Bone collar. Intramembranous osteogenesis forms a bone collar. This cylinder of bone surrounding the cartilage of the diaphysis is the first bone to be formed.

(1) Blood vessels proliferate in the perichondrium around the middle of the diaphysis.

(2) The cambium layer of the perichondrium forms a layer of bone by intramembranous osteogenesis.

(3) The cambium layer of what is now periosteum adds additional bone. Eventually, most of the diaphysis is formed by intramembranous osteogenesis.

b. Primary center. Endochondral osteogenesis is initiated at the primary center of ossification.

(1) Cartilage is destroyed in the middle of the diaphysis, opening channels for ingrowing blood vessels.

(2) Osteoclasts erode holes in the bone collar, allowing blood vessels from the adjacent periosteum to grow into the primary center of ossification.

(3) Osteoprogenitor cells carried on the blood vessels form endochondral bone on the surface of calcified spicules and septa of cartilage.

(4) Continued hypertrophy and programmed death of chondrocytes around the primary center permit radial enlargement of the ossified area.

c. Physeal plates develop between the diaphysis and epiphyses.

(1) Interstitial growth of cartilage continues at the ends of the diaphysis.

(2) **Zones.** When the primary center of ossification fills the diaphysis, the only remaining cartilage is in transverse plates adjacent to the epiphyses. Therefore, endochondral growth is oriented toward the epiphyses. Zones of development can be identified on a longitudinal section through the physeal plate (Figure 7-11).

(a) **Zone of proliferation.** This zone is adjacent to the reserve (resting) hyaline cartilage. Mitotic division of chondrocytes in this zone creates rows of chondrocytes (isogenous groups) parallel to the long axis of the bone.

(b) **Zone of maturing chondrocytes.** Interstitial growth occurs in this zone. The chondrocytes increase in height, and new cartilage matrix is formed, mostly between the cell columns.

(c) **Zone of hypertrophy and calcification.** Chondrocytes are enlarged at the expense of the surrounding matrix.

(i) The matrix between cell columns becomes calcified.

(ii) At the end of the zone of hypertrophy and calcification, a signal causes the chondrocytes abruptly to degenerate and die. The transverse septa are destroyed, leaving only longitudinal septa and spicules of calcified cartilage.

(iii) The zone of hypertrophy and calcification is the most fragile region, most subject to fractures.

(3) Events in the different zones are balanced so that the thickness of the physeal plate remains constant.

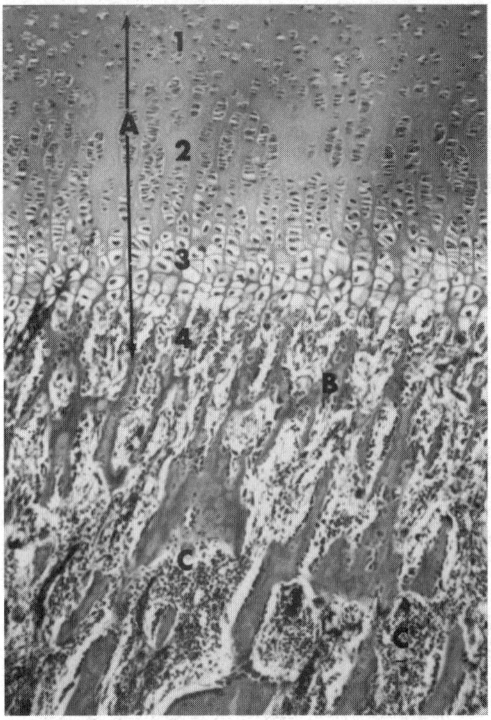

Figure 7-11. Physeal plate of a long bone. The line (*A*) indicates the extent of the growth plate. The reserve zone of hyaline cartilage (*1*), the zone of proliferation (*2*), the zone of maturing chondrocytes (*3*), and the zone of hypertrophy and calcification (*4*) are shown. Newly formed bone (*B*) on septa of calcified cartilage, with bone marrow (*C*) in the spaces between, is visible in the zone of ossification. (Reprinted with permission from Dellmann H-D: *Textbook of Veterinary Histology,* 4th ed. Baltimore, Williams & Wilkins, 1993, p 48.)

d. **Ossification.** At the border of the growth plate, capillary loops grow into the channels created by the death of chondrocytes, and osteoblasts cover the longitudinal spicules and septa of calcified cartilage with newly formed bone.

e. **Continued growth.** The periosteal bone collar, meanwhile, continues to grow.
   - **(1)** It grows at the ends in the direction of the epiphyses, helping to lengthen the bone, as well as radially, increasing the thickness of the bone.
   - **(2)** Collagen fibers and bundles of collagen fibers in the periosteum, ligaments, and tendons become embedded in the matrix during radial appositional growth, thus strengthening their attachments.

f. **Osteoclastic activity.** The marrow space is enlarged by osteoclasts, which are active from the time the primary center of osteogenesis develops.
   - **(1)** Osteoclasts destroy primary bone and the calcified cartilage on which it is formed at the same rate that new bone is formed by endochondral osteogenesis. Therefore, the zone of ossification remains the same thickness during growth.
   - **(2)** Osteoclasts destroy the inner surface of the periosteal bone collar at a slightly slower rate than new bone is formed by intramembranous osteogenesis. Therefore, the diaphysis gradually increases in thickness as it grows.

g. **Physeal closure.** Eventually, growth stops in the physeal plate, and the cartilage is replaced by bone. Closure ages are specific for each physeal plate and vary among species.

h. **Secondary centers.** Secondary centers of osteogenesis form in the epiphyses and some large processes. Endochondral osteogenesis occurs as in the primary centers of osteogenesis; however, the direction of growth remains radial as the epiphyses increase in size.

i. **Bone marrow.** The formation of bone marrow begins in the primary center of osteogenesis and continues as the marrow cavity is enlarged.
   - **(1)** Mesenchyme surrounding the blood vessels differentiates to form reticular tissue.
   - **(2)** The reticular tissue is seeded with blood-forming (hemopoietic) stem cells from the blood.

4. **Nutritional needs** of bone are especially important during growth.
   a. **Calcium** is essential for mineralization.
   b. **Vitamin D** is important for absorption of calcium.
   c. **Vitamin C** is essential for collagen synthesis.

F. **Remodeling** of bone is very active in growing animals (it occurs at a rate of up to 200% per year) and continues through adulthood (at a rate of approximately 1% per year).

1. **Process.** During remodeling, existing bone is partially resorbed by osteoclastic action and then replaced by new bone. For example, remodeling of osteonal compact bone takes place as follows:
   a. Osteoclasts erode a cylindrical channel through existing compact bone, and capillary loops grow into the channel.
   b. When the cavity has reached its ultimate diameter, osteoblasts deposit a lining layer of cementing substance and then form a lamella of secondary bone on its surface.
   c. Additional concentric lamellae are formed central to the first until the central canal is only large enough for its blood vessels. The remaining osteoprogenitor cells form the endosteal lining of the central canal.
   d. As later generations of osteons form, they are smaller and their matrix is more compact.

2. **Applications**
   a. Remodeling is **essential during growth.**
      (1) **Maintenance of shape.** Remodeling permits the shape of a bone to be maintained while it increases in size.
      (2) **Strength.** Remodeling permits primary bone to be replaced with stronger secondary bone. Each generation of reorganization produces bone that is more compact and more highly mineralized.
   b. Remodeling is **essential in adults.**
      (1) **Response to stress.** Remodeling permits bones to respond to mechanical stresses by changing their shape and microscopic structure.
         (a) **Movement of ions.** Compression and decompression of different parts of a bone cause movement of ions, establishing an **electrical potential** that affects cellular activity.
         (b) **Stimulation of osteoblasts and osteoclasts.** Osteoblasts are stimulated in areas that are compressed, and osteoclasts are stimulated in areas that are decompressed, gradually altering the shape of the bone until it is aligned in the direction of the applied force.
      (2) **Reservoir.** Remodeling creates a reservoir of readily available calcium, phosphate, and other ions.

G. **Fracture repair**

1. **Cleanup.** Macrophages remove the blood clot, the damaged matrix, and osteocytes that have died in the tissue adjacent to the break.

2. **Cell proliferation.** The adjacent periosteum and endosteum proliferate to produce many osteoprogenitor cells. These cells surround the damaged region and migrate between the fractured ends.

3. **Cartilage production.** Osteoprogenitor cells in an oxygen-poor environment become chondroblasts. Therefore, until the region is revascularized, small fragments of cartilage are produced.

4. **Bone formation.** The **bone callus** is formed. Bone is produced by endochondral ossification of the cartilage and intramembranous osteogenesis in the surrounding tissue until irregular trabeculae of primary bone join the fractured ends.

5. **Remodeling.** Primary bone is replaced with secondary bone. Normal mechanical stresses cause the new bone to have the same shape as the original organ.

H. **Synovial joints (diarthroses)** permit a wide range of movement, usually between long bones. The **articular cavity** is a sealed structure between bones. It contains synovial fluid. Ligaments and a joint capsule enclose the articular cavity and hold the bones together.

1. The **joint capsule** is composed of an outer fibrous layer and an inner synovial membrane (Figure 7-12).
   a. The **fibrous layer** is dense connective tissue.
   b. The deeply folded **synovial membrane** lines the fibrous layer up to the bare weight-bearing articular cartilage. It has a surface (lining) layer and subsynovial connective tissue.
      (1) The lining layer of the synovial membrane is formed by a discontinuous layer of flattened or cuboidal synovial cells. Some of these cells are phagocytic. The others, which resemble fibroblasts, secrete hyaluronic acid and a lubricating glycoprotein that combine with plasma from capillaries in the membrane to form **synovial fluid**.
      (2) The **subsynovial tissue** between the surface layer and the fibrous layer of the joint capsule can be dense fibrous connective tissue, loose connective tissue, or white adipose tissue. It contains blood and lymph vessels and pressoreceptors.
2. **Synovial fluid** is primarily derived from plasma, but it is more viscous because of a high concentration of hyaluronic acid that is produced by the fibroblast-like lining cells. It lubricates the articular surface and nourishes the articular cartilage.

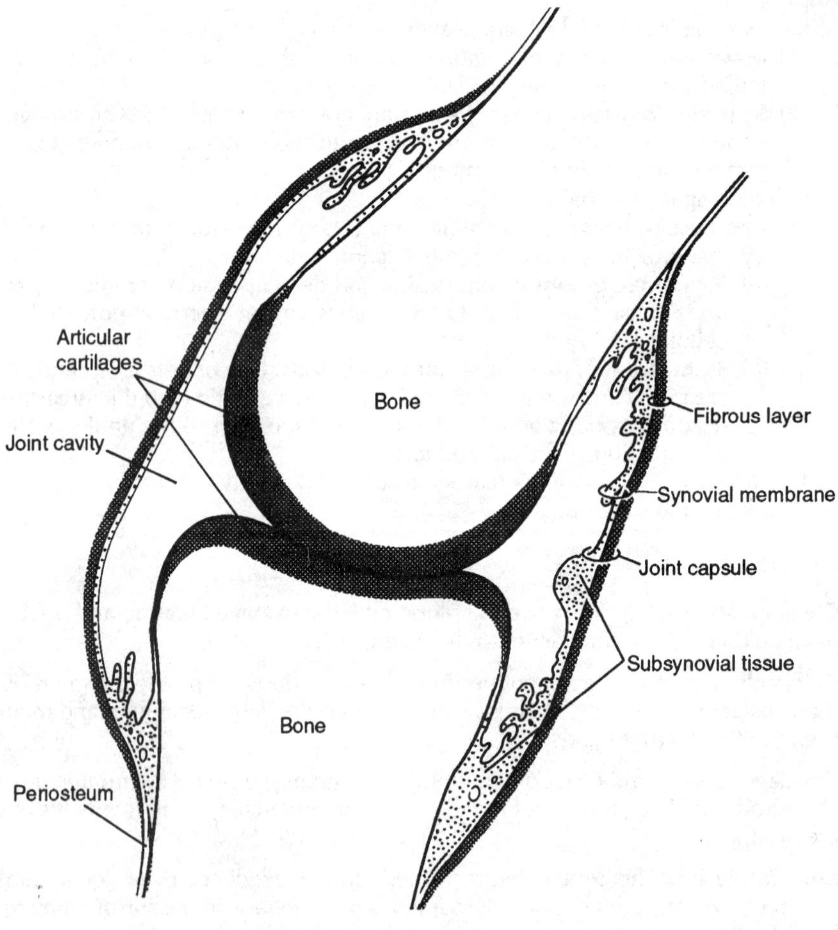

Figure 7-12. Schematic drawing of a synovial joint. (Redrawn with permission from Dellmann H-D: *Textbook of Veterinary Histology,* 4th ed. Baltimore, Williams & Wilkins, 1993, p 51.)

STUDY QUESTIONS

DIRECTIONS: Each of the numbered items or incomplete statements in this section is followed by answers or by completions of the statement. Select the **one** numbered answer or completion that is **best** in each case.

1. Cartilage and bone are similar in that:

(1) their cells do not divide once they are surrounded with matrix.
(2) they both have many immigrant cells from the blood.
(3) they both lack an organ capsule.
(4) the ground substance in their matrices gives them tensile strength.
(5) the primary functions of both are performed by their extracellular matrices.

2. In growing bones, osteoblasts are cells that:

(1) are surrounded by bone.
(2) have very acidophilic cytoplasm.
(3) form a squamous layer on bone surfaces.
(4) are connected to neighboring cells by gap junctions.
(5) release matrix components from all surfaces.

3. Which one of the following is a structural characteristic of compact bone?

(1) Central canals of osteons are joined by communicating and perforating canals.
(2) Collagen fibers in one lamella are parallel to those in adjacent lamellae.
(3) Interstitial lamellae are formed by osteoblasts that remain on the surface after osteons are completed.
(4) Circumferential lamellae surround each central canal.
(5) Periosteum covers its outer surfaces, endosteum lines its marrow space, and endothelium lines its canals.

4. During the formation and growth of cartilage:

(1) the tissue can expand in volume from within.
(2) appositional growth is responsible for the formation of isogenous groups.
(3) processes of chondroblasts retain their contact with other cells.
(4) chondroblasts become chondrocytes when they begin to secrete chondromucoproteins.
(5) chondrocyte cytoplasm is intensely acidophilic.

5. Which of the following is a characteristic of mature hyaline cartilage?

(1) Its repair is mostly by interstitial growth.
(2) Its cells are noticeably uniform in shape.
(3) Isogenous groups of cells are limited to the most superficial region.
(4) Its fibers are visible under the light microscope.
(5) Its tensile strength is derived primarily from collagen type II fibrils.

6. The matrix of bone is characterized by the fact that it:

(1) contains no amorphous ground substance.
(2) contains no organic material.
(3) contains no water.
(4) depends on collagen type II to resist compression.
(5) depends on collagen type I for tensile strength.

7. When a mature bone is fractured:

(1) osteogenesis begins immediately.
(2) the neighboring endosteum atrophies.
(3) osteoprogenitor cells become chondroblasts during early stages of repair.
(4) the osteoprogenitor cells are carried into the region on blood vessels.
(5) the first bone formed is bone callus of secondary bone.

8. Which one of the following statements regarding the function of cartilage is true?

(1) All fibrocartilage is associated with the skeletal system.
(2) All hyaline cartilage is associated with the skeletal system.
(3) Elastic cartilage forms a temporary skeleton in the embryo.
(4) Elastic cartilage forms a resilient articular surface in joints.
(5) Fibrocartilage supports the walls of the upper airways.

9. In which way does primary bone differ from secondary bone?

(1) Primary bone is stronger.
(2) Collagen fibers in primary bone are randomly oriented.
(3) The concentration of organic matrix in primary bone is not as high as it is in secondary bone.
(4) Primary bone is formed only by intramembranous osteogenesis.
(5) Primary bone is not present in adults.

10. Which of the following is the basic pattern in all types of osteogenesis?

(1) An embryonic connective tissue model is replaced by bone.
(2) Matrix granules are the first secretions of the osteoblasts.
(3) Isolated spicules of bone are formed and then grow until they fuse into a continuous tissue.
(4) Osteoid is formed and then undergoes mineralization.
(5) Ingrowth of blood vessels precedes differentiation of osteoblasts.

11. During formation of a long bone, the physeal plate:

(1) remains the same width because of the balance between interstitial growth of cartilage and the death of chondrocytes.
(2) remains the same width because of the balance between growth of the epiphysis and growth of the diaphysis.
(3) has a zone of chondrocytes that gradually degenerate before they die.
(4) is converted to bone by calcification of the cartilage matrix.
(5) is most fragile in the zone of ossification.

12. Which one of the following statements *best* describes a synovial joint?

(1) The articular cartilages are bare.
(2) The synovial membrane is cuboidal epithelium.
(3) The subsynovial tissue is dense connective tissue.
(4) The synovial fluid resembles blood plasma in composition and viscosity.
(5) The articular cartilages are nourished by diffusion from the underlying bone.

13. Which one of the following statements describes how bone is affected by substances carried in the blood?

(1) Vitamin D is essential for collagen synthesis.
(2) Vitamin C is essential for absorption of calcium and mineralization.
(3) Parathormone has a short-term stimulatory effect on osteoblasts.
(4) Calcitonin inhibits loss of calcium from bone.
(5) Calcium is the only ion whose release from bone is regulated.

DIRECTIONS: Each of the numbered items or incomplete statements in this section is negatively phrased, as indicated by an italicized word such as *not, least,* or *except.* Select the **one** numbered answer or completion that is **best** in each case.

14. All of the following are characteristics of mature cancellous bone *except:*

(1) cells are usually supplied by diffusion from the marrow space.
(2) all its surfaces are covered by endosteum.
(3) it is always in contact with compact bone.
(4) it is not organized in lamellae.
(5) processes of its cells remain connected by gap junctions.

15. All of the following statements are true regarding remodeling of bone *except:*

(1) it continues throughout life.
(2) over time, the earliest osteons are replaced with larger and larger osteons.
(3) it can alter the gross form of a bone in an adult animal.
(4) it is affected by an electrical potential.
(5) it is important for maintenance of normal blood ion levels.

ANSWERS AND EXPLANATIONS

1. The answer is 5 *[I]*. The primary function of both cartilage and bone is support, which depends on the rigid extracellular matrix. Chondrocytes in young cartilage can divide, forming isogenous groups. Neither bone nor cartilage contains immigrant cells, which are characteristic of loose connective tissue. The perichondrium of cartilage and periosteum of bone are organ capsules. The tensile strength of cartilage and bone results from the collagen fibrils and fibers in the matrix, not the ground substance.

2. The answer is 4 *[III B 1 a (1)]*. Osteoblasts are connected by gap junctions to osteocytes in the underlying bone and to neighboring osteoblasts. They form a surface layer of polarized cuboidal to columnar cells. Their cytoplasm is intensely basophilic because of their active secretion of the organic matrix of bone, which is released on the surface facing the bone.

3. The answer is 1 *[III C 1 a (1) (a); Figure 7-8A]*. Perforating canals carry blood vessels that supply the capillary branches in central canals, and communicating canals carry small anastomosing vascular branches between central canals. Collagen fibers in one lamella lie parallel to each other but are at approximately right angles to those in adjacent lamellae. This increases the ability of bone to resist tensile forces in a variety of axes, a principle similar to that used in the construction of plywood. Interstitial lamellae are remnants of older osteons that have been partially destroyed by the formation of younger osteons during remodeling. Circumferential lamellae are characteristic of the diaphyses of long bones. Outer circumferential lamellae lie under the periosteum, where they surround the entire shaft, and inner circumferential lamellae lie adjacent to the endosteum, where they surround the marrow space. Osteonal lamellae surround central canals. The canals in compact bone are lined by endosteum, not endothelium.

4. The answer is 1 *[II C 1 a (2)]*. Young cartilage grows both from within (interstitial growth) and by addition of cartilage to the surface (appositional growth). Isogenous groups are formed during interstitial growth, not appositional growth. One of the first events in chondrogenesis is withdrawal of cell processes that contact other cells. Chondroblasts become chondrocytes when they have surrounded themselves with matrix, which consists primarily of chondromucoproteins and collagen. The cytoplasm of chondrocytes in growing cartilage is intensely basophilic because the chondrocytes are very active in protein synthesis.

5. The answer is 5 *[II D 1 a (3) (a)]*. The primary fiber type and the source of tensile strength in hyaline cartilage is collagen type II, which forms slender fibrils. If mature cartilage is damaged, its repair is limited; what replacement of cartilage does occur is primarily by appositional growth. Large deficits are usually replaced, at least in part, by dense connective tissue. The cells near the surface are flattened, while those deeper in the tissue are round. Isogenous groups occur in deeper parts of the tissue, not superficially. The collagen in hyaline cartilage is not visible, both because the collagen is mostly in the form of submicroscopic fibrils and because the refractive index of collagen is similar to that of the surrounding ground substance. The glassy appearance of this type of cartilage results from the apparent homogeneity of its matrix.

6. The answer is 5 *[III B 2 a]*. The organic component of bone, which accounts for approximately half of its dry weight, is primarily collagen type I. The sturdy fibers formed by collagen type I are responsible for the tensile strength of bone. The function of collagen in bone can be compared to that of the steel rods in reinforced concrete. Bone matrix contains a small amount of ground substance, and it also contains water in hydration layers on its mineral crystals. This water is the medium for exchange of ions between bone, the interstitial fluid, and, eventually, the blood. The rigid inorganic matrix, primarily hydroxyapatite, is responsible for resisting compressive forces.

7. The answer is 3 *[III G 3]*. A fracture damages the surrounding tissue, including the capillaries, so the region is poorly perfused with oxygen until debris is removed and capillary regrowth occurs. In that environment, osteoprogenitor cells become chondroblasts instead of osteoblasts. Remodeling of the bone callus can restore the original shape of the bone, provided the broken ends are well aligned. The neighboring endosteum (and periosteum) proliferate, increasing the number of osteoprogenitor cells in the damaged region. The bone callus is formed of primary bone; it is later remodeled with secondary bone.

8. The answer is 1 *[II D 1 c, 2 b, 3 b].* Fibrocartilage occurs at attachments of ligaments and tendons to bones and forms the intervertebral discs and menisci of the stifle. These sites require rigid support with great tensile strength. Hyaline cartilage supports the larger airways, in addition to being associated with the skeletal system. It forms a temporary skeleton in the embryo and is the smooth resilient articular cartilage in synovial joints. Elastic cartilage is associated with structures that are subject to mechanical deformation (e.g., the auricle of the ear, the epiglottis).

9. The answer is 2 *[III D 1–2].* Primary bone is also called woven bone because its collagen fibers are randomly oriented. It is not as strong as secondary bone, in which the collagen fibers are aligned in parallel arrays within each lamella, and in which the ratio of inorganic matrix to organic matrix is higher. Primary bone may be formed by either intramembranous or endochondral osteogenesis. It persists in specific loci, such as the attachments of certain tendons and ligaments and in the attachments of teeth.

10. The answer is 4 *[III E 1 b (1)].* Osteoid, which comprises collagen and ground substance, is secreted by osteoblasts first. Osteoblasts then release matrix granules that contain alkaline phosphatase and calcium phosphate, causing the osteoid to become mineralized. An embryonic model is replaced by bone only in endochondral osteogenesis. Isolated spicules grow until they fuse during formation of bones by intramembranous osteogenesis, but not during endochondral osteogenesis. Ingrowth of blood vessels is necessary to carry osteoprogenitor cells into spaces where cartilage has been destroyed during endochondral osteogenesis, but blood vessels do not grow into regions of intramembranous bone formation until after osteogenesis is under way.

11. The answer is 1 *[III E 3 c (3)].* The physeal plate and zone of ossification remain the same width throughout development because the interstitial growth of cartilage in the zone of maturing chondrocytes occurs at the same rate at which chondrocytes die at the border of the zone of hypertrophy and calcification. The processes across the physeal plate and adjacent zone of ossification are all in balance. Growth of the epiphysis and diaphysis would destroy the physeal plate if interstitial growth did not occur in the physeal cartilage. Chondrocytes in the physeal plate are healthy until approximately 15–20 minutes before they die. The signal that causes their apparently programmed death has not yet been identified. Calcified cartilage is not bone. The most fragile region in the physeal plate is the zone of hypertrophy and calcification, where much of the cartilage matrix has been destroyed but has not yet been reinforced by bone.

12. The answer is 1 *[III H].* The weight-bearing articular cartilages are the only surfaces in the synovial cavity that are not lined by the synovial membrane. The synovial membrane has a surface of phagocytic and fibroblast-like cells, not an epithelial lining. The connective tissue portion of the membrane is often loose connective tissue and white adipose tissue. The fibroblast-like cells of the synovial lining add hyaluronic acid to the synovial fluid; the high concentration of hyaluronic acid increases the viscosity and lubricating properties of the fluid over those of plasma. An additional function of the synovial fluid is nourishing the avascular articular cartilage.

13. The answer is 4 *[III A 3 a–b].* Calcitonin inhibits the calcium-releasing effects of parathormone on osteocytes and osteoclasts, and it also has a short-term stimulatory effect on osteoblasts. Vitamin D is essential for absorption of calcium. Vitamin C is essential for collagen synthesis. Parathormone stimulates osteocytic osteolysis and osteoclastic activity; it does not promote osteoblastic activity. The storage and release from bone of several additional ions, including phosphate, are regulated.

14. The answer is 4 *[III C 2].* Like all mature bone, cancellous bone is organized into lamellae. The arrangements of the lamellae are less orderly than in compact bone, however, and very rarely form osteons. The structural elements of cancellous bone are thin enough that the cells can be nourished by diffusion from blood vessels in the marrow space; therefore, osteons are not needed. Because cancellous bone is always continuous with an outer layer of compact bone, its free surfaces are covered by endosteum. As in all types of bone, osteocyte processes are joined by gap junctions.

15. The answer is 2 *[III F 1 d]*. Later generations of osteons are smaller and smaller, which contributes to the increased strength of remodeled bone. Although remodeling continues throughout life, the rate is only 0.5%–1% as great in the adult as it is during growth. The gross form of bones can be altered in adult animals. Differences in compression and decompression in different parts of the bone cause movement of ions, setting up an electrical potential that stimulates osteoclasts and osteoblasts differentially. Decompression (such as the pull exerted by a tendon during muscular activity) stimulates osteoblasts, enlarging the attachments of heavily used muscles. Remodeling of bone creates a dynamic sink for calcium and other ions, which enables blood levels to be exquisitely regulated.

Chapter 8
Blood

I. INTRODUCTION.

Blood transports cells, solutes, and suspended solids to different parts of the body. Blood comprises plasma and blood cells (Figure 8-1).

A. Plasma

Plasma is the **fluid ground substance** of blood. It is approximately 90% water and 10% solutes and suspended solids.

1. **Plasma proteins,** which help maintain the osmotic pressure of blood, account for 7% of the volume. Plasma proteins include carrier molecules, components of the clotting system, and immunoglobulins (antibodies).
   a. **Fibrinogen** is a plasma protein.
   b. **Fibrin fibers** arise from fibrinogen and appear during clotting.
   c. **Serum** is the fluid remaining after removal of fibrinogen and fibrin from plasma.

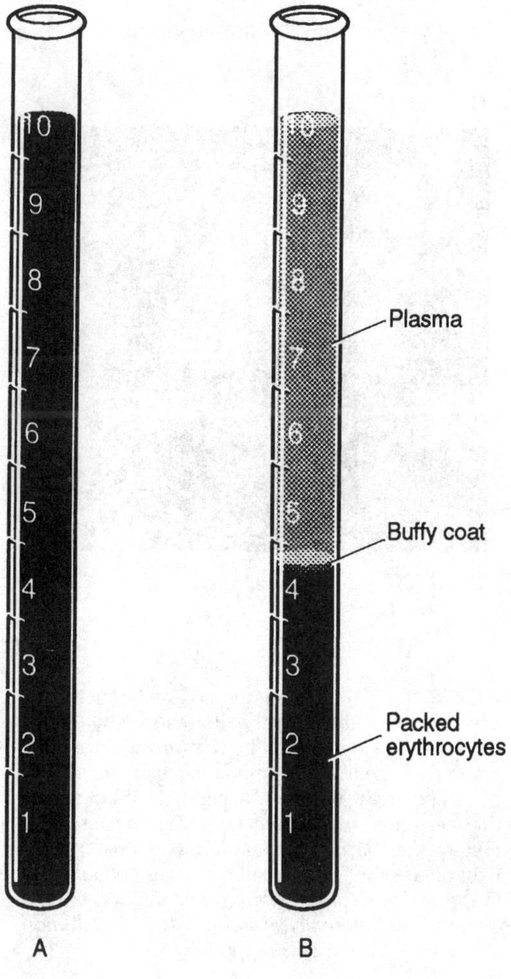

FIGURE 8-1. Blood before (*A*) and after (*B*) centrifugal sedimentation. The buffy coat is a layer of leukocytes with a thin layer of platelets on top of it. The supernatant is plasma. (Redrawn with permission from Dellmann H-D: *Textbook of Veterinary Histology,* 4th ed. Baltimore, Williams & Wilkins, 1993, p 55.)

2. **Nutrients, wastes, hormones,** and **other substances** are also present in plasma.

B. **Blood cells** are classified as **erythrocytes, leukocytes,** and **platelets**.

II. BLOOD CELLS

A. Erythrocytes (red blood cells)

1. **Structure**
   a. **Contents**
      (1) The **nucleus and all organelles are lost** during development in mammals.
         (a) **Howell-Jolly** bodies are nuclear remnants that are present in 1% of erythrocytes in some species (Figure 8-2A).
         (b) Because red blood cells do not contain nuclei, they are sometimes called **blood corpuscles**.
      (2) Erythrocytes are filled with the red gas-carrying pigment, **hemoglobin**.
   b. **Shape.** Their shape, which depends on the species, is usually a **biconcave flattened disk** (see Figure 8-2B).
      (1) The degree of biconcavity varies among species.
      (2) **Poikilocytosis** is the presence of erythrocytes with an abnormal shape.

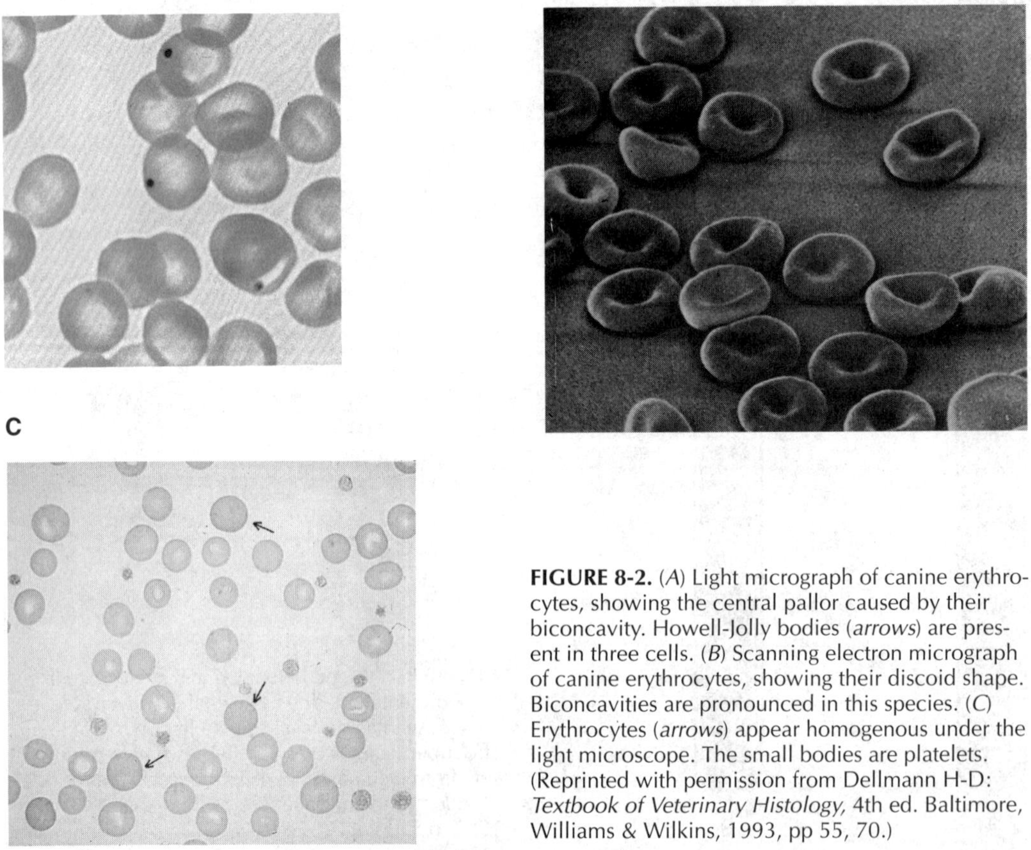

FIGURE 8-2. (*A*) Light micrograph of canine erythrocytes, showing the central pallor caused by their biconcavity. Howell-Jolly bodies (*arrows*) are present in three cells. (*B*) Scanning electron micrograph of canine erythrocytes, showing their discoid shape. Biconcavities are pronounced in this species. (*C*) Erythrocytes (*arrows*) appear homogenous under the light microscope. The small bodies are platelets. (Reprinted with permission from Dellmann H-D: *Textbook of Veterinary Histology,* 4th ed. Baltimore, Williams & Wilkins, 1993, pp 55, 70.)

2. **Function.** The hemoglobin in erythrocytes carries oxygen from the lungs to the tissues and returns carbon dioxide to the lungs.
   a. Gas exchange is facilitated when the cell membrane is pressed against the endothelium as the supple and deformable erythrocytes squeeze through small capillaries.
   b. Erythrocytes function without a nucleus or organelles until their energy-producing enzymes are exhausted.

3. **Microscopic appearance**
   a. **Size.** Erythrocytes in a given species are usually uniform in size, but **anisocytosis** (i.e., variation in erythrocyte size in an individual animal) is normal in some species.
      (1) **Normocytes** are normal-sized erythrocytes.
      (2) **Macrocytes** are erythrocytes that are larger than normal.
      (3) **Microcytes** are erythrocytes that are smaller than normal.
   b. Because they contain hemoglobin, erythrocytes **appear homogenous** under both electron and light microscopes (see Figure 8-2C). Erythrocytes **stain pink** with routine stains.
   c. **Biconcave** erythrocytes exhibit **central pallor** under the light microscope (see Figure 8-2A).
   d. **Rouleaux** are stacks of erythrocytes, which are seen normally in some species.

4. **Distribution and lifespan**
   a. Erythrocytes occupy **45% ±5% of the total blood volume** (see Figure 8-1).
      (1) **Hematocrit** is an estimation of the percentage of blood volume occupied by erythrocytes, based on a centrifuged blood sample.
      (2) **Anemia** is a lower-than-normal number of erythrocytes in a given volume of blood, a below-normal hematocrit (i.e., a low relative volume of erythrocytes in centrifuged blood), or a less-than-normal amount of hemoglobin.
   b. Erythrocytes, which are **nonmotile, live for several months** in the blood.

B. Leukocytes (white blood cells)

1. **General information**
   a. **Classification.** All leukocytes contain **lysosomal azurophilic (primary) granules,** which are often too small to see under the light microscope. **Specific (secondary) granules,** unique to each cell type, are the basis for subdivision of leukocytes.
      (1) **Agranulocytes** contain no specific granules. They include **lymphocytes** and **monocytes.**
      (2) **Granulocytes** contain **specific granules**. Their names are based on the staining reaction of their specific granules in human blood. All of the granulocytes have **segmented (lobulated) nuclei**. Granulocytes include **neutrophils** [heterophils, polymorphonuclear leukocytes (PMLs)], **eosinophils,** and **basophils.**
   b. **Distribution.** Leukocytes, **motile cells** that use the blood for transportation to the connective tissue, leave the blood after only a few minutes to a few days and perform most of their functions in the formed connective tissue.
      (1) **Margination, diapedesis,** and **migration** are leukocyte movements influenced by substances released in injured and inflamed tissue.
         (a) **Margination** is the accumulation and adhesion of leukocytes to the endothelial cells.
            (i) The marginal pool (i.e., the number of marginated neutrophils and monocytes) normally equals or surpasses the number of circulating cells.
            (ii) The marginal pool is in a constant state of flux (i.e., most cells are marginated only temporarily).
         (b) **Diapedesis (emigration)** is the passage of leukocytes through the intact wall of a blood vessel via temporary spaces they form between endothelial cells. Diapedesis is promoted by substances released during inflammation.
         (c) **Migration** through the tissue enables leukocytes to reach sites where they are needed for defense.

(2) Leukocytes account for only **1% of the blood volume** because they leave the blood so quickly (see Figure 8-1). Approximately equal numbers of erythrocytes, neutrophils, and eosinophils are produced. The great difference in their concentrations in blood results from differences in how long they remain in the blood.

2. **Lymphocytes** (see also Chapter 6 II C 2 d). Most circulating lymphocytes are T lymphocytes.
   a. **Structure** (Figure 8-3). Lymphocytes have a spherical to ovoid heterochromatic nucleus surrounded by a small amount of moderately basophilic cytoplasm.
   b. **Functions.** Lymphocytes perform diverse functions, even within the major groups. These functions are covered in more detail in Chapter 12.
      (1) **B lymphocytes** are responsible for **humoral immunity**.
      (2) **T lymphocytes** are responsible for **cell-mediated immunity**.
   c. **Distribution and lifespan**
      (1) Lymphocytes, the most abundant agranulocytes, circulate between the blood and connective tissue, and lymphatic organs.
      (2) Some types are short-lived, but others live many years.

3. **Monocytes**
   a. **Structure** (Figure 8-4; see Figure 8-3B)
      (1) Monocytes, the **largest cells** in circulating blood, have a **kidney-shaped to trilobed nucleus** and **abundant cytoplasm,** which is basophilic and often appears frothy. Compared to lymphocytes, their ratio of cytoplasmic to nuclear volume is greater, and the basophilic cytoplasm appears grayer.
      (2) Monocytes are relatively **rigid,** appearing in smears to indent adjacent cells.
      (3) They often have **pseudopodia**.
   b. **Functions. Monocytes become macrophages** when they enter the connective tissue.
      (1) **Phagocytosis.** Macrophages phagocytose bacteria, viruses, antigen–antibody complexes in the blood, and debris from wounded tissue.
         (a) **Recognition factors** usually initiate phagocytosis.
            (i) **Immunoglobulin G (IgG) receptors** are located on the surface of macrophages. Antigen–IgG complexes attach to the macrophage membrane. In addition, **free IgG** attaches to the surface receptors on macrophages and may then form complexes with free antigens.
            (ii) **Opsonin receptors** are also located on macrophage membranes. Opsonins are antibody-containing recognition factors that are released during immune reactions. They coat foreign particles, such as microorganisms. Macrophages phagocytose some opsonized bacteria that are ignored by neutrophils.
         (b) **Engulfment** of the particle results from a spreading wave of surface interactions between receptors and ligands or antibodies and antigens that draw the macrophage membrane along the surface of the foreign particle until the particle is surrounded.
            (i) **Foreign body giant cells** are formed by fusion of macrophages. If a particle is too large to be engulfed by a single cell, several macrophages may fuse to enclose it. Fusion of macrophages in bone forms osteoclasts.
            (ii) **Epithelioid walls** may be formed by macrophages to isolate a focal infection.
      (2) **Immune responses.** The roles of macrophages in immunity are covered in more detail in Chapter 12.
         (a) Macrophages process ingested antigens and then exhibit fragments of these foreign antigens together with self antigens on their plasma membrane.
         (b) Presentation of **antigenic fragments** and self antigens to lymphocytes is an early step in the immune response.
         (c) **Interleukins** (e.g., IL-1), which stimulate lymphocyte responses, are secreted by macrophages.
      (3) **Secretion.** Macrophages secrete tumor necrosis factor α (TNFα) and they produce (and are acted on by) interferons (e.g., IFN-γ).

A

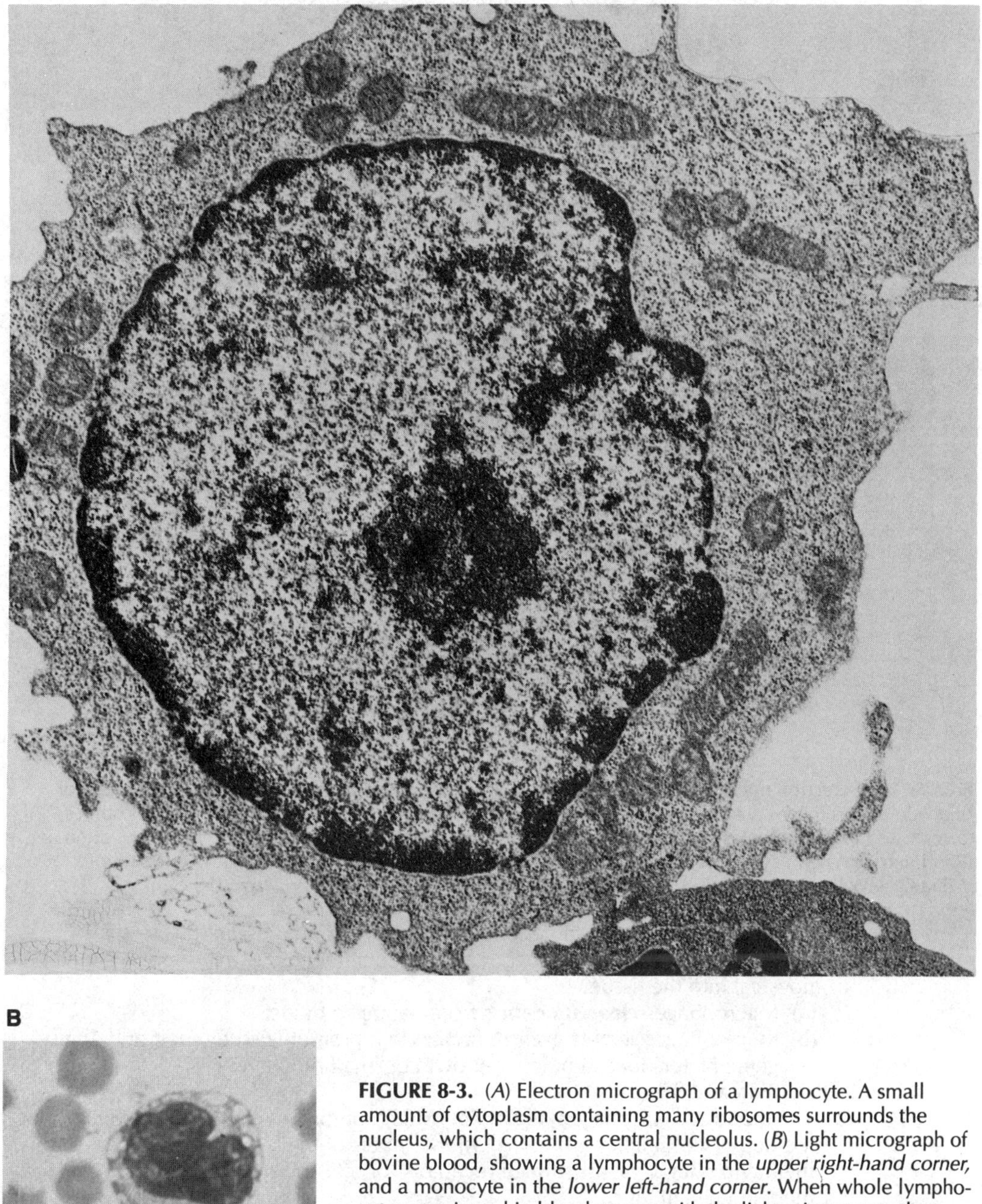

B

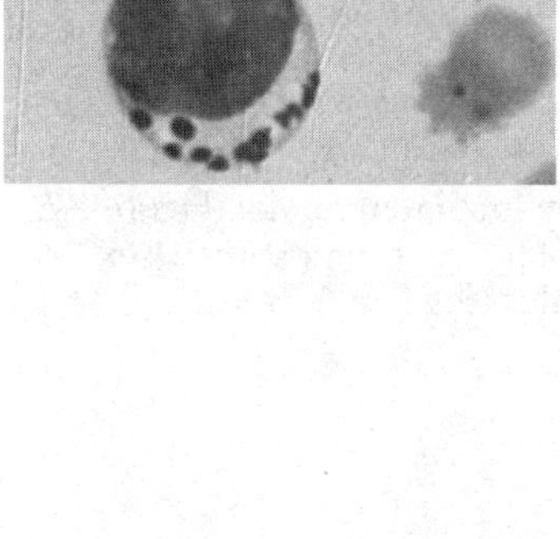

FIGURE 8-3. (*A*) Electron micrograph of a lymphocyte. A small amount of cytoplasm containing many ribosomes surrounds the nucleus, which contains a central nucleolus. (*B*) Light micrograph of bovine blood, showing a lymphocyte in the *upper right-hand corner,* and a monocyte in the *lower left-hand corner.* When whole lymphocytes are viewed in blood smears with the light microscope, the nucleolus is obscured by peripheral heterochromatin. Several large, dark, azurophilic granules, which are present more frequently in bovine species than in most species, are visible in the lymphocyte. Notice the vacuolated cytoplasm of the monocyte. (Reprinted with permission from Dellmann H-D: *Textbook of Veterinary Histology,* 4th ed. Baltimore, Williams & Wilkins, 1993, pp 61, 70.)

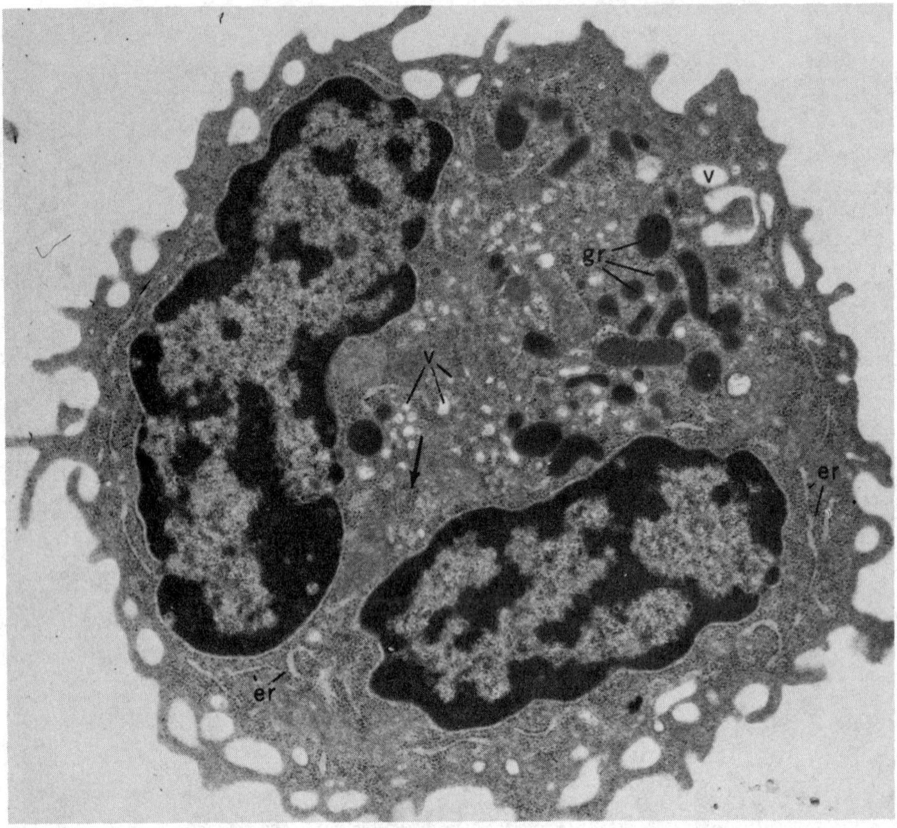

FIGURE 8-4. Electron micrograph of a monocyte. The section passes through the horseshoe-shaped or bilobed nucleus in two places. The cell contains many lysosomal granules (*gr*), vesicles (*v*), ribosomes (*arrow*), and rough endoplasmic reticulum (er) and has a highly irregular surface with many pseudopodia. (Reprinted with permission from Dellmann H-D: *Textbook of Veterinary Histology,* 4th ed. Baltimore, Williams & Wilkins, 1993, p 60.)

(4) **Healing.** Lymphocytes and endothelial cells in injured tissue release lymphokines and cytokines, respectively, which attract tissue macrophages (i.e., histiocytes) into the tissue.
   (a) Macrophages **clean up debris** from damaged tissue.
   (b) Macrophages secrete **growth factors** that promote tissue repair and angiogenic factors that stimulate regrowth of small blood vessels.

c. **Distribution and lifespan**
   (1) The **mononuclear phagocyte system (MPS)** comprises macrophages throughout the body [see Chapter 6 II C 1 g (3)]. Members of the MPS can be identified by their avid phagocytosis, surface receptors for IgG and opsonins, and firm attachment to glass in vitro.
   (2) Monocytes remain in the blood about 40 hours, and may live in the tissue for **several months**. They are normal constituents of specific regions in many organs.

4. **Neutrophils**
   a. **Structure**
      (1) **Nucleus**
         (a) Neutrophils have **very heterochromatic, highly lobulated** nuclei (Figure 8-5).
         (b) A **nuclear appendage** may be formed by one of the X chromosomes (sex chromatin), which remains condensed in females (see Figure 8-5C).

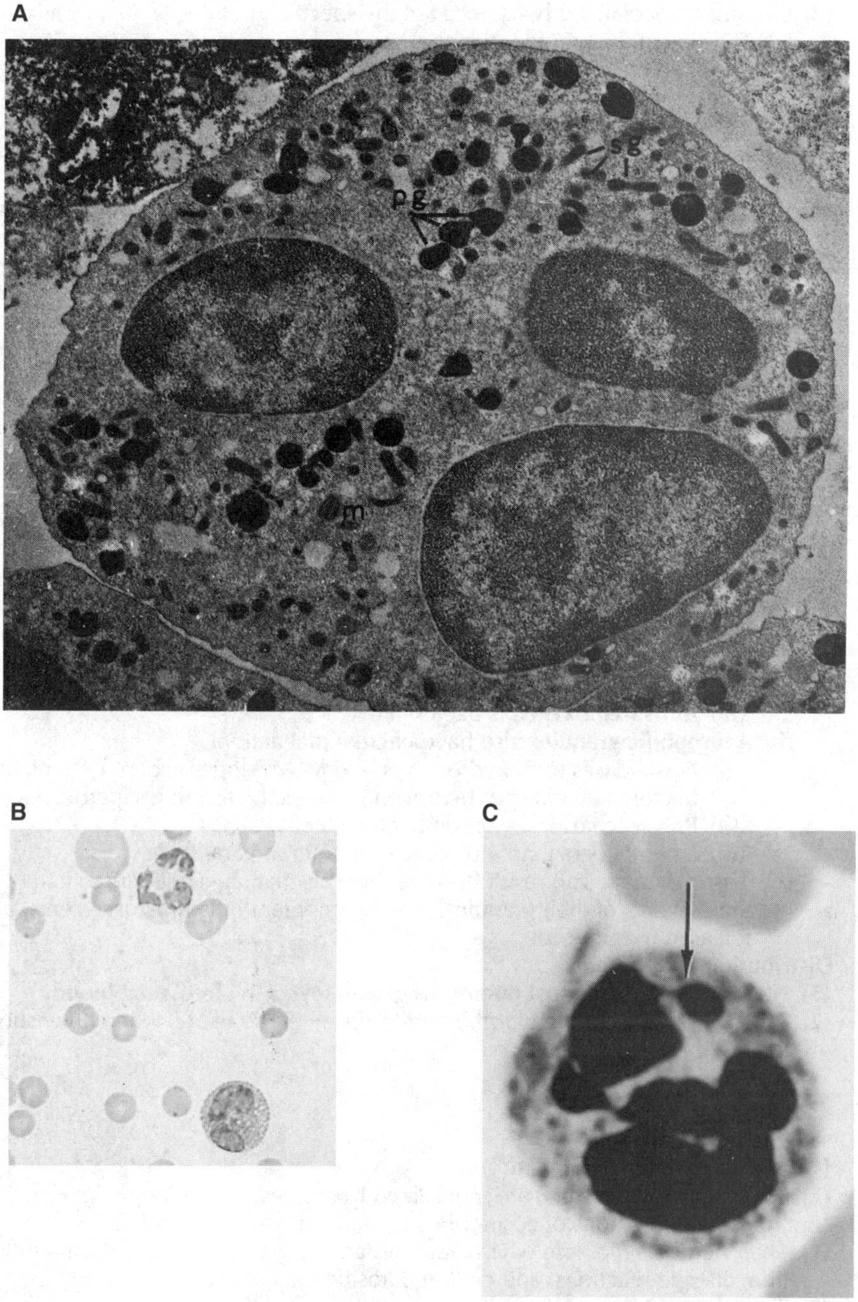

FIGURE 8-5. (*A*) Electron micrograph of a neutrophil. The section passes through three lobules of the heterochromatic nucleus. The large round primary (azurophilic) granules (*pg*) have been stained to demonstrate peroxidase, which makes them very dark. The specific granules (*sg*) are smaller, and their shapes are varied. Some mitochondria (*m*) are present. (*B*) The multiple lobes of a neutrophil (*top*) are visible. An eosinophil (*lower right*) is visible as well. (*C*) A neutrophil from a female animal, showing sex chromatin (*arrow*). (Reprinted with permission from Dellmann H-D: *Textbook of Veterinary Histology,* 4th ed. Baltimore, Williams & Wilkins 1993, pp 10, 58, 70.)

(2) **Organelles.** Some **mitochondria** are found in neutrophils.
(3) **Granules. Specialized lysosomes** are the specific granules of neutrophils.
(a) The size of the granules varies.
(b) The **staining reaction** of granules varies from **light pink to purple,** which is why they are sometimes called **heterophils**. Often the granules are not visible, and the cytoplasm **appears weakly acidophilic**.
(c) In poultry, guinea pigs, and rabbits, the granules are **acidophilic** and the cells may be called **pseudoeosinophils**.

b. **Functions.** Neutrophils are the **first line of defense against pathogenic bacteria**. Antigen–antibody complexes and substances released by bacteria and endothelial cells quickly attract large numbers of neutrophils into the tissues. Once in the tissue, neutrophils become phagocytic. Anaerobic glycolysis enables neutrophils to operate in inflamed or necrotic tissue.
(1) Neutrophils in the tissue are often called **microphages** because they phagocytose smaller particles than do macrophages.
(2) **Both nonspecific** and **specific phagocytosis** can occur. Specific phagocytosis is facilitated by opsonization of the foreign particle. Neutrophils do not process and exhibit antigens.
(3) **Antibacterial activity.** The granular system of neutrophils exposes bacteria to oxygen radicals, nitrous oxide, and enzymes. Phagosomes that contain bacteria fuse first with the specific granules and then with azurophilic granules of the microphage.
(a) **Specific granules** (i.e., **specialized lysosomes**) contain substances specialized to attack bacteria.
(i) **Lysozyme** degrades the bacterial wall.
(ii) **Lactoferrin** binds iron, a crucial element in bacterial nutrition.
(iii) **Activated oxygen** is bactericidal.
(b) **Azurophilic granules** also have bactericidal action.
(i) **Peroxidases** form hydrogen peroxide. Myeloperoxidase potentiates the bactericidal effect of hydrogen peroxide by forming superoxides.
(ii) **Polysaccharidases** act on bacterial cell walls.
(iii) **Low pH** (less than 4.0) kills some microorganisms.
(c) **Tissue damage** can result from neutrophils that have become so active that the contents of their granules, which are potent inflammatory agents, are released from the cell.

c. **Distribution and lifespan**
(1) Neutrophils are the **most numerous granulocytes in circulating blood**.
(2) After **6–10 hours in the blood,** neutrophils enter the **tissue,** where they survive for **1–2 days**.

5. **Eosinophils**

a. **Structure** (Figure 8-6)
(1) **Nuclei** are usually **bilobed**.
(2) **Specific granules,** which are **specialized lysosomes,** are **eosinophilic** (Figure 8-7).

b. **Functions.** The functions of eosinophils are not yet well understood.
(1) Their numbers increase when tissue histamine is elevated (e.g., during inflammation, allergic reactions, and certain parasitic infections).
(2) **Secretion**
(a) Eosinophils secrete enzymes that inactivate some inflammatory substances and reverse certain aspects of allergic reactions.
(b) Other secretions exacerbate certain deleterious effects of allergens.
(3) **Phagocytosis.** Eosinophils are phagocytic, but less so than neutrophils.
(a) They phagocytose granules released from basophils and mast cells.
(b) They phagocytose some opsonized bacteria and antigen–antibody complexes.
(4) **Degranulation.** Eosinophils can degranulate onto the surface of opsonized parasites that they are unable to engulf.

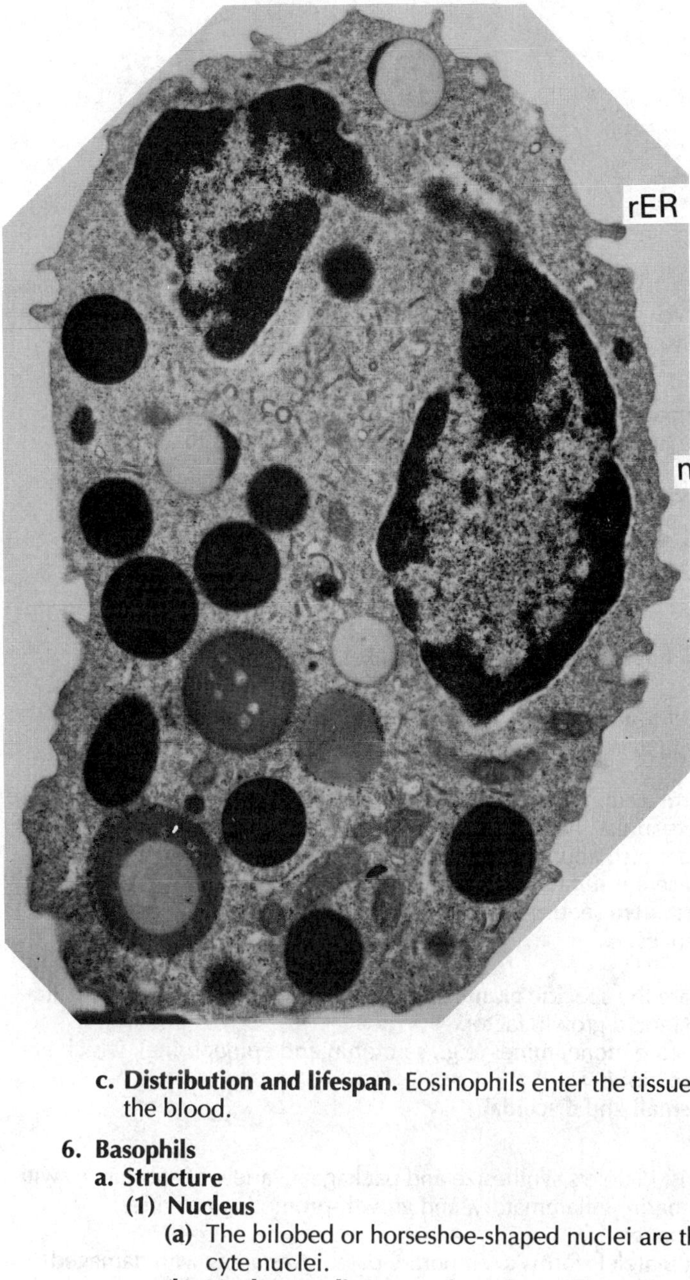

FIGURE 8-6. Electron micrograph of a canine eosinophil. The section passes through two lobes of the heterochromatic nucleus and grazes the strand connecting the lobes. The granules vary in appearance. (Reprinted with permission from Dellmann H-D: *Textbook of Veterinary Histology,* 4th ed. Baltimore, Williams & Wilkins, 1993, p 59.)

c. **Distribution and lifespan.** Eosinophils enter the tissue after approximately 20 minutes in the blood.

6. **Basophils**
   a. **Structure**
      (1) **Nucleus**
         (a) The bilobed or horseshoe-shaped nuclei are the **least lobulated** of the granulocyte nuclei.
         (b) **Nuclear outlines** are **often obscured** by the specific granules.
      (2) **Granules**
         (a) The specific granules of basophils are **basophilic** and **metachromatic** (see Figure 8-7).
         (b) Basophil granules are similar to those of mast cells (see Chapter 6 II C 1 f). Like mast cell granules, they contain **histamine, heparin,** and **other substances** that act on blood vessels, smooth muscle in certain organs, and other leukocytes.
   b. **Functions**
      (1) **Inflammation reaction.** Basophils are attracted to sites of entry of antigens. **Receptor-mediated degranulation** helps initiate the inflammation response by promoting localized edema and movement of other white blood cells into the tissue. **Anaphylactic shock** can result from massive degranulation of basophils and mast cells.
      (2) **Phagocytosis**

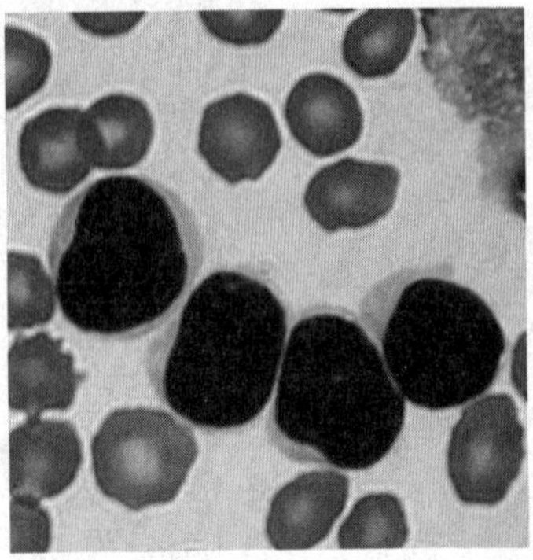

FIGURE 8-7. An equine eosinophil (*left*) and basophil (*right*). The granules in equine eosinophils are very large, causing the cells to resemble raspberries.

c. **Distribution and lifespan**
   (1) Basophils are the **least numerous leukocytes** (comprising less than 1% of the total).
   (2) They live 10–12 days in the blood.

C. Platelets (thrombocytes)

1. **Structure**
   a. **Nucleus**
      (1) **Mammalian platelets** (thrombocytes) are small cytoplasmic fragments (see Figure 8-2C).
      (2) **Avian thrombocytes** are **nucleated** cells that perform the same functions as platelets.
   b. **Organelles**
      (1) **Microtubules** form a supportive ring around the periphery of the platelet in vivo; however, platelets spread out on the glass slide when blood smears are made.
      (2) **Microfilaments** are also abundant at the cell periphery.
      (3) **Canaliculi** increase the surface area for secretion.
      (4) A **dense tubular system** sequesters calcium and may synthesize prostaglandins and other substances.
   c. **Granules**
      (1) **Alpha granules** are the **specific granules** of platelets. They contain clotting factors, antiheparin, and a growth factor.
      (2) **Dense granules** store monoamines (e.g., serotonin and epinephrine), which are taken up from the blood.
   d. **Shape.** Platelets are **small** and **discoidal.**

2. **Functions**
   a. **Storage and synthesis.** Platelets synthesize and package a variety of substances with procoagulant, antiheparin, inflammatory, and growth-promoting activities.
   b. **Endothelium maintenance**
      (1) **Agglutination** of platelets forms a temporary patch over areas with damaged endothelium. Platelets adhere to any exposed basal lamina, collagen, or elastic fibers, forming a **platelet plug**.
      (2) **Clotting**
         (a) **Degranulation releases clotting factors** from alpha granules **and a vasoconstrictor** (serotonin) from dense granules.
         (b) Clotting factors from platelets and damaged tissues initiate **a complex clotting mechanism** that **stimulates the formation of fibrin** from fibrinogen in the blood.
         (c) A **clot** forms from a meshwork of fibrin, trapped erythrocytes (which later disintegrate), and platelets. The platelets become stellate, and their long slender processes attach to the fibrin.
            (i) The peripheral microtubules depolymerize.

(ii) The number of actin filaments increases (by polymerization of G actin), and myosin fibers appear between them.

(iii) **Contraction** of platelets draws in the fibrin to which they are attached and decreases the volume of the clot by as much as 90%.

(3) **Release of growth factor** from alpha granules stimulates proliferation of several different cell types, including smooth muscle and fibroblasts.

(4) **Phagocytosis.** Platelet adherence to bacteria facilitates phagocytosis of bacteria by leukocytes.

3. **Distribution and lifespan.** Platelets, which are nonmotile, live in mammalian blood for 8–10 days.

III. HEMOPOIESIS

A. Introduction

1. **Prenatal hemopoietic organs**

a. **Yolk sac.** Mesodermal cells differentiate to become **hemopoietic stem cells,** forming **blood islands** that produce the earliest blood cells.

b. **Liver, spleen, and bone marrow.** Circulating stem cells are carried in the blood to the reticular tissue of the liver, the spleen, and finally the bone marrow. By the time of birth, most hemopoiesis is in the bone marrow (**myeloid tissue**), which produces **myeloid elements** [i.e., mature erythrocytes, monocytes, granulocytes, platelets, lymphocytic progenitor cells (which develop in the bone marrow but are carried by the blood to lymphatic organs), and, possibly, immunocompetent B lymphocytes].

c. **Thymus.** This is the earliest center of lymphocyte production (**lymphopoiesis**), followed by other lymphatic organs: **lymph nodes, gut-associated lymphatic tissue,** and the **spleen** (see Chapter 12 IV).

2. **Postnatal hemopoietic organs**

a. **Bone marrow**

(1) **Classification.** Bone marrow is classified as red or yellow, based on its gross appearance in the fresh state.

(a) **Red marrow** is active in hemopoiesis. It is the first type of bone marrow formed during development and the only type present in newborns.

(b) **Yellow marrow** contains large amounts of fat.

(i) It gradually replaces red marrow in the diaphyses of most long bones and some short bones during growth.

(ii) Yellow marrow can revert to red marrow when hemopoiesis is stimulated (e.g., by severe anemia).

(2) **Components**

(a) **Stroma.** The stroma is **reticular tissue**. Reticular cells and macrophages are the major stromal cells.

(i) **Reticular cells produce reticular fibers,** some collagen around blood vessels, and **hemopoietic regulating substances**. In yellow marrow, they store large amounts of lipid and resemble white adipose cells.

(ii) **Macrophages** are numerous. Some macrophages are associated with groups of developing erythrocytes called **erythroblastic islands** (Figure 8-8). The macrophages phagocytose nuclei expelled from developing erythrocytes and defective cells. In addition, they may help the nonmotile erythrocytes enter the circulating blood in the sinuses, and they **produce substances that influence hemopoiesis**.

(b) **Parenchyma.** The parenchyma of red marrow comprises stem cells, developing blood cells, and mature cells waiting to be released.

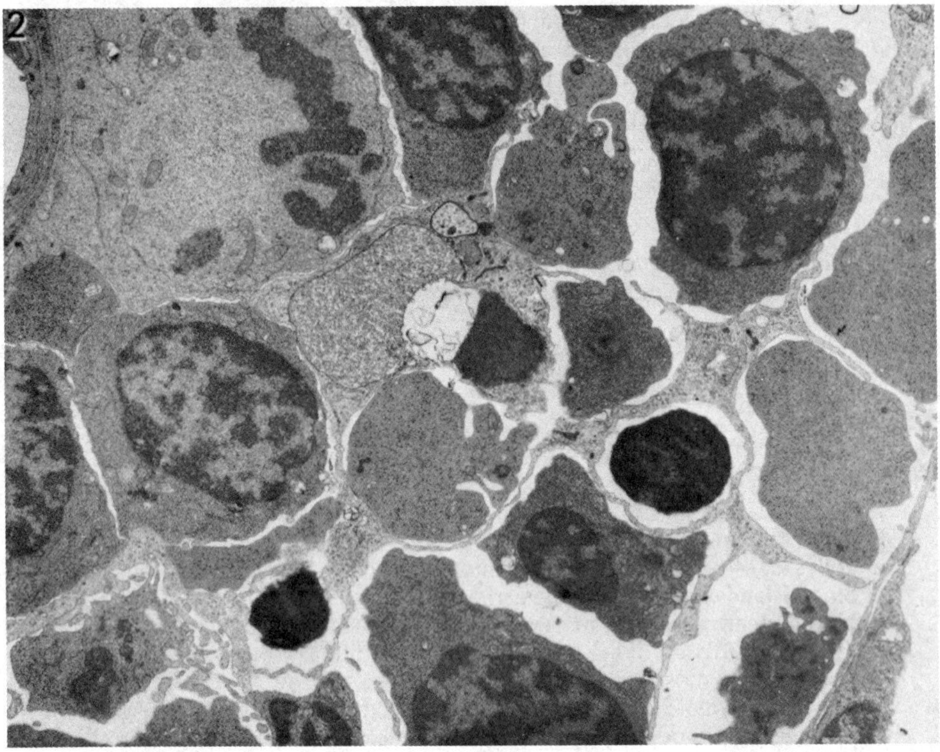

FIGURE 8-8. Electron micrograph of an erythroblastic island in bone marrow. A macrophage (*M*) extends cytoplasmic processes around the erythrocytes that surround it. Two erythrocyte nuclei that it has phagocytosed appear as very dark, roughly round masses in its peripheral cytoplasm. (Reprinted with permission from Dellmann H-D: *Textbook of Veterinary Histology,* 4th ed. Baltimore, Williams & Wilkins, 1993, p 65.)

(c) **Sinuses** are the blood vessels of the bone marrow. Newly formed blood cells enter the circulating blood through sinus walls.

(i) The **endothelium** is highly attenuated in some areas.

(ii) The **basal lamina** is discontinuous.

(iii) The **tunica adventitia** is a net-like layer of reticular cells and fibers that surrounds the sinus.

Reticular cells in the adventitia are contractile, and their processes are retractable. These properties enable them to regulate the rate of entry of newly formed blood cells by adjusting the available surface area.

At a site of entry, reticular cells withdraw and the basal lamina depolymerizes, allowing the new blood cells to press directly against the attenuated endothelium.

Transient migration pores form in the endothelial cytoplasm and close after one or a series of cells has passed through.

b. **Lymphatic organs** are sites of lymphopoiesis from bone marrow progenitor cells (see Chapter 12).

c. The **spleen** and **liver** can temporarily resume hemopoietic activity in severely anemic animals.

3. **Stem cells** (Figure 8-9). Blood cells divide repeatedly during development, giving rise to clones of cells at the same developmental stage.

a. **Pluripotential hematopoietic stem cells** are small cells that resemble lymphocytes. They are capable of unlimited self-replication and can give rise to any type of blood cell.

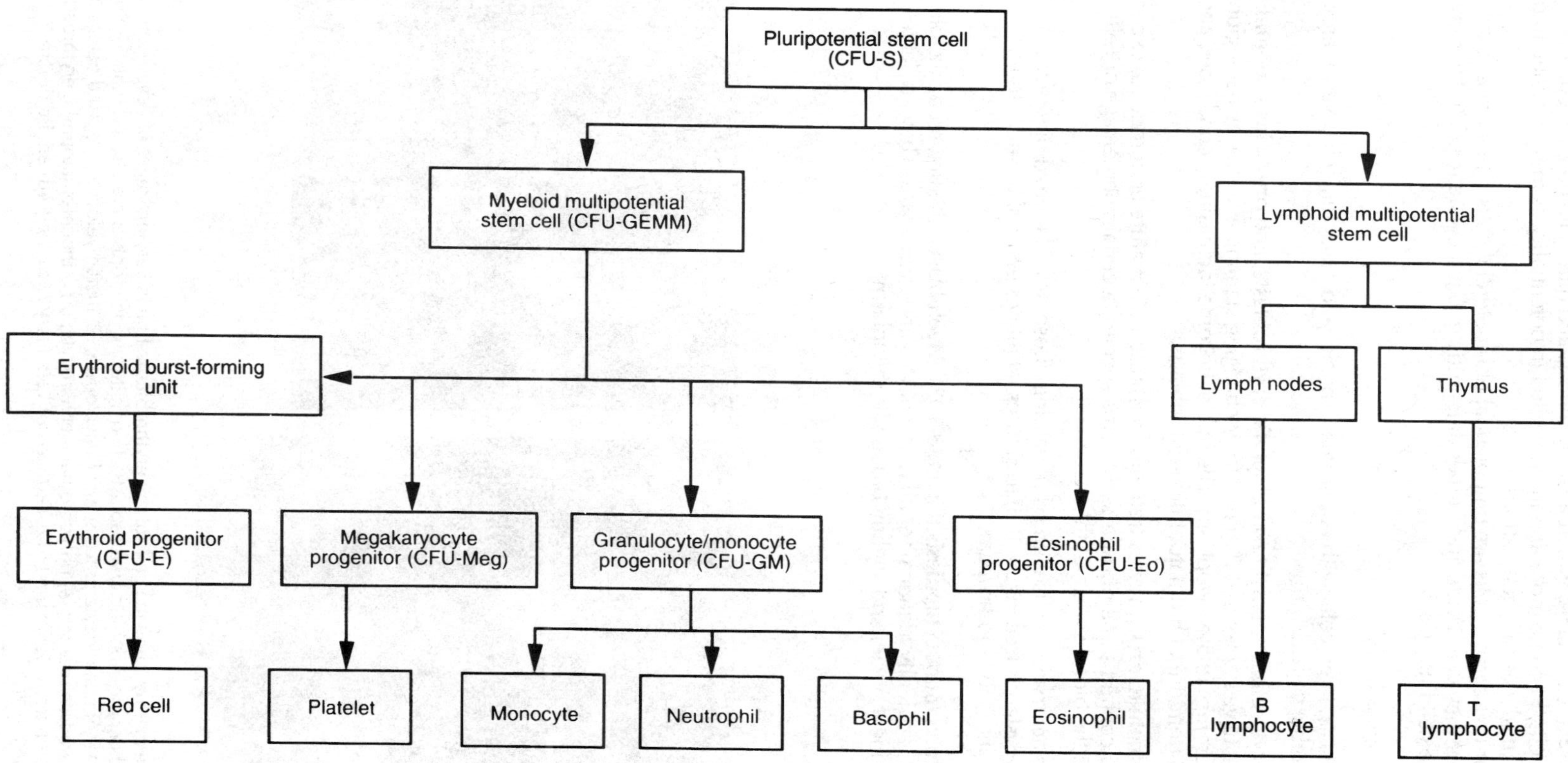

FIGURE 8-9. Stages during the formation of mature blood cells in bone marrow culture. The hemopoietic stem cells and various pluripotential, multipotential, and progenitor cells are represented. Colony-forming units (*CFUs*) are cells that form colonies of specific cell types. *CFU-S* = spleen; *CFU-GEMM* = mixed granulocyte/erythroid/monocyte/megakaryocyte; *CFU-E* = erythrocyte; *CFU-Meg* = megakaryocyte; *CFU-GM* = granulocyte/monocyte; *CFU-Eo* = eosinophil. (Reprinted with permission from Besa EC: NMS *Hematology*. Baltimore, Williams & Wilkins, 1992, p 13.)

   b. **Multipotential stem cells,** which arise by mitosis and differentiation from pluripotential stem cells, become more and more limited in potentiality as they continue to differentiate in succeeding generations.
   c. **Progenitor (precursor) cells** are unipotential or bipotential cells. They are also stem cells in that they can divide and further differentiate, but they are restricted to only one or two cell lineages.

B. Erythropoiesis (Figure 8-10A)

1. **Proerythroblasts,** large cells with euchromatic nuclei and basophilic cytoplasm, are the first recognizable cells.
2. **Basophilic erythroblasts, polychromatophilic erythroblasts,** and **orthochromatophilic erythroblasts** have names that describe their changing staining affinities as hemoglobin replaces ribosomes in the cytoplasm. The nuclei become increasingly condensed and are expelled from orthochromatophilic erythroblasts.
3. **Polychromatophilic erythrocytes** (reticulocytes) resemble mature erythrocytes, except that they still contain some ribosomes. In some species, a certain percentage of cells is released into the blood stream at this stage.
4. **Erythrocytes** are mature cells with no remaining ribosomes. The proximity of the erythroblastic islands (see Figure 8-8) to sinuses facilitates entry of the nonmotile erythrocytes into the blood stream.

C. Granulopoiesis and monocytopoiesis (Figure 8-10B). **Myeloblasts,** the first recognizable cells, are morphologically identical for all granulocytes and monocytes. They are large cells with prominent nuclei and slightly basophilic cytoplasm.

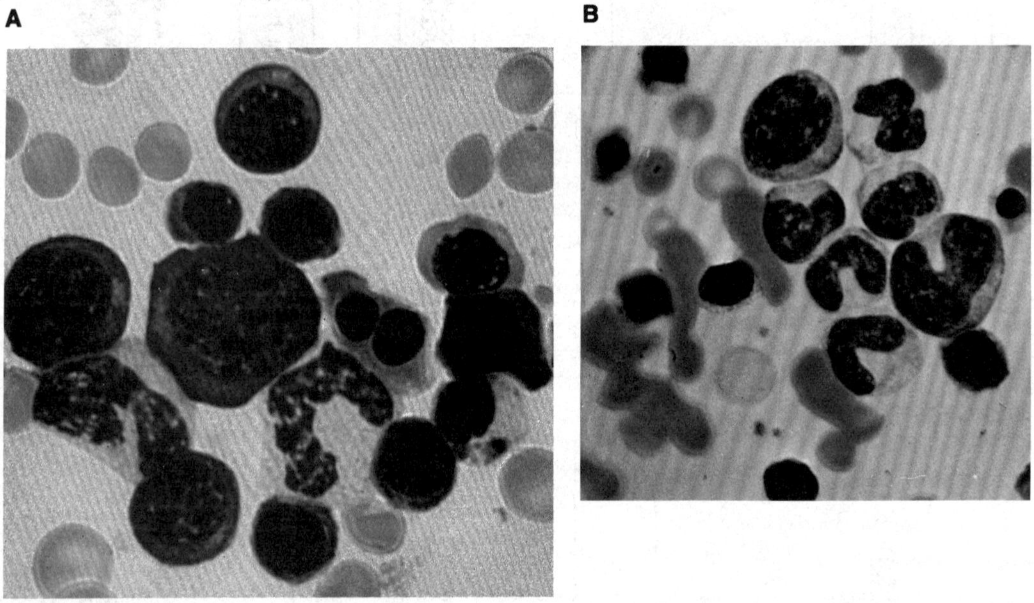

FIGURE 8-10. (*A*) Bone marrow showing cells of the erythroblastic line in varying stages of development from erythroblast to orthochromatophilic erythroblasts. Two maturing neutrophils are also present. (*B*) Bone marrow showing a cluster of granulocyte precursors: (*1*) myelocyte; (*2*) metamyelocyte; (*3*) band neutrophil. Erythrocyte precursors are also present: (*4*) polychromatic erythrocyte; (*5*) orthochromatophilic erythroblast. (Reprinted with permission from Dellmann H-D: *Textbook of Veterinary Histology,* 4th ed. Baltimore, Williams & Wilkins, 1993, p 70.)

1. **Granulopoiesis**
   a. **Promyelocytes** are produced by **granulopoietic myeloblasts**.
   b. **Early myelocytes** follow. They contain specific granules and can be identified as neutrophilic, eosinophilic, or basophilic myelocytes.
   c. **Late myelocytes** and then **metamyelocytes** have increasingly condensed and indented nuclei, and they progressively accumulate granules. An intermediate **band cell** stage, in which the nucleus resembles a curved rod or band, is recognized in developing neutrophils.
   d. **Mature neutrophils, eosinophils,** and **basophils** are characterized by lobulated nuclei and a full complement of granules. Lobulation of the nucleus becomes more pronounced with age.
2. **Monocytopoiesis**
   a. **Promonocytes** are produced by division of **monocytopoietic myeloblasts**.
   b. Mature monocytes are produced after promonocytes undergo two cell divisions.
3. Clones of developing leukocytes lie in the regions between sinuses. Mature leukocytes are motile and can migrate to the sinus wall.

D. Thrombopoiesis

1. **Megakaryoblasts** undergo endomitosis (i.e., nuclear division without cytoplasmic division), giving rise to megakaryocytes.
2. **Megakaryocytes** are huge cells with proportionately large, irregularly shaped nuclei (Figure 8-11) formed by the repeated chromosomal replication. Megakaryocytes lie along the surface of sinuses and extend cytoplasmic projections into the sinus lumen.
3. **Platelets** are formed by **demarcation systems**. Aligned invaginations of the cell membrane delineate compartments of peripheral cytoplasm. These membranes fuse, separating cytoplasmic fragments, the platelets, from the rest of the cell to be carried away in the blood.

E. Changes during maturation. All myeloid elements (except megakaryocytes) undergo common changes during maturation.

1. **Cells decrease dramatically in size** from the large progenitor cells (in which protein synthesis is very active) to the mature cells (in which protein synthesis is minimal). This decrease is nonlinear because of cycles of growth and division.
2. The **nuclei become smaller and more heterochromatic** as synthesis of specific cytoplasmic substances is gradually completed. Nuclei are lost in erythrocytes and become indented or lobulated in leukocytes.
3. The **ratio of nuclear volume to cytoplasmic volume decreases**. This ratio is the most dependable criterion for estimating maturity.
4. The early committed developmental stages (blasts) contain many ribosomes for rapid synthesis of granules or hemoglobin and are very basophilic. **Basophilia is replaced by specific cytoplasmic staining reactions** as the accumulating products gradually replace the organelles that produced them.

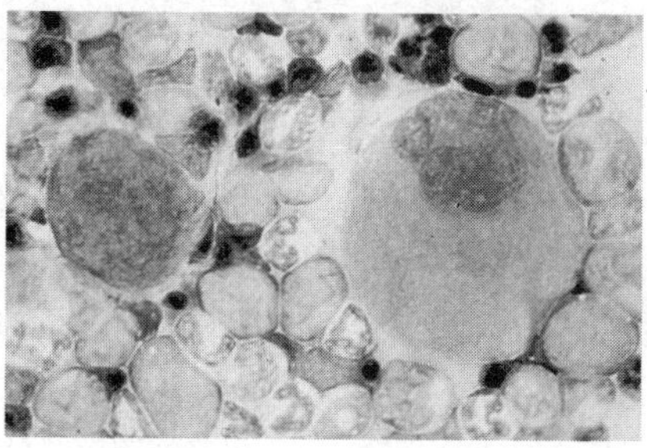

FIGURE 8-11. A megakaryoblast (*right*) and a megakaryocyte (*left*). (Reprinted with permission from Dellmann H-D: *Textbook of Veterinary Histology,* 4th ed. Baltimore, Williams & Wilkins, 1993, p 70.)

F. Factors affecting development and release of blood cells

1. **Development**
   a. **Iron** is essential for the **production of hemoglobin**.
   b. **Erythropoietin** (from the kidney), **granulopoietin** (from macrophages and lymphocytes), **thrombopoietin,** and **factors produced by bone marrow stromal cells** are among a variety of inducers and regulatory factors that regulate development.
   c. **Growth factors** act at three levels, but different factors act most effectively at different developmental stages.
      (1) They **stimulate mitosis of immature (progenitor) cells**.
      (2) They **support differentiation** of maturing cells.
      (3) They **enhance the function of mature cells**.

2. **Release**
   a. **Reserves.** The bone marrow stores a supply of mature leukocytes that far exceeds the number in the circulation.
      (1) Mature cells remain in the bone marrow for several days before they are released to the circulating blood.
      (2) Together, leukocytes in the bone marrow and marginated leukocytes form a ready reserve of defense cells.
   b. **Cell maturity.** The maturity of cells when they enter the blood varies among species.
      (1) Swine release relatively immature forms.
      (2) Horses release only mature cells.
   c. **Environmental stimuli**
      (1) **Stress** or **inflammation reactions** stimulate the release of neutrophils.
      (2) **Elevated blood histamine** stimulates eosinophil release.
      (3) **Gonadal and adrenal steroid hormones,** some **bacterial toxins,** and substances released during **immune responses** also act as releasing factors.

STUDY QUESTIONS

DIRECTIONS: Each of the numbered items or incomplete statements in this section is followed by answers or by completions of the statement. Select the **one** numbered answer or completion that is **best** in each case.

1. The entrance of leukocytes into the connective tissue begins with:

(1) migration.
(2) diapedesis.
(3) deformation.
(4) formation of rouleaux.
(5) margination.

2. Granules in leukocytes include:

(1) azurophilic granules in all types of leukocytes.
(2) specific azurophilic granules in monocytes.
(3) specific azurophilic granules in basophils.
(4) specific granules for each type of leukocyte.
(5) two types that are lysosomes.

3. In what way do lymphocytes resemble other leukocytes?

(1) They have a predictable lifespan in the blood.
(2) They are produced in the bone marrow.
(3) They are motile.
(4) They have a low nucleus-to-cytoplasm volume ratio.
(5) They function primarily in the blood.

4. Which of the following is a characteristic of monocytes?

(1) They are smaller than lymphocytes.
(2) They have the most lobulated of all leukocyte nuclei.
(3) They often have pseudopodia in blood smears.
(4) They have surface receptors for antigens.
(5) They are called microphages in the tissue.

5. Neutrophils can be recognized in any domestic species primarily by:

(1) the fact that their specific granules stain only with neutral dyes.
(2) their many large mitochondria.
(3) the absence of azurophilic granules.
(4) their basophilic cytoplasmic matrix.
(5) their highly lobulated and heterochromatic nucleus.

6. Which leukocytes are most involved in promoting the healing process?

(1) Lymphocytes
(2) Monocytes
(3) Neutrophils
(4) Eosinophils
(5) Basophils

7. Which leukocytes form foreign body giant cells?

(1) Lymphocytes
(2) Monocytes
(3) Neutrophils
(4) Eosinophils
(5) Basophils

8. Peroxidases, iron-binding protein, and polysaccharidases are characteristic of the granules in which cell type?

(1) Lymphocytes
(2) Monocytes
(3) Neutrophils
(4) Eosinophils
(5) Basophils

9. Which one of the following statements *best* describes bone marrow?

(1) The conversion of red bone marrow to yellow is irreversible.
(2) The stroma of red bone marrow is loose areolar connective tissue.
(3) New blood cells enter blood sinuses in bone marrow by passing between the endothelial cells.
(4) Hemopoiesis in bone marrow begins near the time of birth.
(5) Macrophages and reticular cells influence hemopoiesis.

10. Which one of the following statements *best* describes the parenchyma of bone marrow?

(1) Clones of developing cells are randomly distributed in the reticular connective tissue.
(2) The great majority of the cells are developing erythrocytes.
(3) Erythrocytes mature in close proximity to blood sinuses.
(4) Progenitor cells are the largest cells.
(5) Newly formed cells enter the sinuses as soon as they are mature.

11. Which of the following statements describes a pluripotential hemopoietic stem cell?

(1) It can produce only one or possibly two types of blood cells.
(2) It can produce an unlimited number of new copies of itself.
(3) It can produce any of several different types of blood cells, but it cannot reproduce itself.
(4) It can be recognized by its specific cytoplasmic staining.
(5) It can be recognized by its large size and intensely basophilic cytoplasm.

DIRECTIONS: Each of the numbered items or incomplete statements in this section is negatively phrased, as indicated by an italicized word such as *not, least,* or *except.* Select the **one** numbered answer or completion that is **best** in each case.

12. All of the following describe changes common to developing erythrocytes, granulocytes, and monocytes *except:*

(1) the cells become smaller.
(2) the nuclei become smaller.
(3) the nuclei become more heterochromatic.
(4) the nucleus-to-cytoplasm volume ratio increases.
(5) the cytoplasm becomes less basophilic.

13. All of the following statements correctly describe factors that affect the development or release of blood cells from the bone marrow *except:*

(1) iron is essential for hemoglobin production in erythropoiesis.
(2) most growth factors act only at a specific stage of hemopoiesis.
(3) histamine causes release of eosinophils.
(4) stress stimulates release of neutrophils.
(5) in some species, cells are normally released before they are fully mature.

14. All of the following are erythropoietic organs at some stage of development *except* the:

(1) spleen.
(2) yolk sac.
(3) bone marrow.
(4) liver.
(5) thymus.

ANSWERS AND EXPLANATIONS

1. The answer is 5 *[II B 1 b (1)].* Margination (i.e., the accumulation and adhesion of leukocytes to endothelial walls) is the first step in the movement of leukocytes from the blood stream to the connective tissue. Margination is followed by diapedesis, or movement through the wall of the vessel, after which migration may occur. Deformation occurs during diapedesis when the cells squeeze through small temporary gaps in the vessel wall. Rouleaux formation (i.e., "stacking" of erythrocytes) is seen in some species.

2. The answer is 1 *[II B 1 a].* All types of leukocytes contain lysosomal azurophilic granules, although they are often too small to see with the light microscope. Monocytes have no specific granules, and the specific granules in basophils are basophilic. Only the granulocytes (i.e., neutrophils, eosinophils, and basophils) have specific granules; the agranulocytes (i.e., monocytes and lymphocytes) have none. There are three types of lysosomal granules: azurophilic granules and the specific granules in eosinophils and neutrophils.

3. The answer is 3 *[II B 1 b].* All leukocytes are motile. Lifespans of different types of lymphocytes range from hours to years. Lymphocyte stem cells are produced in the bone marrow, but lymphocytes develop in lymphatic organs, unlike all the other leukocytes. Their nucleus-to-cytoplasm volume ratio is high; the nucleus is surrounded by only a small amount of cytoplasm. No type of leukocyte functions primarily in the blood.

4. The answer is 3 *[II B 3].* Monocytes begin to migrate on the glass slide as soon as blood smears are prepared and can often be identified by the pseudopodia that were extended when they died. They are the largest cells in circulating blood; lymphocytes are usually the smallest of the nucleated cells. Monocyte nuclei are less lobulated than those of the granulocytes. They have surface receptors for antibodies, such as immunoglobulin G (IgG), not for antigens. After entering the tissue, they convert to macrophages, not microphages.

5. The answer is 5 *[II B 4 a (1)].* Mature neutrophils in all species have the most lobulated nuclei of any leukocytes. They are named for the staining reaction of their specific granules in humans, which stain with neutral dyes. Although the same staining reaction is seen in many domestic species, the granules are intensely acidophilic in poultry. They are also acidophilic in rabbits and guinea pigs. Neutrophils contain few mitochondria because they derive much of their energy by anaerobic pathways. This permits them to operate effectively in tissues where the blood supply has been compromised or destroyed. All leukocytes have azurophilic granules. The cytoplasmic matrix of neutrophils is acidophilic.

6. The answer is 2 *[II B 3 b (4)].* Monocytes, which become macrophages when they enter tissue, promote healing by phagocytosing the debris of damaged tissue and secreting growth factors that promote tissue repair and revascularization. Lymphocytes are involved with immunity. Neutrophils phagocytose pathogenic bacteria. Eosinophils have some functions that tend to reduce inflammation, but they also secrete substances that contribute to tissue damage. Basophils help initiate the inflammation response.

7. The answer is 2 *[II B 3 b (1) (b) (i)].* Macrophages, formed from monocytes in the tissue, fuse to form multinucleated foreign body giant cells, enabling them to phagocytose large particles. They can also cooperate to wall off focal infections by forming epithelioid walls.

8. The answer is 3 *[II B 4 b (3)].* Peroxidases (which produce bactericidal superoxides), the iron-binding protein lactoferrin (which deprives bacteria of an essential mineral), and polysaccharidases (which break down bacterial cell walls) are among the bacteria-fighting substances in neutrophil granules.

9. The answer is 5 *[III A 2 a (2) (a)].* Both reticular cells and macrophages produce substances that influence hemopoiesis. In addition, macrophages are intimately involved with groups of developing erythrocytes, and they remove defective cells. Yellow bone marrow, which develops in the diaphyses of long and some short bones during growth, can revert to red marrow by resuming its hemopoietic activity when needed. The stroma of bone marrow is reticular connective tissue. New blood cells enter blood sinuses in bone marrow by passing through temporary channels that form in the attenuated cytoplasm of endothelial cells, rather than by passing between the cells. By the time of birth, the bone marrow is already responsible for most hemopoiesis.

10. The answer is 3 *[III B 4]*. Erythroblastic islands (clones of developing erythrocytes surrounding a macrophage) and megakaryocytes are adjacent to sinuses, making it easier for the nonmotile erythrocytes and platelets to enter the circulation. Clones of developing leukocytes are some distance from the sinuses because mature leukocytes can migrate to the blood stream. Approximately equal numbers of developing erythrocytes, neutrophils, and eosinophils are present. Megakaryocytes are by far the largest cells. Mature leukocytes typically are stored in the bone marrow for several days before entering the sinuses.

11. The answer is 2 *[III A 3 a; Figure 8-9]*. A pluripotential hemopoietic stem cell (also called a CFU-S) is capable of unlimited self-replication, and it can produce any type of blood cell. It has no specific cytoplasmic staining. It is a small cell that resembles a lymphocyte. Progenitor cells, in which active synthesis of the characteristic granules of leukocytes or hemoglobin of erythrocytes is underway, are large and basophilic.

12. The answer is 4 *[III E 3]*. During the maturation process, the ratio of the nucleus-to-cytoplasm volume ratio of erythrocytes, granulocytes, and monocytes decreases because the nucleus decreases proportionately more in size than does the rest of the cell. In all myeloid elements (except megakaryocytes), the cells become smaller, the nuclei become more heterochromatic, and the cytoplasm becomes less basophilic.

13. The answer is 2 *[III F 1 c]*. Most growth factors act broadly to increase the number and effect of their target cells. They typically act at three levels: stimulating cell division in progenitor cells, promoting differentiation of cells in intermediate stages of maturation, and enhancing the function of mature cells.

14. The answer is 5 *[III A 1–2]*. The thymus is a site of lymphopoiesis but not of the development of erythrocytes or other blood elements. The spleen, yolk sac, bone marrow, and liver all participate in erythropoiesis.

Chapter 9

Nervous Tissue

I. INTRODUCTION

A. **Nervous tissue** comprises neurons and neuroglial (glial) cells.

1. **Neurons** are excitable cells specialized for the generation, conduction, and transmission of impulses.
2. **Neuroglial cells** play an essential role in support and protection of neurons, regulation of the extracellular environment, immune responses, and damage repair.
   a. In the **central nervous system (CNS),** they include **astrocytes, oligodendrocytes, ependymal cells, choroid plexus cells,** and **microglial cells.**
   b. In the **peripheral nervous system (PNS),** the neuroglial cells are **Schwann cells** (neurolemmocytes).

B. The **CNS** comprises the brain and spinal cord.

1. **Brain**
   a. **Gray matter,** which primarily consists of neurons and neuroglial cells, is present superficially in the **cortex** and deep within the hemispheres as clusters of nerve cell bodies called **nuclei**.
   b. **White matter,** which primarily consists of myelinated axons and neuroglial cells, is present deep to the cortex. It forms tracts that connect different regions of gray matter in the brain and spinal cord.
2. **Spinal cord**
   a. **Gray matter** occupies the center of the cord, forming an H-shape in cross-section.
   b. **White matter** forms tracts that are superficial to the gray matter.

C. The **PNS** includes nerves, ganglia, and efferent and afferent terminals.

1. **Nerves** are composed of **fascicles** of nerve fibers (axons and their associated Schwann cell sheaths) and the connective tissue sheaths that surround the fascicles. Cranial nerves arise from the brain, and spinal nerves arise from the spinal cord.
2. **Ganglia** are accumulations of nerve cells and associated neuroglial cells in the course of a nerve (e.g., spinal ganglion).
3. **Efferent terminals** are axon terminals that contact an effector (e.g., muscle cells).
4. **Afferent terminals** are specialized for reception of various stimuli.

II. NEURONS

A. Components

1. **Perikaryon (cell body).** The perikaryon comprises a nucleus and the surrounding cytoplasm (Figure 9-1).
   a. **Nucleus.** The nucleus of a neuron is usually located in the center of the perikaryon.
      (1) It is **euchromatic** because of the high activity level of the cell.
      (2) A **nucleolus** is prominent.

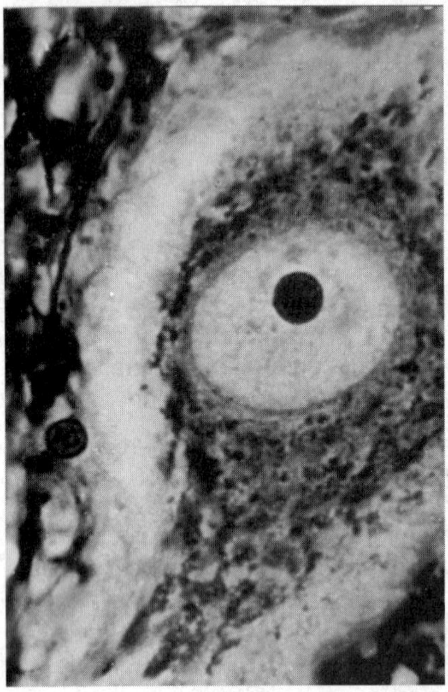

FIGURE 9-1. In this perikaryon of a spinal cord motor neuron, the euchromatic nucleus, containing a large nucleolus, is surrounded by cytoplasm in which the chromatic Nissl substance is evident. Notice that the large dendrite, which leaves the cell toward the lower left corner, also contains chromatophilic substance. (Reprinted with permission from Dellmann H-D: *Textbook of Veterinary Histology,* 4th ed. Baltimore, Williams & Wilkins, 1993, p 3.)

b. Cytoplasm. The cytoplasm is rich in organelles involved in the synthesis of substances for maintenance of the cell and transmitter production.

(1) **Nissl substance (Nissl bodies, chromatophilic substance)** creates intensely basophilic granular areas that occupy most of the perikaryal cytoplasm. It is composed of aggregates of parallel cisternae of rough endoplasmic reticulum (rER), free ribosomes, and polyribosomes.

(a) **rER** is involved in the synthesis of proteins (e.g., secretory, lysosomal, and membrane proteins).

(b) **Free ribosomes** and **polyribosomes** are involved in the synthesis of proteins that help maintain cell structure and function, such as cytoskeletal proteins.

(2) The **Golgi complex** is prominent in all neuronal cell bodies, but it is especially extensive in neurosecretory neurons (e.g., vasopressin- and oxytocin-secreting hypothalamic neurons).

(3) **Mitochondria** and **lysosomes** are prominent.

(4) **Smooth endoplasmic reticulum (sER)** is usually inconspicuous.

(5) **Cytoskeletal elements** include abundant neurofilaments and microtubules. Microtubules play an important role in the cellular transport of membrane-bound organelles (e.g., secretory and synaptic vesicles, mitochondria).

(6) **Lipofuscin** inclusions commonly occur in neurons and become more numerous in aging neurons.

(7) **Melanin** is present in neurons of the substantia nigra.

2. **Dendrites** are thick processes that originate from the perikaryon and divide repeatedly into increasingly thinner branches. Most neurons have multiple dendrites.

a. Cytoplasm. The dendritic cytoplasm resembles that of the perikaryon.

(1) **Ribosomes, polyribosomes,** and **rER** are abundant in large dendrites but are sparse or absent in smaller ones.

(2) A **Golgi complex** is present in the largest trunks but absent in the smaller ones.

(3) **Microtubules** are numerous.

(4) **Neurofilaments** are usually present in low numbers.

(5) **sER** cisternae and tubules are conspicuous, especially at increasing distances from the perikaryon.

(6) **Mitochondria** are especially numerous in small dendrites.

b. Synaptic contacts made on dendrites by axons of other neurons are numerous. Contacts are either directly on the **dendritic trunk** or on **dendritic spines,** small projections of varying structure, shape, and size.

3. **Axons.** Most neurons have only one axon, a cell process with a constant diameter and few to no collateral branches. **Telodendria** are the numerous terminal branches of the axon.
   a. **Structure.** The structure of the axon varies regionally.
      (1) The **axon hillock** is the region in the perikaryon or large dendrite from which the axon originates. It is characterized by the absence of rER and free ribosomes and the presence of fascicles of neurofilaments and microtubules.
      (2) The **initial segment** is adjacent to the axon hillock. This portion of the axon has the lowest threshold for the generation and propagation of an action potential.
         (a) The **axolemma** (cell membrane of axons) contains numerous **ion channels** that function in the transmembrane movements of ions associated with the generation of an action potential.
         (b) A **subaxolemmal layer,** which is thin and electron dense, is characteristically present.
         (c) **Neurofilaments and microtubules** are bundled.
      (3) The **remainder of the axon,** except at synapses, has a rather uniform structure.
         (a) **Microtubules and neurofilaments.** In large axons, microtubules are fewer than in dendrites, and neurofilaments predominate. In small axons, microtubules predominate. Microtubules, together with microtubule-associated proteins, function in **axonal transport.**
            (i) **Slow anterograde transport** moves neurofilaments, microtubules, actin filaments, and proteins for use by the axon at a rate of up to 5 mm/day.
            (ii) **Fast anterograde transport** moves mitochondria and vesicles at a rate of up to 400 mm/day.
            (iii) **Fast retrograde transport** carries aging organelles and endocytic vesicles back to the perikaryon at a rate of 200–300 mm/day.
         (b) **sER** cisternae are common.
         (c) **Mitochondria** are present.
         (d) **Actin filaments** are located underneath the axolemma.

B. Polarization. Neurons are functionally and structurally polarized (Figure 9-2).

1. The **dendritic zone** receives input, which results in excitation (depolarization) of the cell membrane. This zone comprises all dendritic branches of the neuron.

2. The **telodendritic zone** transmits excitation to another cell. The telodendritic zone usually consists of multiple terminal tree-like branches. Neurotransmitters are stored in and released from the dilated branch ends, which are the presynaptic elements of synapses.

3. The **axon** has few or no branches. It conducts the wave of depolarization from the dendritic zone to the telodendritic zone.

C. Anatomic classification of neurons (Figure 9-3) is based on the number of cell processes (i.e., axons, dendrites).

1. **Multipolar neurons.** Most neurons are multipolar.
   a. Large and multiple dendrites originate from almost the entire perikaryal surface, thereby including the perikaryon topographically in the dendritic zone.
   b. A single axon is present.

2. **Bipolar neurons** are present in the ganglion of the vestibulocochlear nerve, the retina, and the olfactory mucosa.
   a. The perikaryon is located in the course of the axon.
   b. The dendritic zone is near the perikaryon.
   c. The telodendritic zone is at a distance from the perikaryon.

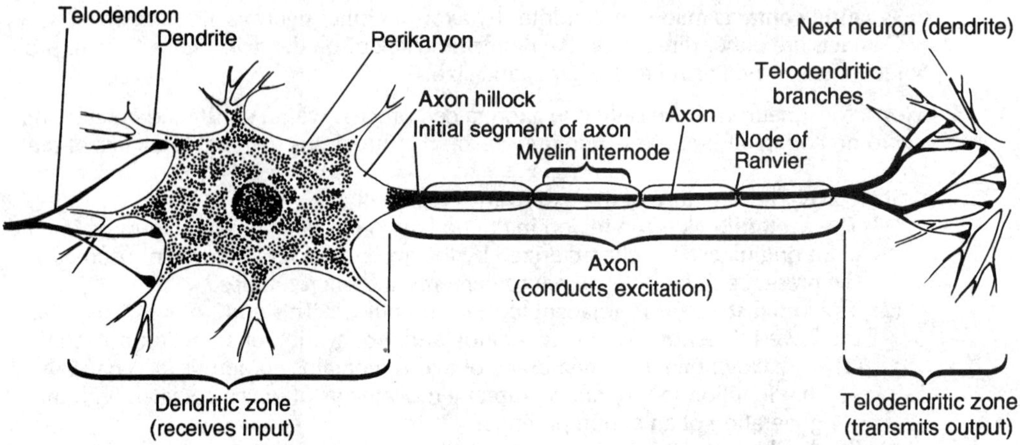

FIGURE 9-2. Schematic drawing of a multipolar neuron in the central nervous system (CNS). Multiple dendrites with many branches originate from the perikaryon and constitute the dendritic zone, which receives synaptic input. Synapses also occur in the perikaryon. A single unbranched myelinated axon connects the dendritic zone and perikaryon to the telodendritic zone (i.e., the terminal branches of the axon), which are in synaptic contact with dendrites and perikaryon of another neuron. (Redrawn with permission from Dellmann H-D: *Textbook of Veterinary Histology,* 4th ed. Baltimore, Williams & Wilkins, 1993, p 88.)

3. **Unipolar (pseudounipolar) neurons** are characteristic of spinal and cranial sensory ganglia.
   - **a.** A single axon originates from the perikaryon and gives rise to two branches.
   - **b.** The dendritic zone is at the end of the longer peripheral branch.
   - **c.** The telodendritic zone is at the end of the shorter central branch.

III. SYNAPSES. A synapse is the site of contact between an axon and another neuron, a muscle cell, or a glandular cell.

A. Components.
Typically, a synapse comprises a presynaptic element, a synaptic cleft, and a postsynaptic element (Figure 9-4), but variations do occur.

1. **Presynaptic element**
   - **a. Terminal bulbs (*boutons terminaux*)** are telodendritic terminal expansions of variable shape (e.g., club, bulb, basket).
   - **b. Preterminal bulbs (*boutons de passage*)** are preterminal axon expansions. The **inner leaflet** of the terminal and preterminal bulb cell membranes is characterized by increased thickness and cone-shaped, electron-dense protrusions.
   - **c. Synaptic vesicles** of varying shapes and sizes are the most conspicuous presynaptic organelles.
     - **(1) Spherical electron-lucent vesicles** (40–50 nm in diameter) are most common. They are characteristic of terminals that contain the neurotransmitter acetylcholine (ACh).
     - **(2) Spherical electron-dense vesicles** (40–60 nm in diameter) are characteristic for monoamine neurotransmitters, such as norepinephrine, dopamine, and serotonin.
   - **d. Other presynaptic organelles** include mitochondria, tubular smooth axoplasmic reticulum, occasional microtubules, and neurofilaments.
2. The **synaptic cleft** is a narrow (15–20 nm) extracellular space that separates presynaptic and postsynaptic elements.

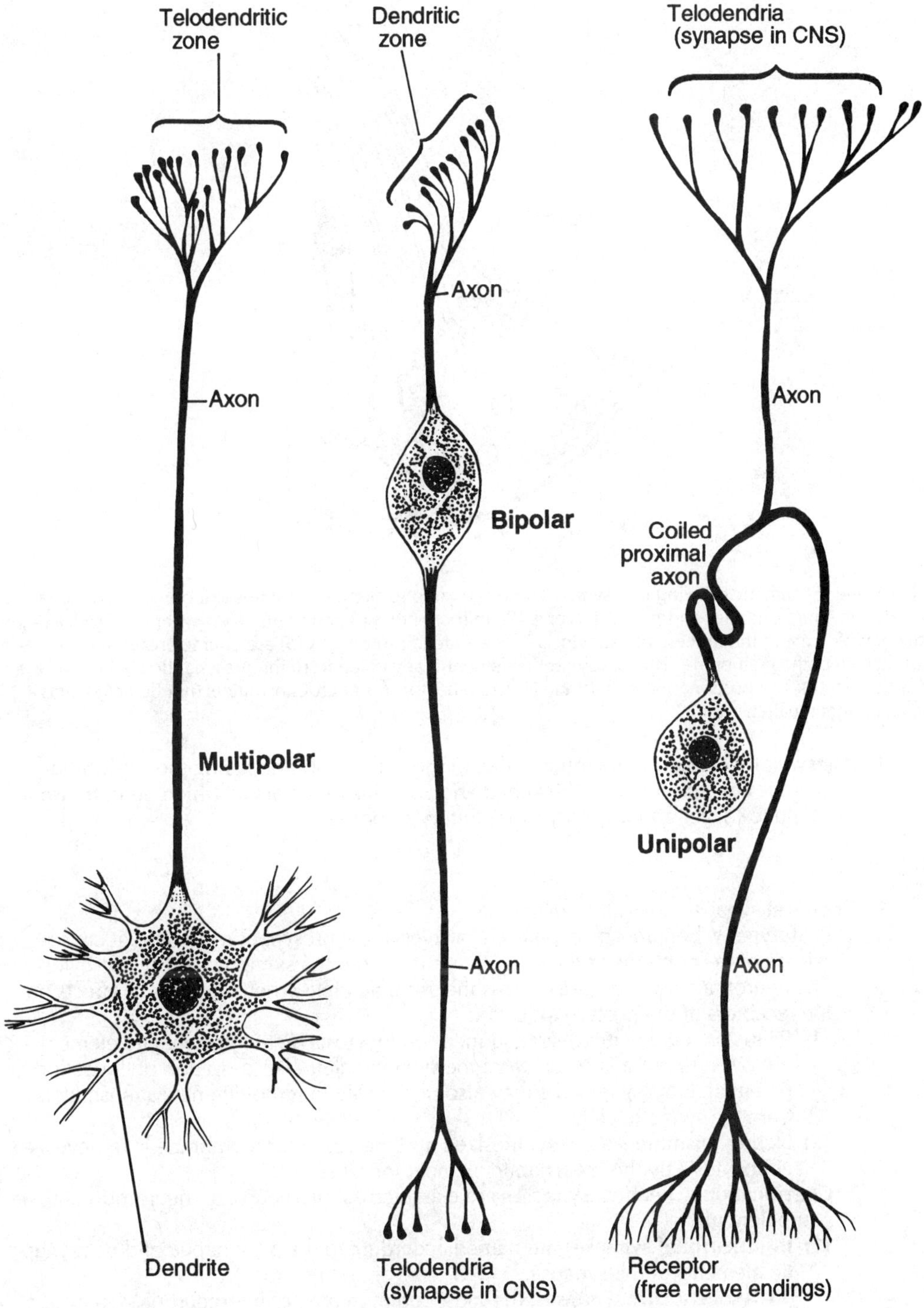

FIGURE 9-3. Schematic drawing of a multipolar neuron, a bipolar neuron, and a unipolar neuron. Classification of neurons is based on the number of cellular processes. Notice the input-receiving dendritic zones and their relationship to the perikarya, the output-transmitting telodendritic zones, and the connecting axons. *CNS* = central nervous system. (Redrawn from Dellmann H-D: *Textbook of Veterinary Histology,* 4th ed. Baltimore, Williams & Wilkins, 1993, p 89.)

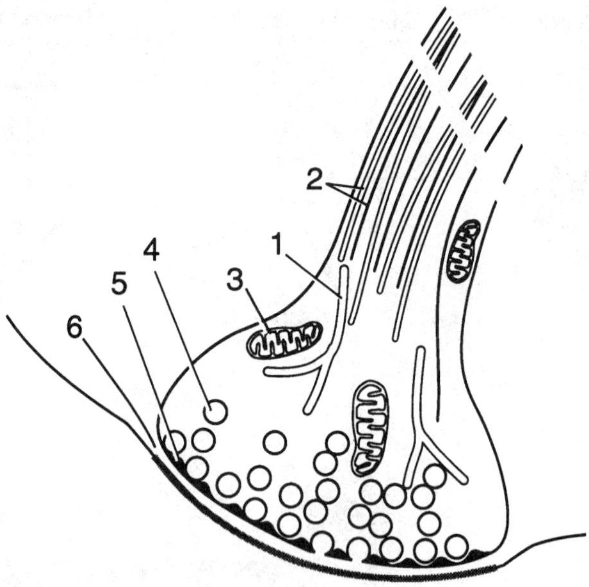

FIGURE 9-4. Schematic drawing of a synapse. The presynaptic element contains smooth axoplasmic reticulum (*1*), a few microtubules and neurofilaments (*2*), mitochondria (*3*), and numerous synaptic vesicles (*4*), some of which are in the process of exocytosis. Cone-shaped protrusions (*5*) are characteristic of the cytoplasmic face of the membrane. The postsynaptic element is separated from the presynaptic element by the synaptic cleft (*6*). The postsynaptic membrane (*7*) has receptors for neurotransmitters (not depicted) and a thickened inner leaflet.

3. **Postsynaptic element.** The inner leaflet of the cell membrane facing the presynaptic element is characteristically thickened and contains receptors to which neurotransmitters bind to trigger an excitatory or inhibitory response.

B. Types

1. **Chemical synapses** prevail in mammals.
   a. **Prototype.** When an action potential arrives at the presynaptic element, it causes release of the contents of the synaptic vesicles into the synaptic cleft by exocytosis. The neurotransmitter diffuses across the synaptic cleft, where it exerts its effects on the receptors of the postsynaptic cleft.
      (1) Diffusion, enzymatic degradation, or endocytosis by the presynaptic element removes neurotransmitters from the synaptic cleft after cessation of the action potential. Neuroglial cells may also play a role in removing neurotransmitters from the synaptic cleft.
      (2) Neurotransmitters are resynthesized and the vesicular membrane is retrieved via endocytosis by the presynaptic element for reuse.
   b. **Classification.** Chemical synapses are classified as interneuronal, neuromuscular, or neuroglandular.
      (1) **Interneuronal synapses** are named according to the presynaptic and postsynaptic elements of the synapse.
         (a) **Axodendritic synapses,** the most common type of interneuronal synapse, occur between an axon and a dendrite.
         (b) **Axosomatic synapses** occur between an axon and a perikaryon.
         (c) **Axoaxonic synapses** usually occur at the initial segment of the axon, where they are most effective in initiating an action potential. When they occur at a terminal or preterminal bulb, they are inhibitory (presynaptic inhibition).
         (d) **Dendrodendritic and dendrosomatic synapses** are relatively rare.

(2) Neuromuscular synapses (myoneuronal junctions). Efferent fibers in the PNS, both somatic and autonomic fibers, end in a synapse on muscle cells.

(a) Components (Figure 9-5)

(i) The **motor end-plate** is composed of short telodendritic branches that terminate as bulbous expansions embedded into troughs in an oval zone of the skeletal muscle fiber, called the **sole plate**.

The surface of the axon that is not in contact with the muscle fiber is covered by a single layer of Schwann cells.

The bulbous expansions contain numerous ACh-containing synaptic vesicles and mitochondria.

(ii) The **synaptic cleft** contains a basal lamina, to which acetylcholinesterase is anchored to ensure rapid removal of ACh.

(iii) The **sole plate** is the postsynaptic element. This area of the sarcoplasm contains many nuclei, mitochondria, rER, free ribosomes, and glycogen, but no myofibrils. At the troughs, the sarcolemma forms deep junctional folds filled with basal lamina.

(b) Locations

(i) Skeletal muscle. The ordinary fibers of the skeletal muscle mass, **extrafusal fibers,** are innervated by motor end-plates. Motor end-plate terminals also occur between efferent fusimotor fibers (gamma motoneurons) and **intrafusal muscle fibers** in **muscle spindles** (see Figure 9-6).

(ii) Cardiac muscle. Autonomic axons form preterminal and terminal bulbs that contact cardiac myocytes, especially in the sinoatrial node.

(iii) Smooth muscle. Neuromuscular synapses are formed on smooth muscle fibers by presynaptic autonomic nerve fibers ensheathed by Schwann cells. Multiple preterminal dilatations closely contact smooth muscle cells, which have no postsynaptic specialization.

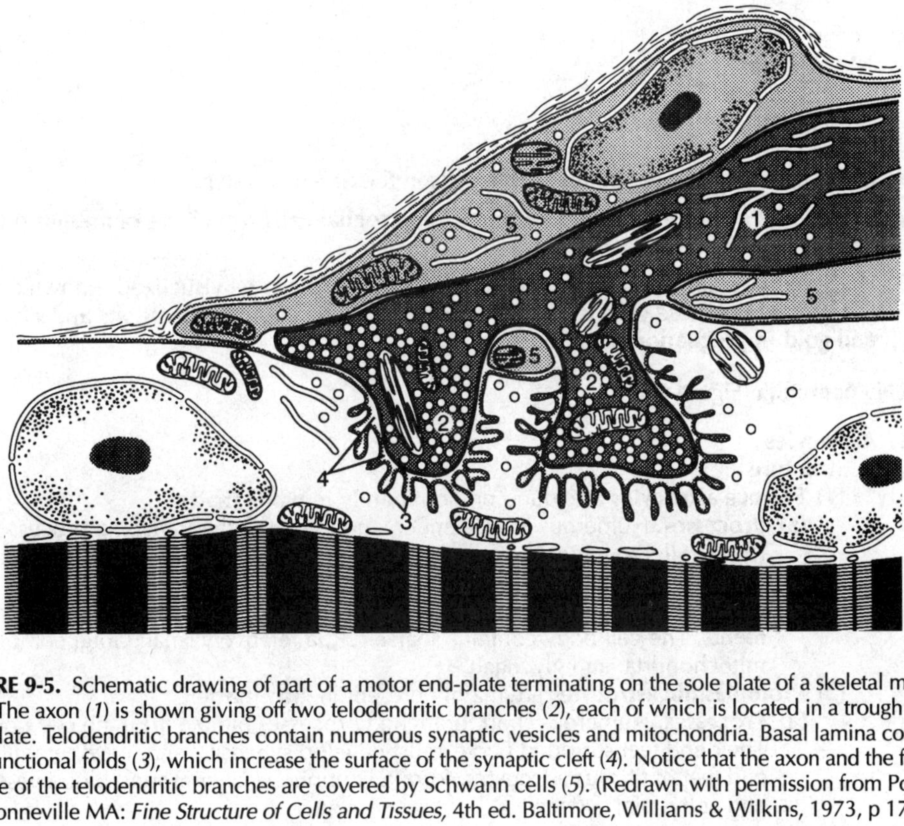

FIGURE 9-5. Schematic drawing of part of a motor end-plate terminating on the sole plate of a skeletal muscle fiber. The axon (*1*) is shown giving off two telodendritic branches (*2*), each of which is located in a trough of the sole plate. Telodendritic branches contain numerous synaptic vesicles and mitochondria. Basal lamina continues into junctional folds (*3*), which increase the surface of the synaptic cleft (*4*). Notice that the axon and the free surface of the telodendritic branches are covered by Schwann cells (*5*). (Redrawn with permission from Porter KR, Bonneville MA: *Fine Structure of Cells and Tissues,* 4th ed. Baltimore, Williams & Wilkins, 1973, p 174.)

(3) **Neuroglandular synapses** have a structure similar to that of neuromuscular synapses.

2. **Electrical synapses** occur mainly in lower vertebrates and invertebrates. Communication among neurons occurs through gap junctions (**electrotonic coupling**).

C. **Receptors** are structures in the dendritic zone of a neuron. They transform stimuli into action potentials, which are transmitted to the CNS by afferent axons.

1. **Classification.** Receptors may be classified according to various criteria:
   a. **Source of stimulus** (e.g., proprioceptors, exteroceptors, interoceptors)
   b. **Type of stimulus energy** (e.g., chemoreceptors, photoreceptors, sound receptors, mechanoreceptors, nociceptors, thermoreceptors)
   c. **Structure** (e.g., free nonencapsulated receptors, encapsulated receptors)
2. **Free nonencapsulated receptors** are the most common type of nerve ending.
   a. This type of receptor, which is almost ubiquitous, includes mechano- and thermoreceptors.
   b. Free nonencapsulated receptors are found among epidermal keratinocytes and between the cells of the external root sheath and in the dermal sheath of hair follicles (see Chapter 20 II C 2).
   c. Tactile disks are formed by the association of free nerve terminals and Merkel cells in the epidermis (see Chapter 20 II A 2 b).
3. **Encapsulated receptors** comprise one or several nerve endings, often associated with nonneuronal cells, that are surrounded by a connective tissue capsule.
   a. Table 9-1 summarizes the characteristics of the most common encapsulated receptors.
   b. A neuromuscular spindle, one of the more complex encapsulated receptors, is illustrated in Figure 9-6.

IV. NEUROGLIA

A. Introduction

1. Neuroglial cells are the **nonexcitable cells** in the nervous system.
2. They are of **ectodermal origin, except for microglial cells,** which are of **mesodermal origin**.
3. With routine stains, only the nuclei of neuroglial cells can be visualized. Knowledge of the structure of these cells is based on **electron microscopic observations** and **silver- and gold-impregnation techniques**.

B. CNS neuroglia (Figure 9-7)

1. **Astrocytes**
   a. **Structure**
      (1) **Fibrous astrocytes** are found predominantly in **white matter**.
         (a) **Processes.** Numerous long, slender, and infrequently branching processes run parallel to nerve fibers in the white matter. They terminate as expansions or **end feet** around blood vessels and at the pial surface.
         (b) **Cytoplasm.** Fibrous astrocytes contain numerous **intermediate (glial) filaments**. The cell body contains sparse rER, a relatively small Golgi complex, mitochondria, and glycogen.
      (2) **Protoplasmic astrocytes** are mainly present in **gray matter**.
         (a) **Processes.** Numerous short, branched processes radiate from the cell body. Their end feet surround nerve cells, envelop synapses, and, together with the end feet of fibrous astrocytes, form a continuous layer around blood vessels and at the pial surface.

TABLE 9-1. Encapsulated Receptors

Receptor	Shape	Capsule	Innervation	Function	Location
Touch (Meissner's) corpuscle	Bulb-shaped	Perineural cells encapsulate horizontally stacked, flattened Schwann cells; delicate collagen fibrils are attached to the perineural cells	Several myelinated axons enter corpuscle at pole opposite the epidermis and give rise to many nonmyelinated dendritic branches that penetrate and terminate within the Schwann cell stack	Touch	Dermis (reticular layer) of hairless skin
Lamellar (pacinian) corpuscle	Ellipsoid	A thin layer of connective tissue encapsulates several concentric layers of flattened fibrocytes; fluid-filled spaces separate the fibrocytic layers	A single nonmyelinated dendritic terminal surrounded by several layers of interdigitating Schwann cells forms the core of the corpuscle	Vibration	Footpads, mesentery, pancreas (particularly in the cat)
Bulbous corpuscle	Various	Perineural cells and a thin layer of connective tissue	Coiled, nonmyelinated dendritic terminals and Schwann cells form the core of the corpuscle	Unknown, possibly thermoreceptors	Various, including genitals, skin, mouth, and conjunctiva
Neurotendinous spindle (Golgi tendon organ)	Elongated	Several lamellae of perineural cells	Dendritic nonmyelinated branches of a single axon contact bundles of collagen fibers that are continuous with the collagen fibers of the tendon	Maintain muscle tension, play a role in proprioception	Junction between muscle and tendon
Neuromuscular spindle	Elongated	Several lamellae of perineural cells; a thin, fluid-filled space separates the lamellae from the thin connective tissue capsule	Afferent Primary: Annulospiral endings surround the center of nuclear chain and nuclear bag (intrafusal) muscle fibers Secondary: Flower-spray endings terminate on nuclear chain fibers Efferent: Fusimotor fibers (gamma motoneurons) terminate on nuclear bag and nuclear chain fibers	Maintenance of posture, regulation of muscle tone, control of the activity of antagonistic muscle groups involved in movement	Skeletal muscle

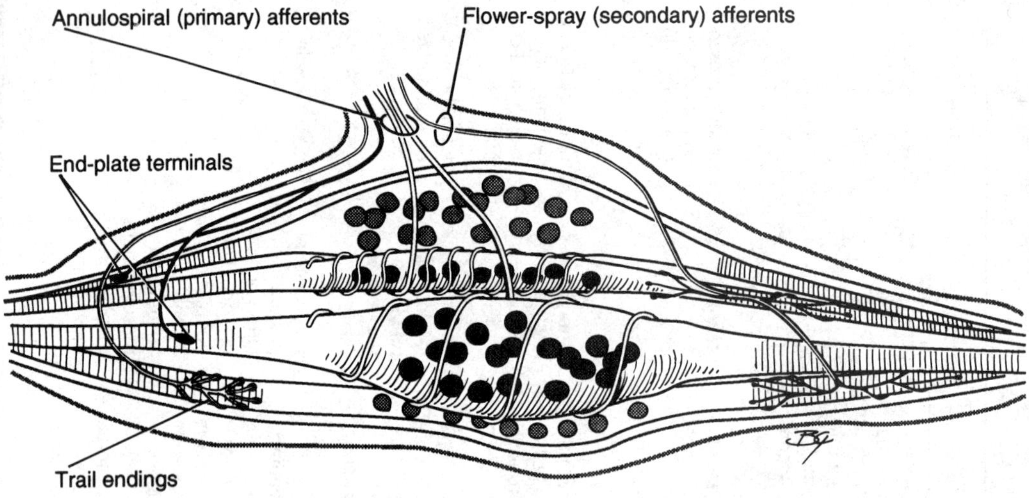

FIGURE 9-6. Schematic drawing of a muscle spindle. The muscle spindle is surrounded by a capsule of perineural cells that are continuous with those of the nerve fascicle whose fibers innervate the spindle. Intrafusal muscle fibers comprise nuclear bag fibers and nuclear chain fibers. Nuclear bag fibers contain numerous nuclei in a central thickened (bag-like) area. Nuclear chain fibers are of uniform diameter and contain nuclei in a chain in their center. The intrafusal fibers are surrounded by a thin connective tissue capsule whose collagen fibers attach to the perineural capsule at the poles of the spindle. Primary (annulospiral) sensory endings spiral around the center of both types of intrafusal muscle fibers; secondary (flower-spray) sensory endings are located more peripherally and prevail on nuclear chain fibers. Fusimotor (gamma motoneurons) form end-plate terminals on nuclear bag fibers and trail endings on nuclear chain fibers. These efferent terminals maintain muscle fibers at a tension just below the threshold of the stretch receptors.

(b) **Cytoplasm.** The cytoplasm of protoplasmic astrocytes is similar to that of fibrous astrocytes, but contains fewer intermediate filaments.

b. Functions

(1) **Support.** Astrocytes provide structural support for the CNS.

(2) **Protection.** Astrocyte end feet and nonexpanded processes together form the **glia limitans** (glial limiting membrane) of the CNS, an uninterrupted layer of neuroglia at the external surface of the CNS and around blood vessels. It is a protective barrier limiting the penetration of substances into the CNS.

(3) **Maintenance of extracellular environment.** Astrocytes help maintain the ionic extracellular environment of the CNS (e.g., by ensheathing synapses).

(4) **Reactive gliosis.** In response to injury, astrocytes proliferate and form a scar to seal off the injured portion of the CNS from the external environment.

(5) **Neuroblast and axon guidance.** Astrocytes play an important role in guiding migrating neuroblasts in the developing CNS and in guiding injured and regenerating axons.

2. Oligodendrocytes

a. Types

(1) **Interfascicular oligodendrocytes** occur in white and gray matter in association **with myelinated nerve fibers.**

(2) **Satellite oligodendrocytes** occur in gray matter in close association with neuronal perikarya.

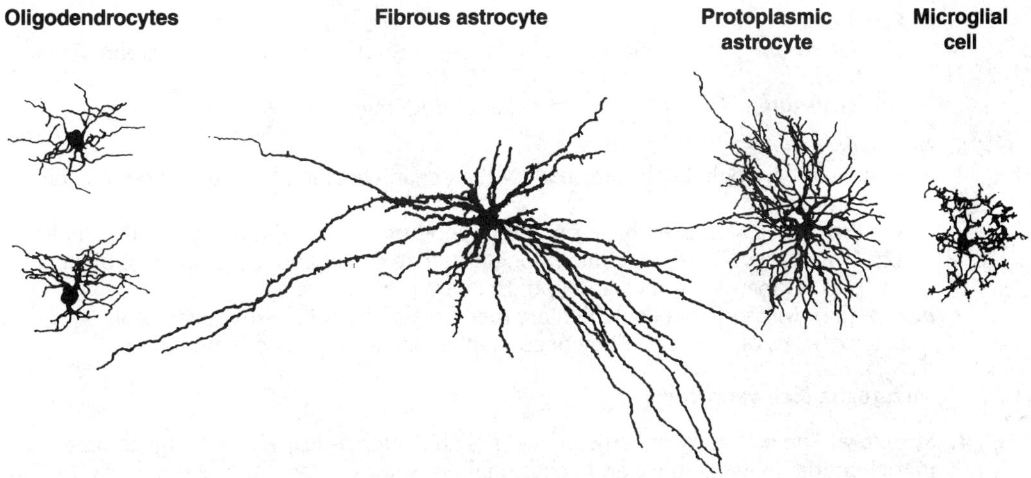

FIGURE 9-7. Drawing of silver-impregnated astrocytes, oligodendrocytes, and microglial cells from the central nervous system (CNS). (Reprinted with permission from Dellmann H-D: *Textbook of Veterinary Histology,* 4th ed. Baltimore, Williams & Wilkins, 1993, p 93.)

b. Structure. Oligodendrocytes are small cells with spherical, heterochromatic nuclei.

(1) Processes. Oligodendrocytes have thin processes that surround CNS axons.

(2) Cytoplasm. The oligodendrocyte cytoplasm contains abundant rER, an extensive Golgi complex, and many mitochondria and microtubules.

c. Function

(1) Insulation. Interfascicular oligodendrocytes **form myelin sheaths** that insulate axons from the environment (see V B 1).

(2) Metabolism. Because of their close relationship to perikarya, satellite oligodendrocytes are believed to play a role in neuronal metabolism.

3. Ependymal cells

a. Location

(1) Ependymal cells line the ventricles of the brain and the central canal of the spinal cord.

(2) Tanycytes are ependymal cells with long processes that terminate on capillaries, neurons, and the brain surface. They are found in certain locations, such as the floor of the third ventricle.

b. Structure. Ependymal cells are mostly **cuboidal or columnar cells** that bear cilia and microvilli on their luminal surfaces.

(1) Junctions. Ependymal cells are joined by gap junctions and tight junctions.

(2) Cytoplasm. Ependymal cells contain the usual set of organelles and conspicuous intermediate filaments.

c. Functions

(1) Propulsion. The ciliary beat of ependymal cells moves cerebrospinal fluid through the ventricles and central canal.

(2) Ependymal cells may also be involved in **secretion** and the **uptake** and **transport** of substances from the cerebrospinal fluid to the blood or neuropil.

4. Choroid plexus epithelial cells

a. Structure. Choroid plexus cells are **cuboidal** with a bulging luminal surface bearing many microvilli and groups of cilia.

(1) Junctions. The blood–cerebrospinal fluid barrier, a selective barrier between blood and cerebrospinal fluid, is formed by zonulae adherentes and tight junctions near the luminal surface of choroid plexus epithelial cells.

(2) Cytoplasm. Numerous mitochondria and clear vesicles, rER, sER, and a Golgi complex are present.

b. Functions

(1) **Secretion.** Choroid plexus epithelial cells secrete components of cerebrospinal fluid.

(2) **Absorption.** They also absorb material from the cerebrospinal fluid.

5. Microglia

a. Structure. Microglial cells are small, with a characteristically heterochromatic, elongated nucleus.

(1) **Processes.** Microglia have numerous short processes with many small branches.

(2) **Cytoplasm.** Microglia contain long cisternae of rER and a prominent Golgi complex. Often, lysosomes and lipofuscin are present.

b. Function. Microglial cells, which are members of the MPS, are the resident macrophages of the CNS. They become phagocytic when stimulated.

C. PNS neuroglia (Schwann cells)

1. Structure. The cell body of Schwann cells is characterized by rER, a Golgi complex, mitochondria, microtubules, and occasional lysosomes.

2. Functions

a. Myelination

(1) **Schwann cells** form the myelin sheath of myelinated axons in peripheral nerves (see V A 1).

(2) **Satellite cells** form a continuous layer around ganglion cells in craniospinal ganglia and a discontinuous layer in autonomic ganglia.

b. Nourishment. Neurolemmocytes are believed to help nourish neurons.

c. Axon guidance. After peripheral nerve transection, neurolemmocytes guide regenerating axons.

V. NERVE FIBERS.

A nerve fiber, which may be myelinated or nonmyelinated, is defined as an axon and its surrounding sheaths.

A. PNS

1. Myelinated nerve fibers. The axon is surrounded by a myelin sheath.

a. Myelin sheath formation is illustrated in Figure 9-8*A*.

b. Myelin sheath structure (Figure 9-9)

(1) **Internodes** are individual segments of myelin sheath, each formed by one Schwann cell.

(a) **Cell membrane.** The internodes consist primarily of concentric layers of Schwann cell membrane without intervening cytoplasm. **External mesaxons** and **internal mesaxons,** respectively, are the beginnings and ends of the spiral wrapping.

(i) **Major dense lines** are formed by close apposition of the inner layers of the cell membrane.

(ii) **Intraperiod lines** are formed by apposition of the outer layers of the cell membrane, which remain separated by a narrow gap.

(b) **Cytoplasm** of Schwann cells is present in the outermost and innermost layers of the myelin sheath.

(i) The **nucleus** of the Schwann cell is contained in the outermost layer.

(ii) **Paranodes** are the regions in which the myelin layers terminate adjacent to the nerve fiber.

(2) **Nodes of Ranvier** are the junctions between adjacent internodes.

(a) At nodes, processes of the outer lamellae of adjacent internodes interdigitate, ensheathing the node.

(b) The axon of a myelinated nerve fiber has the characteristics described under II A 3, but at each node it is thickened, and an electron-dense layer, similar to that of the initial segment of the axon, is present.

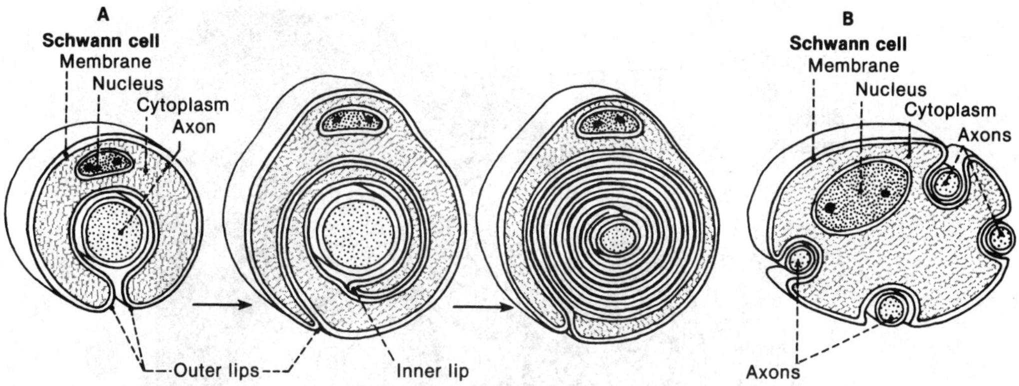

FIGURE 9-8. Schematic drawing illustrating the formation of myelinated and nonmyelinated fibers in the peripheral nervous system (PNS). (*A*) During the formation of a myelinated fiber, Schwann cell forms a furrow to house a single axon. Elongation of one of the Schwann cell processes that forms the furrow leads to the formation of a multilayered sheath. The cytoplasm is extruded (except for the innermost and outermost lamellae) to form the myelin sheath. (*B*) In nonmyelinated fibers, several nonmyelinated axons are supported by each Schwann cell; the axons are located in individual invaginations. (Reprinted with permission from DeMyer W: NMS *Neuroanatomy*. Baltimore, Williams & Wilkins, 1988, p 49.)

2. **Nonmyelinated nerve fibers.** A number of individual axons are located in longitudinal furrows of a Schwann cell, partially or entirely covered by a thin layer of Schwann cell cytoplasm (Figure 9-8*B*).
3. **Peripheral nerves** comprise one or several fascicles, each composed of myelinated or nonmyelinated axons, or both. **Three connective tissue sheaths** are present: epineurium, perineurium, and endoneurium (Figure 9-10).

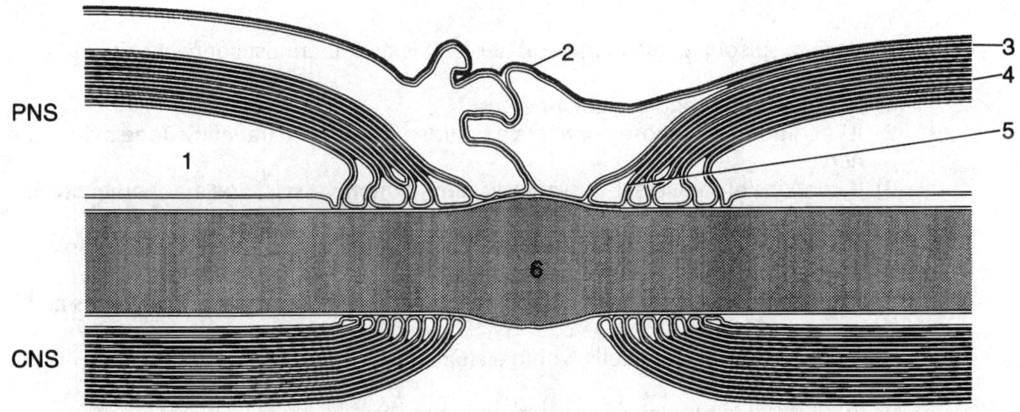

FIGURE 9-9. Schematic drawing of part of a myelinated nerve fiber in the peripheral (*top*) and central (*bottom*) nervous systems (*PNS, CNS*). In the PNS, the innermost lamellae of the myelin sheath contain cytoplasm (*1*). At the node, the outermost lamellae overlap deeper layers and interdigitate with those of adjacent Schwann cells (*2*). In the remaining lamellae, myelin is the apposed membranes of adjacent concentric wrappings, forming major dense lines (*3*) and intraperiod lines (*4*). At the paranode (*5*), cytoplasm-containing lamellae contact the nerve fiber (*6*). In the CNS, the paranode (*7*) is similar to that in the PNS. No overlap occurs between adjacent oligodendrocytes at the node; therefore, the node is exposed to the extracellular space. (Redrawn with permission from Bunge RP: Glia cells and the central myelin sheath. *Physiol Rev* 48:197, 1970.)

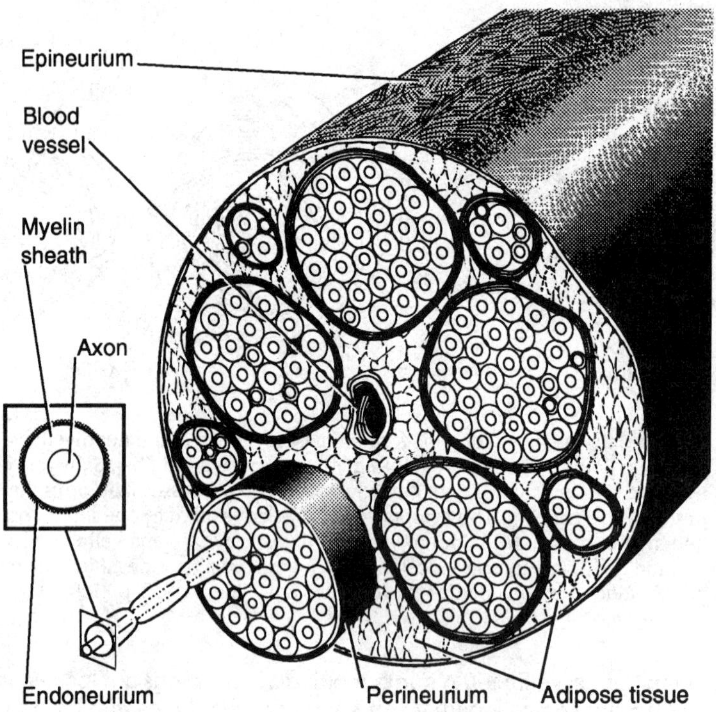

FIGURE 9-10. Schematic drawing of a peripheral nerve consisting of several fascicles. The entire nerve is surrounded by epineurium. Each fascicle is enclosed by perineurium consisting of several layers of flattened perineural cells. Individual myelinated nerve fibers are surrounded by endoneurium. A myelinated nerve fiber comprises an axon and the surrounding internodal myelin sheaths formed by Schwann cells. (Redrawn and modified from Jenkins TW: *Functional Mammalian Neuroanatomy,* 2nd ed. Baltimore, Williams & Wilkins, 1978, p 103.)

a. **Epineurium** surrounds the peripheral nerve. It is the outermost connective tissue sheath.
   (1) It is absent in monofascicular nerves.
   (2) It is composed of loose connective tissue; most fibers parallel the long axis of the nerve.
   (3) It contains blood vessels (**vasa nervorum**), lymph vessels, and autonomic nerve fibers that innervate the vessels.
   (4) The epineurium primarily **provides structural support** to the peripheral nerve.
b. **Perineurium** surrounds each nerve fascicle.
   (1) It is composed of concentric alternating layers of **flattened perineural cells and collagen fibrils.**
      (a) Edges of adjacent cells within a single layer interlock and are **joined by tight junctions.**
      (b) A **basal lamina** encloses each perineural cell layer.
   (2) **As nerves branch, the number of perineural cell layers decreases.** Individual nerve fibers are surrounded by a single perineural cell layer that terminates in an open cuff.
   (3) The perineurium **prevents or restricts access of certain substances** to the endoneurial compartment.
c. **Endoneurium** surrounds Schwann cells, from which it is separated by a basal lamina.
   (1) It is composed of loose connective tissue.
   (2) Endoneurial capillaries, by virtue of endothelial tight junctions, are impermeable to many substances, creating a **blood–nerve barrier.**

B. CNS

1. **Myelinated nerve fibers.**
   a. **Myelin sheath formation**
      (1) An oligodendrocyte forms several processes, each of which contacts a different axon and wraps around a certain length of the axon, the internode.
      (2) Through further elongation, the oligodendrocyte process encircles the axon several times to form lamellae.
      (3) Cytoplasm is lost from the spiral, leading to apposition of the inner surface of the cell membranes, with lines forming as in the PNS [see V A 1 b (1) (a) (i)–(ii)]. Some cytoplasm remains in the innermost and part of the outermost lamellae.
   b. **Myelin sheath structure**
      (1) Internodes. Internodal **myelin sheath structure** is similar to that of the PNS, except the cytoplasm in the outermost myelin lamella is confined to a small area that appears tongue-shaped in cross-section and does not entirely encircle the sheath. **Paranode structure** is identical to that of paranodes in the PNS (see Figure 9-9).
      (2) Nodes of Ranvier are not covered by lamellae of adjacent internodes as in the PNS (see Figure 9-9).
   c. **Axon characteristics** are identical to those in the PNS [see V A 1 b (2) (b)].
2. **Nonmyelinated nerve fibers** are not ensheathed by oligodendrocytes or any other neuroglial cell.

STUDY QUESTIONS

DIRECTIONS: Each of the numbered items or incomplete statements in this section is followed by answers or by completions of the statement. Select the **one** numbered answer or completion that is **best** in each case.

1. Which one of the following statements is true regarding peripheral nerves?

(1) Each internode of a myelinated nerve fiber is surrounded by concentric layers of flattened Schwann cells.
(2) The node is not ensheathed by Schwann cells.
(3) Nonmyelinated nerve fibers are ensheathed by a basal lamina and collagen fibers.
(4) Nonmyelinated nerve fibers are not ensheathed by Schwann cells.
(5) Fascicles are surrounded by concentric layers of flattened perineural cells and collagen fibers.

DIRECTIONS: Each of the numbered items or incomplete statements in this section is negatively phrased, as indicated by an italicized word such as *not, least,* or *except.* Select the **one** numbered answer or completion that is **best** in each case.

2. Which of the following events does *not* take place at a synapse?

(1) Neurotransmitters are released by exocytosis from the presynaptic element into the synaptic cleft.
(2) Neurotransmitters are effectively removed from the synaptic cleft by enzymatic degradation.
(3) Neurotransmitters bind to postsynaptic receptors.
(4) Neurotransmitters are taken up by endocytosis by the postsynaptic element.
(5) Neurotransmitters are removed from the synaptic cleft by diffusion.

3. All of the following are prominent organelles of neuronal perikarya *except:*

(1) rough endoplasmic reticulum (rER).
(2) Golgi complex.
(3) lysosomes.
(4) microtubules.
(5) smooth endoplasmic reticulum (sER).

4. All of the following are part of a neuromuscular synapse *except:*

(1) telodendritic branches of somatic efferent fibers.
(2) sole plate troughs.
(3) tight junctions.
(4) basal lamina in the synaptic cleft.
(5) Schwann cells.

5. Which of the following statements is *not* true regarding free receptive nerve endings?

(1) They are mechanoreceptors.
(2) They are exteroceptors.
(3) They are numerous in the epidermis.
(4) They innervate gland cells.
(5) They innervate hair follicles.

6. Pacinian corpuscles are characterized by all of the following *except:*

(1) they are mechanoreceptors.
(2) they are encapsulated by a connective tissue capsule.
(3) they have a nonmyelinated nerve ending in the center.
(4) they possess many lamellae of Schwann cells separated by fluid-filled spaces.
(5) they possess many lamellae of fibrocytes separated by fluid-filled spaces.

7. Which of the following statements concerning muscle spindles is *not* correct?

(1) They are mechanoreceptors.
(2) They possess two types of muscle fibers.
(3) Two types of afferent endings are present.
(4) They are encapsulated by several lamellae of fibrocytes.
(5) Two types of efferent endings are present.

8. All of the following are characteristic functions of astrocytes *except:*

(1) ensheathment of synapses.
(2) postinjury scar formation.
(3) guidance of migration of neuroblasts during embryonic development.
(4) myelin sheath formation.
(5) formation of the pericapillary glia limitans.

9. All of the following are components of the axon *except:*

(1) smooth endoplasmic reticulum (sER).
(2) ribosomes.
(3) neurofilaments.
(4) mitochondria.
(5) microtubules.

ANSWERS AND EXPLANATIONS

1. The answer is 5 *[V A 3 b]*. Alternating layers of flattened perineural cells and collagen fibers make up the perineurium that surrounds each nerve fascicle in a peripheral nerve. Internodes of myelinated peripheral nerve fibers are surrounded by concentric layers of myelin (i.e., the cell membrane of Schwann cells). At the node, processes of Schwann cells of adjacent internodes overlap and isolate the node from the environment. Nonmyelinated nerve fibers in a peripheral nerve are always associated with Schwann cells and are located in invaginations of the Schwann cell surface. Schwann cells are surrounded by a basal lamina and associated collagen fibrils, which constitute the endoneurium.

2. The answer is 4 *[III B 1 a]*. Endocytosis is not the mechanism by which the postsynaptic element receives neurotransmitters; rather, they attach to receptors on the postsynaptic cell membrane. Neurotransmitters are released into the synaptic cleft by exocytosis from the presynaptic element. When the cell membrane of the presynaptic element ceases to be depolarized (i.e., when neurotransmitter is no longer released), it is imperative that neurotransmitter remaining in the synaptic cleft be removed rapidly so that no further stimulation of the postsynaptic element occurs. This is achieved by diffusion, enzymatic degradation, and probably also uptake by neuroglial cells.

3. The answer is 5 *[II A 1 b]*. Smooth endoplasmic reticulum (sER) is not a prominent organelle of neuronal perikarya but is extensive in both dendrites and axons. Rough endoplasmic reticulum (rER) is abundant in neuronal perikarya and, together with free ribosomes and polyribosomes, constitutes Nissl substance. The Golgi complex is especially prominent in neurosecretory neurons. Lysosomes are also numerous; one of their functions is to participate in the disposal of aging or worn-out organelles. Microtubules are part of the cytoskeleton and function in the transport of membrane-bounded organelles.

4. The answer is 3 *[III B 1 b (2)]*. Tight junctions are not part of a neuromuscular synapse (myoneuronal junction). Telodendritic branches of somatic efferent fibers terminate within troughs of the sole plate. Wherever the telodendritic branches are not in touch with the muscle fiber, they are covered by a single layer of Schwann cells. A basal lamina is present in the synaptic cleft between the axolemma and the sarcolemma, including the junctional folds. The basal lamina plays an important role in the function of the neuromuscular synapse because it contains acetylcholinesterase, which hydrolyzes acetylcholine (ACh).

5. The answer is 4 *[III C 1–2]*. Gland cells are innervated by efferent fibers that participate in the modulation of their secretory activity, not by afferent fibers. Free receptive nerve endings respond to mechanical stimulation. They are located near the body surface and, therefore, are exteroceptors. They are most frequent in the epidermis and innervate hair follicles. They are particularly numerous in tactile hairs (sinus hairs).

6. The answer is 4 *[Table 9-1]*. In pacinian (lamellar) corpuscles, a multilayered sheath of intricately interdigitating Schwann cells surrounds a central nonmyelinated dendritic nerve ending. There are no fluid-filled spaces present between Schwann cells. The central core of the pacinian corpuscle is surrounded by many layers (lamellae) of fibrocytes; a fluid-filled space separates adjacent layers. A thin connective tissue capsule encloses the corpuscle. Lamellar corpuscles are mechanoreceptors (i.e., they respond to mechanical stimulation such as pressure and vibration).

7. The answer is 4 *[Figure 9-6]*. Muscle spindles are surrounded by several lamellae of perineural cells, not fibrocytes. Nuclear bag and nuclear chain fibers are the two types of intrafusal muscle fibers present. They receive efferent input from end-plate terminals and trail endings, and afferent endings are primary (annulospiral) and secondary (flower-spray) in nature. Muscle spindles are mechanoreceptors; they sense muscle tension and, by reflex action, adjust posture, muscle tone, and muscle activity.

8. The answer is 4 *[IV B 1 b]*. Myelin sheaths in the central nervous system (CNS) are formed by oligodendrocytes, not astrocytes. Astrocytes serve as guidance structures along which neuroblasts migrate during embryonic development of the CNS. They ensheath synapses and form the glia limitans, or glial limiting membrane, at the surface of the CNS and around capillaries. In addition, astrocytes proliferate in response to injury, forming a scar and sealing the injured portion of the CNS off from the external environment (reactive gliosis).

9. The answer is 2 *[II A 3 a]*. The axon is devoid of ribosomes, which are abundant in the perikaryon and dendrites. Axonal protein synthesis is thus not possible, and proteins have to be imported from the perikaryon. This is an energy-requiring process involving microtubules and mitochondria. Neurofilaments are especially numerous in large axons.

Chapter 10

Muscle

I. INTRODUCTION

A. Muscle cells. Myocytes are specialized cells that contract to create movement. Muscle cells are also called **muscle fibers** or **myofibers** because of their shape, which is elongated with the long axis parallel to the direction of the force they exert.

B. Contraction

1. Muscle cells, which are excitable, exhibit **action potentials,** self-propagating waves of depolarization initiated by stimulation of the cell membrane.

2. Interdigitating arrays of the **contractile proteins actin** and **myosin** effect contraction of the muscle cells.

C. Classification. There are three types of muscle: **skeletal, cardiac,** and **smooth** (Table 10-1). Skeletal muscle and the skeletal system together form the musculoskeletal system.

TABLE 10-1. Muscle Types

Muscle Type	Appearance (Longitudinal section)	Location	Contraction
Skeletal	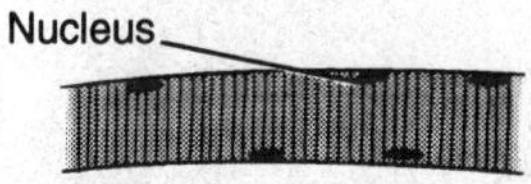 Transversely striated; cells are long and cylindrical with numerous peripherally located nuclei	Body wall, limbs	Mostly voluntary
Cardiac	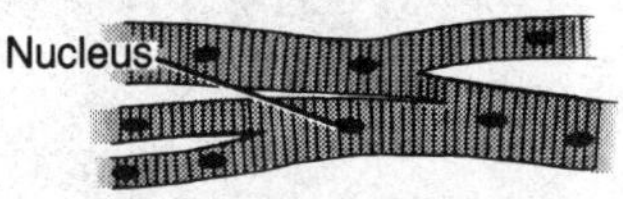 Transversely striated; cells are blunt and bifurcated with one or two centrally located nuclei	Heart, may extend into great vessels	Involuntary
Smooth	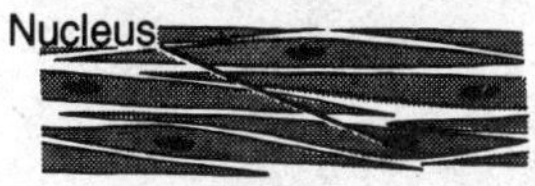 Lacks striations; cells are short and spindle-shaped with one centrally located nucleus; cytoplasm appears homogenous	Walls of hollow visceral organs, blood vessels	Involuntary

II. SKELETAL MUSCLE

A. Light-microscope structure

1. **Skeletal muscle cells**
   a. **Appearance**
      (1) Skeletal muscle cells are **elongated cylinders with tapered ends**.
      (2) They range from **10–100 μm in diameter** and can reach **50 cm in length**.
   b. **Structure**
      (1) Skeletal muscle cells are encased by a cell membrane, the **sarcolemma,** which forms tubular invaginations [**T (transverse) tubules**] that extend into the cells in an anastomosing network.
      (2) Each skeletal muscle cell contains numerous **myofibrils,** long cylinders measuring 1–2 μm in diameter.
         (a) Myofibrils, which are formed by bundles of **thick** and **thin myofilaments** (see II B 1–2), have a striated appearance when viewed in longitudinal section (Figure 10-1).
            (i) **A (anisotropic) bands** are dark. Thick and thin filaments overlap in the A band.
            (ii) **I (isotropic) bands** are light. The I band contains only thin filaments.
            (iii) The A and I bands are in register in adjacent myofibrils and in adjacent cells, giving the entire muscle a striated appearance.
         (b) Myofibrils appear as dark dots in cross-sections of skeletal muscle cells.
      (3) Intermediate filaments, primarily desmin, provide support and attachment for the myofibrils and transmit their conformational changes to the sarcolemma.
      (4) The **cytoplasm (sarcoplasm)** is **acidophilic,** and **nuclei** are **peripherally located**.
   c. **Tissue.** A **syncytium** is formed by the fusion of up to several hundred cells.

A B

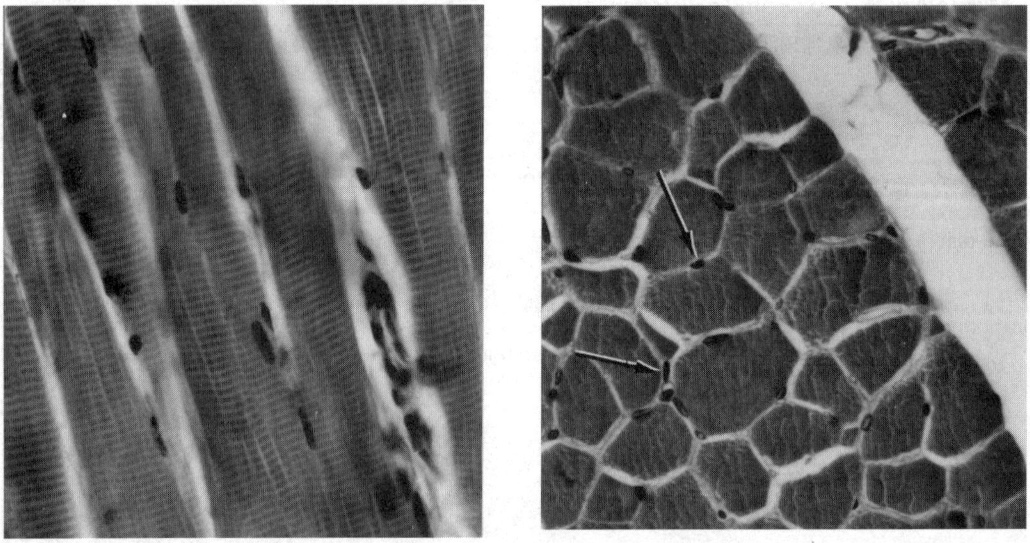

FIGURE 10-1. Skeletal muscle. (*A*) Longitudinal section. Cross-striations are evident. The muscle cell nuclei are in the peripheral cytoplasm. (*B*) Cross-section. The nuclei between muscle cells (*arrows*) belong to fibroblasts in the endomysium. (Reprinted with permission from Dellmann H-D: *Textbook of Veterinary Histology,* 4th ed. Baltimore, Williams & Wilkins, 1993, p 74.)

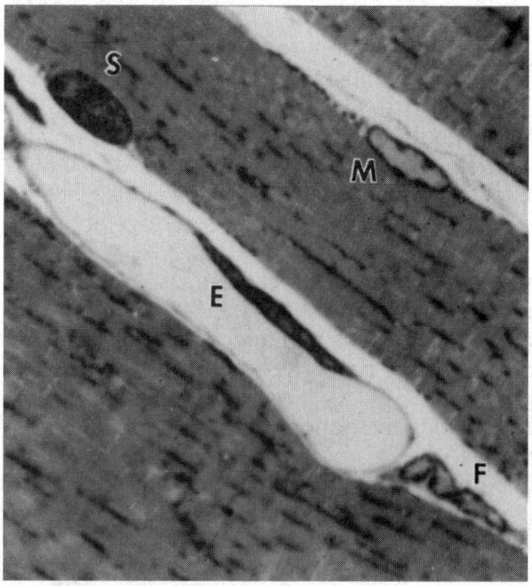

FIGURE 10-2. Longitudinal section through several skeletal muscle cells and a capillary (*E*). A peripherally located muscle cell nucleus (*M*) and a satellite cell nucleus (*S*) are indicated. A fibroblast nucleus (*F*) is in the endomysium. The elongated dark bodies in the muscle cells are mitochondria aligned in rows between myofibrils. (Reprinted with permission from Dellmann H-D: *Textbook of Veterinary Histology,* 4th ed. Baltimore, Williams & Wilkins, 1993, p 76.)

2. **Satellite cells** (Figure 10-2) are spindle-shaped cells with a heterochromatic nucleus. They lie within the basal lamina surrounding the muscle cell and are considered a residual population of inactive myoblasts.
3. The **stroma** of skeletal muscle transmits the forces generated by contraction of individual muscle cells to the muscle attachments. Blood vessels and nerves are abundant in the stroma of skeletal muscle.
   a. **Epimysium** is a capsule of dense irregular connective tissue that surrounds the entire muscle (Figure 10-3).
   b. **Perimysium** comprises thin septa of dense irregular connective tissue that separate and surround fascicles (bundles) of muscle cells (see Figure 10-3).
   c. **Endomysium** consists of a network of reticular fibers (see Figure 10-1) that surrounds individual muscle cells.

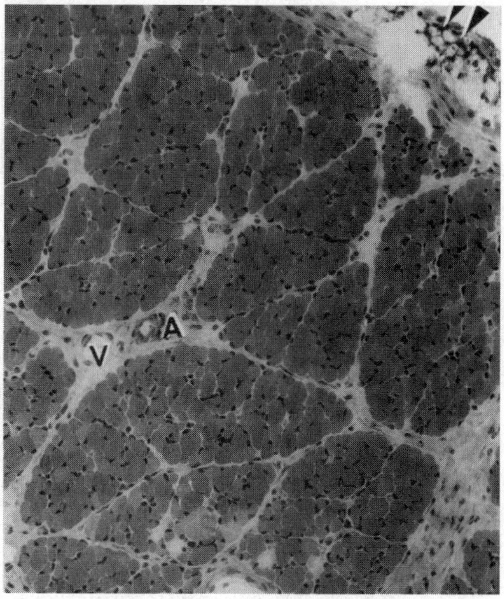

FIGURE 10-3. Cross-section through a portion of a skeletal muscle. A portion of the epimysium is at the upper right-hand corner (*arrowheads*). Perimysium separating fascicles of muscle cells contains a venule (*V*) and an arteriole (*A*). The peripheral location of muscle cell nuclei is noticeable even at this low magnification. (Reprinted with permission from Dellmann H-D: *Textbook of Veterinary Histology,* 4th ed. Baltimore, Williams & Wilkins, 1993, p 75.)

B. Fine structure

1. **Filaments.** The myofibrils of muscle cells contain thin filaments, thick filaments, and intermediate filaments.
   a. **Thin filaments** (Figure 10-4A) are primarily composed of actin, but they also contain tropomyosin and troponin.
      (1) **Actin.** Globular molecules called G-actin polymerize to form filamentous F-actin.
         (a) **F-actin** consists of two strands of polymerized G-actin, twisted together to form a double helix.
         (b) **G-actin** molecules are polar; therefore, F-actin filaments are also polar. Each G-actin molecule has a binding site for myosin.
      (2) **Tropomyosin** molecules, which are filamentous, lie end to end along the groove between the two twisted strands of actin. They cover the binding sites for myosin on the actin filament.
      (3) **Troponin** is spaced at regular intervals along the tropomyosin. It is formed of three globular subunits (see Figure 10-4A).
   b. **Thick filaments** (Figure 10-4B) are formed by overlapping complexes of myosin.
      (1) **Composition.** Each myosin complex consists of a light and heavy fragment.
         (a) The **light fragment (light meromyosin)** is rod-like.
         (b) The **heavy fragment (heavy meromyosin)** is rod-like where it joins the light fragment and globular on the free end. The globular portion is called the **myosin head.**
      (2) **Formation.** Thick filaments are formed when the rod-like tails of several hundred myosin complexes overlap (see Figure 10-4B).
         (a) The head and some of the rod-like portion of the heavy fragment project from the filament.

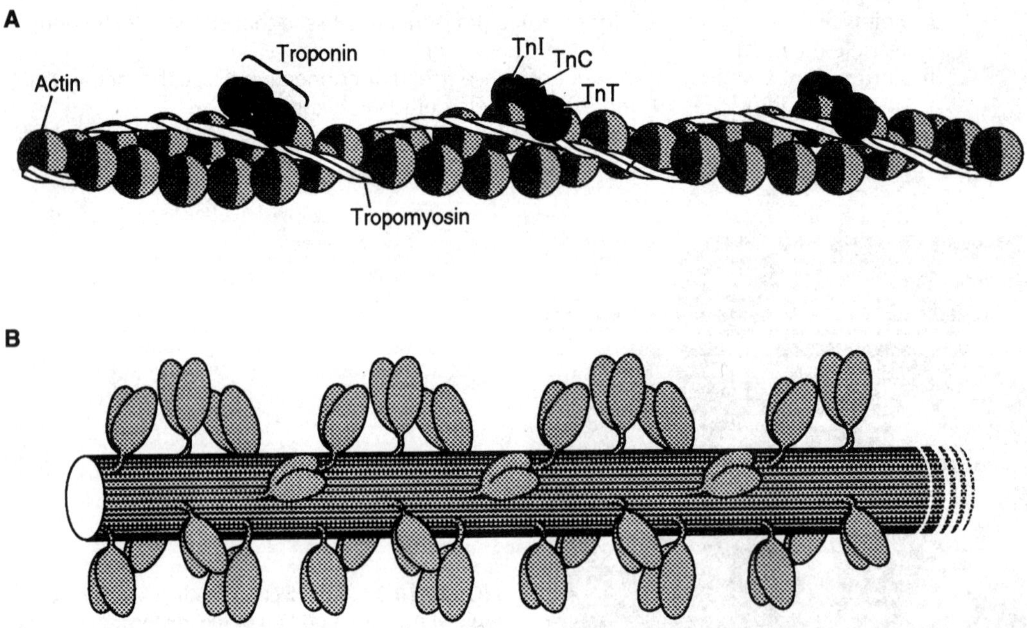

FIGURE 10-4. (*A*) Configuration of the three major proteins that comprise the thin filaments of skeletal muscle. The *shaded portions* of the actin molecules are the myosin binding sites. The three troponin subunits (*TnI, TnC,* and *TnT*) inhibit interaction between actin and myosin, bind calcium, and attach troponin to tropomyosin, respectively. (*B*) Thick filaments are formed by overlapping complexes of myosin that consist of a rod-like tail and a globular head.

(b) The heads point toward the end of the filament to which they are closer. Half of them point one way and half of them point the other way; therefore, the central part of the filament comprises only overlapping tails.

(c) The heads have binding sites for actin and for adenosine triphosphate (ATP). In addition, they have adenosine triphosphatase (ATPase) activity (i.e., the ability to cleave ATP to release its energy).

2. **Sarcomeres** (Figure 10-5) are the smallest repeating units of a myofibril. Each sarcomere extends from the middle of one I band to the middle of the next.
   a. **Z lines** are dark lines that **bisect the I bands;** therefore they mark the ends of each sarcomere.

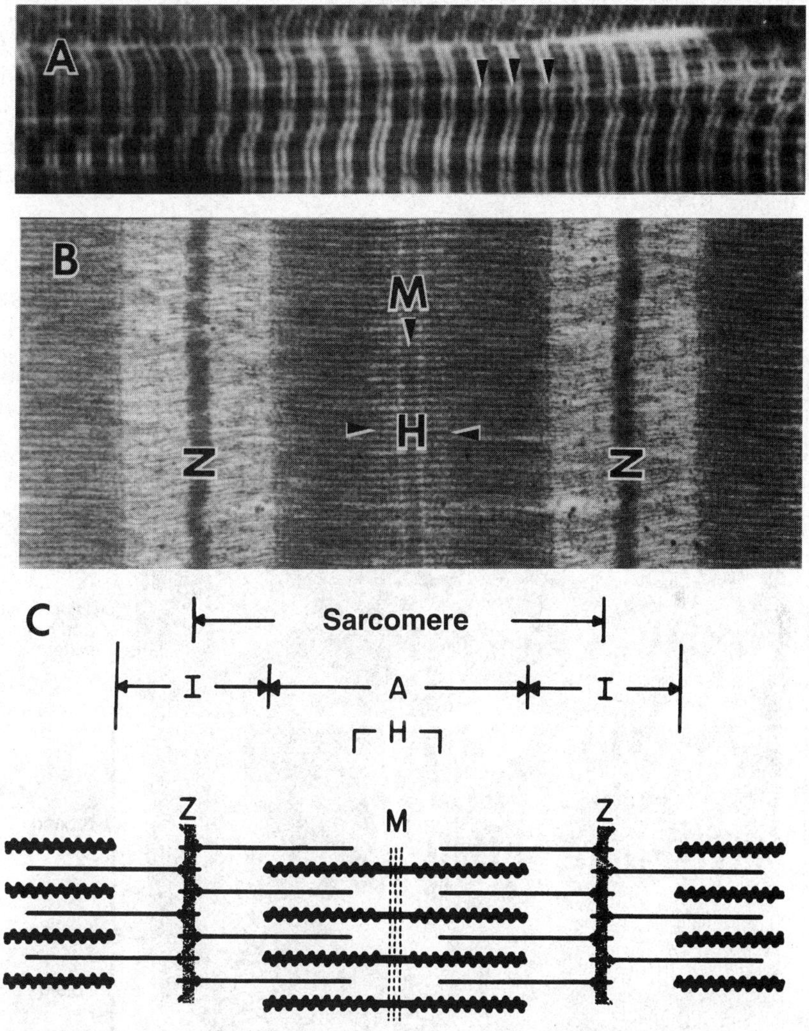

FIGURE 10-5. Longitudinal sections through skeletal muscle. (*A*) Light micrograph. The wider dark bands are A bands, and the lighter I bands are bisected by dark Z lines (*arrowheads*). (*B*) Electron micrograph. This magnification reveals how the arrangement of longitudinal thick and thin filaments causes cross-striations. *Z* = Z line; *M* = M line; *H* = H band. (*C*) Schematic representation. The orientation of thick and thin filaments and their attachments to the Z line (thin filaments) and M line (thick filaments) is illustrated. The H band (between ends of the thin filaments) and I band (between ends of the thick filaments) become narrower when the thick and thin filaments slide past each other during contraction. (Reprinted with permission from Dellmann H-D: *Textbook of Veterinary Histology,* 4th ed. Baltimore, Williams & Wilkins, 1993, p 77.)

(1) **Actin filaments attach to both sides of the Z line.** The polarity of actin filaments on one side of the Z line is opposite that of actin filaments on the other side.

(2) **α-Actinin,** a major component of the Z line, is believed to anchor the actin filaments. It is likely that α-actinin and desmin tie adjacent myofibrils together and keep them aligned.

b. A bands contain thick filaments and the portions of the thin filaments that overlap the thick filaments.

(1) The **H band** is a lighter region in the center of the A band where there are no actin filaments and the thick filaments contain only the rod-like portions of the myosin molecules. The H band narrows during contraction.

(2) The **M line,** which bisects the H band, is formed by lateral connections between thick filaments. **Creatine kinase** in the M line helps maintain adequate ATP for contraction.

c. I bands contain thin filaments and the Z line, to which the actin is attached. I bands narrow during contraction.

3. A **triad** comprises a T tubule and two cisternae of the sarcoplasmic reticulum.

a. T tubules form a transversely oriented network at the level of each A-I junction (Figure 10-6).

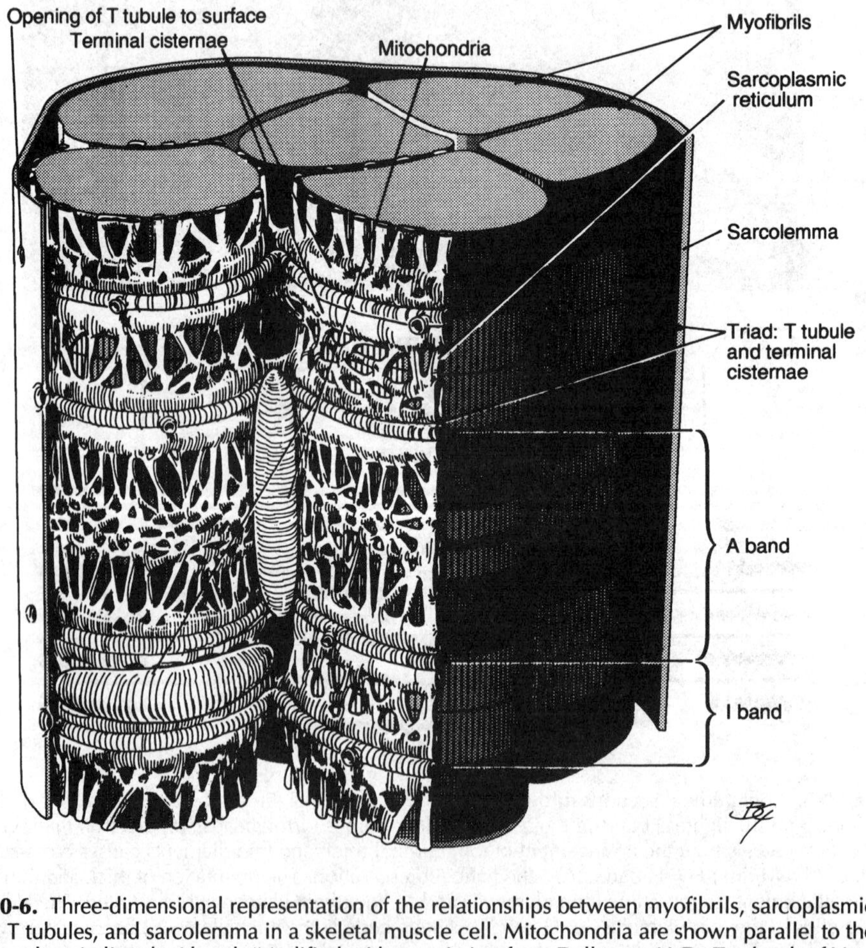

FIGURE 10-6. Three-dimensional representation of the relationships between myofibrils, sarcoplasmic reticulum, T tubules, and sarcolemma in a skeletal muscle cell. Mitochondria are shown parallel to the myofibrils and encircling the I band. (Modified with permission from Dellmann H-D: *Textbook of Veterinary Histology,* 4th ed. Baltimore, Williams & Wilkins, 1993, p 79.)

b. The **sarcoplasmic reticulum** is highly specialized smooth endoplasmic reticulum (sER) that forms a "collar" of anastomosing tubules and cisternae around each A band in the myofibril. Expanded **terminal cisternae** abut each side of the T tubules at the A-I junctions (see Figure 10-6).

4. **Organelles and granules**
   a. **Mitochondria** are numerous near the sarcolemma. They also form rows between myofibrils (see Figure 10-6) and collars surrounding myofibrils at each A band.
   b. **Glycogen granules** are stored carbohydrates that can be oxidized to provide energy during contraction.

5. **Basal lamina.** Each muscle cell is entirely surrounded by its own basal lamina and a small amount of connective tissue.

C. Contraction

1. **Excitation–contraction coupling** is the process by which an action potential initiates contraction.
   a. **Resting state.** In a resting muscle, the tropomyosin–troponin complex covers the myosin binding sites on the actin filament. Myosin heads are bound to ATP, but they hydrolyze it very slowly when they are not bound to actin.
   b. **Activation**
      (1) An action potential spreading over the surface of the sarcolemma is propagated into the network of T tubules. When the wave of depolarization reaches a triad, it causes the sarcoplasmic reticulum to release its stored calcium into the region of the myofibrils.
      (2) The calcium binds to troponin, causing the troponin to undergo a conformational change that moves the tropomyosin molecule deeper into the groove of the actin helix and exposes the myosin binding sites.
         (a) Actin and myosin heads interact, enabling the myosin heads to hydrolyze ATP rapidly.
         (b) The energy released by hydrolysis of ATP is used to bend the head and adjacent part of the myosin complex (the **cross-bridge**). Because the head is bound to actin, its movement pulls the Z line toward the center of the sarcomere.
         (c) Sliding of thick and thin filaments shortens the sarcomere and, because it occurs synchronously in all sarcomeres, the entire cell.
      (3) After the myosin head binds a new ATP molecule, it detaches from the actin filament and the cycle is ready to repeat. If ATP is exhausted, the muscle cannot relax. This is the basis for rigor mortis.
         (a) Hundreds of cycles of bridges forming and breaking occur at different times on different myosin heads of each thick filament during a single contraction.
         (b) In skeletal muscle, enough calcium is released for complete activation of contraction.
   c. **Relaxation.** When depolarization ends, the sarcoplasmic reticulum actively transports calcium back into its cisternae, causing contraction to stop.

2. **Regulation of contraction**
   a. A **motor unit** comprises a nerve fiber and the muscle cells it innervates.
      (1) A motor unit may contain one to several hundred muscle cells.
      (2) Precisely regulated contraction of skeletal muscle is accomplished by varying the number of motor units that contract.
   b. **Neuromuscular junction** [see Chapter 9 III B 1 b (2) (a)]. The axon to a skeletal muscle cell branches out in a spray-like pattern of expanded terminals called a motor end-plate (see Figure 9-5). Each muscle cell is supplied by one or more motor end-plates.
      (1) **Acetylcholine (ACh) release.** When an action potential reaches the motor end-plate, ACh is released. It diffuses across the synaptic cleft to the junctional folds.

(2) **Sodium influx.** ACh binds to receptors in the sarcolemma of the junctional folds. Receptor-gated sodium channels open, allowing sodium to rush into the muscle cell. Excess ACh is hydrolyzed by cholinesterase in the basal lamina.

(3) **Depolarization.** The sodium influx depolarizes the sarcolemma, initiating a wave of depolarization that spreads across the muscle cell membrane.

c. **Muscle spindles** (see Figure 9-6) act as strain gauges in skeletal muscle.

D. Classification. Skeletal muscle can be classified as red, white, or intermediate. Red and white muscle are classified on the basis of their gross appearance in the fresh state.

1. **General considerations**
   a. The myosins in red and white muscle are slightly different.
   b. Most skeletal muscles contain a mixture of muscle cell types.
   c. The innervation of a skeletal muscle cell determines whether it will be red, white, or intermediate. If the innervation of a muscle cell is altered surgically, the cell will change accordingly.

2. **Red muscle cells** are small fibers that depend largely on **oxidative pathways** for energy; therefore, myoglobin and mitochondria are abundant.
   a. Myoglobin is a pigment that stores oxygen used by mitochondria to release energy (ATP) during contraction.
   b. The rich blood supply, the large amount of myoglobin, and the many mitochondria with densely packed cristae give red muscle its characteristic color.
   c. Most red muscle cells are **slow-twitch fibers** (i.e., they contract relatively slowly but are slow to fatigue). Some **fast-twitch** red muscle cells exist, but fast-twitch fibers are more common in white muscle cells (see II D 3 b).

3. **White muscle cells** are larger than red muscle cells. Their energy is derived mainly from **anaerobic glycolysis;** therefore, they contain many high-energy compounds (e.g., ATP, creatinine phosphate).
   a. Neuromuscular junctions on white muscle cells have more synaptic vesicles in the axon terminal than those of red muscle cells. The junctional folds are more extensive and complex, increasing the receptive surface area.
   b. White muscle cells are **fast-twitch fibers** (i.e., they contract rapidly and are more quickly fatigued than red muscle cells).

4. **Intermediate muscle cells** superficially resemble red muscle cells but have structural and functional characteristics between those of red and white muscle cells.

E. Myogenesis, hypertrophy, atrophy, and regeneration

1. **Myogenesis** (development)
   a. **Mesenchymal cells** differentiate into myoblasts.
   b. **Myoblasts** become aligned in rows and then fuse end to end, forming myotubes.
   c. **Myotubes** develop the fine structural characteristics of skeletal muscle cells. Contractile filaments are produced and become organized into **myofibrils**.
   d. Additional myoblasts and myotubes fuse along the periphery of the myotube, and the nuclei migrate to the periphery of the definitive muscle cell.
   e. Satellite cells comprise a reserve population of myogenic cells that remain enclosed in the basal lamina.

2. **Hypertrophy** is growth of muscle cells in response to repeated vigorous exercise. Hypertrophied cells increase in diameter, numbers of nuclei, and numbers of myofibrils.
   a. Satellite cells undergo mitosis, giving rise to two daughter cells. One daughter cell remains as a satellite cell. The other daughter cell fuses with the muscle cell, increasing the number of nuclei. The added nuclei help produce additional myofibrils and other cytoplasmic elements.
   b. No division of muscle cell nuclei occurs.

3. **Atrophy,** which can result from disuse or disease, involves loss of cellular substance. Myofibrils are lost, and the number of nuclei is reduced.

4. **Regeneration** is effected by fusion of satellite cells with each other to form new muscle cells, or with existing cells to repair damaged portions of the muscle. Regeneration is most successful if the endomysium is intact. Extensively damaged muscle may be replaced by connective tissue.

III. CARDIAC MUSCLE

A. Light-microscope structure

1. **Cell appearance** (Figure 10-7)
   a. Cardiac muscle cells are **roughly cylindrical** with **blunt ends,** but they often **bifurcate** longitudinally.
   b. They are usually approximately **15 μm in diameter and 85–100 μm long**.
2. **Cell structure.** Table 10-2 compares structural characteristics of cardiac and smooth muscle to those of skeletal muscle.
   a. Although cardiac muscle cells have a banding pattern identical to that found in skeletal muscle cells, the **myofibrils of cardiac muscle cells anastomose** and are therefore more irregular than the cylindrical myofibrils of skeletal muscle (Figure 10-8).
   b. Unlike skeletal muscle cells, cardiac muscle cells have a **single, centrally located nucleus**. Occasionally, two nuclei are present. As in skeletal muscle cells, the **cytoplasm is acidophilic**.
3. **Tissue**
   a. Complex end-to-end **junctions,** known as **intercalated disks,** join cardiac muscle cells together to form long chains (see Figure 10-7). These chains anastomose to form a tightly woven mass of cells; lateral junctions also join cells in adjacent chains.
   b. Cardiac muscle is **richly vascularized**.

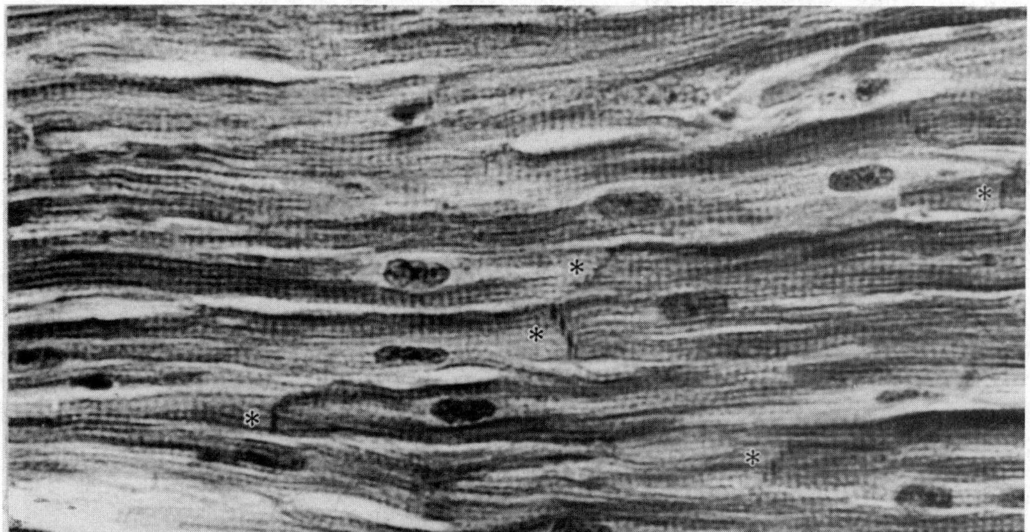

FIGURE 10-7. Cardiac muscle in longitudinal section, showing cross-striations and intercalated disks (*). (Reprinted with permission from Dellmann H-D: *Textbook of Veterinary Histology,* 4th ed. Baltimore, Williams & Wilkins, 1993, p 76.)

TABLE 10-2. Comparison of Skeletal, Cardiac, and Smooth Muscle

Characteristic	Skeletal Muscle	Cardiac Muscle	Smooth Muscle
Striations	Yes	Yes	No
Sarcolemmal specializations	T tubules at A-I junctions	T tubules at Z lines	Caveolae
Junctions	None	Gap junctions between lateral cell membranes; desmosomes, gap junctions, and fasciae adherentes in intercalated disks	Gap junctions between lateral cell membranes in unitary smooth muscle; none in multiunit smooth muscle
Regenerative capacity	Restricted	Nonexistent	Extensive
Distinguishing feature	Peripheral nuclei	Intercalated disks	Lack of striations

B. Fine structure

1. **General characteristics**
   a. **Diads**
      (1) T tubules are larger and more numerous in cardiac muscle than in skeletal muscle, and they are located at the Z line rather than at the A-I junction.
      (2) The sarcoplasmic reticulum is not as regularly arranged, and it is usually located on only one side of the T tubule, forming a diad.
   b. **Organelles and inclusions**
      (1) **Mitochondria** are larger and far more numerous than in skeletal muscle.
      (2) **Lipid droplets** contain stored fatty acids. A small amount of **glycogen** may also be stored.
   c. **Intercellular junctions** are numerous.
      (1) **Gap junctions** are common between adjacent lateral cell membranes and longitudinal portions of the intercalated disks.
      (2) **Intercalated disks.** Transverse portions of the intercalated disks have two types of junctions.
         (a) **Fasciae adherentes** are large junctions that resemble intermediate junctions except for their shape. Actin filaments are attached to the dense material along the cell membrane in these junctions, which function as hemi-Z lines.
         (b) **Desmosomes,** anchored by intermediate filaments, attach the ends of cells between fasciae adherentes.
   d. **Basal lamina.** A basal lamina surrounds each cell, except where intercellular junctions exist.

2. **Specific characteristics.** There are two types of contractile cells, atrial and ventricular, which have some differences in structure. A third cell type is specialized for conduction instead of contraction.
   a. **Contractile cells**
      (1) **Atrial cells** are **smaller** and have **fewer T tubules** than ventricular cells.
      (2) Granules containing **atrial natriuretic factor,** a hormone that causes loss of sodium and water from the kidneys, are present in all cardiac muscle cells, but they are **most abundant in cells of the right atrium**.
   b. **Conducting cells**
      (1) **Purkinje fibers** are the largest of the conducting cells. They form the atrioventricular bundle and its branches in the walls of the ventricles.
      (2) Conducting cells are **larger than other cardiac muscle cells** (especially in ungulates) and have a large **pale area around the nucleus** where stored glycogen has been dissolved.

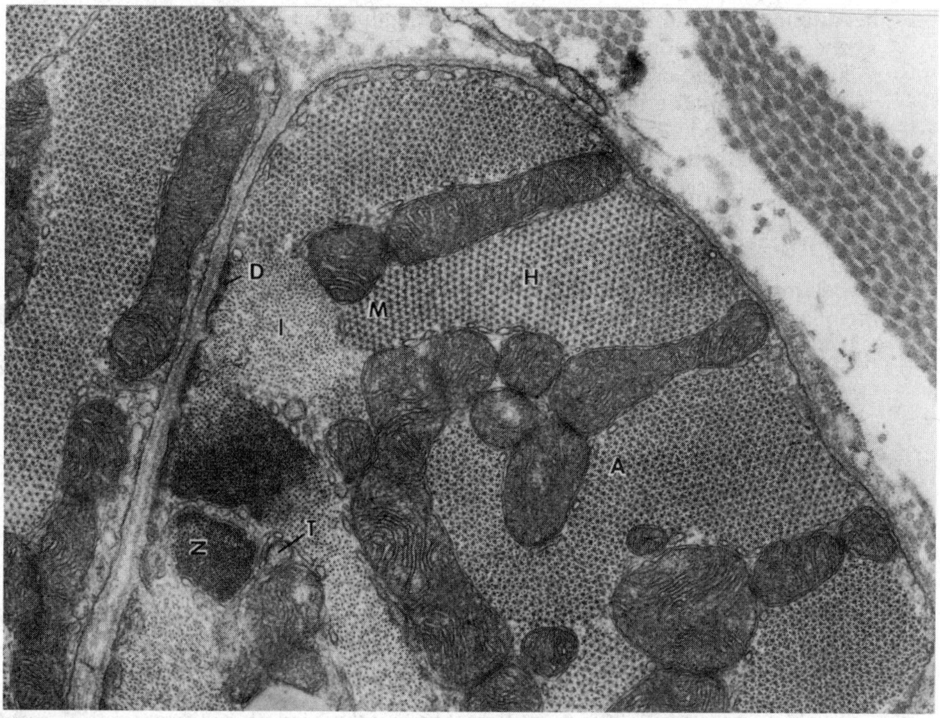

FIGURE 10-8. Electron micrograph of a cross-section through portions of two cardiac muscle cells. The myofibrils are irregular in shape because they separate and anastomose; they are not separate cylinders as they are in skeletal muscle. The plane of section passes through different regions of the myofibril: the Z-line (*Z*), I band (*I*), A band (*A*), M line (*M*), and H band (*H*). Mitochondria are abundant between myofibrils. A T tubule (*T*) and hemidesmosome (*D*) are also visible. (Micrograph courtesy of NP Westmoreland. Reprinted with permission from Dellmann H-D: *Textbook of Veterinary Histology,* 4th ed. Baltimore, Williams & Wilkins, 1993, p 78.)

(3) There are **fewer myofibrils** in conducting cells.
(4) No T tubules are present, and the **sarcoplasmic reticulum is poorly organized**.
(5) Gap junctions between conducting cells **are very large**.

C. Contraction

1. Excitation–contraction coupling. Action potentials spread **electrotonically** from cell to cell via the many gap junctions, allowing the tissue to act as a syncytium.

a. Depolarization of the cell membrane causes the release of calcium from the sarcoplasmic reticulum. In cardiac muscle, calcium also enters the cytosol from the extracellular fluid through the walls of T tubules and other parts of the cell membrane. This source of calcium is relatively slow and long-lasting. The sliding of actin and myosin filaments follows, as in skeletal muscle (see II C 1 b).

b. The **strength of contraction** is related to the:

(1) Amount of calcium that enters the cytosol. Unlike skeletal muscle, not enough calcium is released with every action potential for full activation.

(2) Length of the cells. When cells are stretched (i.e., when the heart is distended), the contractions are stronger.

2. Regulation of contraction

a. Automaticity. Cardiac muscle cells have inherent rhythmicity that is characteristic for different regions of the heart. The fastest rate is generated in a region in the right atrium called the sinoatrial node.

b. Autonomic modulation. The rate and strength of cardiac contractions can be influenced by the autonomic nervous system. Both sympathetic and parasympathetic axons terminate near the sinoatrial node.

(1) Parasympathetic terminals release **ACh,** which reduces the rate of depolarization of nodal cells; therefore, the heart rate is slowed.

(2) Sympathetic terminals release **norepinephrine,** which accelerates the heart rate, probably by enhancing calcium conductance.

D. Hypertrophy and regeneration

1. **Hypertrophy.** When cardiac muscle hypertrophies, individual fibers increase in size but the number of cells and nuclei remains the same.

2. **Regeneration does not occur** after infancy. Damaged cardiac muscle is replaced by connective tissue.

IV. SMOOTH MUSCLE

A. Light-microscope structure

1. **Smooth muscle cells**

a. Appearance

(1) Smooth muscle cells are **spindle-shaped,** with an **elongated central nucleus** (Figure 10-9A).

(2) Most cells are **5–20 μm in diameter,** and their length can vary from **20 μm to 1 mm or more** (e.g., in a gravid uterus).

b. Structure (see Table 10-2). The **cytoplasm is acidophilic** and appears **homogenous** in both longitudinal sections and cross-sections.

c. Tissue

(1) Smooth muscle cells overlap, with their nuclei at different levels in the tissue. In cross-sections, most cells are cut through their narrowed tapered ends, but some are cut through the nucleus in their larger central region (see Figure 10-9B).

(2) The organization of smooth muscle depends on the shape and function of the organ it helps form. Many organs contain two or more layers of smooth muscle, each oriented at a different angle.

2. **Stroma.** A network of reticular fibers forms an endomysium around each cell. The endomysium is continuous with the connective tissue in adjacent layers of the organ. This stroma transmits the forces generated by contraction of individual cells throughout the tissue.

B. Fine structure

1. **Filaments.** Oblique bundles of thick and thin filaments cross the cells in many directions.

a. Thin actin-containing filaments are attached to dense bodies in the cytoplasm and on the cell membrane (Figure 10-10).

(1) The **dense bodies** contain α-actinin; therefore, they are **equivalent to the Z line in skeletal muscle**.

(2) Thin filaments in smooth muscle contain **no troponin**.

b. Thick myosin-containing filaments in smooth muscle are thicker (because the myosin molecules are arranged differently) and longer than those in striated muscle.

(1) These differences in organization permit thick and thin filaments in smooth muscle to slide much farther past each other and to shorten the cell much more.

(2) Each thick filament is associated with 15 thin filaments (versus 6 in striated muscle), which permits smooth muscle to generate much greater force than striated muscle.

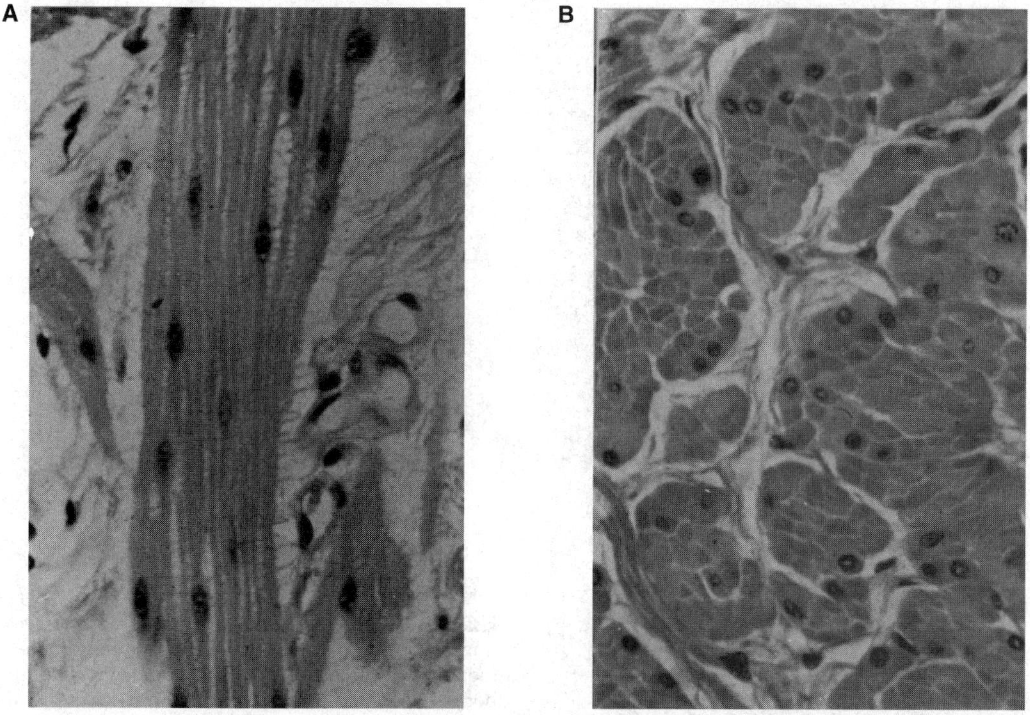

FIGURE 10-9. Smooth muscle. (*A*) Longitudinal section. The spindle shape of the cells can be seen. (*B*) Cross-section. Notice that most cells are sectioned through their elongated terminal portions, so that the centrally located nucleus is not visible. (Micrograph courtesy of RA Kainer. Reprinted with permission from Dellmann H-D: *Textbook of Veterinary Histology,* 4th ed. Baltimore, Williams & Wilkins, 1993, p 73.)

c. **Intermediate filaments,** primarily desmin, support the contractile filaments. They insert into the dense bodies with the thin filaments and help transmit contractile forces to the stroma.

2. **Caveolae.** The cell membrane has many caveolae (pockets), but no T tubules are present. Some sarcoplasmic reticulum can be found adjacent to the caveolae (see Figure 10-10), but most organelles are concentrated at the poles of the nucleus.

3. **Basal lamina.** A basal lamina surrounds each cell between intercellular junctions (see IV D 1 b & Figure 10-10).

C. Contraction

1. **Excitation–contraction coupling** depends, as in other types of muscle, on the influx of calcium. The calcium comes from extracellular and intracellular stores.
   a. **Calcium influx.** Most smooth muscle cells have calcium channels that open when the cell is stimulated.
      (1) Many of these are **voltage-dependent**. Smooth muscle in some organs (e.g., the gut wall) has an unstable membrane potential that fluctuates rhythmically.
      (2) Some are activated by **interaction of neurotransmitters or hormones with receptors**.
      (3) Some are activated by **stretching of the cell membrane**.
   b. Calcium is also released from sarcoplasmic reticulum.
   c. **Actin–myosin interaction** is controlled by the myosin molecule, rather than by the actin molecule (as it is in striated muscle). Smooth muscle myosin is able to interact with actin only when it is phosphorylated.

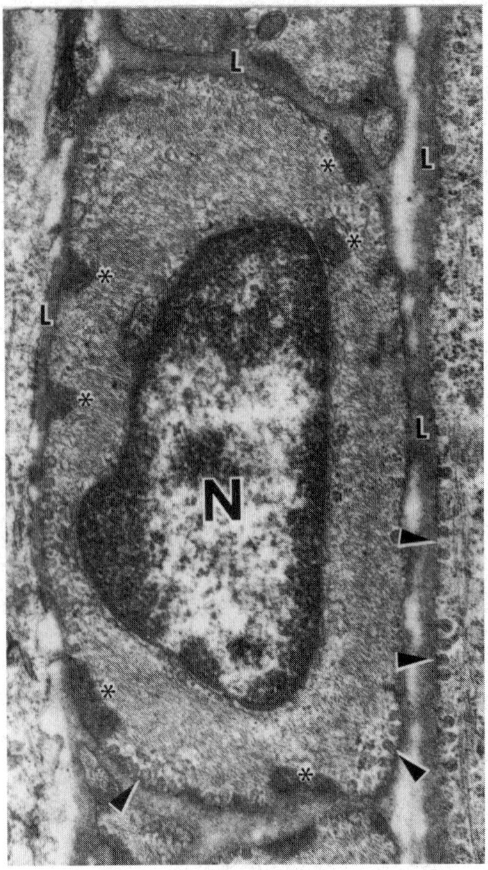

FIGURE 10-10. Electron micrograph of a cross-section through a smooth muscle cell. Bundles of filaments occupy most of the cytoplasm. Several dense bodies (*), which are the attachment sites for thin filaments, are indicated. The *arrowheads* point to caveolae in the cell membrane. A basal lamina (*L*) surrounds the cell. *N* = nucleus. (Micrograph courtesy of WS Tyler. Reprinted with permission from Dellmann H-D: *Textbook of Veterinary Histology,* 4th ed. Baltimore, Williams & Wilkins, 1993, p 74.)

(1) **Calmodulin.** When calcium rushes into the cell, it forms a complex with the calcium-binding protein calmodulin. The calcium–calmodulin complex activates myosin light-chain kinase, an enzyme that causes phosphorylation of myosin.

(2) **Cyclic adenosine monophosphate (cAMP).** Hormones regulate contraction and relaxation by altering intracellular levels of the "second messenger" molecule cAMP. This molecule, like calcium, activates myosin light-chain kinase, causing phosphorylation of myosin.

2. Regulation of contraction

a. Automaticity. Most smooth muscle has spontaneous (autonomous or myogenic) activity, which is modulated, rather than controlled, by the nervous system or by humoral signals.

b. Autonomic modulation. Most smooth muscle receives both parasympathetic and sympathetic input, with the two types of innervation having opposite effects on contractility.

(1) **Neurotransmitters**

(a) **Parasympathetic terminals** release **ACh**.

(b) **Sympathetic** terminals release **norepinephrine**.

(c) In some organs, sympathetic input stimulates motility and parasympathetic input is inhibitory; in other organs, these roles are reversed.

(2) **Neuromuscular junctions** are relatively simple [see Chapter 9 III B 1 b (2) (b) (iii)].

(3) **Nerve endings** may be sparse and lie at some distance from many of the cells, or each cell may be innervated.

D. Classification

1. **Visceral (unitary) smooth muscle** is characteristic of the walls of visceral organs.
   a. **Innervation.** Visceral smooth muscle is **sparsely innervated**.
   b. Because it has **many gap junctions,** visceral smooth muscle acts as a syncytium.
   c. **Regulation of contraction**
      (1) Visceral smooth muscle often has autonomous contractions.
      (2) The cells may have surface receptors for hormones or metabolites.
2. **Multiunit smooth muscle**
   a. **Innervation.** Multiunit smooth muscle is **richly innervated**.
   b. It has **no gap junctions;** therefore, precisely regulated contractions, such as those in the iris of the eye, are possible.

E. Functions

1. **Propulsion.** Smooth muscle contractions change the shape of a hollow organ (e.g., the urinary bladder, uterus), often to move material through it (e.g., peristaltic movement of intestinal contents).
2. **Vascular dynamics.** Contraction of vascular smooth muscle alters blood flow to parts of the body and determines the blood pressure.
3. **Secretion.** Smooth muscle cells secrete collagen, elastin, and proteoglycans.

F. Hypertrophy and regeneration

1. **Hypertrophy** in smooth muscle is accomplished by an increase in the size of individual cells and by hyperplasia, which results from mitosis of existing smooth muscle cells.
2. **Regeneration** of smooth muscle occurs to different degrees in different organs.
   a. Mitosis may occur, or pericytes may differentiate into fibroblasts or smooth muscle cells, contributing to regeneration in certain organs. Both mitosis and pericyte differentiation are stimulated by growth factors released from platelets in damaged tissue.
   b. Regeneration of vascular smooth muscle is necessary for revascularization of damaged tissues.

STUDY QUESTIONS

DIRECTIONS: Each of the numbered items or incomplete statements in this section is followed by answers or by completions of the statement. Select the **one** numbered answer or completion that is **best** in each case.

1. Which one of the following statements is true concerning the structure of skeletal muscle?

(1) The cells may reach a maximum of 50 μm in length.
(2) There are few capillaries.
(3) The A band is anisotropic because it contains both thick and thin filaments.
(4) Skeletal muscle contains many keratin filaments.
(5) Individual myofibrils are too slender to see in light-microscope preparations.

2. Which one of the following statements regarding the components of thin filaments is true?

(1) Tropomyosin binds to calcium.
(2) Troponin inhibits the interaction of actin and myosin.
(3) Tropomyosin is the major component.
(4) G-actin is a filamentous polymer in the form of a double helix.
(5) G-actin molecules are nonpolar.

3. Which one of the following statements regarding satellite cells is true?

(1) They are considered inactive myoblasts.
(2) They lie outside the basal laminae of skeletal muscle cells.
(3) They lie within the basal laminae of capillaries and venules.
(4) They are members of the mononuclear phagocyte system (MPS).
(5) They produce the endomysium.

4. Each sarcomere in a skeletal muscle cell:

(1) is bisected by an M line.
(2) contains a complete I band and halves of two A bands.
(3) maintains the same length during contraction.
(4) is darker in the I band region and lighter in the A band region.
(5) includes two H bands.

5. Which one of the following statements most accurately describes what happens during contraction of skeletal muscle?

(1) Calcium is actively taken up by sarcoplasmic reticulum.
(2) Tropomyosin attaches actin to myosin.
(3) Adenosine triphosphate (ATP) attaches to actin.
(4) Hydrolysis of ATP causes a conformational change in myosin molecules.

6. Which one of the following statements is true regarding the neuromuscular junction?

(1) The neuromuscular junction stimulates an influx of sodium, initiating an action potential in the sarcolemma.
(2) The neuromuscular junction stimulates an influx of calcium, initiating an action potential in the sarcolemma.
(3) Electrotonic transmission of the action potential from the axolemma across the synaptic cleft makes the sarcolemma permeable to sodium.
(4) Activation of the sarcolemma by cholinesterase initiates an action potential.
(5) Cholinesterase in the basal lamina activates acetylcholine (ACh).

7. How does red muscle differ from white muscle?

(1) Red muscle contracts more quickly than white muscle.
(2) Red muscle depends more on anaerobic glycolysis than white muscle.
(3) Red muscle fatigues more rapidly than white muscle.
(4) Red muscle contains more mitochondria than white muscle.
(5) Red muscle has more complex neuromuscular junctions than white muscle.

8. Which one of the following statements is true regarding the development of skeletal muscle?

(1) Mesenchymal cells differentiate into myotubes.
(2) Myotubes fuse end to end to form multinucleated myoblasts.
(3) Myofibrils are first formed in myoblasts.
(4) Pericytes are myogenic cells that remain in the basal lamina after the definitive muscle cells are formed.
(5) The innervation of a muscle cell determines its type.

9. Which one of the following statements is true concerning the arrangement of skeletal muscle stroma?

(1) Endomysium is dense connective tissue.
(2) Perimysium surrounds individual muscle cells.
(3) Epimysium encapsulates fascicles of muscle cells.
(4) The stroma facilitates shortening of the muscle.

10. What is the difference between excitation–contraction coupling in cardiac muscle and skeletal muscle?

(1) Calcium influx causes shortening of the sarcomeres only in skeletal muscle cells.
(2) The amount of calcium released determines the degree of contraction only in skeletal muscle cells.
(3) Depolarization of T tubules causes an influx of calcium only in skeletal muscle cells.
(4) Contraction is not as long-lasting in cardiac muscle cells.
(5) Calcium enters the myofibrils from both T tubules and sarcoplasmic reticulum only in cardiac muscle cells.

11. How do smooth muscle cells differ from other types of muscle cells?

(1) In smooth muscle cells, action potentials can pass from cell to cell via gap junctions.
(2) In smooth muscle cells, the cytoplasm is acidophilic.
(3) Contraction of smooth muscle cells is not initiated by an influx of calcium into the region of the thick and thin filaments.
(4) The cytoplasm of smooth muscle cells looks homogenous under the light microscope.
(5) Smooth muscle cells have no connective tissue stroma.

DIRECTIONS: Each of the numbered items or incomplete statements in this section is negatively phrased, as indicated by an italicized word such as *not, least,* or *except.* Select the **one** numbered answer or completion that is **best** in each case.

12. All of the following occur during hypertrophy of skeletal muscle *except:*

(1) an increase in the diameter of muscle cells.
(2) an increase in the number of nuclei in each muscle cell.
(3) division of muscle cell nuclei.
(4) fusion of satellite cells with muscle cells.
(5) an increase in the number of myofibrils.

13. All of the following statements regarding cardiac muscle cells are true *except:*

(1) sinoatrial node cells are smaller than other cardiac muscle cells.
(2) Purkinje fibers are larger than other cardiac muscle cells.
(3) atrial cells are smaller than ventricular cells.
(4) right ventricular cells are the richest source of a peptide that affects water and salt balance.
(5) cardiac muscle cells contain diads instead of triads.

ANSWERS AND EXPLANATIONS

1. The answer is 3 *[II A 1 b (2) (a) (i)]*. The A band of skeletal muscle is anisotropic (i.e., it exhibits birefringence in polarized light) because it contains two different kinds of parallel filaments: thick filaments and thin filaments. The cells may be 50 cm or more in length, not 50 μm. The tissue is richly vascularized. The cells contain many intermediate filaments, most of which are desmin; keratin is characteristic of epithelial cells. Individual myofibrils are easily seen in both longitudinal section and cross-section in a well-prepared light-microscope specimen.

2. The answer is 2 *[II C 1 b (1)–(2); Figure 10-4]*. One of the three subunits of troponin inhibits the interaction of actin and myosin, another binds to calcium, and the third attaches troponin to tropomyosin. Tropomyosin does not bind to calcium. Actin is the major component of the thin filaments. It is in the form of F-actin, a double-stranded helical polymer of globular G-actin molecules. G-actin molecules are polar, and the orientation of each F-actin filament in a muscle cell is determined by its polarity.

3. The answer is 1 *[II A 2]*. Satellite cells, which are able to fuse with existing skeletal muscle cells or fuse to form new cells in injured tissue, are considered a reservoir of inactive myoblasts. They lie within the basal laminae of skeletal muscle cells. Pericytes lie within the basal laminae of capillaries and venules. Satellite cells are not phagocytic, nor do they produce the endomysial connective tissue between skeletal muscle cells.

4. The answer is 1 *[II B 2]*. The sarcomere runs from Z line to Z line with the A band in the center. The A band, and therefore the sarcomere, is bisected by the M line, which is formed by lateral connections between the middles of thick filaments. A sarcomere contains a complete A band and halves of the two adjacent I bands. The A band does not shorten during contraction, but the I bands and H band do shorten; therefore, the total length of the sarcomere is reduced. The I bands are light and the A bands are dark. Only one H band (in the middle of the A band) is included in a sarcomere.

5. The answer is 4 *[II C 1 b (2) (b)]*. The energy released when adenosine triphosphate (ATP) is broken down causes the head of the myosin molecule to bend toward the center of the thick filament (i.e., toward the H band), taking the actin filament to which it is attached with it. Calcium is released from the sarcoplasmic reticulum during contraction. Its active reuptake causes relaxation. Tropomyosin is a part of the thin filament that does not attach to myosin. ATP attaches to the myosin heads, not to actin.

6. The answer is 1 *[II C 2 b (2)]*. The action potential in the sarcolemma is initiated by an influx of sodium. The sodium influx occurs when acetylcholine (ACh) causes the opening of receptor-gated sodium channels. Calcium influx and electrotonic transmission are not involved in skeletal muscle activation. Cholinesterase, which is located in the basal lamina, breaks down excess ACh. If cholinesterase were not present, the muscle cell would be subjected to continuous stimulation from a single nerve impulse.

7. The answer is 4 *[II D 2–3]*. Red muscle, which relies primarily on oxidative pathways (rather than anaerobic glycolysis), contains more mitochondria, the oxidative machinery of the cell. Moreover, the mitochondrial cristae in red muscle cells are more extensive, and the colored enzymes (cytochromes) in the cristae are partially responsible for the darker color of red muscle cells. White muscle cells contract more quickly than most red muscle cells, and they fatigue more readily. In consonance with their specialization for quick responses, white muscle cells have better-developed neuromuscular junctions with many synaptic vesicles in the axon terminals and more extensive junctional folds.

8. The answer is 5 *[II D 1 c]*. The innervation of a muscle cell determines what type it will be. This has been demonstrated experimentally by surgically altering the innervation of a muscle. The muscle cells change to the type characteristic of the muscle their new nerve supply originally innervated. Mesenchymal cells differentiate into myoblasts, which form a row and fuse end to end to form myotubes. Myofibrils are first seen in myotubes. Satellite cells are residual myogenic cells that are enclosed in the basal laminae of mature muscle cells. They divide and give rise to cells that fuse with muscle cells during hypertrophy, and they also become active during regeneration of damaged tissue.

9. The answer is 4 *[II A 3].* The stroma transmits the forces generated by contraction of individual muscle cells to the muscle attachments, causing shortening of the entire muscle when any of the muscle cells contract. Maximum shortening of the entire muscle occurs only when all the individual muscle cells contract. Endomysium is a network of reticular fibers surrounding individual muscle cells. Perimysium surrounds muscle fascicles. Epimysium, which corresponds to the deep fascia of gross anatomy, encapsulates the entire muscle.

10. The answer is 5 *[II C 1 b (1), III C 1 a].* In cardiac muscle, calcium flows into the region of the myofibrils from T tubules and other extracellular regions as well as from the sarcoplasmic reticulum, which is why the T tubules are larger in cardiac muscle cells. Depolarization of T tubules causes an influx of calcium in both skeletal and cardiac muscle. In skeletal muscle, the influx is entirely from the sarcoplasmic reticulum. Calcium influx causes shortening of the sarcomeres in both cardiac and skeletal muscle. The amount of calcium released is always enough to cause complete contraction in skeletal muscle, but it is a means of varying the strength of contraction in cardiac muscle. Contractions are approximately 20 times longer in cardiac muscle cells than in skeletal muscle cells.

11. The answer is 4 *[II A 1 b; III A 2 b; IV A 1 b; Table 10-2].* Because their actin and myosin filaments are not arranged in parallel arrays to form myofibrils, smooth muscle cells appear homogenous under the light microscope. Action potentials are spread by gap junctions in both cardiac and smooth muscle. The cytoplasm is acidophilic in all types of muscle cells. Contraction is initiated by an influx of calcium into the region of the thick and thin filaments in all types of muscle. Smooth muscle has a connective tissue stroma, which plays an important role in transmitting the forces generated by the cells to cause changes in the shape or dimensions of the organs they form.

12. The answer is 3 *[II E 2 b].* The increase in number of nuclei and diameter of muscle cells is accomplished by fusion with satellite cells; no division of muscle cell nuclei occurs. When skeletal muscle hypertrophies, the cell diameter and the number of nuclei in each cell increase. The extra nuclei produce additional myofibrils and cytoplasmic elements.

13. The answer is 4 *[III B 2 a (2)].* Atrial natriuretic factor, which acts on the kidney to cause loss of water and sodium, is produced primarily by cells in the right atrium, not the right ventricle. Sinoatrial node cells are smaller than other cardiac muscle cells, and Purkinje fibers are larger than most. Atrial cells are smaller than ventricular cells. Cardiac cells contain diads; triads are found in skeletal muscle cells.

Chapter 11

Cardiovascular System

I. INTRODUCTION.

Blood circulates through the body in a closed system of branching and anastomosing tubular organs called the **cardiovascular system**.

II. HEART

A. Function

1. **Right side.** The right atrium receives blood from the systemic circulation. Contraction of the right ventricle pumps the blood into the lungs.
2. **Left side.** The left atrium receives blood from the lungs. Contraction of the left ventricle pumps the blood into the systemic circulation.

B. Structure.

The wall of the heart has **three layers**.

1. **Endocardium** completely lines the atria and ventricles, and it forms the valves (Figure 11-1).
   a. **Endothelium** is a surface layer of simple squamous cells derived from mesoderm.
   b. **Subendothelium** is a layer of dense connective tissue that contains both elastic and collagen fibers. It may also contain smooth muscle cells.
   c. **Subendocardium** is the outer layer, composed of loose connective tissue that contains both elastic and collagen fibers.
      (1) In some areas, this layer is insignificant, but in others, it contains many blood and lymph vessels and adipose cells.
      (2) In the ventricles, the subendocardium also contains impulse-conducting cardiac muscle cells, **Purkinje fibers** (see Figure 11-1).

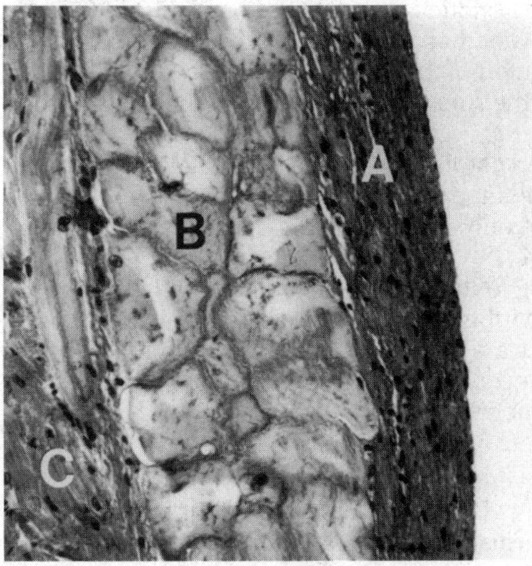

FIGURE 11-1. Horizontal section through part of the ventricle wall in the heart. Most of the field is occupied by endocardium. A thick subendothelial layer of dense connective tissue (*A*) lies under the endothelium at the right. The conducting fibers in the subendocardial layer (*B*) are particularly large and pale because this section is from a large ruminant. A portion of the myocardium (*C*) is visible. (Reprinted with permission from Dellmann H-D: *Textbook of Veterinary Histology,* 4th ed. Baltimore, Williams & Wilkins, 1993, p 116.)

2. **Myocardium,** the thickest layer of the heart, comprises cardiac muscle, the cardiac skeleton, and the conducting system.
   a. **Cardiac muscle**
      (1) Most of the myocardium is composed of interwoven and anastomosing bundles of contractile cardiac muscle cells (see Chapter 10 III).
         (a) **Atria.** Atrial contractions fill the ventricles, which requires relatively little force; therefore, atrial musculature is much less developed than the ventricular musculature. Consequently, the atria have thinner walls than the ventricles.
         (b) **Ventricles.** The wall of the left ventricle is thicker than that of the right because more force is required to push blood through the systemic vasculature than through lung vasculature.
      (2) The muscle cells are supplied by a rich capillary bed in the loose connective tissue stroma of the myocardium. The stroma is continuous with the connective tissue in adjacent layers (i.e., the subendocardium and subepicardium).
   b. **Cardiac skeleton**
      (1) The cardiac skeleton is a layer of connective tissue that separates the contractile muscle cells of the atria from those of the ventricles and forms part of the interventricular septum.
         (a) The atrial myocardium inserts into one side of this layer; the ventricular myocardium inserts into the other.
         (b) Depending on the species and age of the animal, the cardiac skeleton may contain dense irregular connective tissue (in pigs and cats), fibrocartilage (in dogs), hyaline cartilage (in horses), or bone (in large ruminants).
      (2) The cardiac skeleton comprises the:
         (a) Fibrous rings that surround the atrioventricular valves and the valves of the aorta and pulmonary artery
         (b) Triangular connective tissue (**trigonum fibrosum**) between the valves
         (c) Fibrous part of the interventricular septum
   c. **Conducting system.** This system coordinates the contraction of the myocardium so that blood is efficiently pumped out of the chambers with each contraction.
      (1) **Sinoatrial node.** The sinoatrial node in the right atrium acts as the **pacemaker** of the heart. Nodal cells are surrounded by many autonomic nerve endings (see Chapter 10 III C 2 a, b).
      (2) **Atrioventricular node.** Waves of depolarization that begin in the sinoatrial node are passed by gap junctions throughout the entire atrial musculature to the atrioventricular node during atrial contraction. Depolarization does not spread directly from the atrial cells to the ventricular contractile cells because the cardiac skeleton intervenes.
      (3) **Atrioventricular bundle.** These large conductive cells (see Chapter 10 III B 2 b) are arranged in series to form a pathway that arises from the atrioventricular node and penetrates the fibrous skeleton of the heart. The pathway (bundle) then divides into branches that course in the subendocardial layer of the ventricles and branch into the myocardium.
         (a) The conductive cells are modified cardiac muscle cells, specialized for rapid conduction of an action potential rather than for contraction.
         (b) The atrioventricular bundle is the only functional connection between the atrial and ventricular musculature.
         (c) Branches of the bundle extending to the ventricular wall are joined to surrounding contractile cells by gap junctions, through which the action potentials spread. The bundle branches are arranged so that contraction is initiated at the apex of the heart and proceeds toward the aorta and pulmonary artery, forcing the blood out of the chambers.

3. **Epicardium** is the serous membrane that covers the external surface of the heart. In gross anatomical terminology, it is called the **visceral pericardium**. Along with the **parietal pericardium,** it forms the closed **pericardial cavity**.

a. **Subepicardium** is loose connective tissue with numerous elastic fibers. It contains many blood vessels (including the coronary vessels), nerves, and ganglia. It may also contain a large amount of adipose tissue.
b. **Mesothelium** covers the surface.

III. MACROVASCULATURE. The macrovasculature comprises blood vessels that are grossly visible.

A. General structure of blood vessels. The walls of most blood vessels are composed of **three layers (tunics)**.

1. The **tunica interna (intima)** comprises an endothelial lining and subendothelial connective tissue.
   a. Granules in the endothelial cells of all vessels larger than capillaries contain a component of the blood-clotting mechanism.
   b. Smooth muscle cells may be present.
   c. The **internal elastic membrane,** when present, is the outermost layer of the tunica interna.
2. The **tunica media** contains vascular smooth muscle in a circular (tight helix) arrangement around the vessel.
   a. Elastic laminae and elastic and collagen fibers produced by the smooth muscle cells are often present.
   b. The **external elastic membrane,** when present, is a distinct outermost elastic lamina.
3. The **tunica externa (adventitia)** is the outermost connective tissue sheath.
   a. It may contain smooth muscle.
   b. Blood vessels (**vasa vasorum**) and vasomotor nerves (**nervi vasorum**) that supply the vessel wall are present in this layer and may penetrate the outer tunica media in large vessels.

B. Arteries carry blood to the tissues. In general, the walls of arteries, especially muscular arteries, are thick relative to the diameter of their lumens.

1. **Elastic (conducting) arteries** include the aorta and its large branches.
   a. **Function.** These large arteries, closest to the heart, are specialized to reduce fluctuations in blood pressure and blood flow caused by the heartbeat.
      (1) During **systole (ventricular contraction),** the elastic walls are stretched, and the force of the blood pressure is converted to elastic tension.
      (2) During **diastole (ventricular relaxation),** the elastic rebound of the arterial walls maintains the pressure and moves the blood along, acting as an auxiliary pump.
   b. **Structure** (Figure 11-2)
      (1) **Tunica interna**
         (a) The tunica interna is prominent because of its thick subendothelial layer, especially in large animals.
         (b) Smooth muscle cells, usually longitudinally oriented, may be numerous.
         (c) An internal elastic membrane may be present, but is usually not distinct. It is often split into several thin anastomosing elastic laminae.
      (2) **Tunica media**
         (a) The tunica media is the thickest layer.
         (b) It contains smooth muscle cells between abundant thick elastic laminae (see Figure 11-2). The concentrically arranged laminae are fenestrated.
         (c) Elastic and collagen fibers are also present.
      (3) **Tunica externa**
         (a) The tunica externa is thin.
         (b) It contains elastic and collagen fibers.

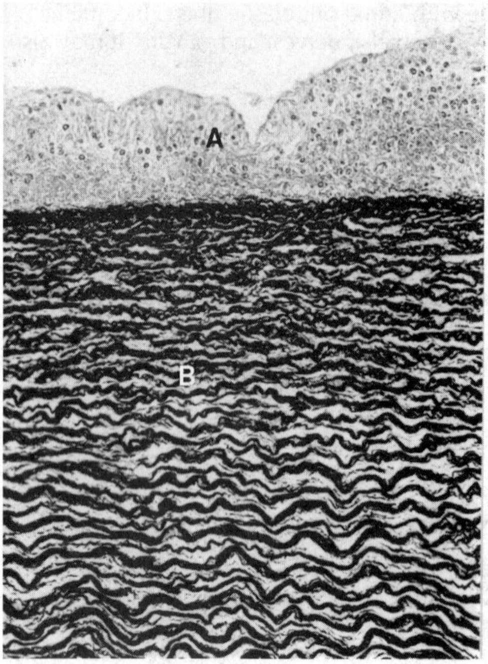

FIGURE 11-2. Cross-section through part of the wall of an elastic artery stained to demonstrate elastin. The subendothelial layer (*A*) is very thick and contains many elastic fibers (cut in cross-section). The tunica media (*B*) contains thick elastic laminae and fibers. (Reprinted with permission from Dellmann H-D: *Textbook of Veterinary Histology,* 4th ed. Baltimore, Williams & Wilkins, 1993, p 109.)

2. **Muscular (distributing) arteries** are the most numerous arteries. They are of smaller diameter than the elastic arteries.
   a. **Function.** The muscular arteries control the blood flow to various organs in response to autonomic regulation or local chemical signals. They are richly innervated.
   b. **Structure** (Figure 11-3)
      (1) **Tunica interna**
         (a) The tunica interna usually has a prominent internal elastic membrane, which typically looks like a wavy line because of contraction of the artery when the specimen is collected (see Figure 11-3).
         (b) A few smooth muscle cells may be present.
      (2) **Tunica media**
         (a) The tunica media consists primarily of smooth muscle with elastic laminae and fibers, reticular fibers, and ground substance.
         (b) An external elastic membrane, similar to that found in elastic arteries, may be present in large muscular arteries.
      (3) **Tunica externa**
         (a) In most cases, the tunica externa is approximately the same thickness as the tunica media.
         (b) It contains collagen and most of the elastin of the artery wall. The amount of elastin gradually lessens as the size of the vessel decreases.
3. **Chemoreceptors** are associated with certain arteries. They contain large spherical or ovoid chemoreceptive cells that are sensitive to low oxygen or elevated carbon dioxide concentrations in the blood and supportive cells.
   a. **Carotid bodies** are chemoreceptors located near the bifurcation of the common carotid.
   b. **Aortic bodies** are chemoreceptors located near the bifurcation of the aorta.

C. **Veins** are capacitance vessels (i.e., their distensibility permits them to accommodate a large increase in blood volume in response to a relatively small increase in blood pressure). They contain 3–5 times the volume of blood in the arteries.

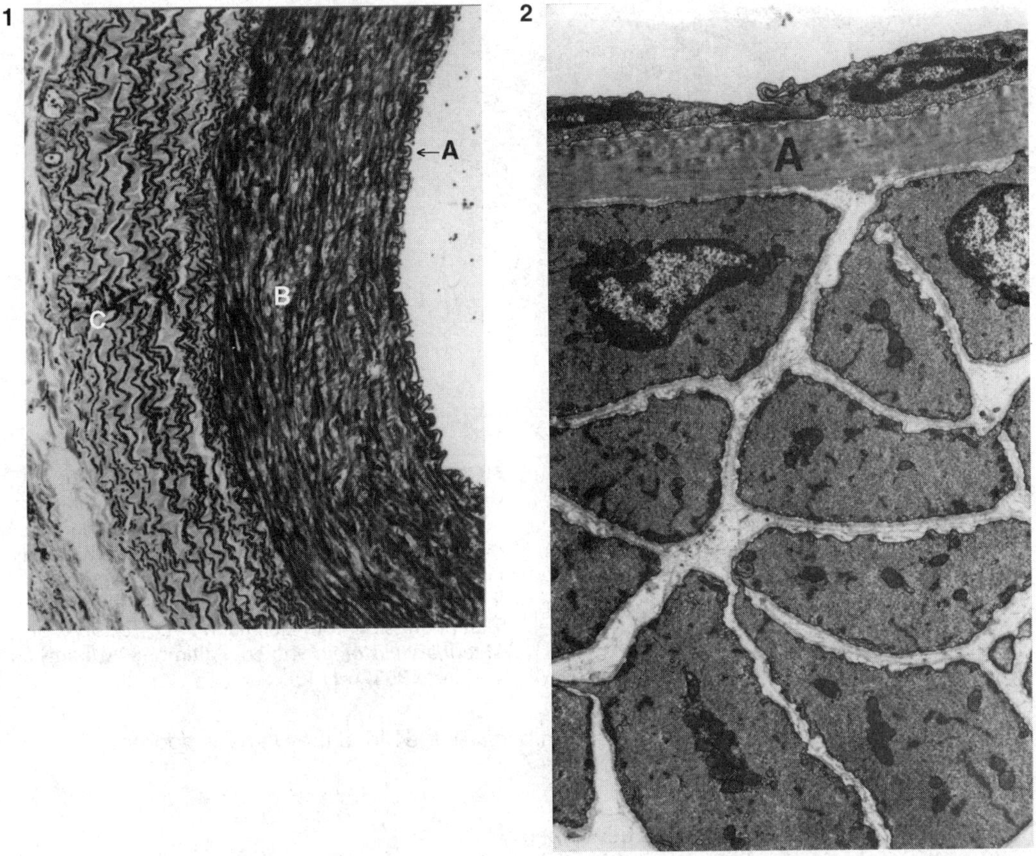

FIGURE 11-3. Sections through part of the wall of a muscular artery. (*1*) Cross-section stained to demonstrate elastin. The tunica interna has a prominent wavy internal elastic membrane (*A*). The tunica media (*B*) is composed primarily of circularly arranged smooth muscle, but elastic laminae are also present. The tunica externa (*C*) is composed primarily of elastic fibers. (*2*) Electron micrograph of a longitudinal section. The thick internal elastic membrane (*A*) lies under the endothelium. Smooth muscle cells in the tunica media are cut in cross-section.

1. Introduction

a. Folds of the tunica interna of veins form **valves,** which allow blood to flow only toward the heart.

(1) Valves are abundant in the extremities, where they prevent gravitational backflow of blood and protect capillary beds from backflow caused by muscular contractions.

(2) Valves are usually absent in veins of the trunk and head.

b. Vein structure varies widely in different parts of the body and among species. It is determined by such local factors as the effects of gravity and the support or pressure provided by adjacent organs.

c. Comparisons with corresponding arteries

(1) The walls of veins are thinner relative to the size of their lumen.

(2) Veins usually contain less muscle; therefore, they are more likely to be collapsed in histologic sections.

(3) In veins, the tunica externa forms a greater portion of the vessel wall, elastin is less abundant, and collagen is more abundant.

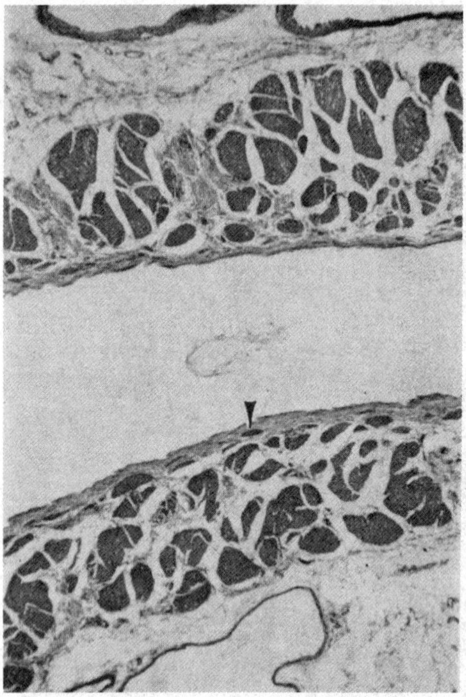

FIGURE 11-4. Low magnification view of a cross-section through part of the vena cava. The tunica media is very thin and contains only a few bundles of smooth muscle (*arrow*). The tunica externa forms the bulk of the wall and contains large bundles of longitudinally oriented smooth muscle. (Reprinted with permission from Dellmann H-D: *Textbook of Veterinary Histology,* 4th ed. Baltimore, Williams & Wilkins, 1993, p 114.)

(4) Veins have more vasa vasorum because the blood they carry is poorly oxygenated.

2. Large veins (Figure 11-4)

a. The **tunica interna** is well developed.

b. The **tunica media** is much thinner in large veins than in arteries and contains significant amounts of connective tissue (see Figure 11-4). Smooth muscle may be absent in the media of large veins.

c. The **tunica externa** is the thickest of the three layers. It contains collagen and elastic fibers; in some veins, it contains large bundles of longitudinally oriented smooth muscle (see Figure 11-4).

3. Small and medium-sized veins

a. The **tunica interna** is thin and may lack a subendothelial layer.

b. The **tunica media** is thin, especially in deep veins.

(1) The tunica media consists mostly of smooth muscle, which may be longitudinally oriented in the inner layers.

(2) Superficial veins that drain dependent limbs have a very well-developed tunica media that helps to offset the influence of gravity on their contents.

c. The **tunica externa,** which is primarily collagen, is usually the thickest layer, except in the superficial veins of the limbs.

4. Portal vessels carry blood from one capillary bed to another. The **portal vein,** which carries blood from the capillary bed in the intestine to sinusoids in the liver, has a thick muscular wall.

IV. MICROVASCULATURE.

The microvasculature comprises blood vessels that are visible microscopically.

A. Arterioles

Arterioles are the smallest branches of the arterial tree.

1. **Functions**
   a. Arterioles deliver blood to capillaries at a low pressure.
   b. They regulate the flow of blood through specific capillary beds in response to local metabolic signals and autonomic innervation. They are the source of half of the total resistance in the circulatory system; therefore, they are the major regulators of blood pressure.

2. **Structure** (Figure 11-5)
   a. The **tunica interna** is very thin but, in the largest arterioles, may include an internal elastic membrane.
   b. The **tunica media** is composed of 1–3 complete layers of smooth muscle.
   c. The **tunica externa** provides a thin covering for the tunica media.

B. **Metarterioles** are small vessels with a discontinuous layer of smooth muscle cells.

1. **Function.** Metarterioles control blood flow through specific capillary beds and give rise to capillaries.

2. **Thoroughfare channels** are alternative routes through which blood can flow directly from the metarteriole to the venule that drains the capillary bed.

3. **Precapillary sphincters** are smooth muscle cells that encircle the openings of the capillaries that branch from the metarteriole. When they contract, blood flows through the thoroughfare channel; when they relax, blood enters the capillaries.

C. **Capillaries** are the smallest blood vessels. Their average diameter is approximately the same as the diameter of erythrocytes in the same species (Figure 11-6).

1. **Function.** Capillaries facilitate the exchange of gasses and other substances between the blood and interstitial fluid.

2. **Structure**
   a. **General structure.** The walls of capillaries are very thin, consisting of as little as an endothelial cell and its basal lamina.
      (1) **Pericytes** (Figure 11-7) may be enclosed within the basal lamina. Pericytes are believed to be contractile, and they constitute a reservoir of cells that can give rise to smooth muscle cells or fibroblasts (see Chapter 6 II C 1 b).

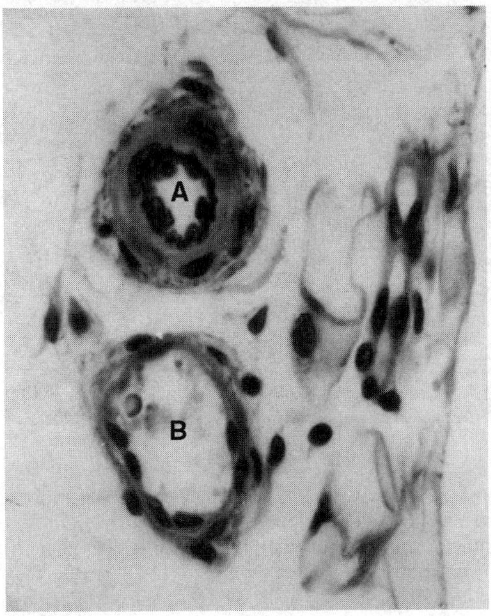

FIGURE 11-5. Cross-sections through an arteriole (*A*) and a venule (*B*). The tunica media of the arteriole contains 2–3 layers of smooth muscle cells.

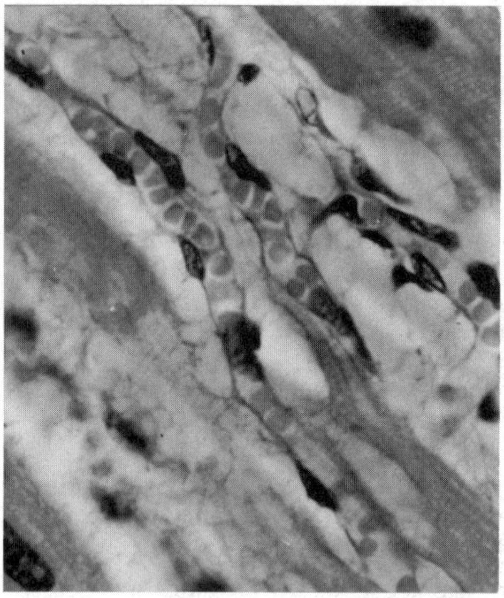

FIGURE 11-6. Capillaries in longitudinal section in the myocardium. Notice that the average diameter of the capillaries is approximately the same as that of the erythrocytes that can be seen in their lumens. (Reprinted with permission from Dellmann H-D: *Textbook of Veterinary Histology,* 4th ed. Baltimore, Williams & Wilkins, 1993, p 112.)

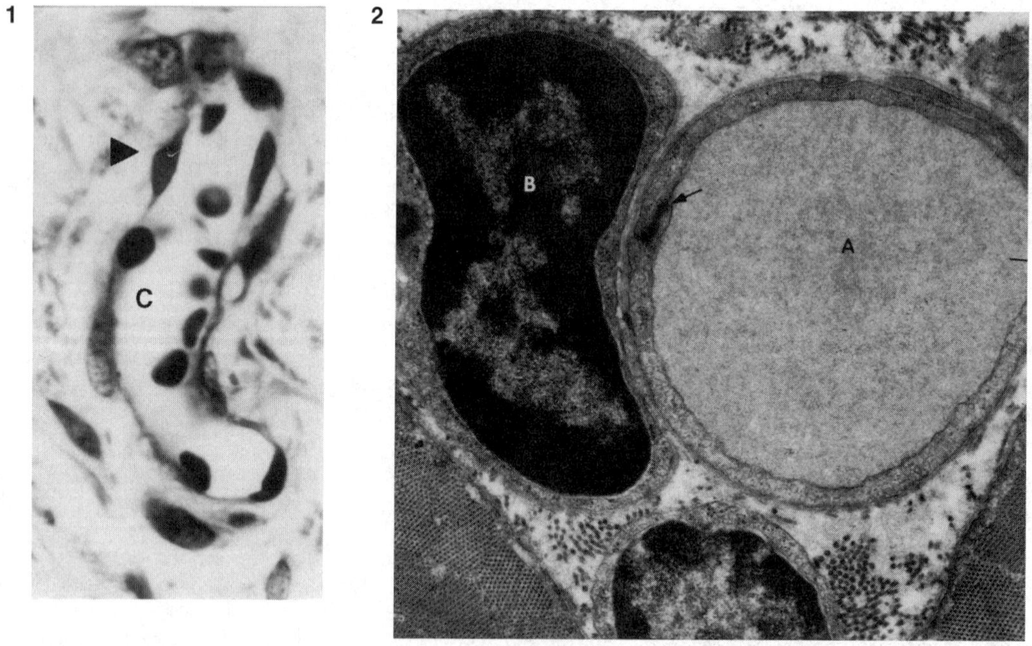

FIGURE 11-7. Capillaries. (*1*) A dilated capillary (*C*) in loose connective tissue. A pericyte nucleus is indicated (*arrow*) in the wall of the capillary. (*2*) Electron micrograph of a continuous capillary (*A*) in skeletal muscle. The endothelial cells are joined by tight junctions (*arrow*) and surrounded by a basal lamina, which also encompasses the adjacent pericyte (*B*). (2 is reprinted with permission from Dellmann H-D: *Textbook of Veterinary Histology,* 4th ed. Baltimore, Williams & Wilkins, 1993, p 112.)

(2) A few **reticular fibers** usually surround the vessel, but these are absent in the central nervous system (CNS).

(3) Many capillaries have **precapillary sphincters** (see IV B 3).

b. Fine structure

(1) Continuous capillaries are found in all organs.

(a) Endothelial cells joined by **tight junctions** form a tube in which the cytoplasm forms a layer that is continuous (see Figure 11-7), although it may be very attenuated.

(b) Transcytotic vesicles

(i) Transcytotic vesicles are common in the capillary endothelium of some organs, such as muscle, and rare in others, such as the brain and spinal cord.

(ii) The paucity of transcytotic vesicles and the integrity of the intercellular tight junctions of the microcirculatory endothelium in the CNS account for the **blood–brain barrier**.

(2) Fenestrated capillaries (Figure 11-8) are common in the lamina propria of the intestine and in endocrine organs. In endocrine organs, they are called **sinusoidal capillaries** (see Figure 19-8B).

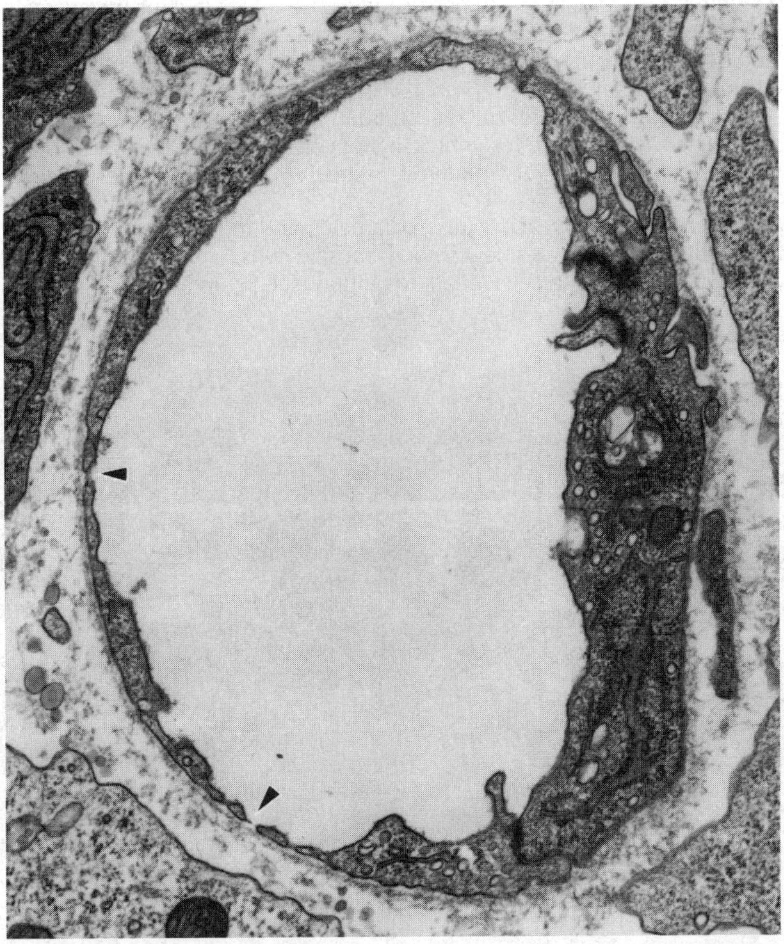

FIGURE 11-8. Electron micrograph of a fenestrated capillary in the lamina propria of the small intestine. Fenestrations (*arrows*) are covered by thin diaphragms. (Reprinted with permission from Dellmann H-D: *Textbook of Veterinary Histology,* 4th ed. Baltimore, Williams & Wilkins, 1993, p 112.)

(a) These capillaries are relatively large, and their walls conform to the shape of surrounding structures rather than forming a cylindrical tube.

(b) Attenuated regions of the cytoplasm have circular fenestrae (windows) 60–80 nm in diameter, which are closed only by a single-layered diaphragm that is thinner than a cell membrane. Fenestrations facilitate passage of substances across the endothelial layer.

(3) **Porous capillaries** (Figure 11-9) are present in the glomeruli of the kidney [see Chapter 15 II B 1 a (1) (a) (i)]. The endothelium has open pores that are not guarded by a diaphragm. Instead, they are underlaid by an unusually thick basal lamina.

(4) **Sinusoids** in the liver are much more permeable than other capillaries because of gaps and open pores in the endothelial cells and discontinuities in the basal lamina. They are large, and their shape and size are determined by the surrounding liver parenchyma.

D. Venules (see Figure 11-5)

1. Postcapillary venules

a. **Function.** Like capillaries, the postcapillary venules are **exchange vessels**. Most of the water and solutes that escape through the capillary walls reenter the blood vascular system through the walls of venules.

b. **Structure**

(1) Postcapillary venules may reach 50 μm in diameter.

(2) Their wall structure resembles that of capillaries, but they are more permeable.

(3) Pericytes may be very numerous, especially in large venules (**pericytic venules**).

2. **Muscular venules** may reach 1 μm in diameter, and their walls are very thin. The smallest muscular venules have a few smooth muscle cells, which gradually increase to 1–2 layers of smooth muscle cells in larger venules (see Figure 11-5).

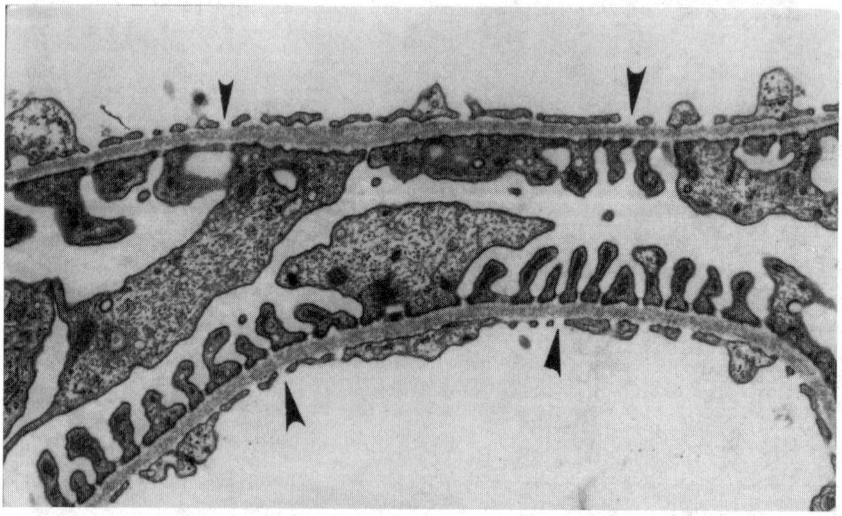

FIGURE 11-9. Electron micrograph of two porous capillaries in the glomerulus of the kidney. The pores (arrows) open directly to the thick basal lamina. (Reprinted with permission from Dellmann H-D: *Textbook of Veterinary Histology,* 4th ed. Baltimore, Williams & Wilkins, 1993, p 113.)

E. Arteriovenous anastomoses

1. **Function.** Arteriovenous anastomoses provide a direct route between the arterial and venous circulation. They usually connect arterioles to venules. Specialized arteriovenous anastomoses are involved in erection, thermoregulation, regulation of blood pressure, and menstruation (in primates).
2. **Structure.** Arteriovenous anastomoses have richly innervated muscular walls, which contract and relax to prevent or permit blood flow through a capillary bed.

V. LYMPHATICS.

LYMPHATICS. Lymph is transported in a one-way system of anastomosing tubular organs called lymphatics. Macromolecules and fluids that escape from the blood into the interstitial fluid are returned to the blood by lymph.

A. Lymph vessels (see Figure 11-10)

1. **Formation.** Lymph vessels start as blind-ending lymph capillaries in the connective tissue. These join to form larger lymph vessels, with at least one lymph node interposed on each lymph vessel. Lymph vessels lead to larger collecting ducts that return the lymph to the venous system.
2. **Structure**
   - **a.** Lymph vessels have the same layers as veins, but the walls are thinner and the layers are not as well organized.
   - **b.** Lymph vessels also contain more valves than veins.

B. Lymph capillaries (Figure 11-11)

1. **Location**
   - **a.** Lymph capillaries are most numerous in loose connective tissue.

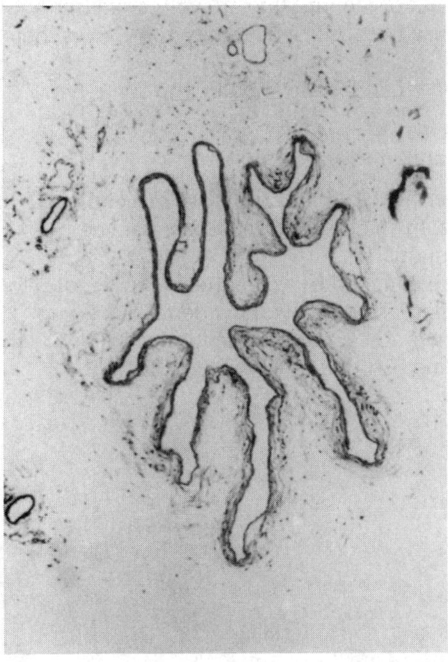

FIGURE 11-10. Cross-section through a large lymph vessel, the thoracic duct of a dog. The wall consists of endothelium, a discontinuous layer of smooth muscle, and a thin tunica externa.

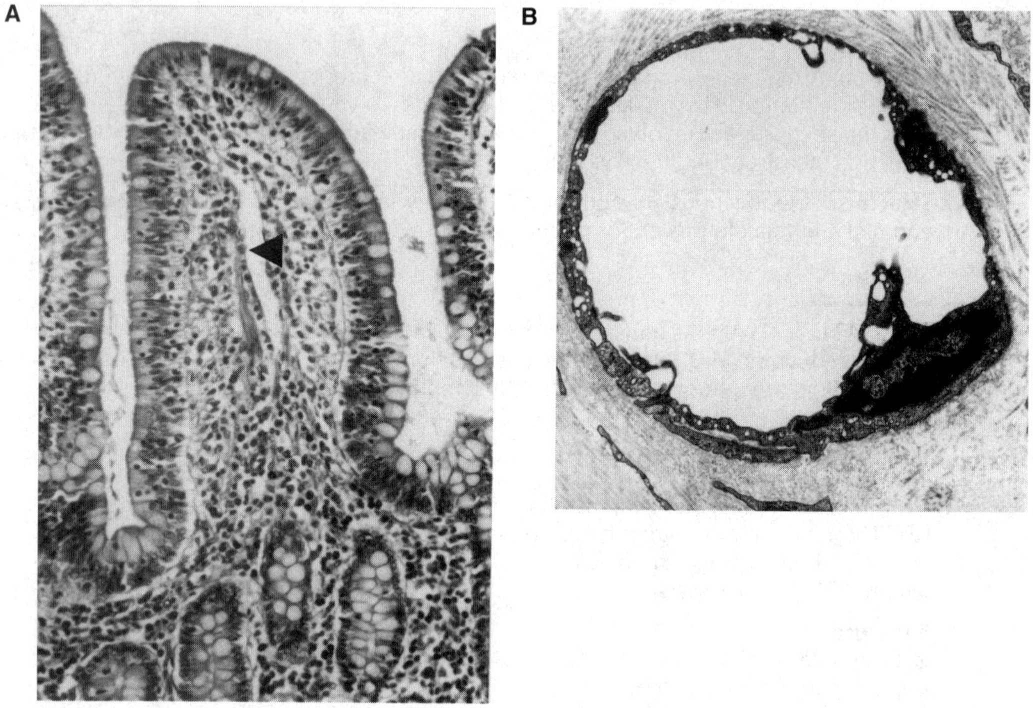

FIGURE 11-11. Sections through lymph capillaries in the small intestine. (*A*) A lacteal (*arrow*) is visible in an intestinal villus. (*B*) Electron micrograph of a lymph capillary. The endothelium contains many pinocytotic vesicles. (*B* is reprinted with permission from Dellmann H-D: *Textbook of Veterinary Histology,* 4th ed. Baltimore, Williams & Wilkins, 1993, p 118.)

b. Lymph capillaries that drain the lamina propria of the intestine are very large (see Figure 11-11). They are called **lacteals** because the absorbed fat they carry gives their contents a milky appearance.

c. Lymph capillaries are absent in the CNS, bone, cartilage, eye bulb, and some lymphatic organs.

2. Size. Lymph capillaries are larger than blood capillaries.

3. Structure. Lymph capillaries are **much more permeable than capillaries or venules**.

a. In the endothelium, the cells merely overlap. In some cases, gaps exist between cells. The basal lamina is absent or discontinuous.

b. The outer surfaces of the endothelial cells are attached by cell adhesion molecules to the surrounding tissue, which holds the capillaries open, even in edematous tissue. Therefore, drainage of their contents into larger vessels lowers the luminal hydrostatic pressure to below that of the surrounding tissue.

STUDY QUESTIONS

DIRECTIONS: Each of the numbered items or incomplete statements in this section is followed by answers or by completions of the statement. Select the **one** numbered answer or completion that is **best** in each case.

1. The walls of the ventricles are characterized by their:

(1) simple cuboidal endothelium.
(2) lack of elastic fibers.
(3) rich innervation.
(4) small cardiac muscle cells (as compared with those of the atrium).
(5) subendocardial layer of loose connective tissue.

2. Which one of the following statements is true of the structure of the myocardium?

(1) The stroma is separated from the endocardium and epicardium.
(2) The cardiac skeleton is a connective tissue layer that separates the contractile cells of the right side of the heart from those of the left side of the heart.
(3) The contractile cells of the atria have no direct connections with those of the ventricles.
(4) The contractile cells are arranged in distinct layers.
(5) No connective tissue is present in this layer.

3. The coronary arteries are located in:

(1) the subepicardium.
(2) the subendocardium.
(3) the subendothelium.
(4) the myocardium.
(5) the mesothelium.

4. Endocrine glands and the intestinal lamina propria both contain:

(1) porous capillaries.
(2) fenestrated capillaries.
(3) sinusoidal capillaries.
(4) sinusoids.

5. Which one of the following statements regarding elastic arteries is true?

(1) Elastic arteries act as auxiliary pumps.
(2) Elastic arteries have little effect on the rate of blood flow.
(3) Elastic arteries have a well-defined internal elastic membrane.
(4) Elastic arteries have a very muscular tunica media.
(5) Elastic arteries generally have the thickest tunica externa of any type of artery.

6. Which one of the following statements correctly describes a structural characteristic of muscular arteries?

(1) The tunica media of muscular arteries is by far the thickest layer.
(2) Muscular arteries rarely have a distinct internal elastic membrane.
(3) Muscular arteries have thick walls relative to the size of their lumens.
(4) There are no elastic laminae in the tunica media of muscular arteries.
(5) There are no elastic elements in the tunica externa of muscular arteries.

7. Which one of the following statements correctly describes a structural feature of veins?

(1) Almost all veins have valves.
(2) Veins are not normally distensible.
(3) The tunica externa of veins is not as well developed as that of the corresponding arteries.
(4) Veins contain more elastin and less collagen than comparable arteries.
(5) The tunica media of veins may not contain smooth muscle.

8. Which one of the following statements is true of arterioles?

(1) The tunica media of arterioles consists of a discontinuous layer of smooth muscle cells.
(2) The tunica externa is the thickest layer.
(3) Arterioles are responsible for 10%–15% of the total resistance in the circulatory system.
(4) Arterioles can be distinguished from small arteries by their lack of an internal elastic membrane.
(5) Arterioles constrict and dilate in response to local metabolic signals.

9. How do lymph vessels differ from veins?

(1) Their contents flow toward the heart.
(2) They have more valves.
(3) They have thicker walls.
(4) The layers in their walls are more organized.
(5) They are less permeable.

DIRECTIONS: Each of the numbered items or incomplete statements in this section is negatively phrased, as indicated by an italicized word such as *not, least,* or *except.* Select the **one** numbered answer or completion that is **best** in each case.

10. All of the following structures are normally present in the walls of capillaries *except:*

(1) a tunica media.
(2) pericytes.
(3) simple squamous endothelium.
(4) a basal lamina.
(5) contractile cells.

11. All of the following types of blood vessels deliver blood to capillaries *except:*

(1) metarterioles.
(2) arteriovenous anastomoses.
(3) arterioles.
(4) portal vessels.

ANSWERS AND EXPLANATIONS

1. The answer is 5 *[II B 1 c]*. The subendocardial layer of loose connective tissue is important because it contains many blood vessels and lymphatics and, in the ventricles, the conducting system. The lining of the entire heart is simple squamous endothelial cells, which appear polygonal when viewed from the surface. Many elastic fibers are present in both the endocardial and epicardial layers. Ventricular myocardium is not innervated, and ventricular muscle cells are larger than those of the atria.

2. The answer is 3 *[II B 2 b 1]*. The cardiac skeleton completely separates the contractile cells of the atria, which insert on one side, from those of the ventricles, which insert on the other side. A connective tissue stroma (sometimes called the endomysium) surrounds the muscle cells and contains the capillary bed that supplies them. The stroma is continuous with the subendocardial layer of the endocardium and the subepicardial layer of the epicardium. More extensive connective tissue surrounds larger vessels and branches of the conductive system. The contractile cells branch and interconnect in a tightly woven mass so that the roughly spherical heart can contract in all dimensions.

3. The answer is 1 *[II B 3 a]*. The coronary arteries are among many blood vessels located in the loose connective tissue of the subepicardium. Most of the fat that accumulates in the wall of the heart is also located in this layer.

4. The answer is 2 *[IV C 2 b (2)]*. Both the intestinal lamina propria and endocrine glands contain fenestrated capillaries (as well as continuous capillaries, which are present in all organs). They do not contain porous capillaries; the fenestrations in their endothelial cells are closed by thin diaphragms. Capillaries in endocrine glands (but not the intestinal lamina propria) are unusually large because their walls lie on the surfaces of surrounding tissues rather than forming cylindrical tubes; therefore, they are called sinusoidal capillaries. Sinusoids are not present in either endocrine organs or the small intestine, but they are characteristic of the liver.

5. The answer is 1 *[III B 1 a]*. The elastic recoil of elastic arteries during diastole (relaxation of the myocardium) keeps the blood moving away from the heart; therefore, the elastic arteries act as an auxiliary pump. This phenomenon also moderates the surges in blood flow caused by the heartbeat. Elastic arteries may have an internal elastic membrane, but it is not usually distinct. The tunica media of elastic arteries is characterized by having more elastic elements (laminae and fibers) than smooth muscle. The tunica interna is unusually thick in elastic arteries, but the tunica externa is thin.

6. The answer is 3 *[III B 2 b]*. Compared with veins, the walls of all arteries are thick, relative to the size of their lumens; this is especially true of muscular arteries. The tunica media and tunica externa are usually about the same thickness in muscular arteries, and muscular arteries often have a distinct internal elastic membrane. Elastic laminae are present between muscle cells in the tunica media, although most of the elastic elements in muscular arteries are in the tunica externa.

7. The answer is 5 *[III C 2 b]*. Smooth muscle may be absent in the tunica media of large veins. They may, however, contain large amounts of muscle (usually oriented longitudinally) in the tunica externa. The tunica externa is usually the thickest portion of the wall. Valves are characteristic of veins that are returning blood to the heart against gravity, such as the veins of the limbs. Many veins have no valves; those in areas that are level with or above the heart, including veins in the thorax and abdomen, usually lack valves. Veins are distensible and compressible. Veins contain more collagen and less elastin than do arteries.

8. The answer is 5 *[IV A 1]*. Arterioles regulate the blood flow to local capillary beds in response to local metabolic signals. The autonomic nervous system also regulates the arterioles. Their tunica media, which is the thickest layer, consists of 1–3 layers of smooth muscle cells. (Metarterioles have only a discontinuous layer.) The tunica externa of arterioles is thin. The small, muscular arterioles are responsible for approximately 50% of the total resistance in the circulatory system. An internal elastic membrane is present in the larger arterioles.

9. The answer is 2 *[V A 2]*. Lymph vessels resemble veins, except that they have more valves, and their walls are thinner and less organized. Both lymphatics and veins carry their contents toward the heart. Lymph vessels are not less permeable than veins.

10. The answer is 1 *[IV C 2]*. Capillaries have no tunica media. They consist, at minimum, of simple squamous endothelium and its basal lamina. Pericytes, which are believed to be contractile, are often enclosed by the basal lamina. In addition, most capillaries are surrounded by a few reticular fibers.

11. The answer is 2 *[IV E]*. Arteriovenous anastomoses are shunts between the arterial and venous system that allow blood to bypass capillary beds. Metarterioles give rise to capillaries but also provide a thoroughfare channel through which blood may bypass the capillaries. Most blood is delivered to capillaries via arterioles. Portal vessels carry blood from one capillary bed to another.

Chapter 12

Lymphatic Organs

I. OVERVIEW OF THE IMMUNE SYSTEM

A. Functions. The immune system is responsible for self-recognition and helps defend the body against disease by producing immunocompetent lymphocytes and strategically placing them where they can monitor the tissue fluid, lymph, and blood. Immunocompetent lymphocytes have the ability to recognize "nonself" and to respond to antigens or abnormal cells.

B. Components

1. **Cells**
   a. **Lymphocytes,** white blood cells that are produced in lymphatic organs by a process called lymphopoiesis, interact with macrophages and other antigen-presenting cells to initiate an immune response (see III).
   b. **Macrophages** are derived from monocytes that have left the blood and entered the tissue.
      (1) Macrophages phagocytose antigens, process them, and present an **epitope** (i.e., an antigenic fragment of the antigen) coupled to a self-identifying **major histocompatibility complex (MHC) molecule** on the surface of their cell membranes.
      (2) **Cytokines** are soluble secretions that affect other cells.
         (a) Monocytes and macrophages secrete **monokines,** such as **interleukin 1 (IL-1)**.
         (b) Secretion of IL-1 by macrophages stimulates lymphocytes to produce **lymphokines,** which affect immune responses and the inflammatory process.
   c. **Other antigen-presenting cells** capture whole antigens and hold them on their surfaces for extended periods. Such cells include **follicular dendritic cells** in nodules of lymph nodes and **Langerhans cells** in the epidermis.
2. **Organs**
   a. **Primary lymphatic (lymphoid) organs** produce immunocompetent T lymphocytes and B lymphocytes.
      (1) Primary lymphatic organs include **bone marrow,** the **thymus,** the **cloacal bursa** in birds, and certain **gut-associated lymphatic tissue (GALT)** in some mammals.
      (2) The lymphocytes produced by primary lymphatic organs are carried in the blood to the secondary lymphatic organs, where they complete their differentiation.
   b. **Secondary lymphatic organs,** which are organized for surveillance, immune response, and immunologic memory, are located where they can monitor the tissue fluid of mucous membranes, the lymph draining from various body parts, and the blood.
      (1) The secondary lymphatic organs include **mucosa-associated lymphatic tissue (MALT), lymph nodes,** the **spleen,** and **hemal nodes**.
      (2) Within each organ, cells are positioned to facilitate interactions that lead to immune responses.
3. The **complement system** is a group of **immunologically active blood proteins,** called **complement components,** that are activated in a series of steps called the **complement cascade**.
   a. The complement cascade can be initiated by an antigen–antibody reaction or by some foreign molecules.
   b. **Functions.** The complement system plays a significant role in host defense and the inflammation process. Specific functions include:
      (1) Lysing of cells and bacteria

(2) Inducing degranulation of mast cells and basophils
(3) Attracting neutrophils
(4) Enhancing phagocytosis

C. **Immune response.** In contrast to the more general inflammation response (see Chapter 6 II C 2), the immune response is highly specific. Recognition of a foreign antigen or its cellular source causes a response that is directed toward elimination of the antigen or its source.

1. **Recognition.** The immune response is based on the recognition of substances or cells as "self" or "nonself."
   a. **Antigens** are foreign substances (proteins or polysaccharides) that evoke a protective response when they contact cells of the immune system.
   b. The immune system recognizes antigens by means of unique combinations of short sequences of amino acids (**epitopes**); therefore, it is a **very selective and specific system.**

2. **Response**
   a. **Activation** causes lymphocytes to enlarge and become intensely basophilic.
   b. **Clonal expansion** (repeated mitotic division, also called **blast transformation**) produces many enlarged cells with the same specificity as the activated cells.
   c. **Differentiation** produces **effector cells. Partial differentiation** produces **memory cells.**

3. **Types**
   a. **Antibody-mediated (humoral) immunity** occurs in response to bacteria that live outside cells of the host and to toxins released by these bacteria. Antibodies are circulating glycoproteins (immunoglobulins) that bind to specific antigens.
      (1) **Immunoglobulin G (IgG)** is the most abundant immunoglobulin in blood and lymph.
         (a) IgG activates the complement system and opsonizes bacteria [see Chapter 8 II B 3 b (1) (a) (ii)].
         (b) It also combines with circulating antigens and binds to the surface receptors on macrophages and some lymphocytes, promoting phagocytosis.
      (2) **Immunoglobulin M (IgM)** has functions similar to those of IgG. It is a potent activator of the complement system.
      (3) **Immunoglobulin A (IgA)** is produced in mucous membranes.
         (a) **Dimeric antibody** (two IgA molecules joined by a protein J piece) is present in intestinal, nasal, bronchial, vaginal, and prostatic secretions, and in saliva, tears, colostrum, and sweat.
         (b) Epithelial cells contribute a protein that is called the **secretory (transport)** component and which may help protect IgA from digestive enzymes. The complex is transported through the epithelium and secreted into the lumen, where IgA is able to inactivate antigens before they enter the tissue.
      (4) **Immunoglobulin E (IgE)** is produced in response to an allergen, and it binds to the surfaces of mast cells and basophils. Subsequent exposure to the same allergen can result in a local allergic reaction or systemic anaphylactic shock when the allergen reacts with the IgE on mast cells or basophils, causing the cells to degranulate.
      (5) **Immunoglobulin D (IgD)** may affect the differentiation of B lymphocytes, but its exact function is uncertain.
   b. **Cell-mediated immunity** is directed against specific antigens that are localized to particular cells in the body.
      (1) Cell-mediated immune responses are initiated by microorganisms that enter the cells of the host, products released by such microorganisms, viruses, fungi, grafted tissue, and certain substances that contact the skin.
      (2) Cells that have undergone malignant transformation also initiate a cell-mediated immune response. Molecular markers on the surface of transformed cells are significantly altered, causing the immune system to recognize them as foreign. If the cellular response fails to destroy such cells, they may metastasize to other organs.

II. LYMPHOCYTES

LYMPHOCYTES circulate in the blood and lymph and occupy characteristic locations in lymphatic organs. They are all similar in appearance (see Chapter 8 II B 2), but three types can be distinguished by their specific functions and distinctive cytochemical markers.

A. B lymphocytes (B cells)

1. **Function.** B lymphocytes and their derivatives, plasma cells, are responsible for humoral immunity.
2. **Markers**
   a. IgD is the predominant immunoglobulin on the surface of B lymphocytes.
   b. IgM is also present on the cell membrane surface.
3. **Activation.** B-cell activation occurs in response to the antigen for which B lymphocytes are specific.
   a. Activation usually requires interaction with an activated T helper lymphocyte with the same specificity [see II B 3 b (2) (b)] and a macrophage or other antigen-presenting cell (or cytokines produced by these cells).
   b. Activated B lymphocytes undergo clonal expansion and differentiation.
      (1) **Plasma cells** (see also Chapter 6 II C 2 e) are **fully differentiated** products of B-cell clonal expansion. They are highly specialized for production of a specific antibody.
      (2) **B memory cells** are B lymphocytes that have stopped at an intermediate stage of clonal expansion and development. They are primed to respond strongly and rapidly by clonal expansion and differentiation upon subsequent exposure to the antigen.

B. T lymphocytes (T cells)

1. **Functions.** T lymphocytes, the most numerous lymphocytes in the blood, are integral to **cell-mediated immunity**. In addition, they play a role in antibody production by B lymphocytes.
2. **Markers.** T lymphocytes are identified by marker molecules on their surfaces and in their interiors. Each T lymphocyte has surface receptors that recognize a specific antigen.
3. **Activation**
   a. T cells are activated when a specific antigen is presented to the T cell by a macrophage or other antigen-presenting cell.
   b. Activated T lymphocytes undergo clonal expansion and differentiation.
      (1) **Cytotoxic (killer) T cells** kill infected, foreign, or abnormal cells (i.e., they are the effectors of cell-mediated immunity).
         (a) When cytotoxic cells encounter a cell with the antigen for which they are specific on its surface, they lyse the cell.
            (i) A classic example of a target cell is a cell that displays glycoproteins of a virus that has infected it on its cell membrane.
            (ii) The cytotoxic T cell establishes intimate cell-to-cell contact with its target cell. It then pierces holes in the cell membrane of the target cell by secreting proteins called **perforins** onto the cell membrane surface.
         (b) Cytotoxic cells are primarily responsible for graft rejection.
         (c) Cytotoxic cells kill certain pathogenic bacteria and fungi.
      (2) **Regulatory T cells** include numerous subsets. Some of the best known are summarized here.
         (a) **Memory T cells** have not completed their differentiation into cytotoxic T cells. Upon subsequent exposure to the same antigen, they mount a secondary reaction that is quicker and more vigorous than the initial response.

(b) **T helper cells** help activate other lymphocytes by direct interaction or by releasing **lymphokines** that promote conversion of B cells to plasma cells and enhance other immune responses.

(i) **Interleukin 2 (IL-2)** is the most important lymphokine produced by T helper cells, because it activates a wide spectrum of cells, including other T helper cells.

(ii) **Other lymphokines** promote the growth and activities of a wide range of cells, both within and without the immune system.

(c) **T suppressor cells** inhibit B-cell formation and suppress other immune responses.

C. **Null cells** are **natural killer (NK) cells.**

1. **Functions.** Null cells are cytotoxic; they secrete perforin directly onto the surface of other cells. Malignant cells are their usual target.
   a. Null cells are not antigen-specific, but some possess antibody receptors and kill any target cells opsonized with antibodies. This process is called **antibody-dependent cellular cytotoxicity (ADCC).**
   b. Other null cells lack antibody receptors. They destroy target cells presented with MHC proteins in an antibody-independent manner.
2. **Markers.** NK cells do not bear the surface markers of either B cells or T cells.
3. It is not known where null cells are formed.

III. PRIMARY LYMPHATIC ORGANS

A. Bone marrow

1. Bone marrow performs **some secondary lymphatic organ functions** and **produces lymphocyte progenitor cells** (see Chapter 8 III A 1 b).
2. In mammals, **differentiation of B lymphocytes** also occurs in bone marrow. However, recent evidence implicates lymphatic tissue associated with the digestive tract as the site of this function in ruminants.

B. **Thymus** (Figure 12-1)

1. **Development.** The thymus arises as an epithelial (entodermal) outgrowth of the pharynx that loses its connection to the pharynx. The epithelial cells become stellate, forming a **cytoreticulum** that attracts circulating T progenitor cells, released first from the fetal liver and later from the fetal and postnatal bone marrow.
2. **Structure.** The thymus is the only lymphatic organ that is lobulated. After puberty, it involutes and its parenchyma is replaced by fat cells; but it can become active again if growth hormone is administered.
   a. **Parenchyma.** Each lobule has an outer **cortex** and an inner **medulla,** but because the division into lobules is incomplete, both cortex and medulla are continuous throughout the organ (Figure 12-2).

      (1) **Cortex.** The densely populated cortex contains developing T cells and many macrophages.

      (2) **Medulla.** The medulla is more loosely organized, and the parenchymal cells are typical of diffuse lymphatic tissue (i.e., T and B lymphocytes, plasma cells, macrophages, and antigen-presenting cells).

   b. **Stroma**

      (1) **Connective tissue** forms a thin **capsule** that continues into septa between the lobules.

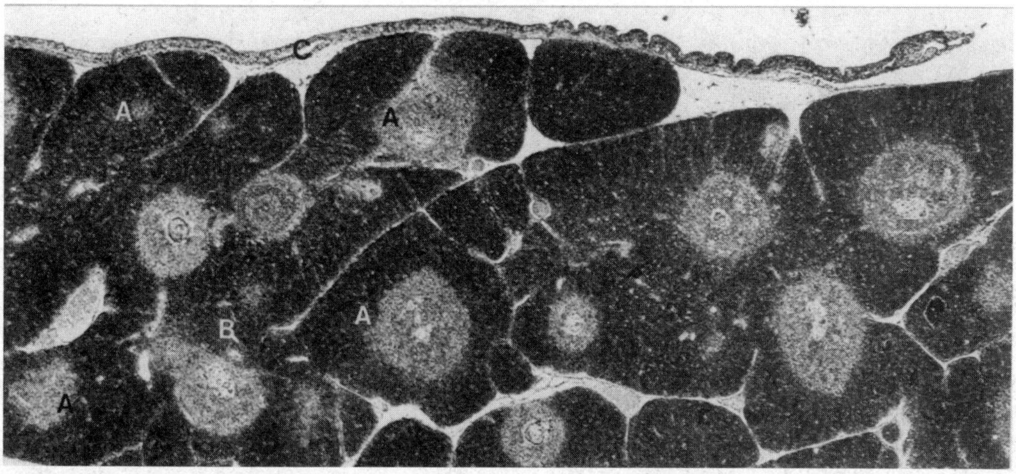

FIGURE 12-1. Survey view of the thymus, showing many lobules (*A*) connected to a central lobe (*B*). The darker outer layer is the cortex, and the light centers are sections through the medulla, which is actually a continuous branching region. The connective tissue capsule (*C*) continues into septa between the lobules. (Reprinted with permission from Dellmann H-D: *Textbook of Veterinary Histology,* 4th ed. Baltimore, Williams & Wilkins, 1993, p 121.)

(2) **Epithelial reticular cells** form the stroma within the cortex and medulla. Their long, slender processes are joined by desmosomes, forming a three-dimensional network that is structurally similar to that of reticular connective tissue but without reticular fibers. Epithelial reticular cells secrete hormone-like substances and contain secretory granules.

(3) **Epithelial cells** that are attached to the cells of the cytoreticulum form a continuous sheet that separates the parenchyma from the connective tissue of the capsule, septa, and perivascular tissue within the organ.

(4) **Thymic corpuscles** (see Figure 12-2), which develop from epithelial-reticular cells in the medulla, are unique to the thymus. They are composed of concentric layers of squamous cells; the central layers degenerate and fill with keratohyalin granules.

3. Functions

a. Production of T cells is the primary function of the thymus.

(1) T progenitor cells from the bone marrow interact by a receptor-mediated process with the walls of capillaries in the outer cortex and enter the parenchyma of the cortex.

(2) The T progenitor cells undergo clonal expansion in the thymus and acquire surface receptors for a specific antigen and for self-recognition. Macrophages and reticular epithelial cells influence T-cell development.

(a) **IL-1,** which stimulates mitosis of developing T cells, is secreted by macrophages.

(b) **Thymosin,** which induces development of T cells, is one of the hormone-like substances produced by reticular epithelial cells.

(3) As the T lymphocytes divide and differentiate, they are gradually moved toward the medulla by the pressure of incoming T progenitor cells. In the thymic cortex, continuous capillaries ensheathed by a sheet of thymic epithelial cells form a **blood–thymus barrier** that limits the entrance of progenitor cells and macromolecules, providing a protected environment for developing T cells.

(4) Two types of selection occur in the thymus.

(a) **Negative selection** is a process that eliminates T cells that are potentially reactive against self-antigens.

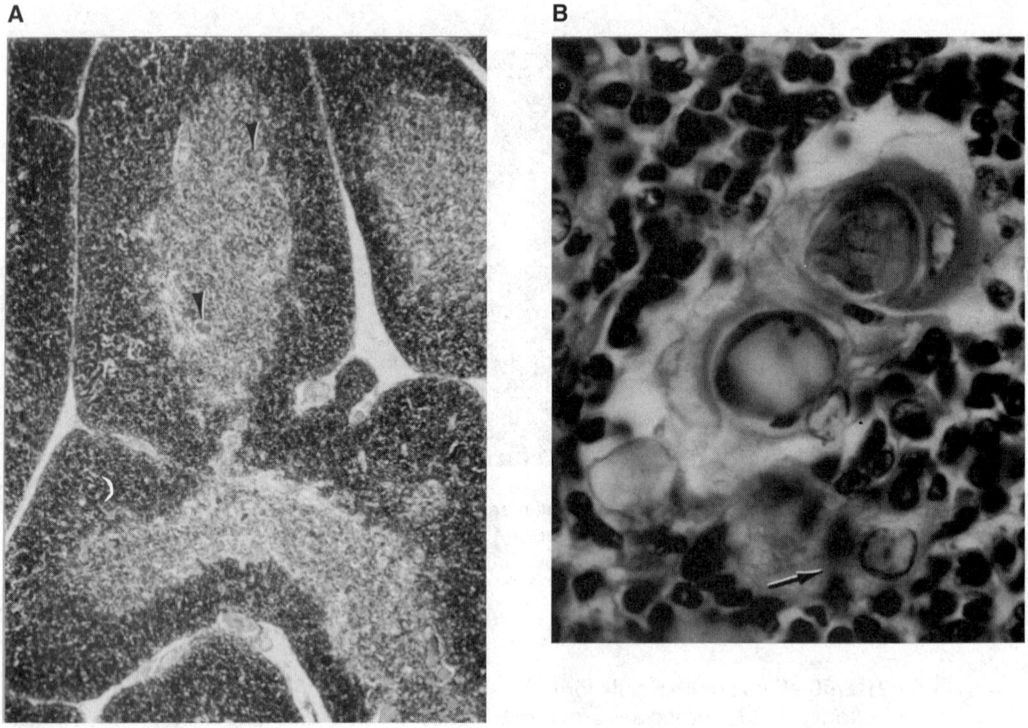

FIGURE 12-2. (*A*) A portion of several thymic lobules showing continuity of the darker cortex and lighter medulla. Thymic corpuscles are indicated by *arrows*. (*B*) Thymic corpuscles in the medulla. At this magnification, the concentric layers of reticular cells forming the corpuscles can be seen. The enlarged reticular cell indicated by the *arrow* is probably at the first stage in formation of a new corpuscle. (Reprinted with permission from Dellmann H-D: *Textbook of Veterinary Histology,* 4th ed. Baltimore, Williams & Wilkins, 1993, p 121.)

(b) **Positive selection** expands the population of T cells that are reactive with MHC molecules but not with self-antigens.

(5) Over 90% of the developing T cells die and are phagocytosed by macrophages. Because the number of deaths exceeds the number of new cells produced by mitosis, the thymus continues to receive T progenitor cells from the bone marrow.

(6) T cells reenter the circulating blood by entering postcapillary venules near the corticomedullary junction. They are carried by the blood to the spleen for their final maturation.

b. **Mast cell differentiation** from progenitor cells is believed to occur in the medulla.

C. The **cloacal bursa** in birds is an epithelial (ectodermal) outgrowth from the proctodeum that retains its connection with the cloaca.

1. **Structure.** The branching lumen of the cloacal bursa is surrounded by nodules of developing B lymphocytes and many macrophages, supported by a reticular epithelial stroma.

2. **Function.** Marrow-derived B progenitor cells divide and differentiate into immunocompetent B lymphocytes in the cloacal bursa. The bursa, like the bone marrow and thymus, has both primary and secondary lymphatic functions.

IV. SECONDARY LYMPHATIC ORGANS

A. General organization

1. **Diffuse** and **nodular regions** are differentiated in lymphatic tissue of secondary lymphatic organs (Figure 12-3).
   a. **Diffuse lymphatic tissue** contains randomly arranged concentrations of lymphocytes, primarily T cells and many other white blood cell-derived cell types. Clonal expansion of T cells occurs in diffuse lymphatic tissue.
   b. **Lymphatic nodules (follicles)** (Figure 12-4) are organized oval concentrations of lymphocytes, primarily B cells, with many macrophages but few other cell types.
      (1) The **stroma** contains follicular dendritic cells (antigen-presenting cells).
      (2) **Germinal centers** are central regions that appear light because they contain enlarged B cells that are undergoing clonal expansion.
         (a) **Primary nodules** lack a germinal center.
         (b) **Secondary nodules** have a germinal center.
2. **Reticular connective tissue** supports the diffuse lymphatic tissue and defines the shape of the nodules.

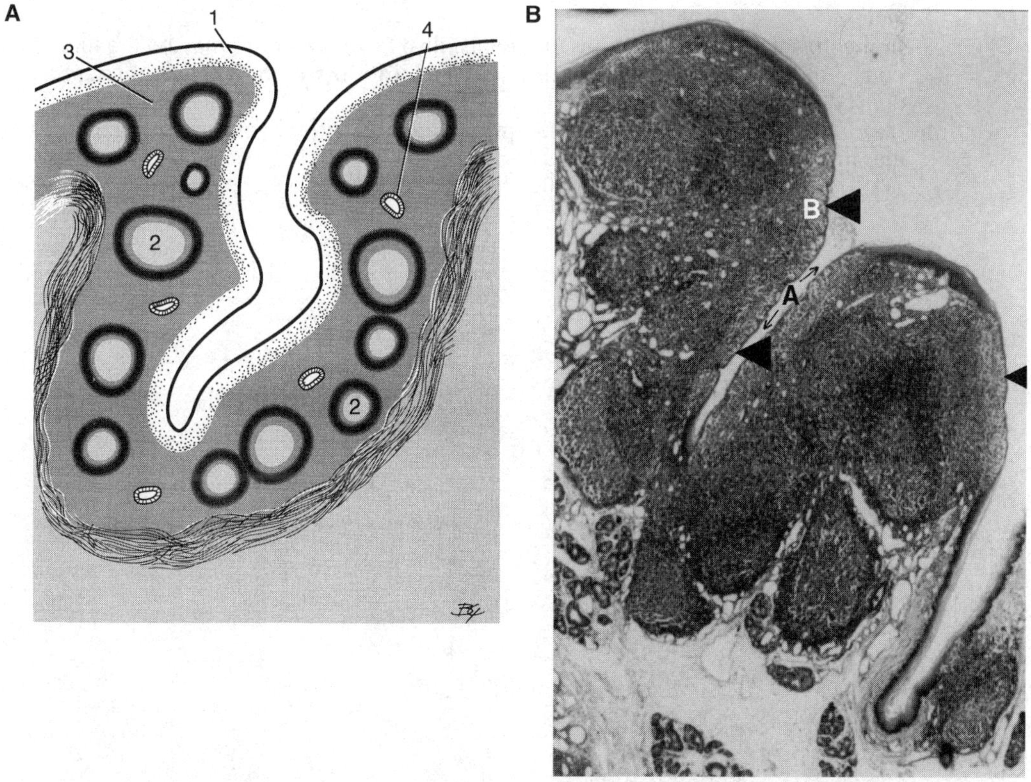

FIGURE 12-3. (*A*) Schematic drawing of the organization of a tonsillar fossula (crypt) in the pharynx. The epithelium (*1*) contains many lymphocytes from the nodular (*2*) and diffuse (*3*) lymphatic tissue. High-endothelium venules (*4*) are in the diffuse lymphatic tissue. Dense connective tissue forms a capsule between the tonsil and the surrounding tissue. (*B*) Portion of a tonsillar fossula (*A*) showing heavy lymphocytic infiltration of the epithelium (*arrows*), diffuse lymphatic tissue (*B*) adjacent to the epithelium, and portions of several nodules.

B. Mucosa-associated lymphatic tissue (MALT)

1. **Location.** Individual lymphocytes and isolated nodules are commonly present in loose connective tissue, especially in the lamina propria of mucous membranes.
   a. Well-defined collections of aggregated nodules occur consistently in certain mucosal regions, and some of these are named.
      (1) **Tonsils** (see Figure 12-3) are located in the pharyngeal region.
      (2) **Peyer's patches** (Figure 12-5) are located in the small intestine, primarily the ileum.
   b. MALT may be specifically named according to its location.
      (1) Gut-associated lymphatic tissue (**GALT**)
      (2) Bronchus-associated lymphatic tissue (**BALT**)

2. **Structure**
   a. **General.** Permanent aggregates of lymph nodules in the lamina propria (sometimes extending into the deeper submucosa) are surrounded by diffuse lymphatic tissue, which contains **high-endothelium venules (HEV)** and many lymph capillaries.
   b. **Peyer's patches. M cells** (see Figure 12-5), specialized epithelial cells in the ileum, lie over clusters of lymphocytes.
   c. **Tonsils.** A concentration of dense connective tissue encapsulates the tonsil and separates it from the surrounding epithelium (see Figure 12-3A).

3. **Functions**
   a. **In sheep,** and probably in other ruminants, ileal Peyer's patches may be the functional equivalent of the cloacal bursa in birds for **formation of B cells** from marrow-derived B progenitors.
   b. MALT **monitors the potentially susceptible mucosal surfaces of the body** and **initiates immune responses.**
      (1) Lymphocytes enter MALT through the walls of HEV by a receptor-mediated process.

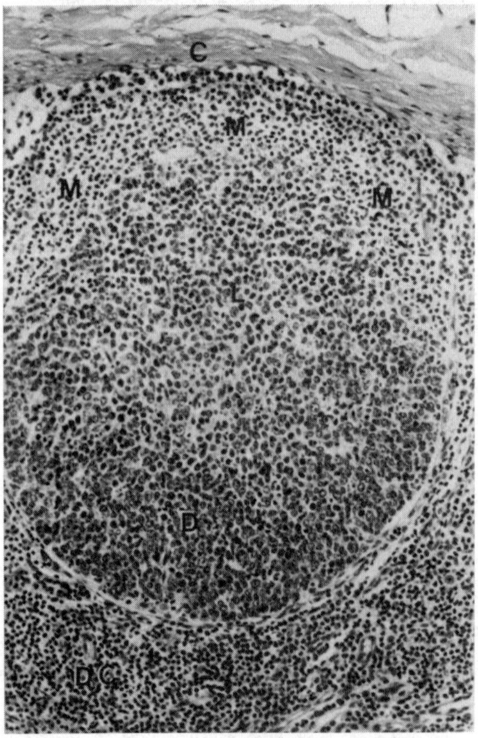

FIGURE 12-4. Micrograph of a lymphatic nodule from a lymph node. The lighter germinal center (*L*) is the site of clonal expansion of B lymphocytes. The mantle (*M*) is a thin layer of small recirculating B lymphocytes. The capsule (*C*) and deep cortex (*DC*) of the lymph node are also visible. (Reprinted with permission from Dellmann H-D: *Textbook of Veterinary Histology,* 4th ed. Baltimore, Williams & Wilkins, 1993, p 126.)

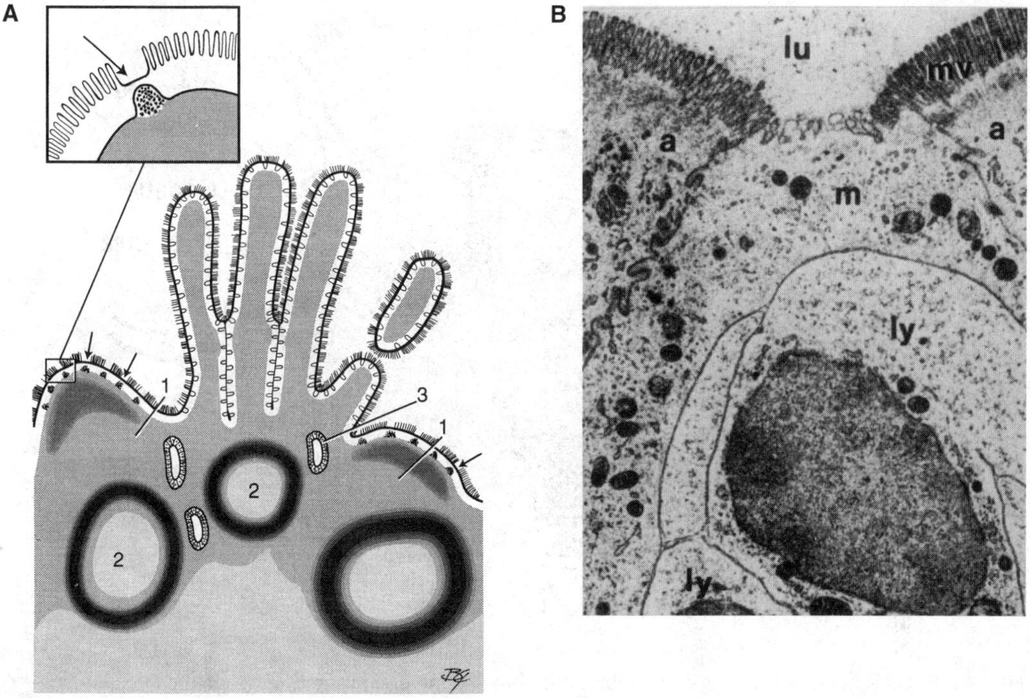

FIGURE 12-5. (*A*) Schematic drawing of part of a Peyer's patch in the small intestine. In dome-shaped regions (*1*) the epithelium contains M cells (*arrows*), under which are clusters of lymphocytes. Nodules (*2*) lie below the domes. Diffuse lymphatic tissue contains high-endothelium venules (*3*). (*B*) Electron micrograph showing a portion of an M cell (*m*) with lymphocytes (*ly*) pressed against its basal surface. The intestinal lumen (*lu*) is at the top, and absorptive cells (*a*) with many microvilli (*mv*) are on each side of the M cell. (Redrawn and reprinted with permission from Dellmann H-D: *Textbook of Veterinary Histology,* 4th ed. Baltimore, Williams & Wilkins, 1993, pp 124, 125.)

(a) The **B cells** are attracted to **lymphatic nodules**.
(b) The **T cells** are attracted to **diffuse lymphatic tissue**.

(2) Most antigens enter MALT by penetrating the epithelium. In Peyer's patches, M cells may capture antigens in the lumen and present them to underlying lymphocytes.

(3) If a lymphocyte encounters its specific antigen and is activated in MALT, it may complete its clonal expansion and differentiation locally; or it may enter a lymph capillary, which carries the lymphocyte to a lymph node to undergo clonal expansion. If clonal expansion occurs in a lymph node, the new cells are carried by lymph to the blood, where they circulate until they recognize HEV in MALT anywhere in the body. They then exit to the MALT parenchyma through the HEV and complete their differentiation in MALT. By this means, the response to an antigen entering the MALT at one point is dispersed throughout the mucous membranes of the entire body.

(4) Lymphocytes that are not activated in MALT may reenter the circulation by entering lymph capillaries.

(5) Some antibodies produced in MALT may act locally, others enter the lymph or the blood, and others are taken up by the epithelium and secreted into the lumen of the organ [see I C 3 a (3)].

C. **Lymph nodes** are distributed along the major lymphatic vessels. Most birds do not have lymph nodes, just loosely organized lymphatic tissue along lymph channels and collections of lymphocytes in the pancreas, liver, and kidneys.

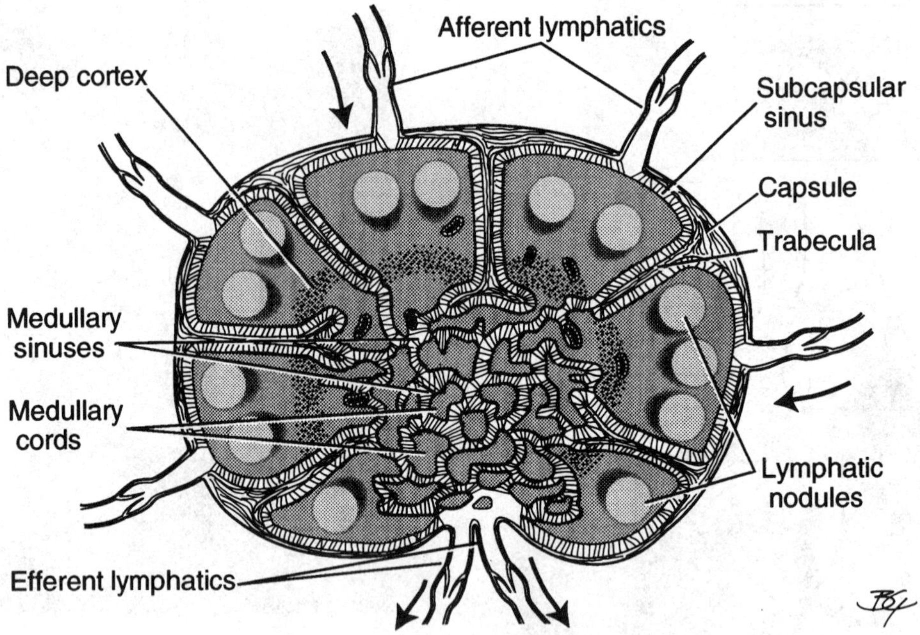

FIGURE 12-6. Schematic drawing of a lymph node showing the organization of lymphatic circulation through the node. The dark cortex along the convex surface is separated from the capsule by the subcapsular sinus. Trabecular sinuses drain into anastomosing medullary sinuses, which converge at the hilus to supply efferent vessels. (Redrawn with permission from Dellmann, H-D: *Textbook of Veterinary Histology*. Baltimore, Williams & Wilkins, 1993, p 125.)

1. **Structure** (Figure 12-6)
   a. A **cortex** and **medulla** are distinguished in lymph nodes.
      (1) The **cortex** contains lymph nodules, diffuse lymphatic tissue, and lymph sinuses.
         (a) The **outer cortex** contains nodules and diffuse lymphatic tissue. In swine, the nodules are more centrally located.
         (b) The **deep (inner, tertiary) cortex (paracortex)** is a layer of diffuse lymphatic tissue between the nodules and the medulla. The deep cortex contains many HEV.
      (2) The **medulla** is composed of anastomosing thick cords of diffuse lymphatic tissue separated by lymph sinuses. It contains many plasma cells.
   b. **Afferent lymph vessels and lymph sinuses,** endothelium-lined channels for the flow of lymph, are present only in lymph nodes.
      (1) **Structure.** The wide lumen is traversed by processes of macrophages and antigen-presenting dendritic cells and by reticular fibers.
      (2) **Lymph flow patterns** (see Figure 12-6). The pattern described here is reversed in swine.
         (a) The **subcapsular sinus** receives afferent lymphatic vessels that penetrate the capsule at several points.
         (b) **Trabecular sinuses** along the connective tissue trabeculae drain the subcapsular sinuses and empty into the medullary sinuses.
         (c) **Medullary sinuses** in the medulla anastomose and fuse.
         (d) **Efferent lymphatic vessels** that drain the medullary sinuses exit at the hilus.
   c. **Stroma**
      (1) **Dense connective tissue** that often contains smooth muscle forms the capsule and trabeculae, which carry blood vessels and nerves from the hilus and other points around the convex surface.

(2) **Reticular tissue** in the parenchymal regions contains many macrophages and dendritic reticular cells that have long, apparently motile processes.

2. **Functions.** Lymph nodes **filter the lymph** and **respond immunologically** to antigens arriving from tissues drained by their afferent vessels.
   a. **Macrophages** associated with the sinuses are important for both functions of lymph nodes.
      (1) **Filtration.** In one passage through a lymph node, 99% of the particulate matter in lymph is removed by macrophages.
      (2) **Immune response**
         (a) Macrophages capture antigens in the lymph, then migrate to present them to lymphocytes in the cortex.
         (b) The probability that antigens in lymph will encounter a macrophage is enhanced by the reticular fibers and cell processes of the sinuses, which slow the flow of lymph and make it turbulent.
   b. **Lymphocytes.** Most lymphocytes enter lymph nodes from the blood via HEV, but some also enter from the lymph (Figure 12-7). Lymphocytes that are not activated within a few hours return to the circulation.
      (1) **B lymphocytes** move to **nodules,** where activated B cells undergo clonal expansion (see Figure 12-7).
         (a) After clonal expansion, the B cells move into the medulla, where they complete their differentiation into plasma cells and live for several days (see Figure 12-7).
         (b) Antibodies secreted by plasma cells are carried by the lymph to the blood.
         (c) Some B lymphocytes do not complete their differentiation. They become B memory cells.
      (2) **T lymphocytes** move to the **deep cortex and internodular diffuse tissue,** where activated T cells undergo clonal expansion.
         (a) Most circulating lymphocytes are T cells, which exercise immunologic surveillance.
         (b) T-cell activation (by antigens from infected cells or abnormal cells) is more likely to occur in lymph nodes than in other secondary organs.
      (3) **MALT-activated lymphocytes** as well as **locally activated lymphocytes** undergo clonal expansion in the **cortex** of lymph nodes.

D. Spleen

1. **Structure**
   a. **Parenchyma.** The spleen is composed of **white pulp** and **red pulp,** named according to their appearance in fresh gross specimens. It has no cortex and medulla.
      (1) **White pulp** consists of diffuse and nodular lymphatic tissue.
         (a) **Diffuse tissue** is arranged in **periarterial lymphatic sheaths (PALS)** around small arteries and arterioles called **arteries of the white pulp (central arteries)**.
         (b) **Nodules** (Figure 12-8) are scattered along the course of the PALS.
      (2) **Red pulp** in most domestic species consists of **pulp spaces,** in which blood percolates through a stroma of reticular tissue. Veins are present, and macrophages are especially numerous in red pulp.
      (3) The **marginal zone** is adjacent to the white pulp. Most blood enters the red pulp in the marginal zone, and sorting of blood elements occurs here.
         (a) Lymphocytes migrate to the white pulp, where they respond to blood-borne antigens.
         (b) Monocytes are sequestered in the marginal zone.
         (c) Other blood cells may remain in the marginal zone for some time before percolating through the red pulp and leaving the spleen.
   b. **Stroma** (Figure 12-9)
      (1) The **heavy capsule** and **trabeculae** contain bundles of **smooth muscle**. The capsule is covered by mesothelium.

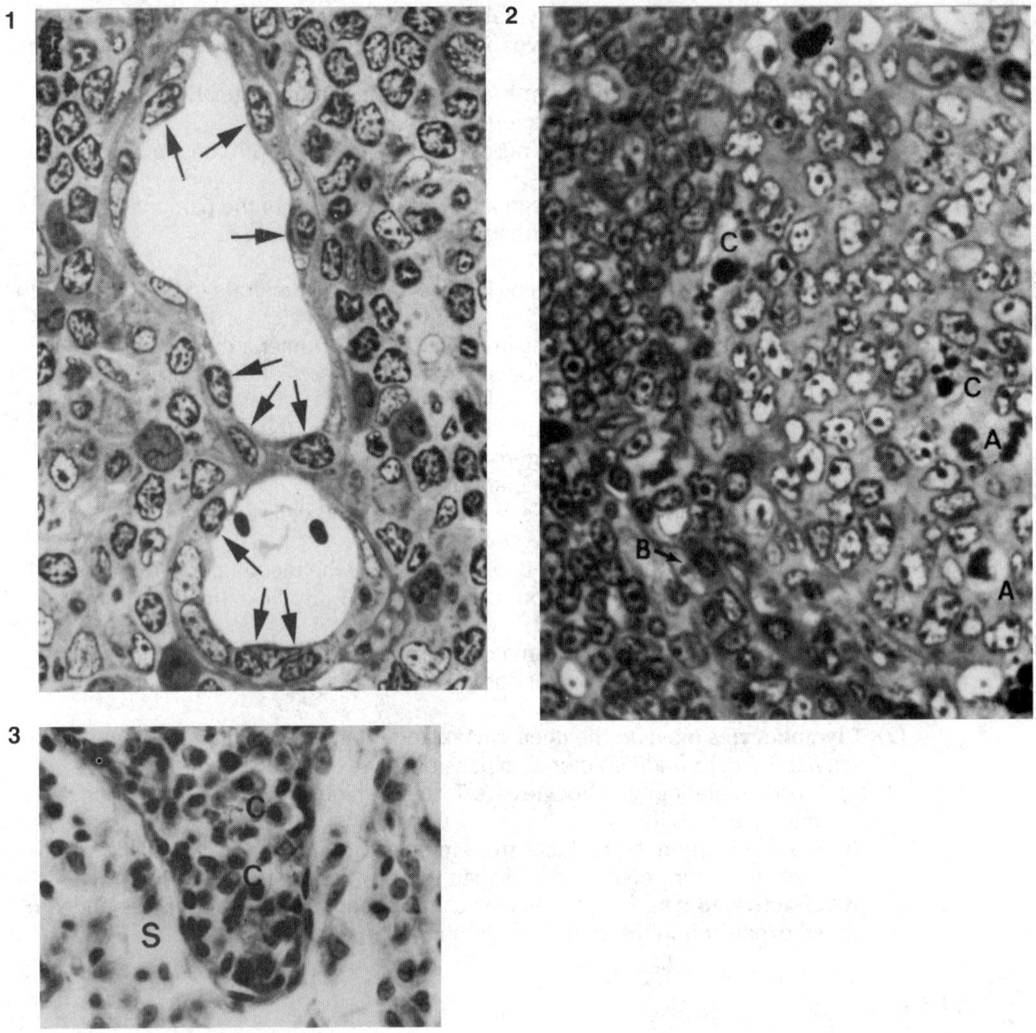

FIGURE 12-7. (*1*) High-endothelium vein (HEV) in lymph node with many migrating lymphocytes (*arrows*). (*2*) After entering the lymph node, B lymphocytes migrate to the lymphatic nodules and undergo clonal expansion. The large cells to the right are undergoing clonal expansion. Several are in mitosis (*A*). The nucleus of a reticular cell (*B*) and macrophages digesting lymphocytes (*C*) can be identified. (*3*) A portion of a medullary cord with several plasma cells (*C*), surrounded by a lymph sinus (*S*). (Reprinted with permission from Dellmann H-D: *Textbook of Veterinary Histology,* 4th ed. Baltimore, Williams & Wilkins, 1993, pp 126, 128, 129.)

(2) **Reticular connective tissue** shapes the PALS and nodules of the white pulp and forms the pulp spaces of the red pulp.

c. **Vasculature** (Figure 12-10)

(1) **Arteries**

(a) **Splenic artery branches** enter the hilus and ramify in the capsule.

(b) **Trabecular arteries** branch from the splenic arteries in the capsule and run in connective tissue trabeculae.

(c) **Arteries of the white pulp** are branches of trabecular arteries that leave the trabeculae.

(2) **Arterioles.** Branches of the arteries of the white pulp deliver blood to pulp spaces in the red pulp.

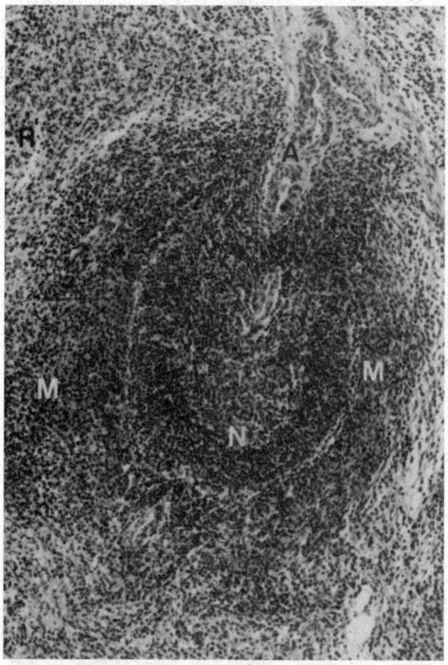

FIGURE 12-8. A splenic nodule (*N*) with its artery (*A*) surrounded by the marginal zone (*M*) and red pulp (*R*). (Reprinted with permission from Dellmann H-D: *Textbook of Veterinary Histology,* 4th ed. Baltimore, Williams & Wilkins, 1993, p 131.)

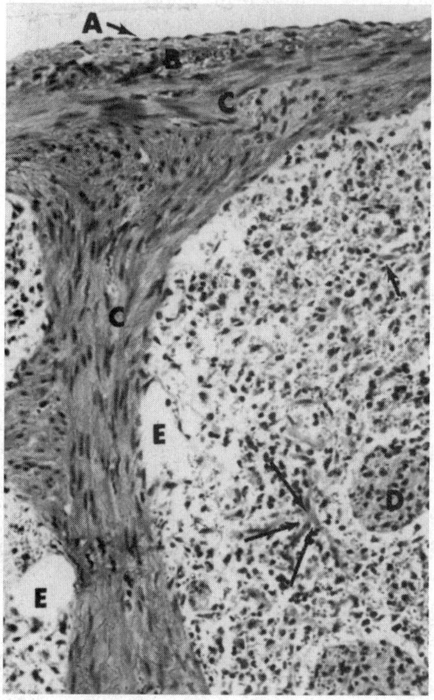

FIGURE 12-9. A portion of the spleen. Mesothelium (*A*) covers the thick capsule (*B*), which contains bundles of smooth muscle (*C*). Dense connective tissue and smooth muscle continue into the trabecula, and isolated smooth muscle cells (*arrows*) are also present in the red pulp. Sheathed capillaries (*D*) and venules (*E*) are also visible. (Reprinted with permission from Dellmann, H-D: *Textbook of Veterinary Histology*. Baltimore, Williams & Wilkins, 1993, p 129.)

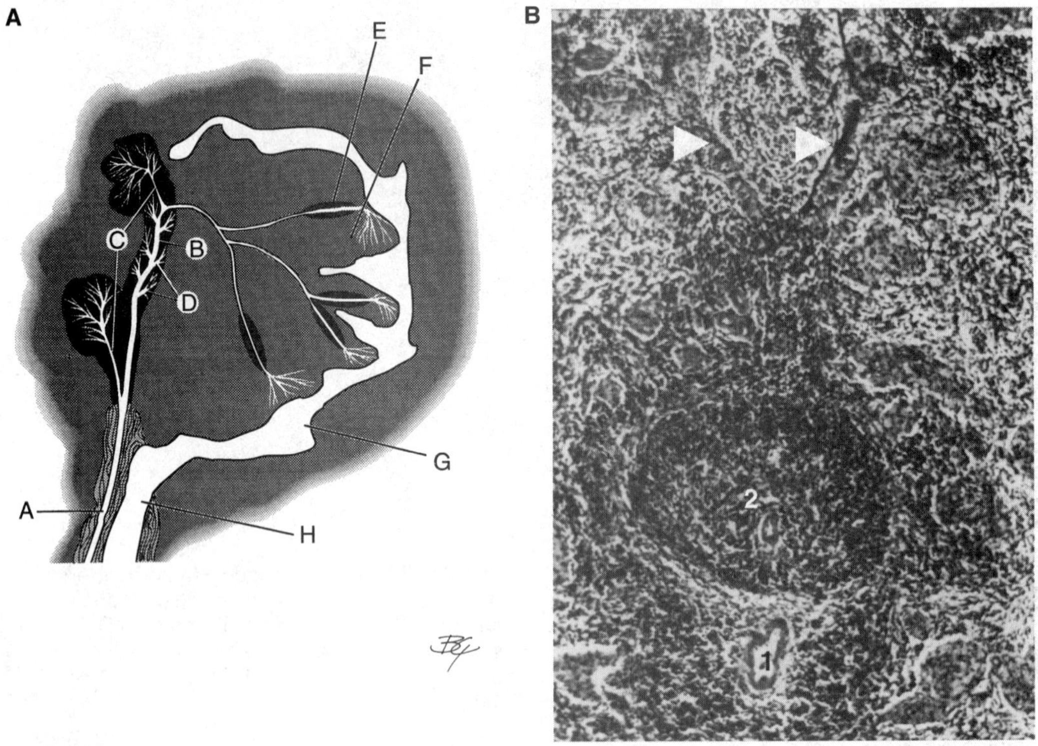

FIGURE 12-10. (*A*) Schematic drawing showing the circulatory pattern of the spleen. (*A*) Trabecular artery; (*B)* artery of the white pulp; (*C*) nodular arteries; (*D*) marginal branches; (*E*) sheathed capillaries; (*F*) pulp spaces; (*G*) pulp vein; (*H*) trabecular vein. (*B*) A portion of a spleen, showing an artery of the white pulp (*1*) surrounded by a periarterial lymphatic sheath (PALS). A nodular artery is present in a lymphatic nodule (*2*) above the PALS. Penicillar arterioles (*arrows*) lead to sheathed capillaries at the top of the field. (A is redrawn with permission from Dellmann H-D: *Textbook of Veterinary Histology,* 4th ed. Baltimore, Williams & Wilkins, 1993, p 132.)

(a) **Nodular arterioles, PALS arterioles,** and **marginal arterioles,** which **empty into the marginal zone,** are all radial branches from the arteries of the white pulp.

(b) **Penicilli** are the brush-like terminations of the arteries of the white pulp. They comprise several straight vessels and their capillary branches.

(3) **Sheathed capillaries (ellipsoids)** are capillaries surrounded by sheaths of macrophages and reticular cells. These are very thick and prominent in some species.

(4) **Sinuses and veins.** A spleen may be either **sinusal** or **nonsinusal,** depending on the type of postcapillary vessel. Dogs (and humans) have sinusal spleens.

(a) In **sinusal spleens,** blood from arterioles and capillaries enters anastomosing strands of reticular connective tissue called **splenic cords**.

(i) Blood cells **exit the cords and enter the sinuses** by negotiating gaps between elements of the highly discontinuous basal lamina and endothelial cells of the sinus wall.

(ii) **Pulp veins** collect blood from the sinuses and drain to **trabecular veins,** which lead to the **splenic vein** at the hilus.

(b) In **nonsinusal spleens,** blood flows directly from arterioles and capillaries into pulp spaces of the red pulp. Pulp spaces are drained by pulp veins.

2. Functions

a. White pulp

(1) The splenic white pulp is **the body's main source of humoral antibodies**.

(a) Activated **B cells** undergo clonal expansion in nodules of the white pulp and then move toward the marginal zone as they begin to differentiate.

(b) Plasma cells arising from splenic B cells are abundant in the marginal zone and adjacent red pulp. The antibodies they produce are continuously carried off in the blood.

(2) Some **T cells** are also activated in the spleen and undergo clonal expansion in the PALS.

(3) Lymphocytes that are not activated reenter the blood circulation.

b. Red pulp

(1) Removal of defective and aged blood cells, especially red blood cells, is the primary function of red pulp. Blood percolates very slowly from the marginal zone through the red pulp, maximizing opportunities for the many macrophages to identify and remove abnormal cells and any suspended particles. Old red blood cells lose sialic acid from their surfaces, exposing antigens that are recognized by phagocytes. In addition, aged cells are not pliant enough to move through the pulp spaces without being damaged.

(a) Macrophages sequestered in the marginal zone are particularly active phagocytes. They are able to phagocytose microorganisms efficiently, even those that have not been opsonized.

(b) Macrophages carrying antigenic fragments on their cell membranes migrate to the white pulp to initiate immune responses.

(2) Iron conservation is accomplished by the spleen. Hemoglobin from exhausted erythrocytes is broken down by macrophages in the red pulp, and the iron, combined with **transferrin,** a carrier molecule, is carried in the blood to erythropoietic tissues. The iron-free heme is metabolized to bilirubin and excreted into the bile by the liver.

(3) Blood cell storage, especially of erythrocytes and platelets (as much as one-third of the total in the circulation), occurs in the red pulp.

(a) Contraction of the smooth muscle forces blood cells out of the red pulp, rapidly increasing the number of circulating erythrocytes and platelets when they are needed because of blood loss or exercise.

(b) The degree to which blood cells are stored in the spleen varies among species.

(i) Cats, dogs, and horses have storage spleens, which have especially large amounts of muscle and red pulp.

(ii) Most domestic animals have an intermediate-type spleen.

(4) Hemopoiesis. The spleen, which is an important hemopoietic organ during fetal life, can resume its erythropoietic activity in severely anemic animals. Megakaryocytes are common in the red pulp of cats and rodents, and in young domestic carnivores and swine.

E. Hemal nodes

1. Locations. Hemal nodes are found primarily in ruminants. They are located along the **vertebral column,** in the **lumbar region** (in cattle), and in the **jugular furrow**. They are also associated with some viscera, including kidneys, especially in sheep and goats.

2. Structure (Figure 12-11)

a. Hemal nodes resemble lymph nodes, but they have blood in their sinuses and are not as well organized. The sinuses are very wide.

b. Nodules may form, but there is no typical medulla.

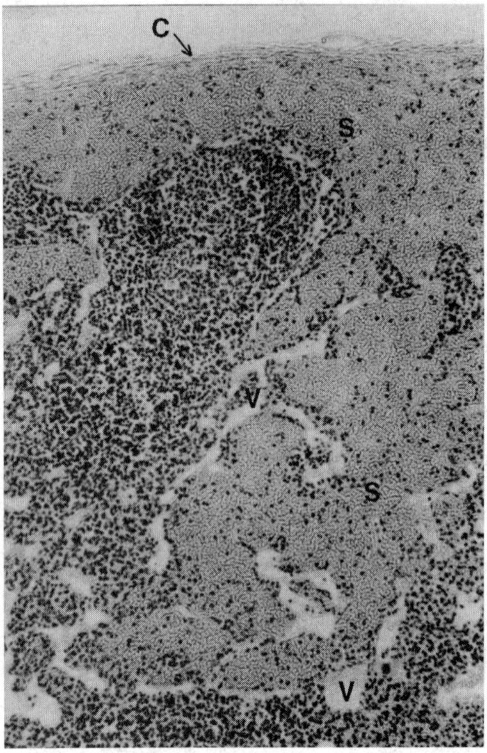

FIGURE 12-11. Survey view of a hemal node. Wide blood-filled sinuses (*S*) are under the capsule (*C*) and adjacent to veins (*V*). There are many small venules in the lymphatic tissue.

   c. No lymph vessels are present. Hemal nodes have only afferent and efferent blood vessels.

   d. No HEV are present, but lymphocytes and erythrocytes pass into and out of blood vessels.

3. Function. Their function is uncertain.

STUDY QUESTIONS

DIRECTIONS: Each of the numbered items or incomplete statements in this section is followed by answers or by completions of the statement. Select the **one** numbered answer or completion that is **best** in each case.

1. Primary lymphatic organs are organs in which:

(1) lymphocytes interact with antigen-presenting cells.
(2) antibodies are produced.
(3) T lymphocytes and B lymphocytes are produced.
(4) tissue fluids, lymph, and blood are monitored for antigens.
(5) T cells, B cells, and macrophages are organized to facilitate interactions.

2. Which one of the following characteristics is true for immune responses?

(1) Immune responses occur most often in primary lymphatic organs.
(2) Individual lymphocytes normally respond to a wide variety of antigenic substances.
(3) The first step is recognition of "self" and "nonself."
(4) The first step is activation of a T lymphocyte.
(5) Lymphocytes undergo clonal expansion and then become activated.

3. Which one of the following statements correctly describes a major class of antibodies (immunoglobulins)?

(1) Immunoglobin G (IgG) is used to identify B cells.
(2) Immunoglobulin M (IgM) on the cell membranes of mast cells and basophils is involved in degranulation.
(3) Immunoglobulin E (IgE) is normally the most abundant antibody in the blood.
(4) Immunoglobulin D (IgD) is the primary activator of the complement system.
(5) Immunoglobulin A (IgA) is secreted into the intestine.

4. Which one of the following statements is true regarding T cells?

(1) T-cell activation usually requires interaction with an activated B cell and a macrophage or other antigen-presenting cell.
(2) Memory T cells are derived from cytotoxic T cells.
(3) Some T cells suppress the immune response.
(4) T cells are unable to respond to a virus if it gains access to the interior of one of the host's cells.
(5) T helper cells release antibodies.

5. An important function of null cells is:

(1) secretion of antibodies.
(2) destruction of malignant cells.
(3) activation of B cells.
(4) suppressing the inflammation response.
(5) phagocytosis of foreign microorganisms and cells.

6. Which one of the following statements is true regarding the development and structure of the thymus?

(1) The reticular stroma of the thymus is derived from pharyngeal mesenchyme.
(2) The thymus is first "seeded" with T progenitor cells from the bone marrow within a few days after birth.
(3) T cells enter the thymic cortex via high-endothelium venules (HEV).
(4) Thymic corpuscles are unique features of the thymic cortex.
(5) The parenchyma of the thymic cortex is completely separated from its connective tissue stroma by a sheet of epithelial-reticular cells.

7. Which one of the following statements is true of mucosa-associated lymphatic tissue (MALT)?

(1) High-endothelium venules (HEV) are not present.
(2) Lymphocytes activated in MALT may undergo clonal expansion elsewhere.
(3) Afferent and efferent lymph vessels are present.
(4) MALT is located in the epithelium.
(5) Its stroma is epithelial.

8. Which one of the following statements regarding lymph sinuses is true?

(1) They are lined by reticular connective tissue.
(2) They are present only in the cortices of lymph nodes.
(3) Lymph is filtered and antigens are captured in the sinuses.
(4) Subcapsular sinuses drain into efferent lymph vessels in most species.
(5) Lymph sinuses have wide, uninterrupted lumina.

9. The spleens of domestic animals are characterized by:

(1) the presence of tissue that behaves as a secondary lymphatic organ, along with tissue designed for a completely separate function.
(2) a well-developed cortex and medulla.
(3) blood sinuses in the red pulp.
(4) a thin connective tissue capsule and septa.
(5) the subcapsular sinus.

DIRECTIONS: Each of the numbered items or incomplete statements in this section is negatively phrased, as indicated by an italicized word such as *not, least,* or *except.* Select the **one** numbered answer or completion that is **best** in each case.

10. All of the following are components of the immune system *except:*

(1) complement blood proteins.
(2) fibrinogen.
(3) follicular dendritic cells.
(4) macrophages.
(5) Kupffer cells.

11. All of the following statements are true regarding the cloacal bursa *except:*

(1) it is a site of T-cell production.
(2) it is not present in mammals.
(3) it resembles the thymus in having an epithelial reticular stroma.
(4) it has a lumen that opens to the cloaca.
(5) it contains nodules of differentiating B cells.

12. Secondary lymphatic organs share all of the following structural characteristics *except:*

(1) diffuse lymphatic tissue.
(2) reticular connective tissue.
(3) nodular lymphatic tissue.
(4) macrophages.
(5) lymph sinuses.

13. All of the following are true of the circulatory system of the spleen *except:*

(1) arteries of the white pulp are branches of trabecular arteries.
(2) marginal arterioles empty blood directly into the reticular connective tissue of the marginal zone.
(3) pulp veins are drained by trabecular veins.
(4) sheathed capillaries are surrounded by diffuse lymphatic tissue.
(5) blood in the red pulp of dog spleens flows from splenic cords into splenic sinuses.

ANSWERS AND EXPLANATIONS

1. The answer is 3 *[I B 2 a]*. Primary lymphatic organs produce T and B lymphocytes. The other functions listed all occur in secondary lymphatic organs.

2. The answer is 3 *[I C 1]*. An immune response is initiated when a substance or cell that is foreign (nonself) is recognized. This usually occurs in a secondary lymphatic organ, but it can also occur in loose connective tissue. An individual lymphocyte responds only to a specific antigen. Therefore, the immune response is very specific, in contrast to the inflammation response, which is nonspecific. After recognition, lymphocytes become activated before they undergo clonal expansion.

3. The answer is 5 *[I C 3 a (1)–(5)]*. Dimers of immunoglobulin A (IgA, secretory immunoglobulin) are taken up by intestinal epithelial cells, bound with a transport protein synthesized in the epithelium, and released into the intestinal lumen, where the IgA can inactivate antigens before they have a chance to enter the tissue. Immunoglobulin M (IgM) is used to identify B cells. Immunoglobulin E (IgE) is concentrated on the cell membranes of basophils and mast cells and causes degranulation when it complexes with its specific antigen. IgM and immunoglobulin G (IgG), the most abundant immunoglobulin in the blood, are potent activators of the complement system. The function of immunoglobulin D (IgD) is not well understood.

4. The answer is 3 *[II B 3 b (2) (c)]*. Regulatory T cells include suppressor cells, which have a variety of different immunosuppressive effects, as well as helper cells and cells that promote more specific aspects of the immune response. T-cell activation does not require interaction with a B cell. Memory cells do not arise from cytotoxic T cells; they may give rise to cytotoxic cells. An important function of T cells is recognizing cells that are infected with a virus and then destroying both the cell and the virus. This recognition is based on the presence of foreign (virus-induced) glycoproteins on the infected cell's surface. Antibodies are released primarily by plasma cells, which are derived from B lymphocytes.

5. The answer is 2 *[II C 1]*. Malignant cells are the usual target of natural killer cells, a category of null cells. Null cells do not secrete antibodies (as B cells do), nor are they involved in activation of B cells or suppression of the immune response (as certain T cells are). No lymphocytes are phagocytic.

6. The answer is 5 *[III B 1, 2 b (3)]*. In the thymus, a layer of epithelial reticular cells forms a continuous layer separating the cortical parenchyma from the connective tissue of the capsule, trabeculae, and perivascular tissue. The reticular stroma is composed of epithelial cells derived from the pharyngeal entoderm. The thymus is the first organ in which fetal lymphopoiesis occurs; it is first "seeded" with T progenitor cells that arrive from the fetal liver. They enter through the walls of capillaries just under the capsule; there are no high-endothelium venules (HEV) in the thymus. Thymic corpuscles are unique features of the thymus, but they are found only in the medulla.

7. The answer is 2 *[IV B 3 b (3)]*. Lymphocytes activated in mucosa-associated lymphatic tissue (MALT) commonly enter lymph capillaries, to be carried to lymph nodes and to undergo clonal expansion there. Their clones then reenter the circulation and return to MALT anywhere in the body. MALT contains high-endothelium venules (HEV). The HEV provide access for lymphocytes entering MALT, because MALT has no afferent lymph vessels. Afferent lymph vessels are unique to lymph nodes. MALT is located in subepithelial connective tissue; however, individual lymphocytes often infiltrate the epithelium. Its stroma is reticular connective tissue.

8. The answer is 3 *[IV C 1 b, 2 a]*. The wide lumina of lymph sinuses are interrupted by many reticular fibers and processes of macrophages and antigen-presenting cells. The macrophages are effective filters, removing 99% of the particulate matter in the lymph as the lymph percolates through one node. The macrophages also capture antigens in the lymph flow and carry the antigenic information to lymphocytes in the lymphatic tissue of the node. The sinuses are lined by endothelium (which is discontinuous on the side toward the parenchyma). In most species, lymph from afferent vessels is emptied into subcapsular sinuses and then flows through trabecular sinuses to anastomosing medullary sinuses. The sinuses in the medulla are drained by efferent vessels, which leave the node at the hilus. The pattern is reversed in swine, in which afferent lymph vessels enter the hilus near centrally located nodules, and anastomosing sinuses similar to medullary sinuses (except for their more peripheral location) are drained from the convex surface of the node by efferent vessels.

9. The answer is 1 *[IV D 2].* The spleen is composed of a secondary lymphatic organ, the white pulp, interdigitated with an organ that removes abnormal blood cells, the red pulp. The arrangement allows sharing of macrophages and a filter-like structure. The spleen is not organized into a cortex and medulla; both red and white pulp may occur anywhere in the organ. Most domestic species (dogs are the exception) have nonsinusal spleens. The thick capsule and trabeculae are composed of fibrous connective tissue and smooth muscle. There are no septa, nor is there a subcapsular sinus (or any other type of lymphatic sinus).

10. The answer is 2 *[I B].* Fibrinogen is a blood protein that is involved in the clotting reaction. Complement blood proteins, follicular dendritic cells, macrophages, and Kupffer cells are components of the immune system.

11. The answer is 1 *[III C].* The cloacal bursa is the site where marrow-derived B progenitor cells develop into immunocompetent B cells (not T cells) in birds. The cloacal bursa is not present in mammals. Like the thymus, the cloacal bursa has an epithelial-reticular stroma. It is an ectodermal outgrowth from the proctodeum that retains its connection with the cloaca. Its branching lumen is surrounded by nodules of B cells undergoing clonal expansion.

12. The answer is 5 *[IV C 1 b].* Lymph sinuses are present only in lymph nodes. All secondary lymphatic organs contain both nodular and diffuse lymphatic tissue, reticular connective tissue, and macrophages.

13. The answer is 4 *[IV D 1 c (3); Figure 12-9].* Sheathed capillaries are surrounded by concentric layers of macrophages and reticular cells. Arteries of the white pulp are surrounded by diffuse lymphatic tissue called the periarterial lymphatic sheath (PALS). The arteries of the white pulp are branches of the trabecular arteries. Marginal arterioles empty blood directly into the reticular connective tissue of the marginal zone. Pulp veins are drained by trabecular veins. Dogs have sinusal spleens; therefore, blood in the red pulp flows from splenic cords into splenic sinuses.

Chapter 13
Digestive System

I. INTRODUCTION

A. Components and functions

1. **Oral cavity**
   a. **Components**
      (1) Lips
      (2) Cheeks
      (3) Palate
      (4) Tongue
      (5) Teeth
      (6) Salivary glands
   b. **Functions.** The functions of the oral cavity are prehension, crushing, moistening, and lubrication of food.

2. **Oropharynx.** The oropharynx connects the oral cavity and the esophagus.

3. **Esophagus.** The esophagus conveys boluses of ingesta to the stomach (or forestomach in ruminants).

4. **Stomach**
   a. **Glandular stomach.** The glandular stomach is a muscular digestive reservoir where ingesta are mixed and their enzymatic and hydrolytic breakdown is initiated. A variety of hormones with primarily paracrine (i.e., local) actions are synthesized in the stomach and intestine.
   b. **Forestomach.** In **ruminants,** a forestomach precedes the glandular stomach. The forestomach breaks down ingesta mechanically and chemically (via microbial fermentation).

5. **Intestines**
   a. In the **small intestine,** the **ingesta** are **broken down** by bile and digestive enzymes secreted by the pancreas and intestinal glands, and **absorption takes place**.
   b. In the **large intestine,** water, vitamins, and electrolytes are absorbed. In herbivores, microbial breakdown of ingesta occurs in the large intestine.

6. **Liver**
   a. **Digestion-related functions**
      (1) Bile secretion
      (2) Metabolite storage
      (3) Gluconeogenesis (carbohydrate formation)
   b. **Other functions**
      (1) Synthesis of plasma proteins
      (2) Detoxification and inactivation of many lipid-soluble substances

7. **Pancreas.** The pancreas has an **exocrine component** and an **endocrine component**.
   a. The **exocrine component synthesizes** and **secretes major digestive enzymes** (e.g., pancreozymin, amylase, lipase, and trypsin).
   b. The **endocrine component produces hormones** that affect glucose metabolism.

B. General histologic organization. In the tubular organs of the digestive system, **four layers** are distinguished. From the lumen out, they are the **tunica mucosa, tela submucosa, tunica muscularis,** and **tunica serosa** or **adventitia**.

1. **Tunica mucosa (mucosa, mucous membrane).** The tunica mucosa has three layers.
   a. **Lamina epithelialis.** The epithelium that lines the lumen is stratified squamous or simple columnar.
      (1) **Stratified squamous epithelium lines cutaneous mucous membranes.**
         (a) A cutaneous mucous membrane is present:
            (i) From the **oral cavity** through the **forestomach** in **ruminants**
            (ii) From the **oral cavity** through the **nonglandular** portion of the **stomach** in horses and pigs
            (iii) In the **anal canal** and **anus**
         (b) The stratified squamous epithelium varies.
            (i) It is **keratinized in ruminants** for protection from the abrasive action of the ingesta.
            (ii) It is **nonkeratinized in carnivores**.
            (iii) It is **moderately keratinized** in horses and pigs.
      (2) **Simple columnar epithelium** lines the **remainder of the digestive system**.
   b. **Lamina propria (propria).** The lamina propria is a layer of **connective tissue**. It contains glands in the oral cavity, esophagus, stomach, and intestine.
      (1) **Dense irregular connective tissue** characterizes the lamina propria in areas where the **epithelium is stratified squamous**.
      (2) **Loose connective tissue** characterizes the lamina propria in areas where the **epithelium is simple columnar**.
   c. **Lamina muscularis.** The lamina muscularis is a layer of smooth muscle, which appears longitudinal but is actually arranged in a loose spiral around the lumen.

2. **Tela submucosa (submucosa).** The tela submucosa is a layer of **loose connective tissue** that connects the tunica mucosa to the tunica muscularis.
   a. Where there is no lamina muscularis, the lamina propria and tela submucosa form a continuous connective tissue layer that is referred to as the **propria–submucosa**.
   b. The tela submucosa permits shifting of the tunica mucosa relative to the rest of the wall (i.e., the tunica muscularis).
   c. Large blood vessels and nerves course through it. Autonomic (parasympathetic) fibers and ganglia (the **submucosal plexus**) are present.

3. **Tunica muscularis**
   a. In most areas, this tunic comprises **two layers of smooth muscle**.
      (1) The **inner layer** consists of muscle fibers arranged in a circle or tight spiral.
      (2) The **outer layer** consists of muscle fibers arranged longitudinally or in a loose spiral.
   b. Between the two layers, autonomic (parasympathetic) fibers and ganglia (the **myenteric plexus**) are present.
   c. In certain areas, **skeletal muscle** is present.

4. **Tunica serosa** or **tunica adventitia**
   a. A **tunica serosa** comprises **mesothelium** over **loose connective tissue,** which often contains numerous adipocytes. It surrounds the pancreas, liver, caudal esophagus, forestomach, stomach, and most of the intestine, which lie in the **peritoneal cavity**.
   b. A **tunica adventitia** is a layer of **loose connective tissue** that permits limited independent movements of adjacent organs. It surrounds those parts of the digestive system that are not suspended in the large body cavities (e.g., the oral cavity, pharynx, most of the esophagus).

II. MAMMALIAN DIGESTIVE SYSTEM.

Only variations from the general histologic organization discussed in I B 1–4 are described.

A. Oral cavity

1. **Lips and cheeks.** The lips function in the **prehension** of food in horses and small ruminants.
   a. The **oral surface** is lined by stratified squamous epithelium that is anchored by extremely well-developed connective tissue papillae.
      (1) Caudally oriented **conical papillae,** which assist in the caudad movement of ingested food, are visible macroscopically in ruminants.
      (2) The **propria–submucosa** contains **labial** and **buccal salivary glands** [see II A 5 c (2)].
   b. A **middle layer** contains skeletal muscle fibers (e.g., orbicularis oris muscle, buccalis muscle) in a loose connective tissue matrix.
   c. **Externally,** the lips and cheeks are covered by typical skin.

2. **Palate and pharynx**
   a. **Hard palate**
      (1) **Tunica mucosa.** The **oral surface** of the hard palate is covered by a **cutaneous mucous membrane** that forms the **ridges (rugae)** characteristic of the hard palate.
      (2) The **propria–submucosa** blends with the periosteum of the overlying (supporting) bone.
         (a) The propria–submucosa contains a **dense venous network,** which functions as a cushioning device.
         (b) **Mucous** or **mixed** (i.e., **mucoserous**) **palatine salivary glands** are present caudally.
      (3) **Dental pad (pulvinus).** In ruminants, a rostral prominence, the dental pad or pulvinus, is present in place of upper incisor teeth. It is formed by pronounced thickening of both the epithelium and the propria–submucosa.
   b. **Soft palate and oropharynx**
      (1) **Soft palate**
         (a) **Tunica mucosa**
            (i) The **oral (ventral) surface** is covered by a cutaneous mucous membrane.
            (ii) Most of the **nasal (dorsal) surface** is covered by respiratory mucosa (i.e., ciliated pseudostratified columnar epithelium), but caudally, a cutaneous mucous membrane is present.
         (b) **Propria–submucosa.** The propria–submucosa of the soft palate contains mucous and mixed glands, solitary lymphatic nodules, and diffuse lymphatic tissue.
         (c) **Core.** The core of the soft palate contains bundles of skeletal muscle fibers.
      (2) **Oropharynx**
         (a) **Tunica mucosa.** The oropharynx is lined by a cutaneous mucous membrane.
         (b) **Propria–submucosa.** The propria–submucosa of the oropharynx also contains lymphatic tissue and mucous glands.
         (c) **Tunica muscularis.** Skeletal muscle fibers form a distinct tunica muscularis in the oropharynx.

3. **Tongue**
   a. **Tunica mucosa.** The tongue is a muscular organ covered by a cutaneous mucosa.
      (1) The **dorsal lingual surface** is covered by keratinized stratified squamous epithelium, which is especially thick in herbivores. It bears macroscopic **mechanical** and **gustatory papillae,** each of which is supported by a core of dense irregular connective tissue.
         (a) **Mechanical papillae**
            (i) **Filiform papillae** are thread-like or cone-shaped, highly keratinized papillae with a caudally directed apex (Figure 13-1). Filiform papillae assist in:
               The prehension of food in large ruminants
               The uptake of fluids in carnivores
               Grooming in cats

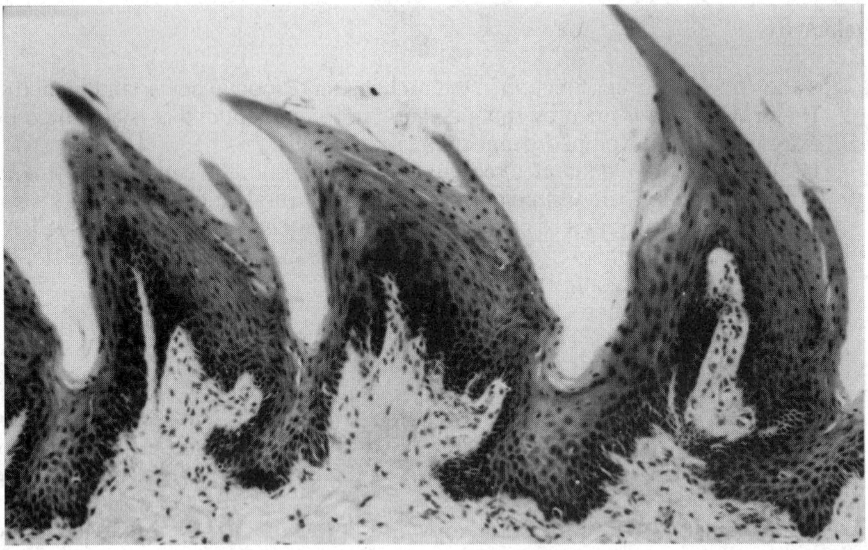

FIGURE 13-1. Filiform papillae of the canine tongue with long and short caudally directed thorn-like apices.

- **(ii) Conical papillae,** similar to those of the cheek, are noticeable on the base of the tongue of ruminants.
- **(iii) Lenticular papillae,** which occur mainly in ruminants, are lens shaped. Together with conical papillae, they help move food toward the pharynx.
- **(iv) Marginal papillae** are temporary structures at the lateral edge of the tongue of newborn carnivores and newborn swine. They are long, flat papillae that contribute to a tight seal around the teat during suckling.

(b) Gustatory papillae contain **taste buds** (i.e., elliptical clusters of supportive, secretory, and chemoreceptor cells) in their surface epithelium. Taste bud cells, which are short lived (10 days), are replenished from the surrounding epithelium.

- **(i) Fungiform papillae** are **mushroom shaped**. They are covered by slightly keratinized stratified squamous epithelium. Their thin epithelium and highly vascularized connective tissue core are responsible for their distinct pink color when observed in the live animal.
- **(ii) Vallate (circumvallate) papillae** are surrounded by a **moat (furrow)**. Taste buds are located on the sides of the papillae. Ducts of serous gustatory glands open into the moat, releasing secretions that dissolve substances for taste perception and flushing the moat.
- **(iii) Foliate papillae** consist of a **series of parallel mucosal folds** with taste buds on the sides. Ducts of serous gustatory glands open into the furrows separating the folds (Figure 13-2).

(2) On the **ventral lingual surface,** the stratified squamous epithelium is less keratinized than dorsally and may even be nonkeratinized. No papillae are present.

b. The **propria–submucosa** contains scattered lingual glands [see II A 5 b 2 (b)].

c. Special structures

(1) A cord-like **dorsal lingual cartilage** (composed of hyaline cartilage, skeletal muscle fibers, and adipose tissue) is present in **horses**.

(2) A **dorsal prominence (torus linguae)** in **ruminants** is rich in adipose tissue.

(3) A **lyssa** is present in the ventral midline in **carnivores** and **pigs**. The functional significance of the lyssa is unknown.

- **(a)** In dogs, the lyssa is a cord of skeletal muscle fibers and adipose tissue surrounded by a capsule of dense irregular connective tissue.
- **(b)** In cats and pigs, the lyssa contains mainly adipose tissue.

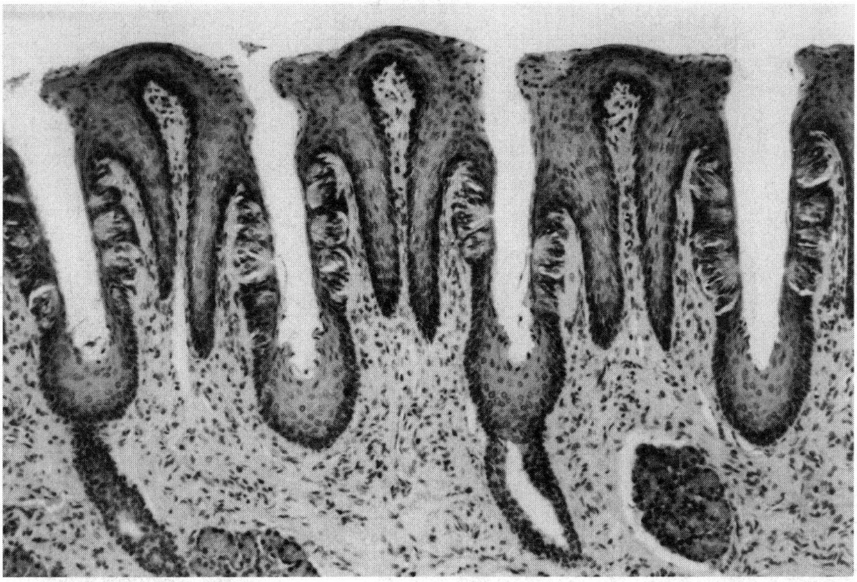

FIGURE 13-2. Taste buds are located in the epithelium on the sides of the folds that make up the foliate papillae. Gustatory glands are present in the propria–submucosa.

4. **Teeth** are used in the **prehension** and **grinding** of food.
   a. **Types.** Teeth in domestic animals are either **brachydont** or **hypsodont**.
      (1) **Brachydont teeth**
         (a) Brachydont teeth have a **crown,** a **neck,** and **one or several roots** (Figure 13-3A).
         (b) All carnivore teeth, the incisors of ruminants, and the teeth of pigs (except the tusks of boars) are brachydont.
      (2) **Hypsodont teeth** have a rough occlusal surface that is well suited for crushing and grinding food.
         (a) Hypsodont teeth are characterized by an **elongated body** and lack a **crown** and **neck** (Figure 13-3B).
         (b) All teeth of horses, the cheek teeth of ruminants, and the tusks of boars are hypsodont teeth.
   b. **Structure**
      (1) The **outer portion** of the tooth is **highly mineralized** and is composed of enamel, dentin, and cementum.
         (a) **Enamel.** Enamel covers the crown of brachydont teeth and almost the entire body of hypsodont teeth, in which it invaginates the occlusal surface to form **infundibula,** and the sides to form **enamel plicae (folds)**.
            (i) **Composition.** Enamel consists of highly ordered crystals (i.e., enamel rods and the interrod enamel) of the inorganic compound **hydroxyapatite,** plus a small amount of organic material.
            (ii) **Ameloblasts** form enamel during tooth development. In brachydont teeth, the ameloblasts degenerate at the time of eruption, but in hypsodont teeth, they may continue to actively synthesize enamel at the root (i.e., on the proximal body) of the tooth.
         (b) **Dentin.** Dentin underlies the enamel of the crown and the cementum of the root in brachydont teeth, and the enamel of the body in hypsodont teeth.
            (i) **Composition.** Dentin is 70% inorganic (mineral) substances and 30% collagen and glycoproteins.
            (ii) **Odontoblasts** located at the pulp–dentin border produce dentin throughout the life of the tooth. Odontoblast processes extend into **dentinal tubules,** which radiate through the dentin from the odontoblast layer in the pulp cavity to the enamel or cementum junction.

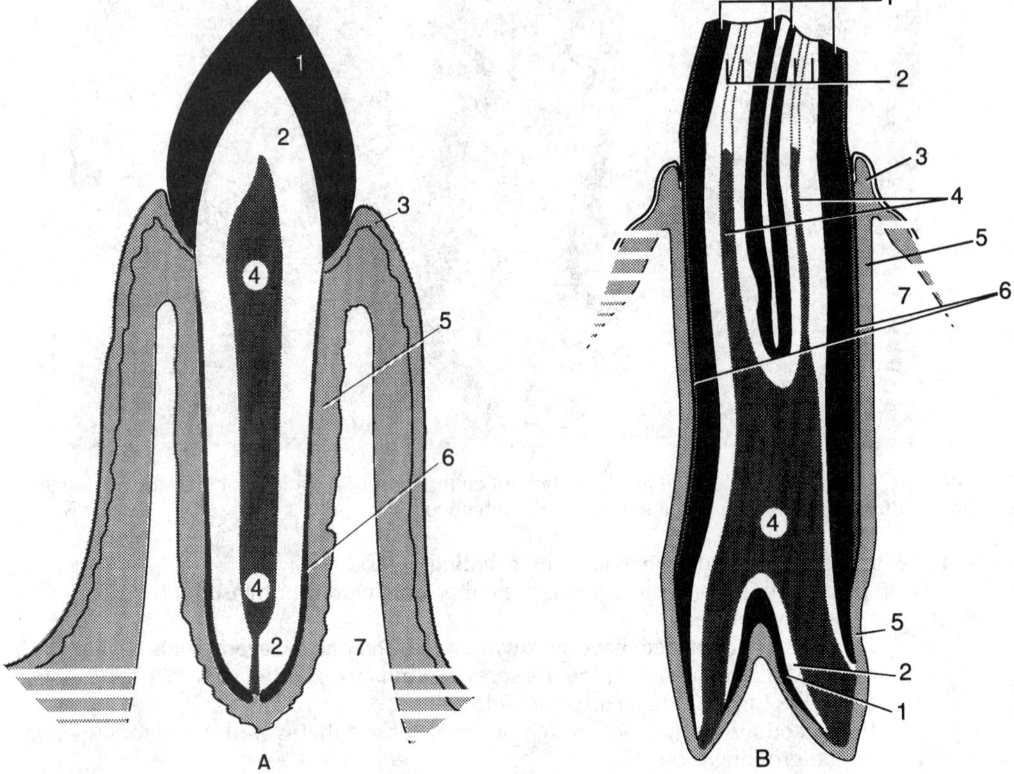

FIGURE 13-3. (*A*) Brachydont tooth. (Redrawn and modified from Dellmann H-D: *Veterinary Histology: An Outline Text–Atlas.* Baltimore, Williams & Wilkins, 1971.) (*B*) Hypsodont tooth. (Redrawn and modified from Weinreb MM and Sharav Y: Tooth development in sheep. *Am J Vet Res* 25: 905, 1964.) (*1*) Enamel; (*2*) dentin; (*3*) gingiva; (*4*) pulp cavity; (*5*) periodontal ligament; (*6*) cementum; (*7*) alveolar bone.

(c) Cementum. Cementum resembles woven bone, but it is frequently acellular.

(i) In brachydont teeth, cementum surrounds dentin in the root.

(ii) In hypsodont teeth, it covers the entire body, where it fills enamel plicae and infundibula.

(2) The **central core** of the tooth is called the **dental pulp** (see Figure 13-3). Dental pulp consists of very cellular loose connective tissue that contains a few collagen fibers, capillaries, nerve fibers, and lymphatics.

(3) The **periodontal ligament** consists of diversely oriented bundles of collagen fibers that extend from the bone socket (i.e., the alveolus) into the cementum, firmly anchoring the tooth (see Figure 13-3).

5. Salivary glands

a. General structural features

(1) Secretory units, which are either acinar or tubuloacinar, may be lined by serous cells, mucous cells, or a combination of both cell types (see also Chapter 5 IV B 4).

(2) **Myoepithelial cells** surround secretory acini and excretory ducts. Their contraction helps to move saliva out of acini and ducts.

(3) **Ducts.** Major salivary glands [see II A 5 b (1)] have intercalated and striated intralobular ducts, interlobular ducts, and main excretory ducts (called the parotid, mandibular, and sublingual ducts).

b. Types

(1) Major salivary glands

(a) **Parotid salivary gland.** This gland has exclusively serous acini in most domestic mammals, but in dogs, mucous acini occur singly or in groups.

(b) **Mandibular salivary gland.** The secretory units consist of tubules that comprise exclusively mucus-secreting cells and terminal acini that comprise mucus-secreting cells and peripheral serous demilunes.

(c) **Sublingual salivary gland.** Mucous cells predominate in cows, sheep, and pigs. Cells that elaborate both mucous and serous products are present in dogs and cats.

(2) **Minor salivary glands** are morphologically and functionally similar to the major salivary glands.

(a) Minor salivary glands are **mixed** (i.e., **mucoserous**) **glands**.

(b) Minor salivary glands are **named according to their location** (i.e., **labial, buccal, molar, lingual, palatine,** and **zygomatic**).

c. **Function.** Salivary gland secretions contain enzymes that **initiate carbohydrate digestion,** water that **moistens food,** and glycoproteins that **lubricate food,** thus **facilitating deglutition**.

B. Esophagus.
The esophagus is a conduit for boluses of ingesta. In ruminants, the presence of skeletal muscle facilitates **eructation** (i.e., belching) and **regurgitation** (Figure 13-4).

1. Tunica mucosa

a. The **lumen** is lined by **stratified squamous epithelium**. The degree of keratinization is related to the texture of the diet [see I B 1 a (1)].

b. The **lamina propria** contains **numerous elastic fibers**. Solitary lymphatic nodules are present in pigs.

c. The **lamina muscularis** consists of primarily longitudinally oriented **smooth muscle bundles**. It is absent cranially in pigs and dogs.

2. **Tela submucosa.** The submucosa contains **numerous mucous glands,** which are located:

a. Along the entire length of the esophagus in dogs

b. In the cranial half of the esophagus in pigs

c. In the cranial third of the esophagus (i.e., in the cervical region) in all other domestic mammals

3. Tunica muscularis

a. The tunica muscularis is **skeletal muscle,** which is located:

(1) Along the entire length of the esophagus in ruminants and dogs

(2) In the cranial two-thirds of the esophagus in horses and pigs

(3) In the cranial four-fifths of the esophagus in cats

b. **Smooth muscle** forms the remainder of the tunica muscularis in horses, pigs, and cats.

C. Forestomach.
The ruminant forestomach comprises three compartments (i.e., the **rumen, reticulum,** and **omasum**) with special functions that are reflected in their structural differences. The stratified squamous lining epithelium possesses absorptive capabilities and, therefore, has special structural characteristics.

1. Rumen

a. Tunica mucosa

(1) Epithelium

(a) **Transepithelial transport** of short-chain fatty acids (i.e., sodium salts, the microbial breakdown product of cellulose) is highest in the many areas where swollen-looking epithelial cells are present in the strata granulosum and corneum (Figure 13-5).

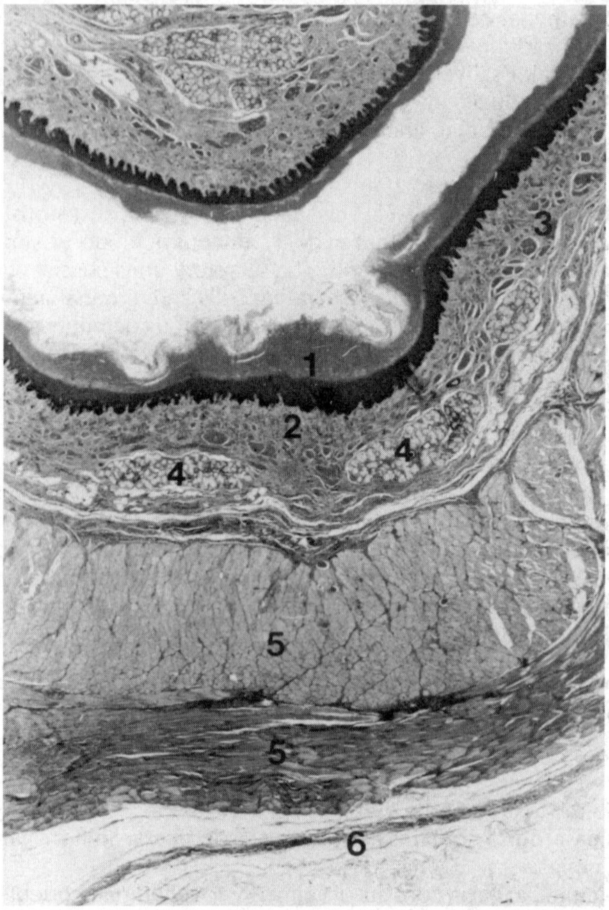

FIGURE 13-4. Esophagus. (*1*) Epithelium; (*2*) lamina propria; (*3*) lamina muscularis; (*4*) esophageal glands in the tela submucosa; (*5*) tunica muscularis; (*6*) tunica adventitia.

(b) **Tight junctions** join the cells of the upper stratum granulosum and the lower stratum corneum.

(2) **Papillae.** The tunica mucosa forms papillae with highly vascularized connective tissue cores (Figure 13-6A).

(3) **No lamina muscularis** is present.

b. Tunica muscularis. The tunica muscularis is particularly thick in the **pillars** of the rumen (i.e., the folds of the ruminal wall).

2. Reticulum

a. Tunica mucosa

(1) The **stratified squamous epithelium** is modified in some areas as it is in the rumen.

(a) Arrays of **perpendicular mucosal folds (laminae)** delineate roughly square compartments, called **cells**.

(b) The mucosa bears **conical papillae** (Figure 13-6B).

(2) The **lamina muscularis** is strands of smooth muscle near the margin of the folds.

b. Function. The reticulum functions in the **regurgitation, mixing** (via interaction with the rumen), and **movement** (to the omasum) of ingesta. In addition, the **uptake of short-chain fatty acids** continues in the reticulum.

3. Omasum

a. Parallel laminae of variable lengths are formed by **folds of the cutaneous mucosa** and **portions of the tunica muscularis** (Figure 13-6C).

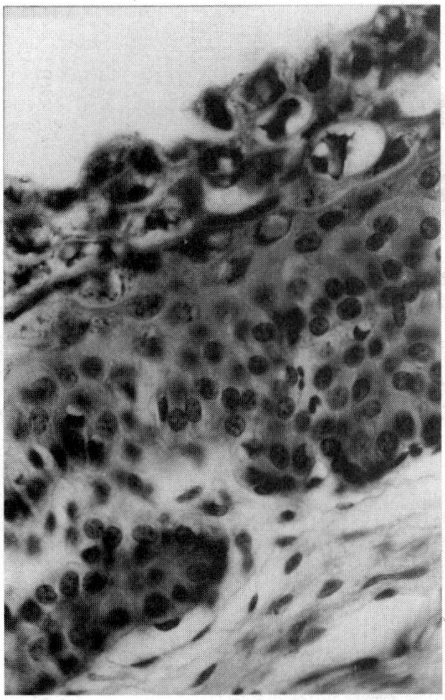

FIGURE 13-5. Swollen cells are present in the strata granulosum and corneum of the ruminal epithelium.

(1) **Papillae** are present on the surface of the laminae.

(2) The laminae contain **three layers of smooth muscle**.

(a) **Two outer layers** are derived from the **lamina muscularis**. Their fibers parallel the free edge of the laminae.

(b) The **single inner layer** is derived from the **tunica muscularis**. Its fibers are perpendicular to those of the lamina muscularis.

b. As ingesta pass between the laminae, they are crushed by the bidirectional movements of the laminae. Ingesta become more solid because water is absorbed in the omasum. The ingesta are then moved into the abomasum (i.e., the glandular stomach of ruminants).

D. Stomach

1. A **nonglandular region** that is lined with a cutaneous mucosa is present near the esophageal–gastric junction in **horses** and **pigs**. It is considered to be **nonabsorptive**.

2. Glandular region

a. Tunica mucosa. The glandular region of the stomach has permanent elevations, referred to as **gastric areas,** which are indented by **gastric pits**. **Gastric glands** open into the bottom of gastric pits (Figure 13-7).

(1) **Epithelial lining.** Simple columnar surface epithelial cells secrete mucous continuously.

(2) **Lamina propria.** The loose connective tissue of the lamina propria contains diffuse lymphatic tissue and occasional lymph nodules as well as **glands**.

(a) **Cardiac** and **pyloric glands** are branched tubular mucous glands. These glands, together with surface epithelial and mucous neck cells in the fundic glands, **produce gastric mucus,** which protects the gastric mucosa from autodigestion.

(b) **Fundic glands** are branched tubular glands in which several types of secretory cells are present (see Figures 13-7A & B).

(i) **Mucous neck cells** occupy the neck of the gland. **Undifferentiated epithelial cells** in the neck region of the gastric glands divide and give rise to both glandular and surface epithelial cells.

(ii) **Chief cells,** which are particularly concentrated at the base of the gland, **secrete pepsinogen**. In the ruminant abomasum, they secrete rennin.

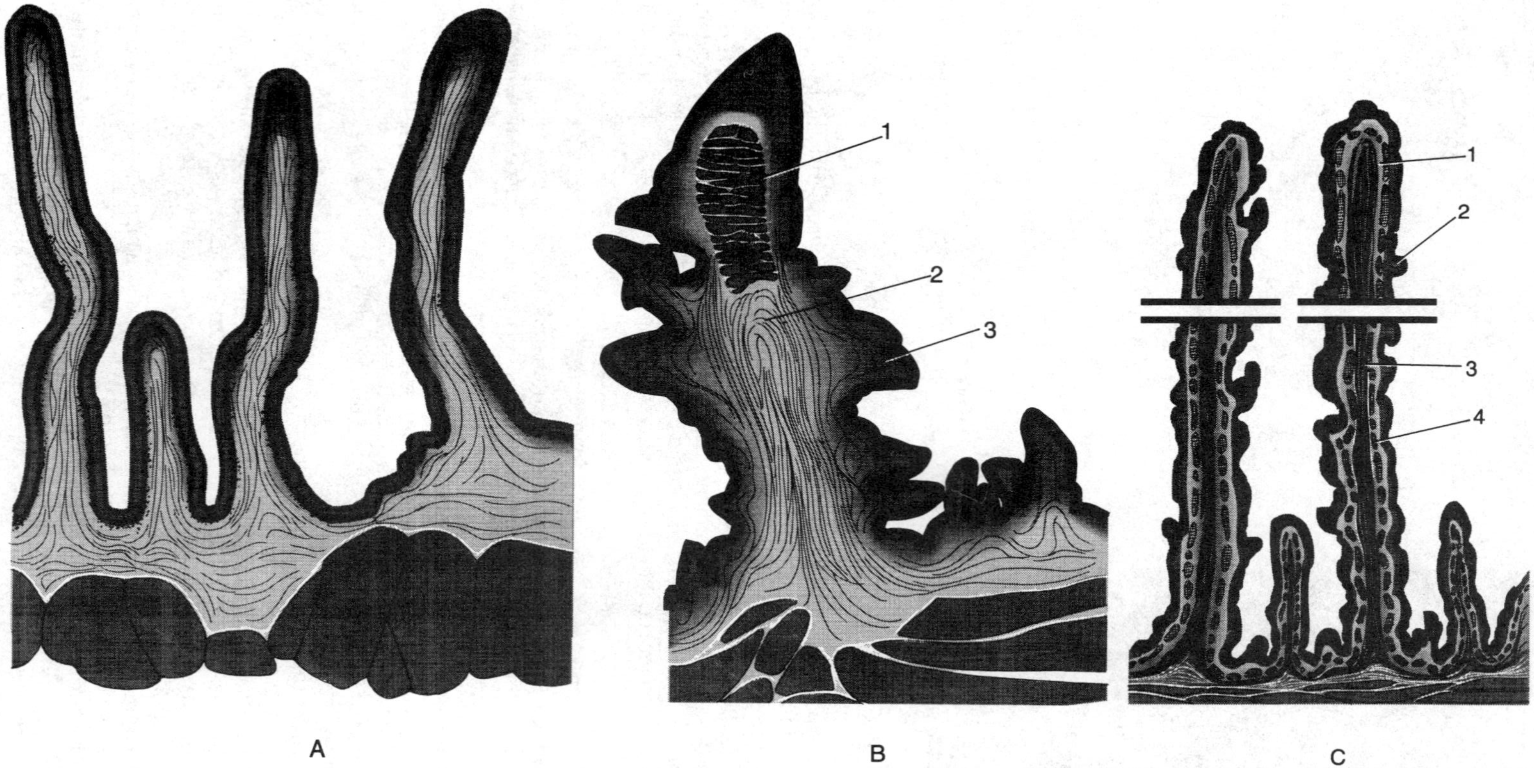

FIGURE 13-6. (*A*) Rumen. Papillae are characteristic of the ruminal mucosa. (*B*) Reticulum. (*1*) Lamina muscularis; (*2*) reticular fold; (*3*) papillae. (*C*) Omasum. (*1*) Omasal lamina; (*2*) papillae; (*3*) tunica muscularis; (*4*) lamina muscularis.

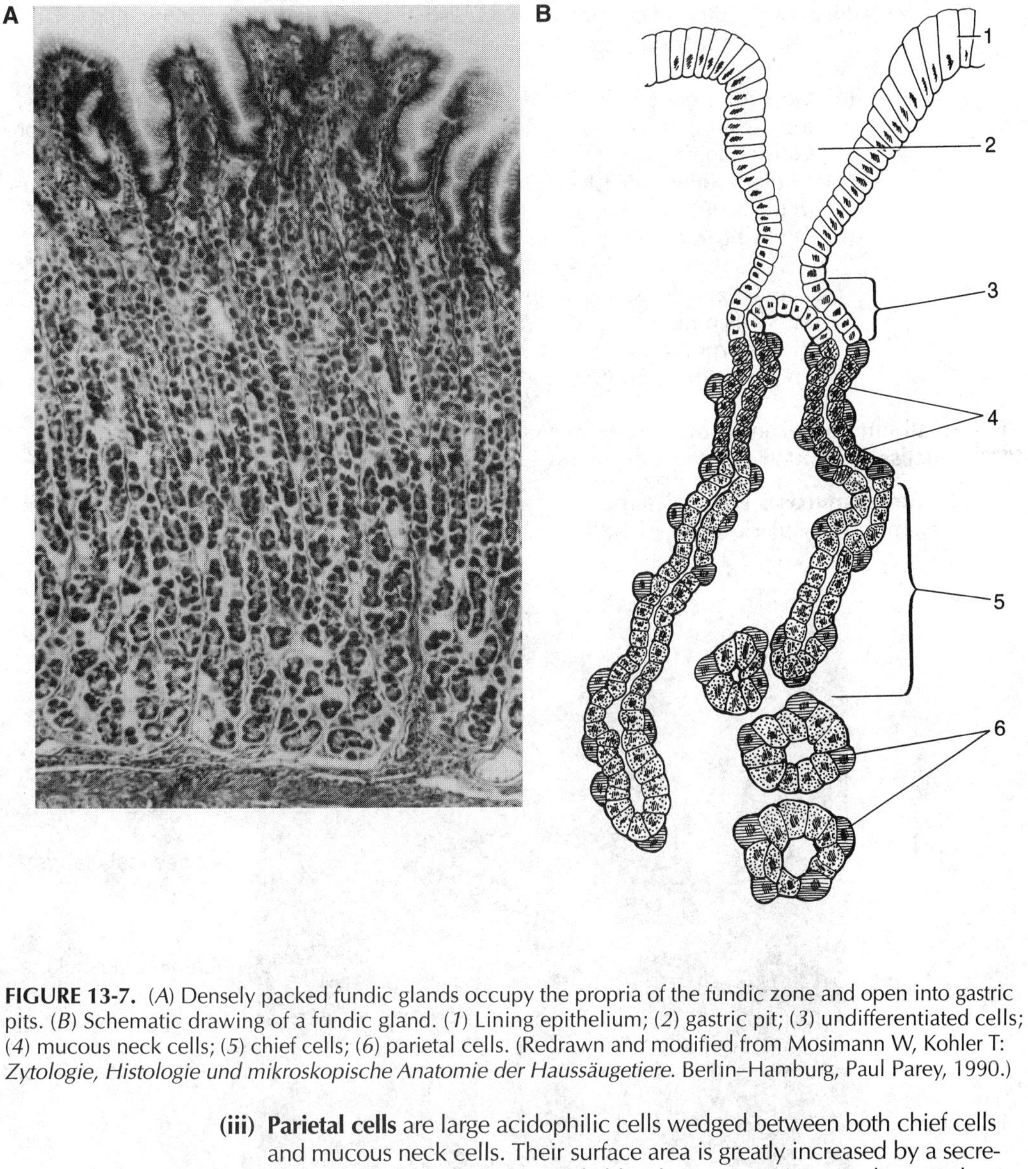

FIGURE 13-7. (*A*) Densely packed fundic glands occupy the propria of the fundic zone and open into gastric pits. (*B*) Schematic drawing of a fundic gland. (*1*) Lining epithelium; (*2*) gastric pit; (*3*) undifferentiated cells; (*4*) mucous neck cells; (*5*) chief cells; (*6*) parietal cells. (Redrawn and modified from Mosimann W, Kohler T: *Zytologie, Histologie und mikroskopische Anatomie der Haussäugetiere.* Berlin–Hamburg, Paul Parey, 1990.)

(iii) **Parietal cells** are large acidophilic cells wedged between both chief cells and mucous neck cells. Their surface area is greatly increased by a secretory canaliculus. Hydrogen and chloride ions are transported across the parietal cell membranes into the lumen, where hydrochloric acid is formed.

(3) Stratum compactum. A **stratum compactum,** composed of collagen and elastic fibers, may be present between the bases of the glands and the lamina muscularis. It is often present in carnivores.

(4) **Lamina muscularis.** The lamina muscularis is prominent and often comprises two or three layers.

b. **Tunica muscularis.** The tunica muscularis has a third muscle layer, the inner oblique layer, in the body (corpus) and fundus of the stomach.

3. **Gastric secretion and motility**

a. **Neural control.** The **vagus nerve** conveys impulses that stimulate gastric secretion.

b. **Hormonal control. Enteroendocrine cells** secrete **gastrointestinal hormones,** which primarily act locally to regulate digestive activity and carbohydrate metabolism.

(1) **Location.** Enteroendocrine cells are located throughout the stomach and intestine, either singly or in groups.

(2) **Structure.** Enteroendocrine cells are usually not in contact with the glandular lumen; their **secretory granules** are in the **basal cytoplasm.**

(3) **Secretory products**

(a) **Gastrin,** produced in the stomach (pylorus) and intestine (duodenum, rectum), stimulates secretion of both pepsinogen and hydrochloric acid and promotes contraction of the gastric musculature.

(b) **Cholecystokinin (CCK)** and **secretin,** produced in the duodenum in response to the arrival of chyme, inhibit gastric secretion and motility.

(c) **Other hormones** produced by the enteroendocrine cells include:

(i) **Pancreatic polypeptide,** produced in the fundus stomach

(ii) **Enteroglucagon,** produced in the pylorus

(iii) **Histamine,** produced throughout the stomach

(iv) **Serotonin,** produced in the stomach and intestine

(v) **Somatostatin (SST),** produced in the stomach and intestine

E. **Small intestine.** The **absorptive surface** of the small intestine is increased by circular **mucosal–submucosal folds, intestinal villi,** and **microvilli** on the absorptive cells.

1. **Tunica mucosa.** The tunica mucosa comprises epithelium, the lamina propria, and the lamina muscularis (Figure 13-8).

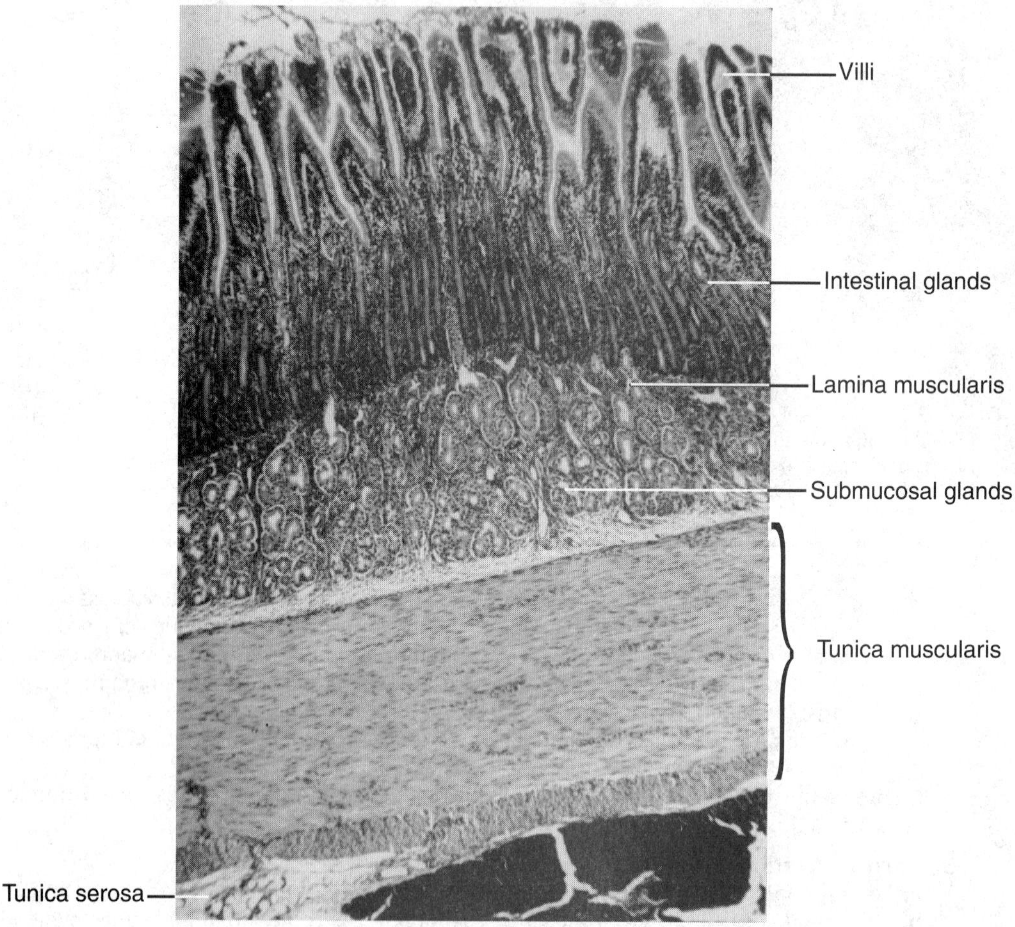

FIGURE 13-8. Small intestine (duodenum of the cat). Straight and parallel intestinal glands open into the intestinal lumen at the base of the villi. Notice the thick layer of submucosal glands with ducts that pierce the lamina muscularis. The two layers of the tunica muscularis and the tunica serosa are visible. The intensely stained organ is the pancreas.

a. Epithelium. The epithelium covering the **villi** is composed of columnar absorptive cells and goblet cells. The **intestinal glands (crypts)** are lined by undifferentiated cells, goblet cells, eosinophilic granular (Paneth) cells, and enteroendocrine cells.

(1) Columnar absorptive cells are by far the most numerous cells of the small intestine epithelium.

(a) Structural characteristics

(i) Columnar absorptive cells are joined at their apices by **tight junctions** that form a seal separating the lumen from the intercellular space.

(ii) The **luminal surface** of the columnar absorptive cells is covered with **microvilli** and has pronounced enzymatic activity (e.g., alkaline phosphatase, peptidase, lipase, disaccharidase). The microvilli form a **striated border** visible with the light microscope.

(b) Function. Absorptive cells **absorb the breakdown products of digestion**.

(i) Amino acids (resulting from the digestion of proteins) and **monosaccharides** (from carbohydrates) are absorbed by active transport.

(ii) Immunoglobulins from colostrum are absorbed by endocytosis.

(iii) Lipids that have been hydrolyzed by pancreatic lipase to monoglycerides and fatty acids diffuse through the apical plasma membrane to be resynthesized to **triglycerides** by the abundant apical smooth endoplasmic reticulum (sER). Triglycerides are then transported to the Golgi complexes to be covered with glycoproteins, after which they are called **chylomicrons**. The chylomicrons move to the lateral plasma membrane, where they are released by exocytosis. They subsequently enter lymph capillaries.

(2) Goblet cells are progressively more numerous caudally.

(3) Undifferentiated cuboidal to columnar cells in the intestinal glands divide mitotically and differentiate into absorptive and goblet cells, which migrate toward the tips of the villi (and, presumably, to enteroendocrine cells as well).

(4) Eosinophilic granular cells, which are pyramid-shaped cells that occur singly or in small clusters, produce **lysozyme,** an antibacterial compound. Eosinophilic granular cells are present in horses and ruminants.

(5) Enteroendocrine cells occur in all domestic mammals (see II D 3 b].

b. Lamina propria

(1) Free cells (especially plasma cells, mast cells, lymphocytes, eosinophils, and globular leukocytes) are numerous.

(2) Scattered diffuse lymphatic tissue and **solitary lymphatic nodules** occur.

(3) Smooth muscle cells in the lamina propria cause periodic shortening of the villi.

(4) Each villus contains a rich capillary plexus and a single central lymph capillary called a **lacteal** (see Figure 11-11A).

2. Tela submucosa

a. The initial portion of the small intestine contains serous, mucous, or mixed simple tubuloalveolar submucosal glands in all domestic mammals (see Figure 13-8). These glands are present in the duodenum and may continue into the jejunum.

b. Solitary lymphatic nodules are present throughout, and aggregated lymphatic nodules (**Peyer's patches**) are most numerous in the ileum.

F. Large intestine

1. Tunica mucosa. The tunica mucosa has **no villi** (Figure 13-9).

a. Goblet cells are usually **more numerous** than absorptive cells in the epithelium of the large intestine.

b. Absorptive cells prevail toward the gland openings and in the intestinal luminal surface.

(1) They absorb water, electrolytes, and vitamins in all domestic mammals.

(2) In pigs and horses, and to a lesser degree in ruminants, absorption of short-chain fatty acids from microbial digestion of cellulose also occurs.

c. Undifferentiated cuboidal to columnar cells are identical to those in the small intestine [see II E 1 a (3)].

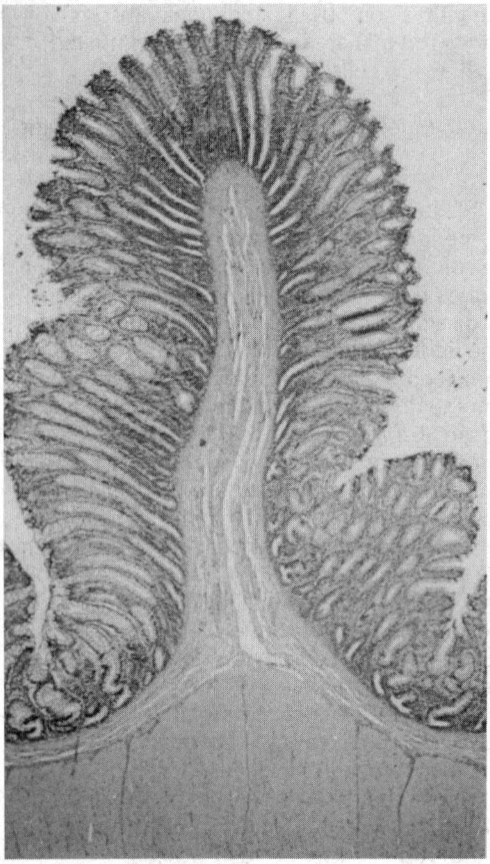

FIGURE 13-9. Longitudinal fold of the large intestinal mucosa, in which villi are lacking.

d. **Eosinophilic granular cells** are **absent**.
e. **Enteroendocrine cells** are present [see II E 1 a (5)].

2. **Tela submucosa.** The **intestinal glands** are longer than those of the small intestine, and there are more lymphatic nodules.

3. **Tunica muscularis**
   a. **Outer muscle layer.** The outer layer forms longitudinal muscle bands (**taeniae**) in the colon and rectum of horses and pigs.
   b. **Inner muscle layer**
      (1) At the recto–anal junction, the inner circular muscle layer forms the **internal anal sphincter**.
      (2) Circularly arranged skeletal muscle forms the **external anal sphincter**.

4. **Special structures**
   a. **Anal glands** (modified tubuloalveolar sweat glands) are present in the anal canal of **pigs** and **carnivores**.
   b. **Bilateral anal sacs** are present in **carnivores**.
   c. **Circumanal glands** are present in **dogs** and less frequently in cats (see Chapter 20).

G. Liver

1. **General organization**
   a. **Stroma and vascularity.** The **stroma** of the liver comprises primarily a thin connective tissue capsule and its continuations into **portal canals** between **liver lobules** (Figure 13-10). The liver receives its **nutrient blood supply from the hepatic artery** and its **functional blood supply from the portal vein**.

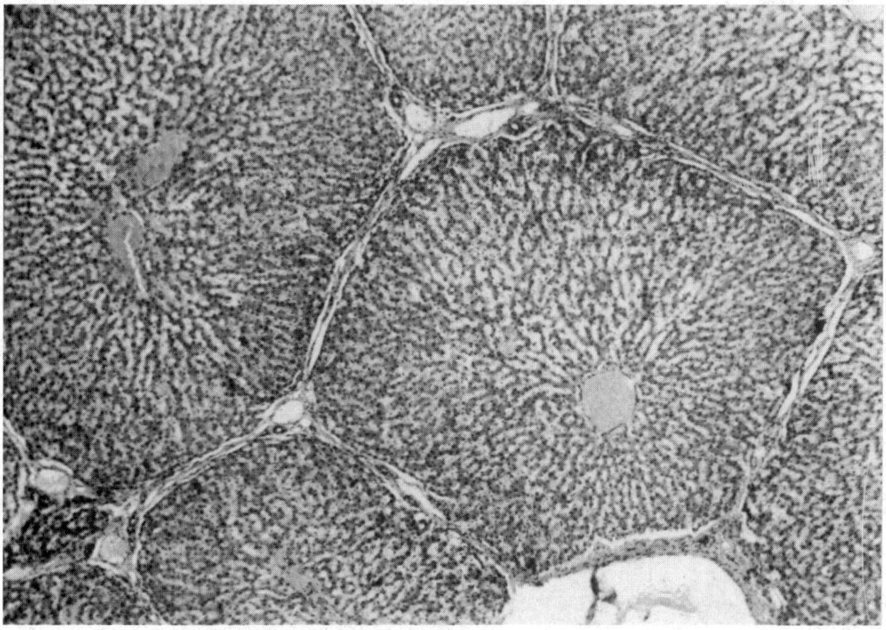

FIGURE 13-10. In this porcine liver, the lobules are delineated by connective tissue. Portal canals are located at the corners of the lobules. Radial liver cell plates alternate with sinusoids.

(1) **Portal canals** contain branches of the hepatic artery and portal vein, lymph vessels, and interlobular bile ducts.

(a) **Interlobular portal venules** in portal canals connect to **sinusoids** (see II G 2 b) via distributing venules.

(b) **Interlobular hepatic arterioles** give rise to capillaries that supply the interlobular connective tissue. They also give rise to capillaries that connect with the sinusoids.

(c) **Lymph vessels** that drain lymph capillaries located in the interlobular connective tissue run in parallel with the blood vessels.

(d) **Interlobular bile ducts** [see II G 2 c (2)] are a regular feature of portal canals.

(2) Distinct interlobular septa are present only in pigs.

b. Liver lobules

(1) Liver lobules have been defined in different ways (Figure 13-11).

(a) **Hepatic lobules** are roughly **hexagonal** columns **drained by one central vein**. **Portal canals** lie **at** the **angles** of the lobule (see Figure 13-10).

(b) **Portal lobules** are **triangular** columns **drained by the bile duct in a portal canal**. The portal canal is in the center, and a central vein lies at each corner.

(c) A **liver acinus** comprises the roughly **diamond-shaped** column supplied by a terminal branch of the hepatic artery and a corresponding branch of the portal vein.

(2) Within each **hepatic lobule,** the polyhedral parenchymal cells are arranged in anastomosing plates that radiate from a central vein (see Figure 13-10). These plates are separated by sinusoids, which receive blood from branches of both the hepatic artery and the portal vein, and which drain into the central vein.

2. Histologic organization. The histologic organization of the liver reflects the organ's many functions.

a. Hepatocytes

(1) **Organelles and inclusions.** Hepatocytes contain numerous mitochondria, abundant rough endoplasmic reticulum (rER) and sER, extensive Golgi complexes, lysosomes, peroxisomes, lipids, and glycogen.

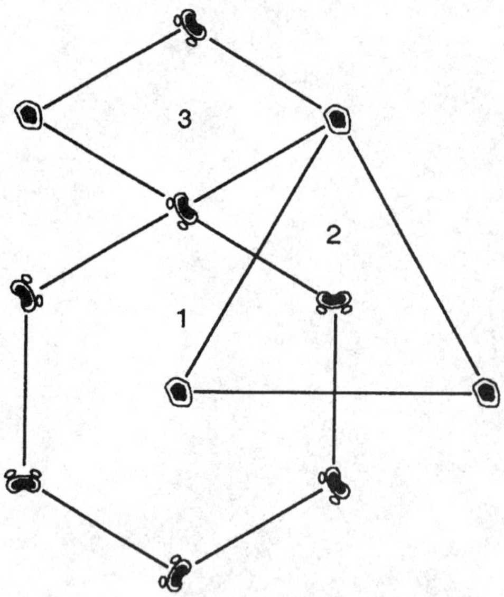

FIGURE 13-11. Schematic drawing of liver lobules. (*1*) Hexagonal hepatic lobule containing a central vein. (*2*) Portal lobule with a portal canal in the center and a central veinat each corner. (*3*) Diamond-shaped liver acinus receiving its blood supply from terminal branches of the hepatic artery and portal vein. (Modified and redrawn from Rappaport AM, Borowy ZJ, Laugheed WM, Lotto WN: Subdivision of hexagonal liver lobules into a structural and functional unit; role in hepatic physiology and pathology. *Anat Rec* 119:11, 1954, Figure 1.)

(a) **Storage**
   (i) **Carbohydrates** are stored in close association with the sER in the form of glycogen, which is broken down to glucose when the need arises.
   (ii) **Lipids** are stored as triglycerides in lipid droplets.

(b) **Detoxification and inactivation** of a variety of lipid-soluble drugs and substances, such as barbiturates, antihistamines, and steroids, are performed by the sER.

(c) **Bile secretion** by hepatocytes involves absorption of blood-borne components, their conjugation in the sER, and excretion into the bile canaliculi [see II G 2 a (2) (b)].

(d) **Synthesis of plasma proteins** (e.g., albumin and fibrinogen) and lipoproteins involves the sER, rER, and Golgi complex.

(2) **Cell surfaces.** Hepatocytes have three types of surfaces.
   (a) **Microvillous surfaces** that face **perisinusoidal spaces** are bathed by blood plasma and function in absorption and secretion.
   (b) **Microvillous surfaces** that face **bile canaliculi** provide a secretory surface for release of bile salts. A **canaliculus** is an expanded intercellular space between contiguous hepatocytes. It is created by a pair of parallel tight junctions that seal off its lumen from the rest of the extracellular space.
   (c) **Contact surfaces** between adjacent hepatocytes are joined by gap junctions.

b. Sinusoids

(1) **Exchange between blood and parenchyma.** Sinusoids are lined by a **discontinuous and porous endothelium** with a **basal lamina** that is **discontinuous or absent**. Thus, the fluid portion of blood has free access to the perisinusoidal space, into which hepatocyte microvilli project.

(2) **Stellate macrophages (Kupffer cells)** are present among the endothelial cells.

(3) **Perisinusoidal stellate cells,** also called **fat-storage cells,** are present in the perisinusoidal space. They are believed to store vitamin A and give rise to fibroblasts.

c. **Biliary system**

(1) **Intralobular bile ductules,** which are lined with simple squamous epithelium, drain the bile canaliculi.

(2) **Interlobular bile ducts** in portal canals are lined by cuboidal to columnar epithelium and drain the intralobular ductules.

(3) **Extrahepatic bile ducts**

(a) The **hepatic duct, cystic duct,** and **bile duct** are lined by simple columnar epithelium, which may contain goblet cells in ruminants. Mucous glands are present in the lamina propria.

(b) The **gallbladder** has a highly folded mucosa–submucosa that forms gland-like **crypts**.

(i) The simple columnar epithelium has a microvillous surface and contains goblet cells in pigs and ruminants.

(ii) Mucous or mixed glands are present in ruminants.

(iii) Diffuse or nodular lymphatic tissue is often present.

H. Pancreas. The pancreas comprises an exocrine and an endocrine portion.

1. **Exocrine pancreas.** The **exocrine portion** is a **compound serous gland**.

a. **Exocrine secretory units** are tubuloacinar or acinar. They contain secretory and centroacinar cells.

(1) **Secretory cells** have a spherical basal nucleus surrounded by basophilic cytoplasm containing abundant rER and mitochondria. Acidophilic zymogen granules containing proenzymes (e.g., trypsinogen) and enzymes (e.g., amylase) fill the apical cytoplasm.

(2) Flat **centroacinar cells** in the acinar lumen form the beginnings of intercalated ducts.

b. The **duct system** comprises intercalated ducts, intralobular ducts, interlobular ducts, and pancreatic ducts, all lined by simple cuboidal to columnar epithelium.

(1) Goblet cells and simple branched tubuloalveolar mucous glands may be present in the larger ducts.

(2) Intralobular ducts secrete bicarbonate, which renders the pancreatic fluid alkaline and neutralizes the acid chyme that enters the duodenum.

2. **Endocrine pancreas.** Pancreatic islets (see Chapter 19) are the endocrine portion of the pancreas; they are surrounded by the exocrine secretory units (Figure 13-12).

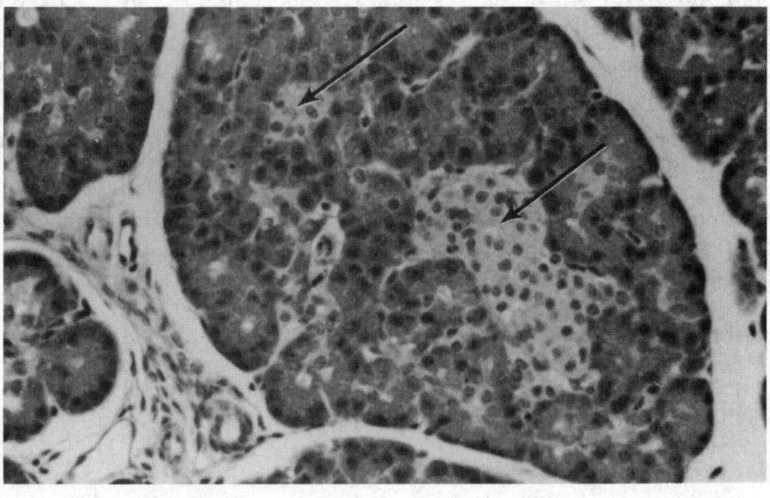

FIGURE 13-12. Exocrine secretory units surround pancreatic islets (*arrows*).

III. AVIAN DIGESTIVE SYSTEM

A. Oral cavity

1. The **oral surface** is lined by stratified squamous epithelium, which is variable in thickness and degree of keratinization.
2. The **tongue** is covered by thick stratified squamous keratinized epithelium, which forms a transverse row of papillae caudally. It contains an entoglossal (i.e., within the tongue) bone, striated muscle bundles, and lingual salivary glands.
3. The **salivary glands** are either simple branched tubular or compound tubular mucous glands.

B. Esophagus

1. **Epithelial lining.** The esophagus is lined with a thick stratified squamous epithelium.
2. **Lamina propria.** The lamina propria contains branched tubular mucous glands, which are frequently associated with solitary lymphatic nodules.
3. **Lamina muscularis.** A thick lamina muscularis is present.

C. Crop.

The crop is structurally similar to the esophagus, but glands are present only at its opening into the esophagus.

D. Proventriculus.

Macroscopic papillae are the most prominent feature of the proventriculus. At the apex of each papilla is the opening of a duct of a submucosal gland, surrounded by concentrically arranged mucosal folds.

1. **Tunica mucosa.** The **lining epithelium** is simple cuboidal to columnar mucigenous cells, and the underlying **lamina propria** contains many lymphocytes. The **lamina muscularis** is discontinuous.
2. **Tela submucosa.** The **submucosal glands** are compound tubular glands lined with simple cuboidal to columnar epithelial cells that are believed to secrete both pepsinogen and hydrochloric acid.

E. Ventriculus.

The ventriculus (gizzard) is specialized for grinding and mixing of ingesta.

1. The **innermost layer,** which is the secretory product of the gizzard glands, is a thick, hard, and keratin-like layer covering the epithelium.
2. The simple columnar **surface epithelium** continues into pits and into simple tubular glands that open into the pits.
3. The **loose connective tissue** of the **propria–submucosa** and thick **tunica muscularis** is surrounded by a dense regular connective tissue layer.

F. Small intestine.

The structure of the small intestine of birds differs from that of domestic mammals in that intestinal villi are long and leaf shaped, and the lamina propria and tela submucosa contain more diffuse and nodular lymphatic tissue.

G. Large intestine.

The large intestine differs from the mammalian pattern in that villi are present in the ceca (although they decrease in size distally, where they may be absent) and in the rectum. Solitary and aggregated lymphatic nodules and diffuse lymphatic tissue are more plentiful in avian lamina propria and tela submucosa than they are in the mammalian counterparts.

H. **Cloaca.** The cloaca comprises the terminal portions of the digestive system (i.e., the **coprodeum**) and the urinary and reproductive systems (i.e., the **urodeum**), and a caudodorsal compartment (i.e., the **proctodeum**).

1. **Villi** are present in the coprodeum and urodeum.
2. The **cloacal bursa** (i.e., the **bursa of Fabricius**), a lymphoepithelial diverticulum of the dorsal wall, is located in the proctodeum (see Chapter 12 III C).
3. The simple columnar epithelial lining of the cloaca changes to stratified squamous epithelium at the **vent** (i.e., the opening of the cloaca).

I. **Liver and pancreas.** The structure of the avian liver and pancreas is similar to that of the mammalian liver and pancreas.

STUDY QUESTIONS

DIRECTIONS: Each of the numbered items or incomplete statements in this section is followed by answers or by completions of the statement. Select the **one** numbered answer or completion that is **best** in each case.

1. Which of the following statements *best* describes lingual papillae?

(1) Filiform papillae occur only in carnivores.
(2) Conical papillae are characteristic of swine.
(3) Fungiform papillae are easily distinguished macroscopically by their pink color.
(4) Marginal papillae are present in all newborn domestic mammals.
(5) Vallate papillae are highly keratinized mechanical papillae.

2. Which of the following statements *best* describes the structure of teeth?

(1) Dentin covers the body of hypsodont teeth.
(2) Enamel covers the root of brachydont teeth.
(3) Enamel is produced throughout the life of both brachydont and hypsodont teeth.
(4) The periodontal ligament is predominantly collagen and anchors the tooth to the socket.
(5) The dental pulp is relatively avascular and sparsely innervated loose connective tissue.

3. Which of the following statements *best* describes salivary glands?

(1) Centroacinar cells form the beginnings of intercalated ducts.
(2) Secretory acini are lined by secretory cells and myoepithelial cells.
(3) In mixed salivary glands, a single cell type produces both mucous and serous secretory products.
(4) Basophilic secretory granules are prominent in serous cells.
(5) Acidophilic secretory granules are prominent in mucous cells.

4. Which of the following statements *best* describes the canine esophagus?

(1) Serous glands are prominent in the lamina propria.
(2) Submucosal lymphatic nodules are numerous.
(3) The lining epithelium is keratinized stratified squamous.
(4) The tunica muscularis is skeletal muscle throughout.
(5) Mixed submucosal glands are present throughout the entire esophagus.

5. Ruminal lining epithelial cells are:

(1) simple columnar absorptive.
(2) simple columnar mucus-secreting.
(3) nonkeratinized stratified squamous absorptive.
(4) keratinized stratified squamous nonabsorptive.
(5) keratinized stratified squamous absorptive.

6. Which one of the following cells produces gastric mucus?

(1) Eosinophilic granular (Paneth) cells
(2) Parietal cells
(3) Pyloric glandular cells
(4) Gastric enteroendocrine cells
(5) Chief cells

7. Which one of the following statements concerning the tunica mucosa of the large intestine in domestic mammals is correct?

(1) Eosinophilic granular (Paneth) cells are absent.
(2) Villi are larger than in the small intestine.
(3) Goblet cells are less numerous than in the small intestine.
(4) Enteroendocrine cells are absent.
(5) Lymphatic nodules are less numerous than in the small intestine.

8. Which one of the following is characteristic of hepatocytes?

(1) Abundant smooth endoplasmic reticulum (sER)
(2) Microvillous projections into the sinusoidal lumen
(3) Sparse rough endoplasmic reticulum (rER)
(4) Few lysosomes
(5) Small Golgi complexes

9. Which one of the following cells is present in cardiac glandular epithelium?

(1) Serous cells
(2) Goblet cells
(3) Parietal cells
(4) Chief cells
(5) Mucous cells

10. Which one of the following statements characterizes hepatic sinusoids?

(1) They are surrounded by a basal lamina.
(2) They have a continuous endothelium.
(3) They have a fenestrated endothelium.
(4) Their lining includes hepatocytes.
(5) Their lining includes hepatic stellate macrophages (Kupffer cells).

11. Which of the following is a *complete* list of cells present in a pancreatic acinus?

(1) Mucous acinar cells, serous acinar cells, myoepithelial cells
(2) Mucous acinar cells, myoepithelial cells
(3) Serous acinar cells, myoepithelial cells
(4) Serous acinar cells, centroacinar cells
(5) Serous acinar cells, centroacinar cells, myoepithelial cells

DIRECTIONS: Each of the numbered items or incomplete statements in this section is negatively phrased, as indicated by an italicized word such as *not, least,* or *except.* Select the **one** numbered answer or completion that is **best** in each case.

12. Each of the following statements concerning the structure of the ruminant forestomach is correct *except:*

(1) The great absorptive capacity of the rumen is evidenced by the presence of numerous highly vascularized papillae.
(2) A bundle of smooth muscle running along the edge of reticular folds is characteristic of the reticulum.
(3) The tunica muscularis gives rise to three layers of muscle in the omasal laminae.
(4) Papillae are present in all three compartments of the forestomach.
(5) The rumen is the only compartment of the forestomach that lacks a lamina muscularis.

13. All of the following statements regarding hypsodont teeth are true *except:*

(1) Cementum covers the body and surrounds root dentin.
(2) Enamel covers the oral surface of the tooth.
(3) Enamel forms folds and infundibula.
(4) Enamel may continue to be produced after tooth eruption.
(5) Cementum fills infundibula.

14. Each of the following statements concerning the small intestine is true *except:*

(1) The epithelium comprises absorptive cells, goblet cells, enteroendocrine cells, and undifferentiated cells.
(2) Intestinal villi periodically shorten and lengthen.
(3) Aggregated lymphatic nodules are rarely found in the ileum.
(4) Submucosal glands are present in the duodenum.
(5) Epithelial cells on the villi are replaced by mitotic division and differentiation of cells in the intestinal glands.

ANSWERS AND EXPLANATIONS

1. The answer is 3 *[II A 3 a (1) (a)–(b)]*. Fungiform papillae, which are a type of gustatory papilla, have a distinct pink color because of their thin epithelium and highly vascularized core. Filiform papillae are present in all domestic mammals, but their size, shape, and degree of keratinization vary considerably. Conical papillae occur only in ruminants. Marginal papillae are present only in newborn (suckling) carnivores and pigs. Vallate papillae are gustatory, not mechanical, papillae.

2. The answer is 4 *[II A 4 b (3)]*. The periodontal ligament is predominantly collagen; it anchors the tooth to the alveolus (i.e., the bone socket). The body of hypsodont teeth (i.e., the visible and alveolar portions of the tooth) is covered by cementum, not dentin. Cementum, not enamel, covers the root of brachydont teeth, but enamel covers the crown. Enamel production ceases in brachydont teeth at the time of eruption, but it continues in hypsodont teeth throughout the tooth's lifetime. On the other hand, dentin continues to be produced throughout the life of both types of teeth. The loose connective tissue of the dental pulp contains a dense capillary network and is highly innervated by afferent nerve fibers.

3. The answer is 2 *[II A 5 b; H 1 a (2)]*. Both secretory and myoepithelial cells make up secretory acini. Myoepithelial cells are also present in the salivary duct system. Centroacinar cells are cells of intercalated ducts that protrude into the acinar lumen; they are characteristic of the pancreas and are absent in salivary glands. Serous cells are characterized by acidophilic secretory granules in the apical cytoplasm, which contrast with the basophilic cell base. In mucous cells, the cytoplasm has a spongy appearance due to the dissolution of mucous granules during histologic processing. In mixed salivary glands, both mucous cells and serous cells coexist in secretory acini.

4. The answer is 4 *[II B 1–3]*. The tunica muscularis is skeletal muscle cranially in all domestic species. It is skeletal muscle throughout the entire esophagus in ruminants and dogs, whereas smooth muscle is present caudally in horses, pigs, and cats. Esophageal glands are mucous submucosal glands present cranially in all domestic species and extending caudally to the stomach in dogs. The tela submucosa does not contain lymphatic nodules; however, they do occur in the lamina propria of the porcine esophagus.

5. The answer is 5 *[I B 1 a (1) (a) (i); II C]*. The rumen is lined with keratinized stratified squamous epithelium that has absorptive capacities for short-chain fatty acids. Nonabsorptive keratinized stratified squamous epithelium is present in the nonglandular portion of the stomach in horses and pigs. The glandular stomach is lined by simple columnar mucus-secreting epithelium. Absorptive simple columnar epithelium occurs in the intestine.

6. The answer is 3 *[II D 2 a (2); E 1 a (4)]*. Secretory cells in the pyloric and cardiac glandular regions, mucous neck cells in fundic glands, and surface epithelial cells secrete gastric mucus. Parietal cells and chief cells in fundic glands produce hydrochloric acid and pepsinogen, respectively. Gastric enteroendocrine cells secrete a variety of hormones (see II D 3 b). Eosinophilic granular (Paneth) cells are absent from the stomach; they occur in the small intestine of horses and ruminants and produce lysozyme.

7. The answer is 1 *[II F 1]*. Eosinophilic granular (Paneth) cells do not occur in the large intestine of any domestic mammal. In domestic mammals, only the small intestine has villi. The large intestine is devoid of villi. In birds, however, villi are present in both the small and large intestine. Goblet cells are more numerous in the large intestine than in the small intestine. Enteroendocrine cells are consistently present in the large intestine. The large intestine has more lymphatic nodules than the small intestine.

8. The answer is 1 *[II G 2 a]*. Hepatocytes possess an abundant smooth endoplasmic reticulum (sER) that participates in a variety of functions (e.g., detoxification, cholesterol synthesis, bile salt synthesis). Golgi complexes and rough endoplasmic reticulum (rER) are extensive in hepatocytes and are both involved in the synthesis of numerous substances. The numerous lysosomes play a role in the breakdown of hepatocyte organelles (autophagy) and endocytosed substances.

Microvillous projections into the perisinusoidal space, not the sinusoidal lumen, ensure maximal exchange between the hepatic parenchyma and the blood supply.

9. The answer is 5 *[II D 2 a (2) (a)]*. Cardiac glandular epithelium comprises mucus-secreting cells, undifferentiated cells, and enteroendocrine cells. Chief cells and parietal cells, located in the fundic glands, produce pepsinogen and hydrochloric acid, respectively. Goblet cells do not occur in the stomach.

10. The answer is 5 *[II G 2 b]*. Stellate macrophages (Kupffer cells) are present among the endothelial cells of the sinusoidal lining. Liver sinusoids are lined by a discontinuous and porous endothelium and often have incomplete or absent basal laminae as well. These modifications allow the sinusoids to communicate with the surrounding perisinusoidal space. Hepatic microvilli project into this space, where they are bathed in the blood plasma. Capillaries in muscle and the central nervous system are examples of vessels lined by continuous endothelium; fenestrated endothelium is present in the capillaries of the endocrine glands, and in the intestinal tunica mucosa.

11. The answer is 4 *[II H 1 a]*. Pancreatic acini contain exclusively serous (zymogen-secreting) cells and centroacinar cells, which are present in the acinar lumen and represent the beginning of the duct system. Myoepithelial cells are not present in pancreatic acini.

12. The answer is 3 *[II C 3 a (2)]*. Even though three layers of smooth muscle characterize the omasal laminae, only the central one is derived from the tunica muscularis. The peripheral layers are derived from the lamina muscularis. The rumen is the only compartment of the forestomach that lacks a lamina muscularis; in the reticulum, the lamina muscularis forms a bundle of smooth muscle near the margin of each mucosal fold (lamina). Papillae are present in all three compartments of the forestomach and are particularly numerous in the rumen.

13. The answer is 2 *[II A 4; Figure 13-3A & B]*. The oral surface of the hypsodont tooth (i.e., that portion of the body of the tooth protruding above the gingiva) is covered by cementum except at the occlusal surface, where cementum, enamel, and dentin are all exposed. After tooth eruption, enamel production ceases in brachydont teeth but may continue in hypsodont teeth.

14. The answer is 3 *[II E 1 a, b (2), 2]*. Aggregated lymphatic nodules are more numerous in the tela submucosa of the ileum than in any other portion of the small intestine. The tela submucosa of the duodenum contains mucous, serous, or mixed glands. The epithelium of the small intestine comprises absorptive cells, goblet cells, enteroendocrine cells, and undifferentiated cells. Epithelial cells on the villi are replaced by mitotic division and differentiation of cells in the intestinal glands. Smooth muscle cells in the lamina propria cause periodic shortening of the villi.

Chapter 14

Respiratory System

I. INTRODUCTION.

The respiratory system comprises the conducting airways and the gas exchange area.

A. Conducting airways

1. **Components**
   - **a.** Nasal cavity, paranasal sinuses, and vomeronasal organ
   - **b.** Nasopharynx
   - **c.** Larynx
   - **d.** Trachea
   - **e.** Bronchi and terminal bronchioles
2. **Functions.** The conducting airways provide for:
   - **a.** Moving air to and from the gas exchange area in the lungs
   - **b.** Conditioning the air (e.g., by cleansing, heating or cooling, humidifying or dehumidifying)
   - **c.** Sound production
   - **d.** Olfaction

B. Gas exchange (respiratory) area

1. **Components**
   - **a.** Pulmonary alveoli
   - **b.** Air passages into which pulmonary alveoli open
     - **(1)** Respiratory bronchioles
     - **(2)** Alveolar ducts
     - **(3)** Alveolar sacs
2. **Functions**
   - **a.** Respiratory gas exchange
   - **b.** Removal of particles (e.g., dust) and bacteria
   - **c.** Secretion of pulmonary surfactant

II. MAMMALIAN RESPIRATORY SYSTEM

A. Nasal cavity, paranasal sinuses, and vomeronasal organ

1. The **nasal cavity** is divided into **three regions**.
   - **a. Vestibular (cutaneous) region**
     - **(1)** The **epithelial lining** of the nasal vestibule changes from the rostral region to the caudal region.
       - **(a)** It is keratinized stratified squamous rostrally, except in horses, where the rostral nasal vestibule and the nasal diverticulum are lined by typical skin.
       - **(b)** It is nonkeratinized stratified squamous in the midsection.
       - **(c)** It is stratified cuboidal or pseudostratified columnar caudally.
     - **(2) Lamina propria**
       - **(a)** Small **serous glands** are present.
       - **(b)** The **lateral nasal gland** is a compound gland that moistens the vestibular mucosa and, in dogs, the planum nasale. It is absent in large ruminants.

b. Respiratory region

(1) The **epithelial lining** is **respiratory epithelium,** which is pseudostratified columnar epithelium with ciliated cells, brush cells, secretory cells, and basal cells (Figure 14-1).

(a) **Ciliated cells** are columnar with numerous cilia and microvilli on their apical surfaces.

(b) **Brush cells** are columnar with numerous apical microvilli.

(c) **Secretory cells** may exhibit constitutive secretion or regulated secretion.

(i) **Columnar cells** with apical microvilli secrete glycoproteins.

Mucous cells secrete acid glycoproteins.

Serous cells secrete neutral glycoproteins.

(ii) **Goblet cells,** which have a narrow base and a wide supranuclear apical portion, accumulate masses of mucous secretory granules (sulfated glycoproteins).

(d) **Basal cells** are polyhedral cells located along the basal lamina. They divide and differentiate into the other types of epithelial cells.

(2) The **propria–submucosa** is loose connective tissue.

(a) **Serous** or **mixed nasal glands** secrete products that moisten the inspired air.

(b) A **cavernous stratum,** in which large, thin-walled veins predominate, is extensive. The degree of engorgement determines the thickness of the mucosa and, hence, the degree of nasal patency.

c. Olfactory region

(1) The epithelial lining is pseudostratified columnar and comprises sustentacular cells, neurosensory olfactory cells, and basal cells (Figure 14-2).

(a) **Sustentacular cells** are columnar **supporting cells**.

(i) The nuclei of the sustentacular cells form the most superficial nuclear layer in the olfactory epithelium.

(ii) Their apical surfaces are covered with microvilli.

(iii) Apical junctional complexes attach sustentacular cells to each other and to adjacent neurosensory cells.

(b) **Neurosensory olfactory cells** are bipolar neurons.

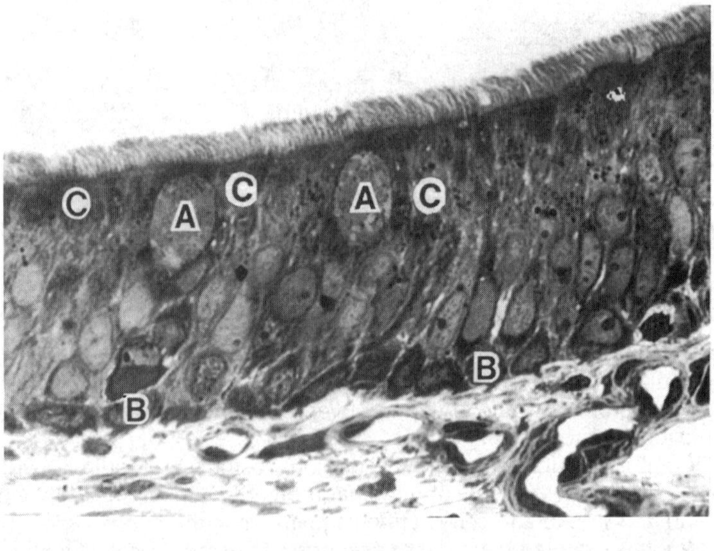

FIGURE 14-1. In this micrograph of a 1-µm thick resin section of typical respiratory mucosa, three epithelial cell types are easily identified: (*A*) Goblet cells; (*B*) basal cells; (*C*) ciliated columnar cells. (Reprinted from Dellmann H-D: *Textbook of Veterinary Histology,* 4th ed. Baltimore, Williams & Wilkins, 1993, p 137.)

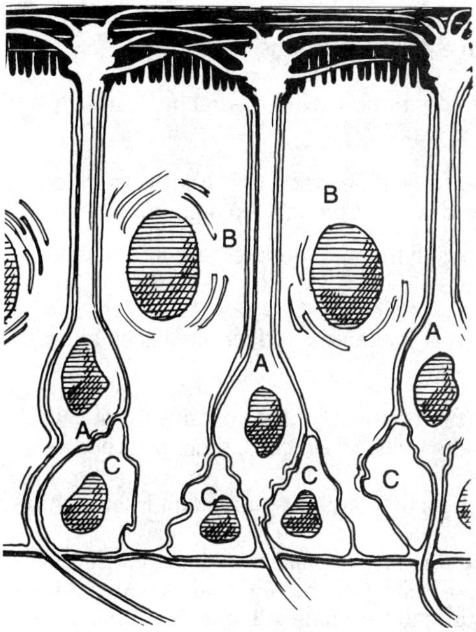

FIGURE 14-2. Schematic drawing of olfactory epithelium. (*A*) Neurosensory olfactory cells with basal axons and apical dendritic bulbs that give rise to tapered cilia. (*B*) Sustentacular cells. (*C*) Basal cells. (Redrawn with permission from Dellmann H-D: *Textbook of Veterinary Histology,* 4th ed. Baltimore, Williams & Wilkins, 1993, p 139.)

(i) **Cell bodies. Neuronal perikarya** are located in the basal epithelium. Their nuclei form a distinct middle layer of nuclei between the more superficial nuclei of the sustentacular cells and the nuclei of the basal cells.

(ii) **Dendrites.** Each neuron has a thin **apical dendrite** extending to the lumen. There it expands to form a **dendritic bulb** from which long (50–80 μm), tapered cilia arise (see Figure 14-2). These cilia are **neurosensory receptors.**

(iii) **Axons.** The axon originates from the cell base and passes into the lamina propria, where it joins other axons to form **nonmyelinated bundles.**

(c) **Basal cells** are **stem cells** similar to those in the respiratory region. They divide and differentiate into neurosensory cells and sustentacular cells.

(2) **Propria–submucosa. Mixed olfactory glands** provide the moisture required for the perception of odoriferous substances.

2. **Paranasal sinuses**
   a. The **epithelial lining** is pseudostratified columnar with ciliated cells and a few goblet cells.
   b. **Propria–submucosa.** Glands are scarce in the propria–submucosa of the paranasal sinuses.

3. **Vomeronasal organ.** The vomeronasal organ is a bilateral, blind-ending tubular organ that opens into the **incisive duct,** which connects the nasal and oral cavities. It acts as a **chemoreceptor** for substances of low volatility. Detection of such substances is important for male and female sexual behavior [e.g., maternal behavior; the Flehman action (upper lip curling by male mammals) is associated with sampling substances in the urine of the female].
   a. The **epithelial lining** is olfactory epithelium medially and respiratory epithelium laterally.
   b. The **propria–submucosa** contains numerous **vessels,** similar to those of the cavernous stratum in the respiratory region of the nasal cavity, and **serous glands.**
   c. **Cartilage** supports the tunica mucosa and tunica submucosa.

B. Nasopharynx. The nasopharynx, which lies dorsal to the soft palate, connects the nasal cavity to the laryngopharynx.

1. The **epithelial lining** of the nasopharynx is respiratory epithelium rostrally and nonkeratinized stratified squamous epithelium caudally.

2. The **propria–submucosa** is loose connective tissue containing mixed glands and lymphatic nodules, which may aggregate to form a pharyngeal tonsil.

C. **Larynx.** The larynx is a cartilage-supported organ continuous with the trachea caudally and the nasopharynx rostrally.

1. The **epithelial lining** of the epiglottis, laryngeal vestibule, and vocal folds is stratified squamous. The remainder of the larynx is lined with respiratory epithelium.

2. The **propria–submucosa** contains mixed glands, lymphatic nodules, and the vestibular and elastic vocal ligaments.

D. **Trachea.** The trachea is a flexible tube that begins at the larynx and terminates by bifurcating into the two primary (extrapulmonary) bronchi.

1. The **epithelial lining of the** trachea is respiratory epithelium that contains **Clara cells** and **neuroendocrine cells** in addition to ciliated cells, brush cells, secretory cells, and goblet cells (see II A 1 b).
   a. **Clara cells** are relatively sparse in the trachea; they are most abundant in bronchioles [see II E 1 b (1)].
   b. **Neuroendocrine cells** belong to the amine precursor uptake and decarboxylation (APUD) system (see Chapter 19 IV C). These cells, which are usually small and pyramidal, secrete catecholamines that act locally to stimulate goblet cells, glands, and ciliated cells.

2. The **propria–submucosa** is composed of loose connective tissue. It contains:
   a. A prominent layer of longitudinally oriented elastic fibers, which abuts the epithelium
   b. Tubuloacinar mucoserous glands
   c. An abundance of lymphocytes, plasma cells, macrophages and mast cells

3. **Tracheal cartilages** are C-shaped pieces of hyaline cartilage. Their dorsal free ends are connected by smooth muscle, which is attached to the outside of the cartilage in carnivores and to the inside in all other domestic mammals.

4. The **tunica adventitia** is loose connective tissue, which permits changes in the relative position of the trachea and adjacent structures during movements of the neck and swallowing.

E. **Lung**

1. **Intrapulmonary conducting airways**
   a. **Bronchi** arise from the primary bronchi and branch into several generations. The total cross-sectional diameter of each generation of bronchi is larger than that of the preceding generation.
      (1) **Epithelial lining.** Respiratory epithelium lines the bronchi.
         (a) Proximodistally, goblet cells decrease and Clara cells increase in number.
         (b) The height of the epithelium progressively decreases.
      (2) **Propria–submucosa.** Glands that are similar to tracheal glands are contained in the thin propria–submucosa. They are less abundant distally.
      (3) **Tunica muscularis.** Smooth muscle forms a circular layer that gradually decreases in thickness proximodistally.
   b. **Bronchioles** arise from bronchi and branch into several generations, the most distal of which are referred to as **terminal bronchioles** (Figure 14-3).
      (1) **Epithelial lining.** Bronchioles are lined by simple columnar or cuboidal epithelium comprising ciliated cells and Clara cells (here called **bronchiolar exocrine cells**).
         (a) Bronchiolar exocrine cells, which are most abundant in terminal bronchioles, secrete proteins of unknown functional significance and metabolize xenobiotic (exogenous) compounds.

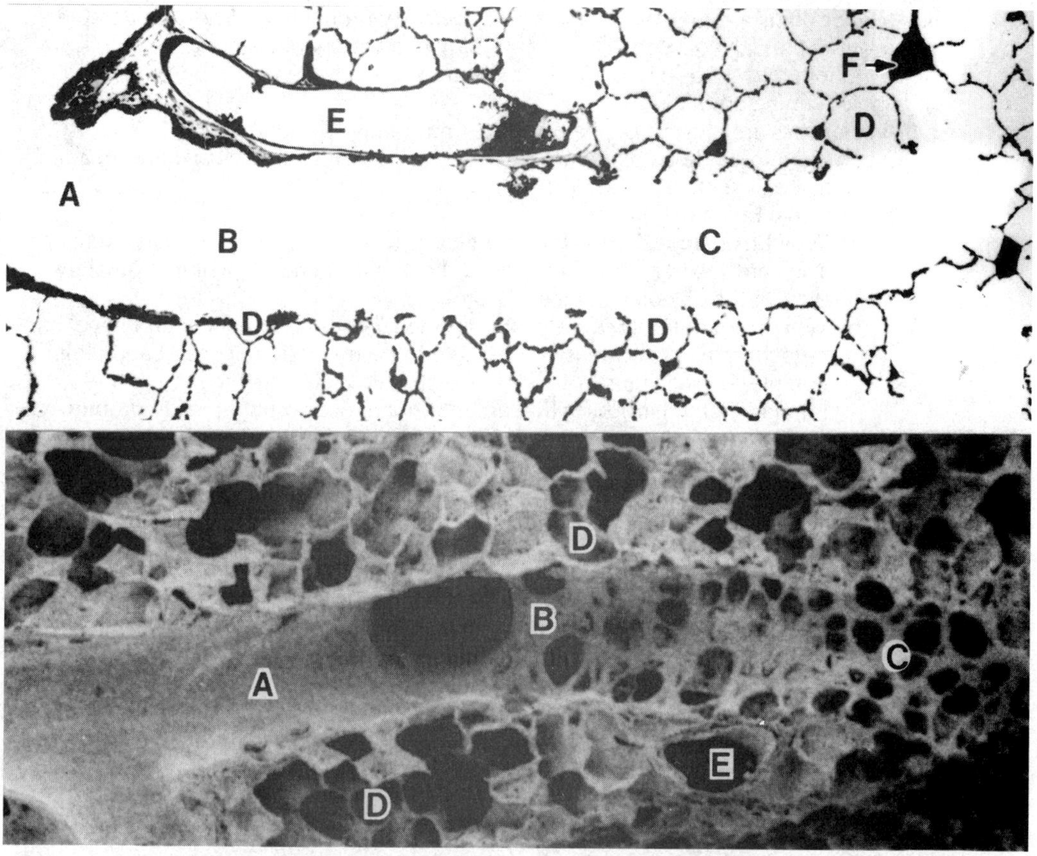

FIGURE 14-3. These two micrographs illustrate the light microscopic and scanning electron microscopic appearance of a terminal bronchiole and the gas exchange area of the feline lung. (*A*) Terminal bronchiole; (*B*) respiratory bronchiole into which open a few alveoli; (*C*) alveolar duct that is completely surrounded by alveoli; (*D*) alveoli; (*E*) pulmonary arteriole; (*F*) pulmonary venule. (Reprinted with permission from Dellmann H-D: *Textbook of Veterinary Histology,* 4th ed. Baltimore, Williams & Wilkins, 1993, p 146.)

(b) Bronchiolar exocrine cells are characterized by:
- **(i)** Secretory granules
- **(ii)** Numerous mitochondria
- **(iii)** Smooth endoplasmic reticulum (sER), particularly abundant in horses and sheep
- **(iv)** Glycogen, abundant in large ruminants and carnivores

(2) The **propria–submucosa** is composed of loose connective tissue. Glands are absent.

(3) **Tunica muscularis.** Smooth muscle is arranged in circular and oblique fascicles.

(4) The **tunica adventitia** is loose connective tissue rich in elastic fibers.

(5) Cartilage is absent.

2. Gas exchange area of the lung. Acini are the functional units of the lung. They are composed of the respiratory bronchioles, alveolar ducts, alveolar sacs, and alveoli distal to one terminal bronchiole.

a. Respiratory bronchioles are similar in structure to terminal bronchioles, but alveoli open directly into them (see Figure 14-3).

(1) They are numerous and branch frequently in carnivores.

(2) They are occasionally present in horses.

(3) They are short or absent in ruminants and pigs.

b. **Alveolar ducts** are the continuations of respiratory bronchioles. They are completely surrounded by alveoli (see Figure 14-3). Between the openings of the alveoli, spiraling smooth muscle cells and elastic fibers are present underneath the simple cuboidal lining epithelium.

c. **Alveolar sacs** are clusters of alveoli at the ends of alveolar ducts.

d. **Alveoli** are thin-walled, epithelium-lined semispherical structures that are separated by interalveolar septa (see Figure 14-3).

(1) **Epithelial lining** (Figure 14-4)

(a) **Type I (squamous) alveolar epithelial cells** are specialized for gas exchange. They have extremely thin attenuated cytoplasm and cover approximately 97% of the alveolar surface.

(b) **Type II (granular, great) alveolar epithelial cells** are cuboidal and have many mitochondria and extensive rough endoplasmic reticulum (rER) and Golgi complexes (see Figure 14-4). They elaborate characteristic membrane-bounded lamellar bodies that are the source of phospholipids in **pulmonary surfactant**.

(2) **Alveolar macrophages** are present in the alveolar lumen, where they phagocytose dust particles and other foreign material. They belong to the mononuclear phagocyte system (MPS) [see Chapter 6 II C 1 g (3)].

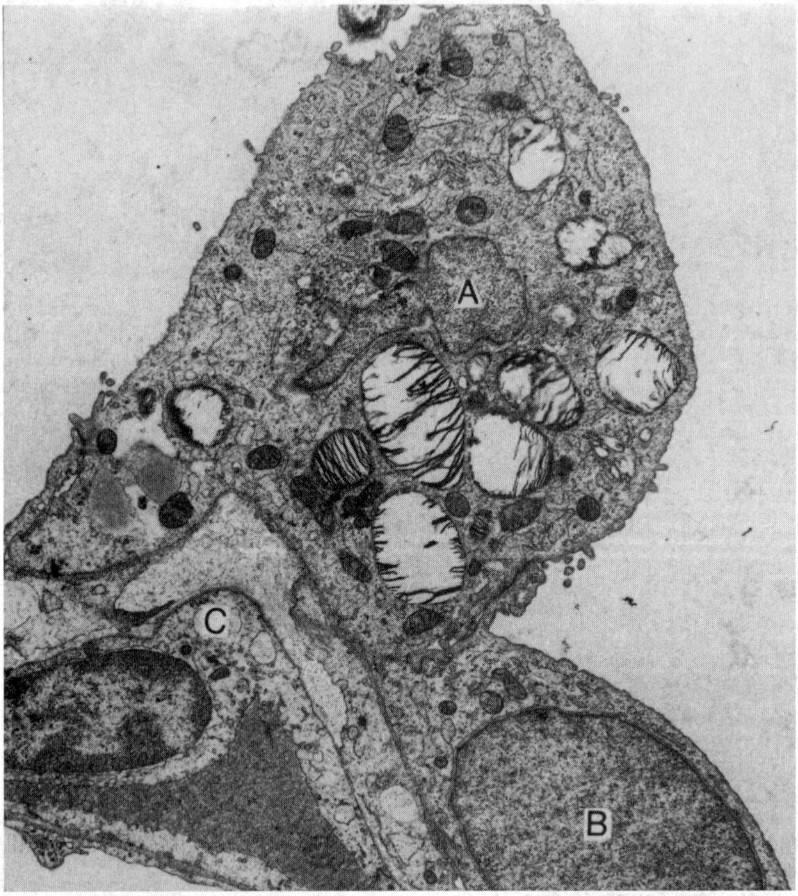

FIGURE 14-4. Electron micrograph of (*A*) a type II alveolar epithelial cell protruding into the alveolar lumen and containing many membrane-bounded lamellar bodies; (*B*) a type I alveolar epithelial cell; and (*C*) a capillary endothelial cell. (Reprinted with permission from Dellmann H-D: *Textbook of Veterinary Histology,* 4th ed. Baltimore, Williams & Wilkins, 1993, p 149.)

TABLE 14-1. Components of the Blood–Air Barrier

Components
Pulmonary surfactant layer
Type I alveolar epithelial cell
Basal lamina of type I alveolar epithelial cell
Interstitial connective tissue*
Basal lamina of capillary endothelial cell
Capillary endothelial cell

*In the thinnest regions of the barrier, the interstitial connective tissue is missing and the two basal laminae fuse, creating a barrier less than 0.2 μm thick.

(3) **Interalveolar septa** contain interstitial connective tissue and capillaries. **Alveolar pores** in the septa connect lumina of adjacent alveoli.

(a) **Interalveolar connective tissue** is an extremely thin layer of elastic and collagen fibers and associated fibrocytes.

(b) **Capillary endothelial cells** usually have attenuated cytoplasm at points adjacent to type I alveolar epithelial cells (Figure 14-5). The **blood–air barrier** separates the alveolar lumen from the capillary lumen (Table 14-1; see Figure 14-5).

e. Pulmonary lobules are clusters of acini separated by interlobular septa.

(1) Pulmonary lobules are particularly well developed in ruminants and pigs.

(2) They are incomplete in horses.

(3) They are absent in carnivores.

3. Pleura and interstitium

a. The **visceral (pulmonary) pleura** surrounds the lung. It consists of simple squamous to cuboidal mesothelium on a layer of loose to dense irregular connective tissue that is rich in elastic fibers.

b. The **parietal pleura** resembles the visceral pleura, from which it is separated by only a very narrow, serous fluid–filled space (the pleural cavity). This disposition allows for smooth movements of the two surfaces against each other during inspiration and expiration.

c. The **interstitial connective tissue** of the lung is continuous with the visceral pleura.

(1) Around the pulmonary alveoli and alveolar capillaries, this tissue is an extremely thin layer of collagen and elastic fibers and associated fibrocytes.

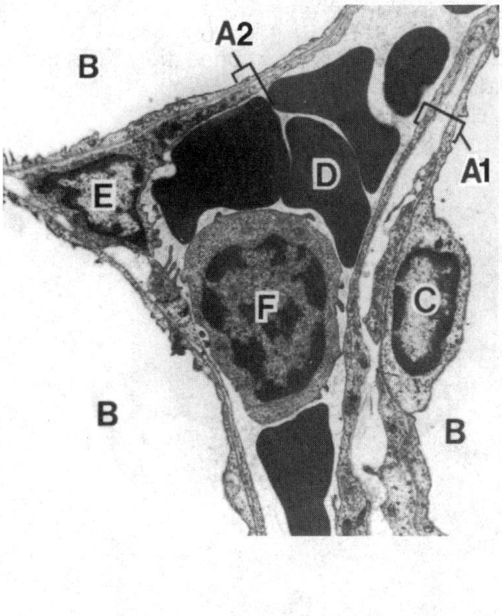

FIGURE 14-5. This electron micrograph illustrates the blood–air barrier components that separate the lumen of a capillary from that of three adjacent alveoli. (*A1*) Blood–air barrier with sparse interstitial connective tissue. (*A2*) Blood–air barrier without interstitial connective tissue; the basal laminae of the alveolar epithelial cells and endothelial cells have fused. (*B*) Alveolar lumen. (*C*) Type I alveolar epithelial cell. (*D*) Erythrocytes in the capillary lumen. (*E*) Endothelial cell. (*F*) A lymphocyte in the capillary lumen. (Reprinted with permission from Dellmann H-D: *Textbook of Veterinary Histology,* 4th ed. Baltimore, Williams & Wilkins, 1993, p 147.)

(2) Around the airways, blood vessels, and pulmonary lobules, loose connective tissue rich in elastic fibers is more abundant.

III. AVIAN RESPIRATORY SYSTEM.
In many respects, the histology of the avian respiratory system is similar to that of mammals. Notable differences are described.

A. **Nasal cavity.** The **respiratory region** is lined with pseudostratified ciliated columnar epithelium, in which goblet cells cluster to form intraepithelial glands.

B. The **trachea** is supported by cartilaginous rings. Adjacent rings overlap and interlock. The lining epithelium is similar to that of the nasal cavity.

C. The **syrinx** is a diverticulum near the tracheobronchial junction. It functions in vocalization. Its structure is species-dependent.

D. The **lungs** comprise **primary bronchi (mesobronchi), secondary bronchi,** and **tertiary bronchi (parabronchi)**. **Atria** arising from tertiary bronchi continue into air **capillaries,** the actual gas exchange areas.

1. **Primary bronchi** continue the trachea and connect the lungs, which are not expandable, to expandable **air sacs**.
   - **a.** The **epithelial lining** is pseudostratified columnar ciliated epithelium, which has both goblet cells and simple alveolar intraepithelial mucous glands.
   - **b.** The **lamina propria** is rich in elastic fibers and frequently contains lymphatic nodules.
   - **c.** A **lamina muscularis** and **cartilage plaques** are present.
2. **Secondary bronchi** branch from primary bronchi and may also lead to air sacs.
   - **a.** The **epithelial lining** is simple ciliated columnar with goblet cells.
   - **b.** The **lamina propria** is similar to that of the primary bronchi, but it usually has no lymphatic nodules.
   - **c.** The **lamina muscularis** is spirally arranged.
3. **Tertiary bronchi** interconnect secondary bronchi.
   - **a.** **Epithelial lining.** They are lined by simple cuboidal or simple squamous epithelium.
   - **b.** A spiraling **lamina muscularis** is present.
4. **Atria** are lined by simple squamous epithelium.
5. **Air capillaries** have walls similar to those of mammalian alveoli.

E. **Air sacs** are lined by simple squamous epithelium, except near their connections with the bronchi, where the epithelium is simple cuboidal and ciliated.

STUDY QUESTIONS

DIRECTIONS: Each of the numbered items or incomplete statements in this section is followed by answers or by completions of the statement. Select the **one** numbered answer or completion that is **best** in each case.

1. Most conducting airways are lined by:

(1) pseudostratified cuboidal epithelium.
(2) simple squamous epithelium.
(3) pseudostratified columnar epithelium.
(4) stratified squamous epithelium.
(5) stratified columnar epithelium.

2. Which of the following *best* describes the respiratory epithelium of nasal conducting airways?

(1) Columnar ciliated cells, goblet cells, basal cells, sustentacular cells
(2) Columnar ciliated cells, brush cells, goblet cells, basal cells, sustentacular cells
(3) Columnar ciliated cells, brush cells, goblet cells, sustentacular cells, columnar secretory cells
(4) Columnar ciliated cells, brush cells, goblet cells, basal cells, columnar secretory cells, Clara cells
(5) Columnar ciliated cells, brush cells, goblet cells, basal cells, columnar secretory cells

3. The propria–submucosa of the respiratory region of the nasal cavity differs from that of the olfactory region in that:

(1) solitary lymphatic nodules are present.
(2) afferent nerve fibers are more numerous.
(3) there is a pronounced cavernous stratum.
(4) glands are absent.
(5) glands are present.

4. Which one of the following airways lacks multicellular glands in the propria–submucosa?

(1) Nasal cavity
(2) Trachea
(3) Larynx
(4) Bronchioles
(5) Bronchi

5. Which one of the following characteristics pertains to type I alveolar epithelial cells?

(1) Cuboidal
(2) Secretory
(3) Phagocytic
(4) Specialized for gas exchange
(5) Ciliated

DIRECTIONS: Each of the numbered items or incomplete statements in this section is negatively phrased, as indicated by an italicized word such as *not, least,* or *except.* Select the **one** numbered answer or completion that is **best** in each case.

6. Which one of the following structures is *not* found in the interalveolar septum?

(1) Collagen fibers
(2) Elastic fibers
(3) Fibrocytes
(4) Endothelial cells
(5) Smooth muscle cells

ANSWERS AND EXPLANATIONS

1. The answer is 3 *[II A, B 1, C 1, D 1, E 1].* Most conducting airways are lined by pseudostratified columnar epithelium comprising many cell types that perform a variety of functions (e.g., capture and removal of dust particles). The most rostral portion of the conducting airways and part of the larynx (e.g., vocal folds) are subjected to strong frictional forces; therefore, they are lined by stratified squamous epithelium. Pseudostratified cuboidal epithelium is occasionally present in the prostate gland. Simple squamous epithelium occurs in a variety of locations, such as the endothelium of the cardiovascular and lymphatic systems, the mesothelium of the serosal cavities, and the gas exchange area in the lung (type I alveolar epithelial cells). Stratified columnar epithelium lines interlobular salivary ducts and main excretory ducts.

2. The answer is 5 *[II A 1 b (1)].* The typical respiratory epithelium of the nasal conducting airways comprises columnar ciliated cells, brush cells, goblet cells, basal cells, and columnar secretory cells. Sustentacular cells are present in the epithelium of the olfactory region but not in the respiratory epithelium of the conducting airways. Clara cells (bronchiolar exocrine cells) are present in the trachea, bronchi, and bronchioles.

3. The answer is 3 *[II A 1 b (2) (b)].* The respiratory region is characterized by a thick cavernous stratum, primarily composed of thin-walled veins. The degree of venous engorgement regulates the width of the nasal passages and thereby the degree of heating and moisturizing of the inhaled air. Solitary lymphatic nodules are not normally present in the respiratory region. An abundance of afferent nerve fiber bundles, which convey sensory information from the olfactory cells to the brain, is characteristic of the olfactory mucosa. Glands are present in both regions; their secretory products moisten the air and include an odorant-binding protein, an immunoglobulin (IgA), and a bactericidal compound (lysozyme).

4. The answer is 4 *[II E 1 b (2)].* Bronchioles have neither supporting cartilage nor multicellular glands in the propria–submucosa. However, Clara cells (called bronchiolar exocrine cells in the lining epithelium) are secretory cells; they play an important role in metabolizing potentially damaging exogenous (xenobiotic) compounds.

5. The answer is 4 *[II E 2 d (1) (a)].* Type I (squamous) alveolar epithelial cells are the predominant cell type in pulmonary alveoli and are the cells through which gas exchange takes place. Cuboidal cells in pulmonary alveoli, which are called type II, great, or granular alveolar cells, synthesize and secrete pulmonary surfactant. Ciliated cells are not present in the most distal airways; they are generally not found beyond the respiratory bronchioles. Alveolar macrophages, which are found in the alveolar lumen, phagocytose dust particles and other foreign material.

6. The answer is 5 *[II E 2 d (3)].* Smooth muscle cells are not found in the interalveolar septa, although they do occur around the openings of alveoli from alveolar ducts. Adjacent epithelium-lined alveoli are separated by interalveolar septa, which are primarily composed of capillaries, collagen and many elastic fibers, and associated fibrocytes. The capillaries are lined by endothelial cells. Plasma cells, lymphocytes, pericytes, and monocytes may also be present.

Chapter 15

Urinary System

I. INTRODUCTION

A. Components.

The urinary system comprises the kidneys, ureters, urinary bladder, and urethra.

B. Functions

1. The **main functions** of the urinary system are:
   a. Excretion of metabolic waste products and salts
   b. Elimination of toxic substances
   c. Regulation of fluid, salt, and acid–base balance
   d. Modulation of blood pressure
2. The urinary system **accomplishes its functions** by the **production, storage,** and **elimination** of urine.
   a. An ultrafiltrate of blood is produced in the renal corpuscles and is subsequently substantially modified by selective reuptake in uriniferous (renal) tubules to produce urine.
   b. The renal calyces, pelvis, and ureter conduct the urine from the kidney to the urinary bladder.
   c. Urine is stored in the urinary bladder and is eliminated through the urethra.

II. KIDNEY

A. General organization

1. The kidney has an **outer cortex** surrounded by a connective tissue capsule and an **inner medulla** projecting into renal calyces or a renal pelvis (Figure 15-1).
   a. The **renal cortex** is composed of the cortical labyrinth and medullary rays (Figures 15-2, 15-3).
      (1) The **labyrinth** contains renal corpuscles, proximal and distal convoluted tubules, and arched collecting ducts.
      (2) The **medullary rays** are groups of parallel straight proximal tubules, straight distal tubules, and collecting ducts.
   b. The **renal medulla** is subdivided into an outer and inner zone (see Figure 15-3).
      (1) The outer zone contains proximal and distal straight tubules, thin tubules, and collecting ducts.
      (2) The inner zone contains only thin tubules and collecting ducts.
   c. The sparse cortical and medullary interstitial **connective tissue,** which surrounds the renal tubules and blood vessels, consists of fibrocytes and reticular fibers.
2. A **renal lobe** comprises a renal medullary pyramid and its associated cortical tissue. A unilobar kidney is present in cats, dogs, horses, sheep, and goats; bovine and pig kidneys are multilobar.

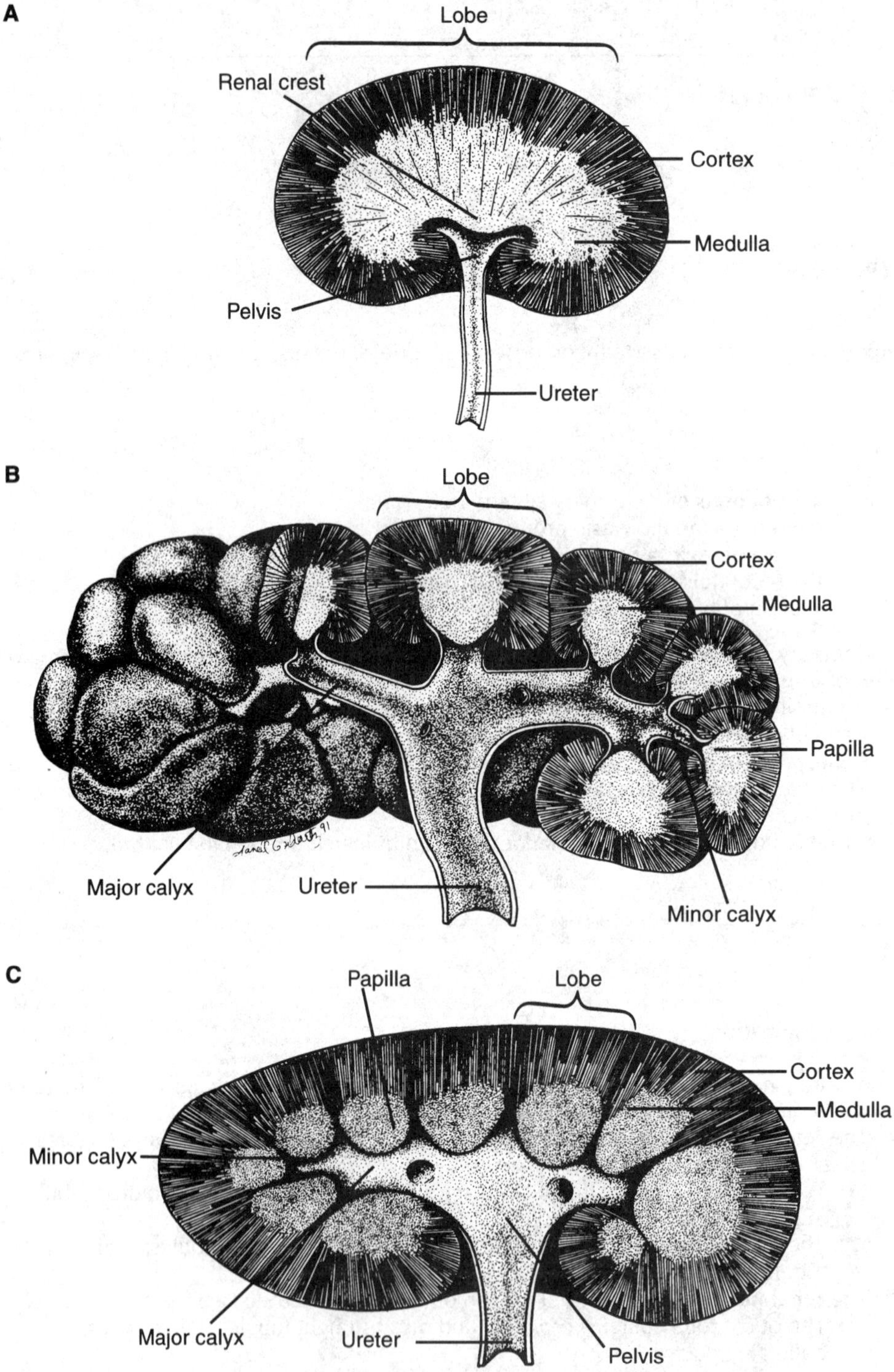

FIGURE 15-1. Depiction of the gross anatomical structure of the three types of kidneys occurring in domestic mammals. (*A*) Unilobar kidney found in carnivores, small ruminants, and horses. (*B*) Multilobar kidney found in large ruminants. Note that the lobation is distinctly visible at the surface. (*C*) Multilobar kidney with a smooth surface, as found in pigs. (Reprinted with permission from Dellmann H-D: *Textbook of Veterinary Histology,* 4th ed. Baltimore, Williams & Wilkins, 1993, p 195.)

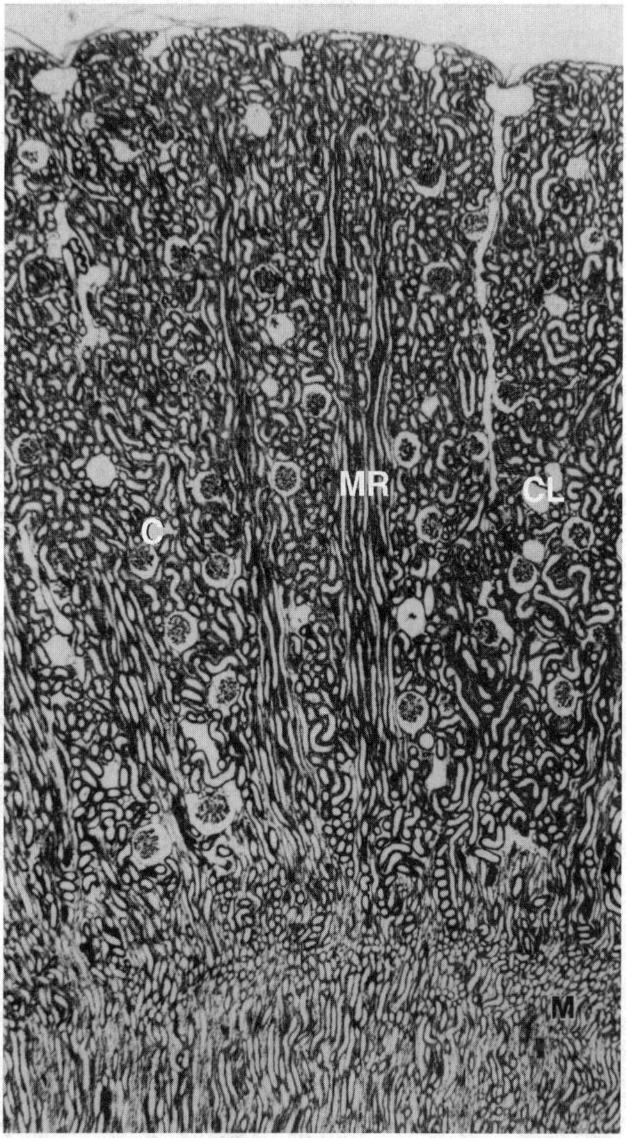

FIGURE 15-2. Light micrograph of the cortex (*C*) and part of the outer medulla (*M*) of the kidney. The cortical labyrinth (*CL*) contains renal corpuscles, proximal and distal convoluted tubules, and arched collecting ducts. Medullary rays (*MR*) are made up of proximal and distal straight tubules and collecting ducts. (From Dellmann H-D: *Textbook of Veterinary Histology,* 4th ed. Baltimore, Williams & Wilkins, 1993, p 196.)

B. **Renal (uriniferous) tubules.** The **structural and functional units of the kidney** are the renal tubules. Each tubule has **two components:** the tubular **nephron** and the **collecting duct** into which it empties.

1. **Nephron.** The nephron starts as the renal corpuscle and continues in the proximal convoluted tubule, proximal straight tubule, thin tubule (i.e., the thin segment of the renal tubule), and distal straight and convoluted tubules. The straight portions of the proximal and distal tubule and the thin tubule form a hairpin loop in the medulla, the loop of the nephron (i.e., Henle's loop; see Figure 15-3).

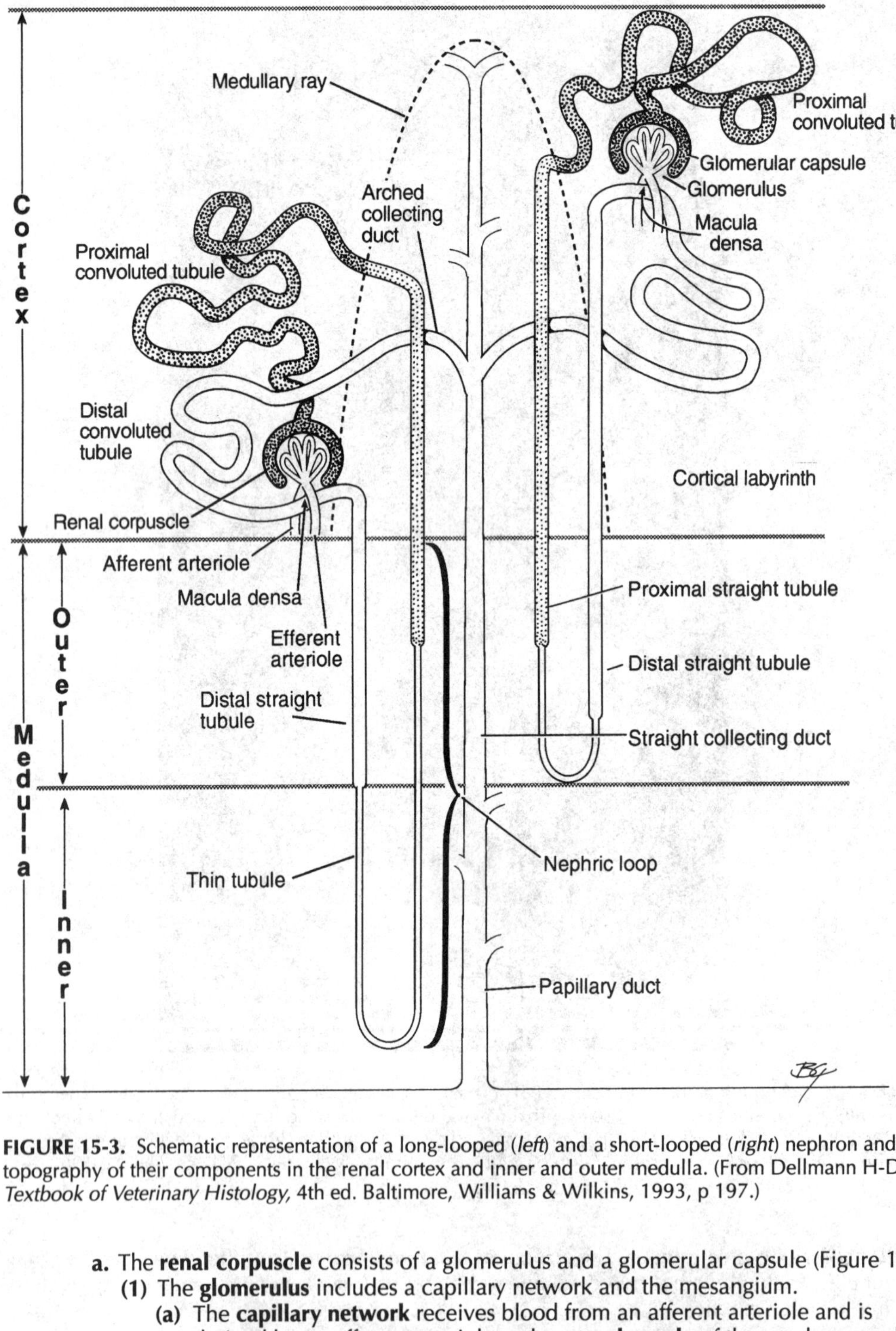

FIGURE 15-3. Schematic representation of a long-looped (*left*) and a short-looped (*right*) nephron and the topography of their components in the renal cortex and inner and outer medulla. (From Dellmann H-D: *Textbook of Veterinary Histology,* 4th ed. Baltimore, Williams & Wilkins, 1993, p 197.)

a. The **renal corpuscle** consists of a glomerulus and a glomerular capsule (Figure 15-4).

(1) The **glomerulus** includes a capillary network and the mesangium.

(a) The **capillary network** receives blood from an afferent arteriole and is drained by an efferent arteriole at the **vascular pole** of the renal corpuscle.

(i) The capillaries are lined by a **porous endothelium** on an unusually thick basal lamina (the **glomerular basement membrane**) that is shared with the podocytes [Figure 15-5; see II B 1 a (2) (a); Figure 11-9].

(ii) The porous endothelium and glomerular basement membrane are the **first two components of the filtration barrier.**

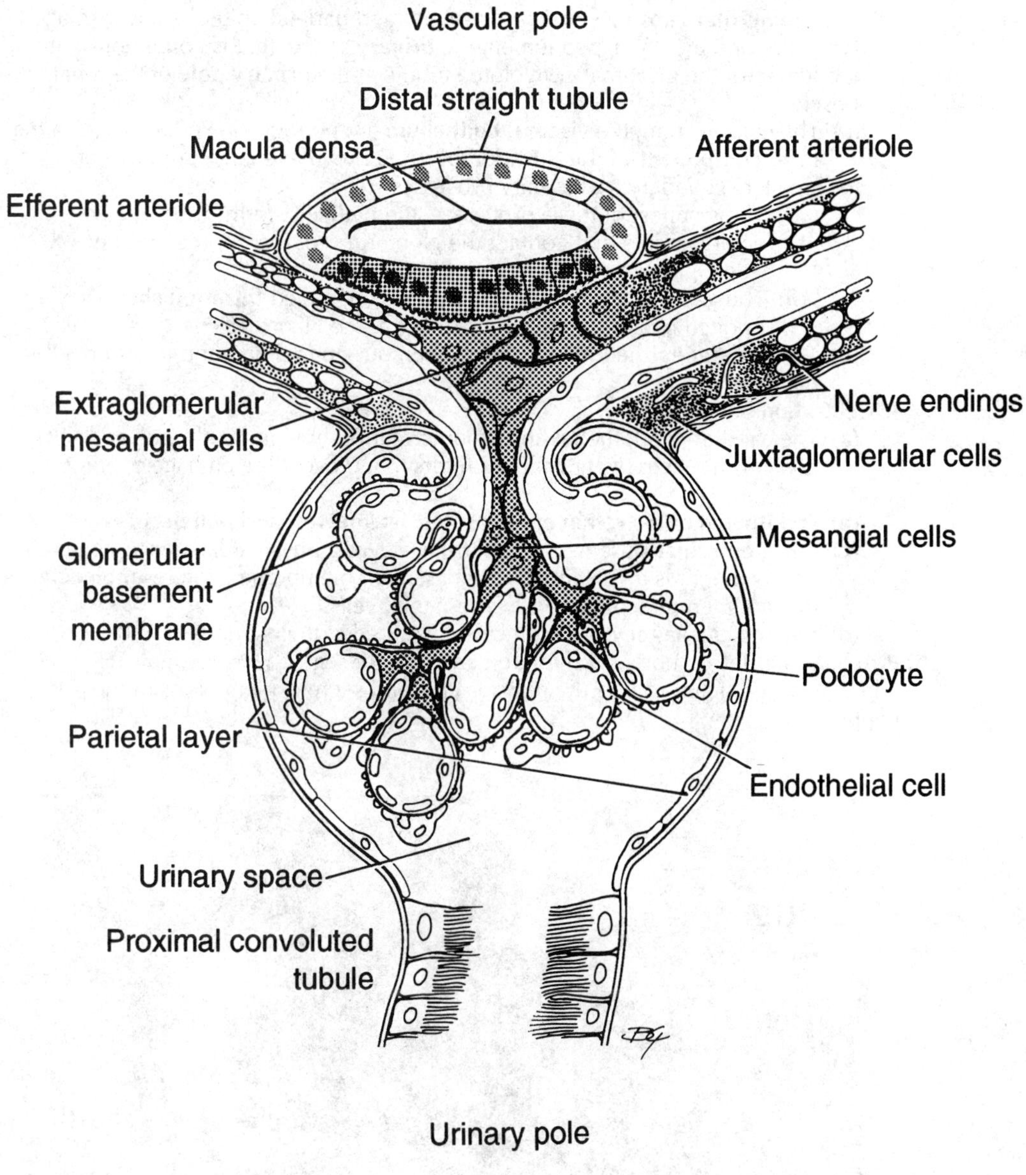

FIGURE 15-4. Schematic drawing of a renal corpuscle and juxtaglomerular apparatus. The glomerular capillaries receive blood from the afferent arteriole and are drained by the efferent arteriole. The capillary endothelium has pores. Glomerular mesangial cells are located on the same side of the glomerular basement membrane as the endothelial cells. The glomerular capillaries are surrounded by the visceral layer of the glomerular capsule, which consists of podocytes whose pedicels contact the glomerular basement membrane and are separated by filtration slits. The parietal layer of the glomerular capsule is formed by flattened epithelial cells. It is separated from the visceral layer by the urinary space, which is continuous with the lumen of the proximal convoluted tubule. The juxtaglomerular apparatus comprises juxtaglomerular cells (which are modified smooth muscle cells), extraglomerular mesangial cells, and the macula densa, which is part of the distal straight tubule. Nerve endings are present in the vicinity of the juxtaglomerular cells. (Redrawn with permission from Koushanpour E and Kriz W: *Renal Physiology: Principles, Structure and Function.* New York, Springer-Verlag, 1986.)

(b) The cells and matrix that occupy the spaces between the capillary loops are called **mesangium**.

(2) The **glomerular capsule** consists of visceral and parietal epithelial layers that, together, form a cup-shaped lumen, the **urinary space,** that is continuous with the lumen of the proximal convoluted tubule at the **urinary pole** of the renal corpuscle.

(a) The cells forming the **visceral epithelium** are **podocytes**. Podocytes form the **third component of the filtration barrier**. They have large primary and smaller secondary and tertiary processes.

(i) The smallest of these processes, the **pedicels,** forms foot-shaped enlargements that contact the glomerular basement membrane (see Figure 15-5).

(ii) The gaps between adjacent pedicels are called **filtration slits**. They are bridged by a filtration slit diaphragm (see Figure 15-5).

(b) The **parietal epithelium** is simple squamous epithelium, and it lies on a thick basal lamina.

(3) **Filtration barrier**

(a) The capillary endothelial cells, glomerular basement membrane, and pedicels are **negatively charged filters** that prevent the passage of anionic molecules.

(b) **Endothelial pores retain erythrocytes, leukocytes,** and **platelets**.

(c) The **glomerular basement membrane** acts as a **physical barrier** to large molecules (i.e., it is a **size filter**). The basement membrane captures **molecules** that are then **phagocytosed by mesangial cells**.

(d) **Podocytes phagocytose molecules** captured at their surfaces.

b. **Proximal tubules** comprise convoluted and straight segments (see Figure 15-3) and play a significant role in the reabsorptive and secretory functions of the nephron.

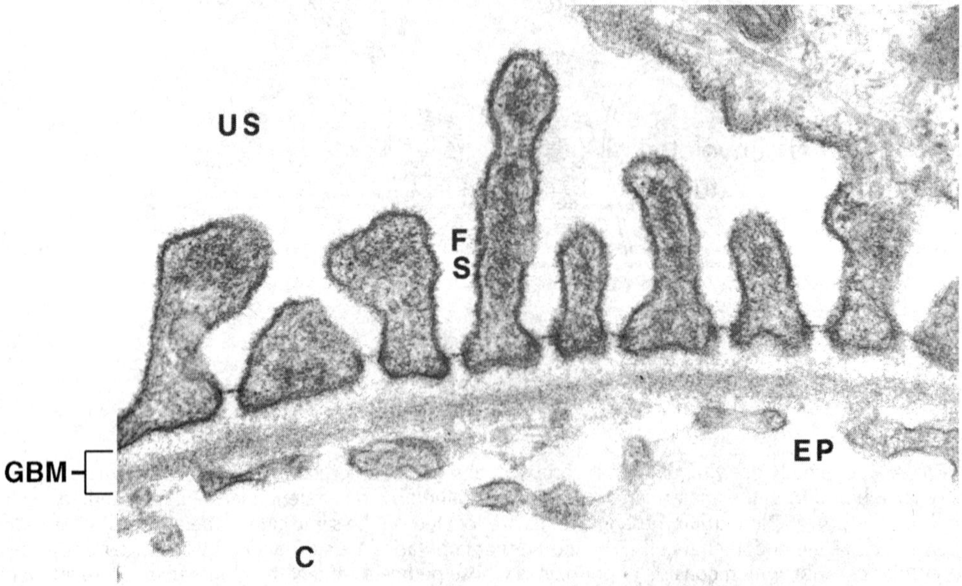

FIGURE 15-5. Electron micrograph of the glomerular filtration barrier comprising endothelial pores (*EP*) of the glomerular capillaries (*C*), a glomerular basement membrane (*GBM*), and filtration slits (*FS*) between podocyte pedicels. Blood filters from the glomerular capillary through these structures and enters the urinary space (*US*). (Courtesy of J.W. Verlander. From Dellmann H-D: *Textbook of Veterinary Histology,* 4th ed. Baltimore, Williams & Wilkins, 1993, p 198.)

(1) **Histologic organization**

(a) **Proximal convoluted tubules** are **major components of the cortical labyrinth**. They are lined by simple cuboidal epithelium with an apical microvillous brush border.

(i) Junctional complexes join cells at the luminal border.

(ii) The lateral cell surfaces and basal cell processes of adjacent cells interdigitate intricately, increasing the surface area for ion transport.

(iii) Numerous long mitochondria within these processes provide energy for ion transport across the basal cell membrane.

(iv) Lysosomes and apical endocytotic vesicles are abundant.

(b) In the **proximal straight tubule,** which is a component of the medullary rays and the outer medulla, the epithelial cells are lower, microvilli are shorter and much less numerous, the lateral and basal intercellular interdigitations are less elaborate, and mitochondria are shorter and less numerous.

(2) **Function**

(a) The renal tubules process the ultrafiltrate of the blood that is formed in the renal corpuscle. There is extensive **reabsorption** (66%–75%) of the glomerular filtrate in the **proximal tubule**.

(i) Active transport of sodium ions into the basolateral extracellular space is followed by passive diffusion of water and chloride ions.

(ii) Amino acids, glucose, bicarbonate, phosphate, and potassium are also reabsorbed.

(iii) Proteins and large polypeptides are reabsorbed by endocytosis and metabolized by lysosomes for reuse.

(b) Reabsorbed glomerular filtrate is cleared from the extracellular space by a dense peritubular capillary network derived from efferent arterioles of superficial and midcortical nephrons.

c. The **thin tubule** has a **descending limb** that courses into the medulla and an **ascending limb** that returns to the cortex. The thin tubule makes a hairpin loop in the medulla. Together with the proximal and distal straight tubules, which it connects, it forms the loop of the nephron (**Henle's loop**).

(1) **Histologic organization.** The thin tubule is lined by simple squamous epithelium.

(2) **Function.** A **countercurrent multiplier system** is operative in the thin tubule.

(a) The interstitial tissue is increasingly hypertonic toward the renal papilla.

(b) The descending limb is highly permeable to water but has low permeability for most solutes; urea diffuses into the tubule from the interstitial tissue.

(c) The ascending limb is impermeable to water but sodium and chloride ions diffuse passively into the interstitial tissue and urea diffuses from the interstitial tissue into the tubule.

(d) As the filtrate descends through the medulla, it becomes increasingly concentrated (because water moves out into the hypertonic interstitial tissue and solutes remain); as it ascends, it becomes less concentrated (because water is retained and solutes enter the interstitial tissue).

d. **Distal tubules** comprise straight and convoluted segments (see Figure 15-3). The straight segment begins in the medulla and ascends in a medullary ray, runs adjacent to the vascular pole of the renal corpuscle of origin, where part of its wall is modified to form the **macula densa** (part of the juxtaglomerular apparatus; see II C 1 c), and then becomes a convoluted segment, located in the cortical labyrinth.

(1) **Histologic organization.** The distal tubule is lined by simple cuboidal epithelium. Its lining cells are noticeably smaller than those of the proximal tubule.

(a) Only a few apical microvilli are present.

(b) Cells are joined by tight junctions at the luminal border.

(c) Basolateral folds are associated with elongated mitochondria.

(2) **Functions**

(a) The **distal straight tubule** is impermeable to water. Sodium is actively reabsorbed, and chloride, calcium, and magnesium ions are passively reabsorbed.

(b) In the **distal convoluted tubule,** sodium and chloride ions (under aldosterone influence) and water are reabsorbed, and potassium and hydrogen ions are secreted.

(c) Reabsorbed substances are removed from the interstitial tissue by peritubular capillaries [see II B 1 b (2) (b)].

2. **Collecting duct system.** The collecting duct system begins with the **arched collecting duct** in the cortical labyrinth. It continues as the **straight collecting duct** within a medullary ray, joins other collecting ducts in the medulla to form a **papillary duct,** which opens on the renal papilla or calyx (see Figure 15-3).

a. **Components and histologic organization**

(1) **Arched collecting ducts** (connecting tubules) connect the distal convoluted tubules and straight collecting ducts. The lining epithelium is transitional between the two tubules.

(2) **Straight collecting ducts** are lined with a simple epithelium comprising principal cuboidal cells and intercalated cells of varying shapes.

(3) **Papillary ducts** are lined by simple or stratified columnar or transitional epithelium.

b. **Function.** Collecting ducts play an important role in the **final composition of urine**.

(1) Sodium is reabsorbed actively, and chloride and urea are reabsorbed passively [under the influence of antidiuretic hormone (ADH) in the outer and inner medulla]. Potassium, hydrogen, and bicarbonate are secreted.

(2) In the presence of ADH, water is osmotically transferred into the hypertonic medullary interstitial tissue, where it is reabsorbed by the **vasa recta**.

(a) **Vasa recta** are blood vessels from efferent arterioles of the juxtamedullary nephron; they loop into the medulla and return to veins at the corticomedullary junction.

(b) The **course** of vasa recta permits a blood supply to the medulla to be maintained without altering the hypertonicity of the deeper medulla or the final tonicity of the blood. Water moves into the interstitial tissue from the descending vasa recta, and sodium and urea enter the blood, but in the ascending vasa recta the opposite occurs, and excess water and solutes are removed.

(c) The descending and ascending vasa recta are interconnected by a peritubular capillary bed that supplies medullary structures.

(3) When ADH levels are low, collecting ducts are less permeable to water; consequently, a more dilute urine is produced.

(4) Increased excretion of sodium is induced by atrial natriuretic hormone.

C. The **juxtaglomerular apparatus** is located at the vascular pole of the renal corpuscle and comprises juxtaglomerular cells, extraglomerular mesangial cells, and the macula densa.

1. **Components and histologic organization**

a. **Juxtaglomerular cells** are epithelioid modified smooth muscle cells, primarily in the wall of the afferent arteriole (see Figure 15-4). They are secretory cells that have a baroreceptor function (i.e., monitoring blood pressure).

b. **Extraglomerular mesangial cells (lacis cells)** are located between the macula densa and the two glomerular arterioles (see Figure 15-4). Their function is not known.

c. The **macula densa** is a group of thin, tall, and tightly packed epithelial cells of the distal tubule. The protein-synthesizing organelles of these cells are polarized toward the basal cell surface. The macula densa may act as a sensor, monitoring tubular concentration of sodium and chloride.

2. **Function.** In response to various stimuli (e.g., hemorrhage that leads to decreased blood pressure, or a change in the sodium and chloride concentration in the distal tubule), juxtaglomerular cells **secrete renin**. Renin acts on plasma angiotensinogen to form angiotensin I, which is converted by an enzyme of pulmonary origin to angiotensin II.

a. **Angiotensin II** increases blood pressure by causing arteriolar constriction and by stimulating ADH secretion.

A

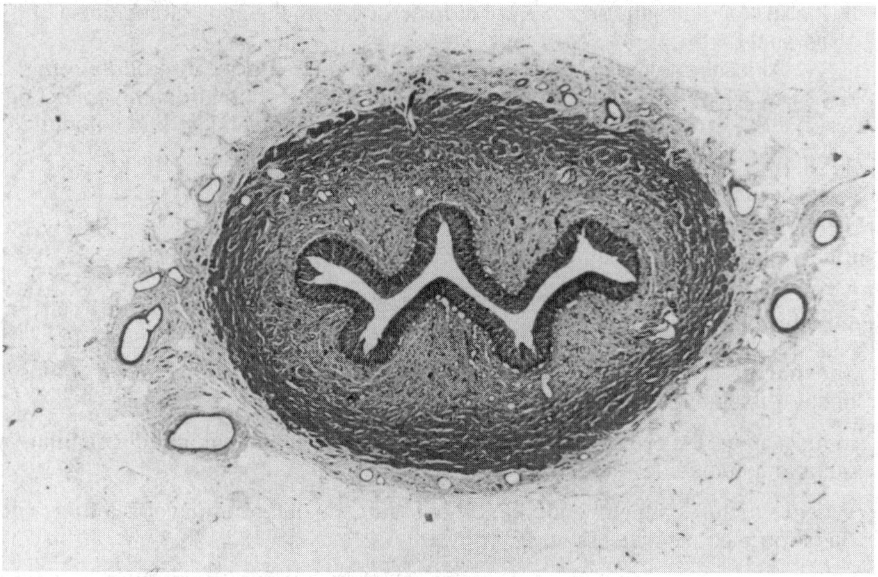

B

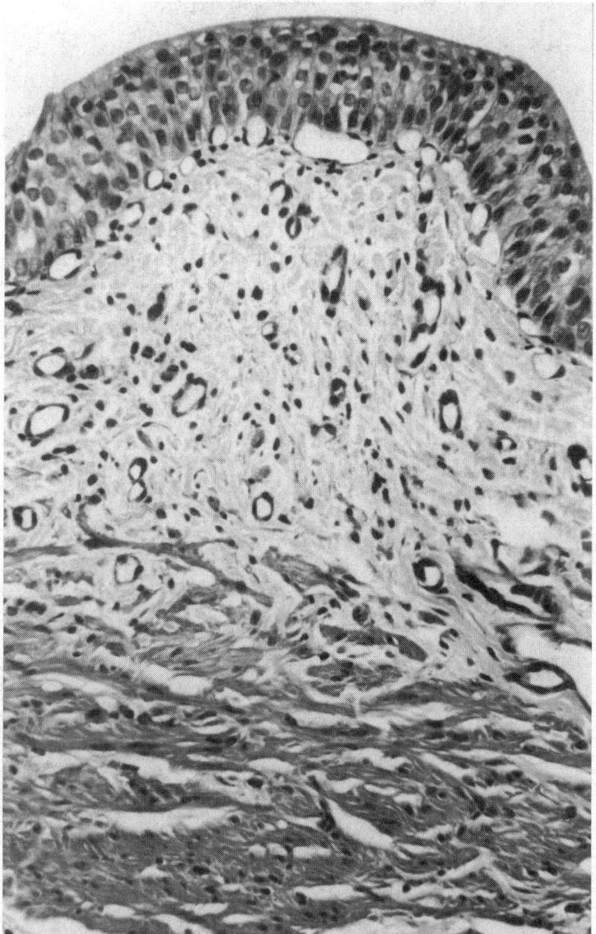

FIGURE 15-6. (*A*) Light micrograph of a cross-section through the canine ureter. Notice the transitional epithelial lining, underlying propria–submucosa, tunica muscularis, and the surrounding adventitia. (*B*) This light micrograph shows part of the ureteral mucosa of (*A*) at higher magnification. Underneath the transitional epithelium lining of the mucosa is the loose connective tissue of the propria–submucosa. Capillaries are numerous and contact the epithelium. (From Dellmann H-D: *Textbook of Veterinary Histology,* 4th ed. Baltimore, Williams & Wilkins, 1993, p 210.)

b. It also stimulates the secretion of **aldosterone** from the zona glomerulosa of the adrenal cortex.
  (1) Aldosterone induces increased sodium and chloride reabsorption from the distal convoluted tubule and increased sodium reabsorption from the collecting ducts.
  (2) Both events, in turn, cause expansion of the extracellular fluid volume.

III. URINARY PASSAGES.

The urinary passages include the calyces, renal pelvis, ureters, urinary bladder, and urethra.

A. General histologic characteristics

1. The **mucosa** is lined by transitional epithelium on a propria–submucosa of loose connective tissue (Figure 15-6).
2. In most areas, the **tunica muscularis** has an inner longitudinal, middle circular, and outer longitudinal layer.
3. Where structures are embedded in other tissue, the outermost layer is a **tunica adventitia** of loose connective tissue.
4. Where structures project into the peritoneal cavity, they are surrounded by a **tunica serosa** of loose connective tissue with a peritoneal mesothelial covering.

B. Special organ characteristics

1. **Mucous glands** are present in the **calyces** and **proximal ureter** of the **equine**.
2. **Contraction** of the **tunica muscularis** results in a **stellate profile of the ureteral lumen** in most histologic sections.
3. In the **urinary bladder,** the appearance of the transitional epithelium varies with the degree of filling. Small bundles of smooth muscle form a discontinuous lamina muscularis in all domestic mammals except the cat. The tunica muscularis consists of an irregular network of smooth muscle bundles rather than distinct layers.
4. Near the external urethral orifice, the **female urethra** is lined by a stratified squamous epithelium. Endothelium-lined caverns form an erectile plexus in the propria–submucosa.
5. The **male urethra** is described in Chapter 18.

STUDY QUESTIONS

DIRECTIONS: Each of the numbered items or incomplete statements in this section is followed by answers or by completions of the statement. Select the **one** numbered answer or completion that is **best** in each case.

1. The macula densa is an aggregation of densely packed epithelial cells in the:

(1) proximal tubule.
(2) distal tubule.
(3) afferent arteriole of the glomerulus.
(4) thin tubule.
(5) efferent arteriole of the glomerulus.

2. Medullary rays are *best* described as:

(1) groups of collecting ducts in the renal medulla.
(2) groups of blood vessels in the renal cortex.
(3) straight proximal and distal tubules and collecting ducts in the renal cortex.
(4) arched collecting ducts and thin tubules in the renal cortex.
(5) groups of descending and ascending thin tubules.

3. The glomerular filtration barrier is *best* described as being composed of:

(1) endothelial cells, glomerular basement membrane, and podocytes.
(2) podocytes, mesangial cells, and juxtaglomerular cells.
(3) endothelial cells, glomerular basement membrane, and mesangial cells.
(4) glomerular basement membrane, mesangial cells, and mesangial matrix.
(5) endothelial cells, parietal capsular epithelial cells, and podocytes.

4. The distal tubule can *best* be described as:

(1) helping to form the loop of the nephron (Henle's loop).
(2) being lined by a simple squamous epithelium.
(3) descending into the inner medulla.
(4) secreting sodium and chloride ions.
(5) reabsorbing potassium and hydrogen ions.

5. Which statement *best* describes the function of the collecting ducts in the final composition of urine?

(1) Urine from the nephron is collected and conveyed to the renal pelvis without further modification.
(2) Sodium is reabsorbed under the influence of atrial natriuretic hormone.
(3) Water reabsorption depends on the availability of antidiuretic hormone (ADH).
(4) Water reabsorption is directly influenced by aldosterone.
(5) Proteins in the ultrafiltrate are endocytosed and metabolized.

6. The function of juxtaglomerular cells is to:

(1) secrete angiotensin II.
(2) secrete renin.
(3) secrete angiotensinogen.
(4) secrete angiotensin I.
(5) sense sodium concentration in the distal tubule.

DIRECTIONS: Each of the numbered items or incomplete statements in this section is negatively phrased, as indicated by an italicized word such as *not, least,* or *except.* Select the **one** numbered answer or completion that is **best** in each case.

7. The renal cortical labyrinth contains all of the following structures *except:*

(1) renal corpuscles.
(2) straight collecting ducts.
(3) proximal convoluted tubules.
(4) distal convoluted tubules.
(5) afferent arterioles.

8. The renal corpuscle comprises all of the following structures *except:*

(1) visceral capsular epithelium.
(2) glomerular endothelium.
(3) glomerular mesangial cells.
(4) mesangial matrix.
(5) macula densa cells.

9. Each of the following statements concerning renal vasa recta is correct *except:*

(1) They form a loop in the renal medulla.
(2) They play an important role in renal tubular physiology.
(3) They form a countercurrent multiplier system.
(4) They remove water that is reabsorbed from the straight collecting ducts.
(5) They remove excess solutes from the renal interstitium.

10. Each of the following phrases concerning the urinary passages is correct *except:*

(1) They are lined by transitional epithelium.
(2) They have many structural similarities.
(3) They participate in the concentration of urine.
(4) They store urine and convey it out of the organism.
(5) They change urine composition in the horse by adding mucus.

ANSWERS AND EXPLANATIONS

1. The answer is 2 *[II C 1 c; Figure 15-4].* Cells lining the distal tubule are tightly packed, tall, and thin, forming the macula densa at the point where the distal tubule is wedged between the afferent and efferent arterioles at the vascular pole of the renal corpuscle. Epithelioid smooth muscle cells in the afferent and (more rarely) efferent arterioles are referred to as juxtaglomerular cells and are part of the juxtaglomerular apparatus, as is the macula densa.

2. The answer is 3 *[II A 1 a (2); Figure 15-3].* The medullary rays are part of the renal cortex. They are called medullary rays because they look like an extension of the medulla into the cortex. In the medullary rays, the straight portions of the proximal and distal tubules and the straight collecting ducts are grouped together. Arched collecting ducts are in the labyrinth. Descending and ascending thin tubules are major components of the inner medulla, and are not considered part of the medullary rays.

3. The answer is 1 *[II B 1 a (1) (a) (i), (2) (a); Figure 15-4; Figure 15-5].* The glomerular filtration barrier comprises porous endothelial cells of the glomerular capillaries, the glomerular basement membrane, and podocytes. Mesangial cells and the mesangial matrix provide support for the glomerulus. Mesangial cells are phagocytic cells and are believed to phagocytose material captured (filtered) by the glomerular basement membrane. The parietal capsular epithelium is part of the glomerular capsule and forms the parietal wall of the capsular space. Juxtaglomerular cells are renin-secreting cells located primarily in the afferent arteriole of the glomerulus.

4. The answer is 1 *[II B 1 c, d (1)–(2); Figure 15-3].* The proximal and distal straight tubules and the thin tubule that connects them form the loop of the nephron. The distal straight tubule continues the ascending thin tubule in the outer medulla, ascends in the medullary ray, and continues into the distal convoluted tubule. At its point of contact with the glomerulus of origin, the distal tubular epithelium is modified to form the macula densa. The inner medulla contains only thin tubules and straight collecting ducts. Sodium and chloride ions are reabsorbed in the distal convoluted tubule, and potassium and hydrogen ions are secreted. A simple squamous epithelial lining is characteristic of the thin tubule; the distal tubule is lined by a simple cuboidal epithelium.

5. The answer is 3 *[II B 2 b].* One of the primary functions of the collecting ducts is the reabsorption of water; therefore, urine reaches its final concentration in the collecting ducts. That process requires antidiuretic hormone (ADH), which renders the cells permeable to water and urea. Aldosterone does not directly induce increased water reabsorption but rather that of sodium ions, whereas atrial natriuretic hormone, as its name implies, increases sodium excretion in the urine. Proteins are reabsorbed by endocytosis and metabolized in the proximal tubule.

6. The answer is 2 *[II C 2].* The juxtaglomerular cells, primarily located in the afferent arteriole, secrete renin. Angiotensinogen is a plasma protein that is converted to angiotensin I through the action of renin. An enzyme of primarily pulmonary origin converts angiotensin I to angiotensin II. The cells of the macula densa in the distal tubule are believed to be sensors of the sodium concentration in that tubule.

7. The answer is 2 *[II A 1 a].* The renal cortical labyrinth is composed of the convoluted proximal and distal tubules, renal corpuscles and their afferent and efferent arterioles, and arched collecting (connecting) ducts. The straight collecting ducts, together with the straight proximal and distal tubules, are located in the medullary rays.

8. The answer is 5 *[II B 1 a (1)–(2)].* The macula densa cells are not part of the renal corpuscle. The visceral capsular epithelium (or podocytes), glomerular capillary endothelium, glomerular mesangial cells, and mesangial matrix are part of the renal corpuscle. A complete list of components would also include the parietal capsular epithelium.

9. The answer is 3 *[II B 2 b (2) (a)–(b)].* A countercurrent multiplier system is functional in the thin tubule, not the vasa recta. Vasa recta are vessels that form hairpin loops in the renal medulla. Blood in vasa recta becomes more hypertonic as it descends into the inner medulla and less hypertonic as it ascends toward the corticomedullary junction. Thus, the high osmolarity of the renal medullary interstitium, which is necessary for reabsorption of water from the straight collecting ducts, is not upset. The ascending vasa recta remove the reabsorbed water and excess solutes from the renal medullary interstitium.

10. The answer is 3 *[III A–B]*. The urinary passages do not participate in the concentration of urine. All of the urinary passages, which are also structurally similar in other respects, are lined by transitional epithelium. Stratified squamous epithelium is found only in the vicinity of the external urethral orifice. In the horse (and other solipeds), mucus produced in the renal calyces and in the proximal ureter accounts for the stringy nature of equine urine. No other modifications of urine take place in these organs.

Chapter 16

Female Reproductive System

I. INTRODUCTION.

INTRODUCTION. Components of the female reproductive system include the **ovaries, uterine tubes, uterus** (i.e., uterine horns, body, and **cervix**), **vagina, vestibule,** and **external genitalia** (i.e., vulva and clitoris). **Functions** of the female reproductive system include the following:

A. Cyclic production of oocytes and corpora lutea in the ovarian cortex

B. Capture of ovulated oocytes by the uterine tubes

C. Transport of spermatozoa to the uterine tubes, where fertilization of the captured oocytes occurs

D. Transport of the fertilized oocyte (zygote) to the uterus and implantation in the endometrium (i.e., placentation)

E. Nutrition of the conceptus in the uterus until birth

F. Cyclic endometrial changes in nonpregnant adults

G. Synthesis and secretion of hormones (e.g., estrogens, progesterone, androgens, relaxin) by the ovaries and placenta

II. MAMMALIAN FEMALE REPRODUCTIVE SYSTEM

A. Ovary. The ovary provides an environment for the maturation of oocytes, and it produces hormones that induce changes in the endometrium in preparation for pregnancy.

1. **General organization.** The ovary has an **outer cortex** and an **inner medulla** (Figure 16-1). In mature mares, this relationship is reversed. Medullary tissue surrounds most of the cortical tissue, which remains on the surface only in an indentation known as the **ovulation fossa**.

   a. Ovarian cortex

   (1) A cuboidal **surface epithelium** is continuous with the peritoneal mesothelium at the attachment of the mesovarium.

   (2) Underneath the surface epithelium is a **tunica albuginea** of dense, irregular connective tissue.

   (3) In bitches, short tubules of unknown significance are present immediately underneath the tunica albuginea. They are lined with simple cuboidal epithelium and occasionally open onto the ovarian surface.

   (4) The **cortical stroma** is loose connective tissue that surrounds follicles and corpora lutea and, in carnivores, clusters or cords of interstitial endocrine cells.

   (5) Ovarian **follicles** in various developmental stages are abundant in young animals and decrease drastically in number with advancing age (see II A 2).

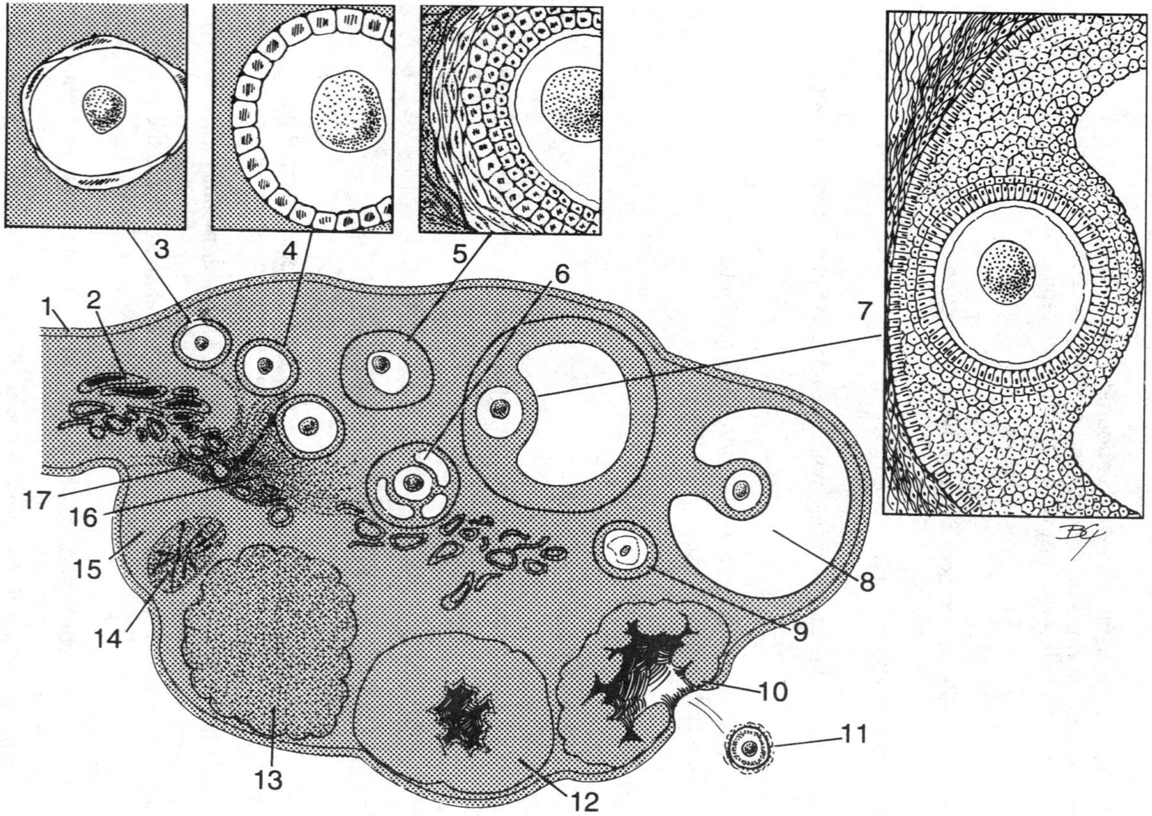

FIGURE 16-1. Schematic drawing of a mammalian ovary. (*1*) Surface epithelium. (*2*) Ovarian rete. (*3*) Primordial follicle with a primary oocyte surrounded by a simple squamous follicular epithelium. (*4*) Primary follicle with a primary oocyte surrounded by a simple cuboidal follicular epithelium. (*5*) Secondary follicle, in which the oocyte is surrounded by a zona pellucida, a stratified follicular epithelium, and a distinct theca. (*6*) Late secondary follicle. (*7*) More advanced tertiary follicle in which a distinct corona radiata of columnar follicular cells is present, surrounded by the cells of the cumulus oophorus; a theca externa and a theca interna enclose the follicle. (*8*) Late tertiary follicle. (*9*) Atretic primary follicle. (*10*) Corpus hemorrhagicum. (*11*) Ovulated oocyte. (*12*) Early and (*13*) mature corpora lutea. (*14*) Corpus albicans. (*15*) Stroma. (*16*) Interstitial endocrine cells. (*17*) Blood vessels. (Adapted from Dellmann H-D: *Textbook of Veterinary Histology,* 4th ed. Baltimore, Williams & Wilkins, 1993, p 234.)

(6) In animals with regular estrous cycles, **corpora lutea** in various stages of development and regression are present.
(7) Branches from large medullary blood vessels form dense **capillary networks** around ovarian follicles and within corpora lutea. Lymph capillaries parallel these networks.

b. Ovarian medulla

(1) Large blood vessels, lymph vessels, and nerves occupy the **stroma** of loose connective tissue.
(2) An ovarian **rete,** which may be formed by epithelium-lined, anastomosing tubes or epithelial cords, is present in ruminants and carnivores (see Figure 16-1). The rete is a developmental remnant without functional significance.

2. **Ovarian follicles** consist of an oocyte (or, rarely, two or three oocytes) surrounded by one to several layers of follicular epithelium. Follicles are either resting (i.e., primordial follicles) or growing (i.e., primary, secondary, tertiary follicles). During the estrous cycle, one or several ovarian follicles undergo changes that lead to ovulation at estrus.

a. **Primordial follicles** consist of a primary oocyte (see II A 3) and a surrounding simple squamous follicular epithelium (see Figure 16-1).

b. In **primary follicles,** the follicular epithelium is simple cuboidal or simple columnar (see Figure 16-1).

c. **Secondary follicles** develop further and are located deeper in the ovarian cortex (see Figure 16-1).

(1) The **primary oocyte** is larger than in primary and primordial follicles.
(2) The **follicular epithelial** cells are stratified, and are referred to as the **granulosa**.
(3) The granulosa cells and the oocyte participate in the elaboration of a glycoprotein layer, the **zona pellucida,** which surrounds the oocyte. Microvilli from the oocyte penetrate the zona pellucida, where they contact microvilli from granulosa cells. Gap junctions join the microvilli of the oocyte and the granulosa cells.
(4) Advanced secondary follicles become surrounded by a **theca,** which is composed of several circularly arranged layers of spindle-shaped cells that are derived from the surrounding stroma. The theca is highly vascularized.
(5) During advanced stages, small pools of **follicular fluid** (liquor), which is secreted by the granulosa cells and contains high concentrations of estrogen, form between these cells.

d. **Tertiary (antral) follicles** develop gradually from secondary follicles (see Figure 16-1).

(1) The **primary oocyte** further increases in size.
(2) Intercellular pools of follicular fluid coalesce to form one large cavity—the **antrum**.
(3) The granulosa cells form a peripheral, stratified epithelial layer—the **stratum granulosum**.
    (a) The **cumulus oophorus** is an accumulation of granulosa cells that protrudes into the antrum and surrounds the oocyte.
    (b) Radially disposed columnar cells immediately adjacent to the zona pellucida form the **corona radiata**.
(4) The theca surrounding tertiary follicles differentiates into the **theca interna** and **theca externa**.
    (a) **Theca interna**
        (i) **Structure.** The theca interna consists of spindle-shaped fibroblasts and epithelioid cells with characteristics of steroid hormone–synthesizing cells.
        (ii) **Function.** The epithelioid cells of the theca interna synthesize and secrete androgens. The androgens are taken up by granulosa cells, which metabolize them to estrogens and secrete them into the follicular fluid.
    (b) The **theca externa** is highly cellular connective tissue whose fibroblasts are arranged concentrically around the follicle.
(5) As the follicle matures, the antrum continues to enlarge. The growing follicular wall approaches the surface of the ovary, causing it to bulge.

3. **Oocyte maturation**
   a. Prenatally, each **primordial germ cell** in the ovarian cortex becomes surrounded by a layer of follicular cells and is then termed an **oogonium**. Oogonium subsequently enlarge to become **primary oocytes**.
   b. Before birth, **primary oocytes** begin the **first meiotic division,** which is arrested at the end of the prophase.
   c. When the first meiotic division is completed, a **secondary oocyte** and the **first polar body** are formed near the time of ovulation.
      (1) Completion of the first meiotic division occurs immediately after ovulation in the bitch and mare.
      (2) It occurs before ovulation in all other domestic mammals.
   d. The **second meiotic division** begins immediately after the first meiotic division is completed. The second meiotic division is arrested in metaphase and is completed only if fertilization occurs.
   e. On completion of the second meiotic division, the secondary oocyte becomes an **ovum** and a second polar body is formed. At this time, the first polar body also divides; thus, a total of three polar bodies is formed.
   f. The diameter of the oocyte ranges from approximately 20 μm in primordial follicles to 300 μm in tertiary follicles.

4. **Ovulation** is the release of the oocyte from the follicle.
   a. **Increase in follicular size.** Increased secretion of follicular fluid leads to an increase in size of the antral follicle.
   b. **Stigma formation.** The follicular wall at the ovarian surface becomes extremely thin at a point called the **stigma.**
   c. **Changes in granulosa.** Intercellular attachments between granulosa cells loosen, and the oocyte may separate from the follicular wall.
   d. **Rupturing of follicular wall.** Collagenases, prostaglandins, and histamine induce rupture of the follicular wall at the stigma.
   e. **Ovulation.** Follicular fluid and the oocyte surrounded by the zona pellucida corona radiata and cells of the cumulus oophorus are released onto the ovarian surface (see Figure 16-1).

5. **Follicular atresia and interstitial endocrine cells**
   a. **Atresia.** Most ovarian follicles degenerate and regress before reaching maturity. This process, which is called atresia, may occur at any stage of follicular development.
      (1) In **primordial, primary, and secondary follicles,** atresia involves shrinkage and vacuolization of the oocyte and separation and pyknosis of the follicular epithelial cells, followed by their degeneration and resorption. Subsequently, stromal fibrocytes invade and fill the remaining cavity.
      (2) In **tertiary follicles** undergoing atresia, visible changes in the oocyte are preceded by pyknosis, shrinkage, and separation of the follicular epithelial cells. The follicular basal lamina commonly thickens and is then referred to as the **glassy membrane.**
         (a) In **obliterative atresia,** the granulosa and theca fold into the follicular antrum. Eventually, granulosa and theca cells degenerate, are disposed of by macrophages, and replaced by stromal cells. The resulting structure is called a **corpus atreticum.**
         (b) In **cystic atresia,** the antrum enlarges through continued accumulation of follicular fluid. The granulosa cells atrophy but the theca may or may not atrophy.
   b. **Interstitial endocrine cells,** which are derived from epithelioid theca interna cells of atretic tertiary follicles or hypertrophied follicular cells of primary and secondary follicles, are particularly prominent in carnivores (see Figure 16-1). These cells **secrete androgens.**

6. **Corpus luteum**
   a. After rupture of the follicle at ovulation, the follicle wall collapses into folds. The remaining follicular fluid coagulates and, together with blood from torn capillaries, fills the antrum. The collapsed follicle with its contents is a **corpus hemorrhagicum** (see Figure 16-1).

b. **Blood vessels** invade the granulosa.
c. Granulosa cells divide and enlarge under the influence of luteinizing hormone (LH); they are then referred to as large lutein cells or **granulosa lutein cells**.
   (1) They differentiate, acquiring all the characteristics of steroid hormone-producing cells.
   (2) They secrete progesterone and, in the corpus luteum of gestation, relaxin.
   (3) A yellow pigment (i.e., lutein) in the cow, mare, and carnivores confers the characteristic color to the corpus luteum.
d. Cells of the theca interna become incorporated into the corpus luteum, especially at its periphery, as **small lutein cells** or **theca lutein cells**. They continue to synthesize androgens.
e. **Regression of the corpus luteum** begins late in diestrus, or after parturition in the case of the corpus luteum of gestation.
   (1) Lipid inclusions become larger.
   (2) The lutein pigment condenses, which changes its color to red.
   (3) Cells undergo autolysis, and the perivascular connective tissue proliferates, forming a scar—the **corpus albicans** (see Figure 16-1).

7. **Cyclic ovarian changes**
   a. **Growth and maturation of ovarian follicles,** as well as the secretion of androgens and their conversion to estrogens, are under the influence of hypophysial follicle-stimulating hormone (FSH) and LH. Follicular growth begins during late diestrus and continues during proestrus and estrus (see II B 3).
   b. **Ovulation** is triggered by an estrogen-dependent surge of LH, which peaks on the day of estrus.
   c. **Corpus luteum formation** is induced by LH, which causes differentiation of the granulosa cells into progesterone-secreting large lutein cells during diestrus.
   d. Endometrial release of prostaglandin $F_{2\alpha}$ ($PGF_{2\alpha}$) in late diestrus causes a drastic decrease in progesterone synthesis and **regression of the corpus luteum**.

B. Uterine tubes

1. **Regional differences.** On the basis of morphologic differences, three segments can be distinguished.
   a. The **infundibulum** is the funnel-shaped, thin-walled cranial end of the tube. It is closely apposed to the ovary, fringed with **fimbriae,** and openly communicates with the abdominal cavity.
   b. The **ampulla,** which is the longest segment, has a wide, thin-walled lumen (Figure 16-2).
   c. The **isthmus** is a short segment that connects to the uterus.

2. **Histologic structure**
   a. The **mucosa–submucosa** has thin primary, secondary, and tertiary **folds** in the infundibulum and ampulla (see Figure 16-2) and thicker primary folds in the isthmus.
      (1) The **epithelium** is composed of simple columnar cells or pseudostratified columnar cells.
         (a) Ciliated cells are more numerous in the infundibulum and ampulla than in the isthmus, and they are most numerous at estrus.
         (b) Synthesis and release of nutrients from secretory cells are particularly pronounced during estrus.
      (2) The **propria–submucosa** is loose connective tissue with many plasma cells.
   b. The **tunica muscularis,** which comprises an inner circular layer and an outer longitudinal layer, is thin in the infundibulum and ampulla and thicker in the isthmus.
   c. The **tunica serosa** is highly vascularized, loose connective tissue covered by peritoneal mesothelium.

3. **Cyclic changes**
   a. At **estrus,** the fimbrial blood vessels become congested and render the infundibular fimbriae more rigid. Muscular contractions cause sweeping motions over the ovary surface, which capture the ovulated oocyte on the ciliated fimbrial surface for transport into the tubal lumen.

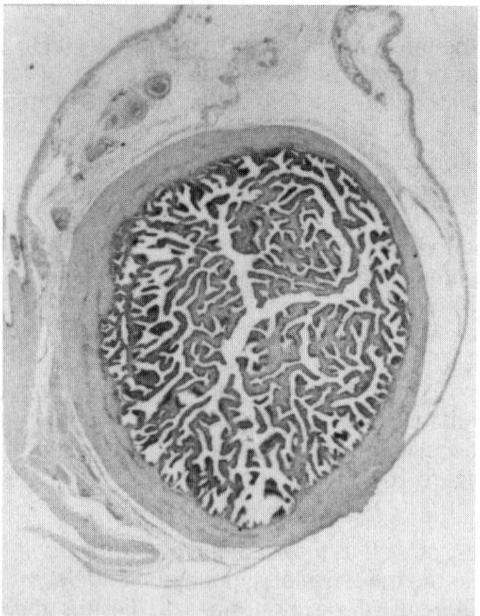

FIGURE 16-2. Cross-section through the ampulla of the porcine uterine tube. Notice the elaborate mucosal folds and the narrow lumen.

b. During **metestrus** and **early diestrus,** secretions of the tubal epithelial cells provide nutrients for the oocyte.

c. Fertilization, if it occurs, takes place in the ampulla during **early diestrus**. The zygote or the unfertilized oocyte is moved toward the isthmus and uterus by peristaltic contractions.

C. Uterus. The bicornual uterus of domestic mammals is composed of the uterine horns, body, and cervix.

1. Histologic structure of the **uterine horns** and **body**. Three layers are present in the uterine horns and body: the endometrium (mucosa–submucosa), the myometrium (tunica muscularis), and the perimetrium (serosa).

a. Endometrium

(1) The uterine **epithelium** is simple columnar in mares and carnivores, but it ranges from simple cuboidal to pseudostratified columnar in ruminants and sows.

(2) Two zones are distinguished in the propria–submucosa—a superficial functional zone and a deep basal zone (Figure 16-3).

(a) The **functional zone** is highly vascularized, loose connective tissue.

(i) It contains many free cells in the vicinity of the epithelium (**cellular stratum**) and fewer cells in its deep portion (**reticular stratum**).

(ii) It contains the upper portions of the simple branched coiled tubular **uterine glands**.

(iii) In ruminants, glandless and highly vascularized local thickenings of the propria–submucosa containing numerous fibrocytes are referred to as **caruncles**. They are sites of attachment of fetal placental cotyledons.

(b) The **basal zone,** which is adjacent to the myometrium, is a thin layer of loose connective tissue surrounding the blind ends of the uterine glands.

b. The **myometrium** consists of two spirally arranged muscle layers, with predominantly circular orientation in the inner layer and more longitudinal orientation in the outer layer (see Figure 16-3). Between these layers is a **vascular layer** (stratum vasculare) from which the functionally important endometrial blood supply is derived.

c. The **perimetrium** is highly vascular, loose connective tissue covered by peritoneal mesothelium.

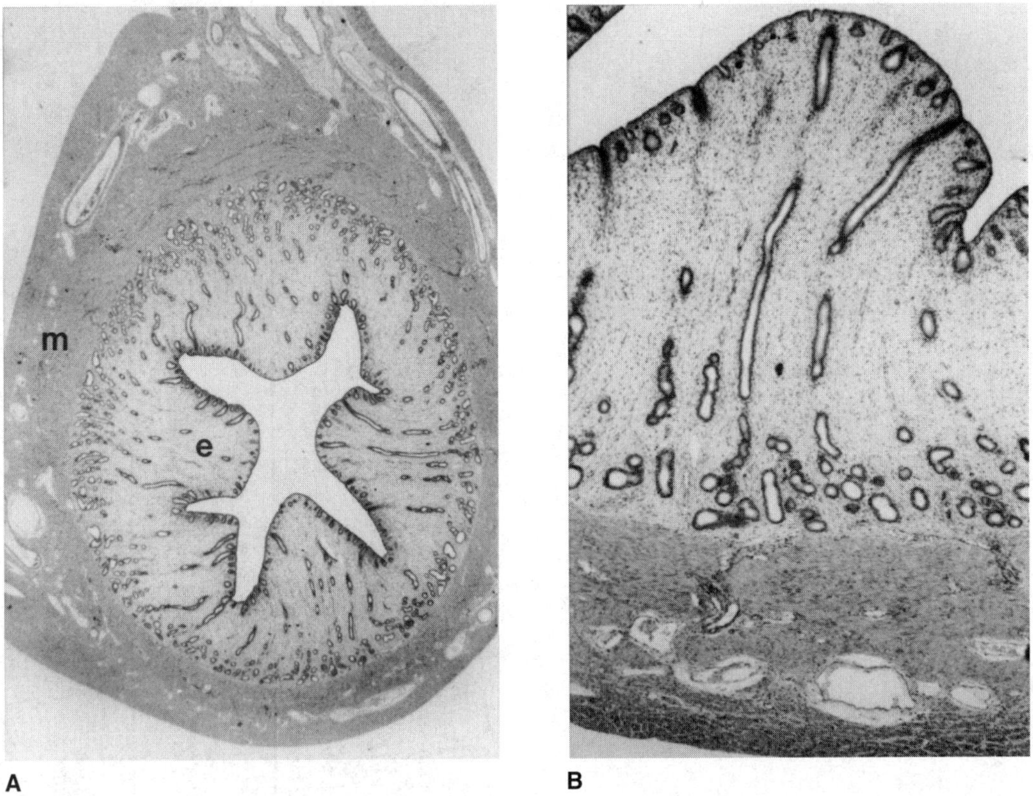

FIGURE 16-3. Cross-section through a canine uterine horn. (*A*) The endometrium (*e*) is highly glandular. The myometrium (*m*) is composed of two layers between which there is a distinct vascular stratum. (*B*) The superficial functional zone of the endometrium contains the upper portions of the uterine glands; the basal zone contains their terminal portions.

2. **Cyclic changes** in the **uterine horns** and **body**. Endometrial changes are influenced primarily by estrogens during proestrus and estrus, by estrogen and progesterone during metestrus, and by progesterone during diestrus (Figure 16-4).
   a. **Cyclic changes in cows**
      (1) During **proestrus,** while progesterone levels decrease, FSH secretion by the adenohypophysis increases and promotes ovarian follicular growth and estrogen secretion.
         (a) The **endometrium** becomes thickened, congested, and edematous.
         (b) The **uterine glands** elongate.
         (c) The **height** of uterine and glandular epithelial cells increases.
      (2) At **estrus,** estrogen levels are maximal, and a short surge of LH induces ovulation.
         (a) The **uterine mucosa** increases further in thickness.
         (b) The **uterine glands** elongate further and branch, and glandular and surface epithelia continue to increase in height.
         (c) Small hemorrhages (**metrorrhagia**) occur in the functional zone shortly before ovulation.
         (d) The **myometrium** is highly contractile.
      (3) During **metestrus,** estrogen levels decline, and progesterone levels begin to rise (initial development of the corpus luteum).
         (a) The **uterine mucosa** is at its maximal height.
         (b) **Uterine glands** continue to branch.
         (c) **Metrorrhagia** ceases at around mid-metestrus.

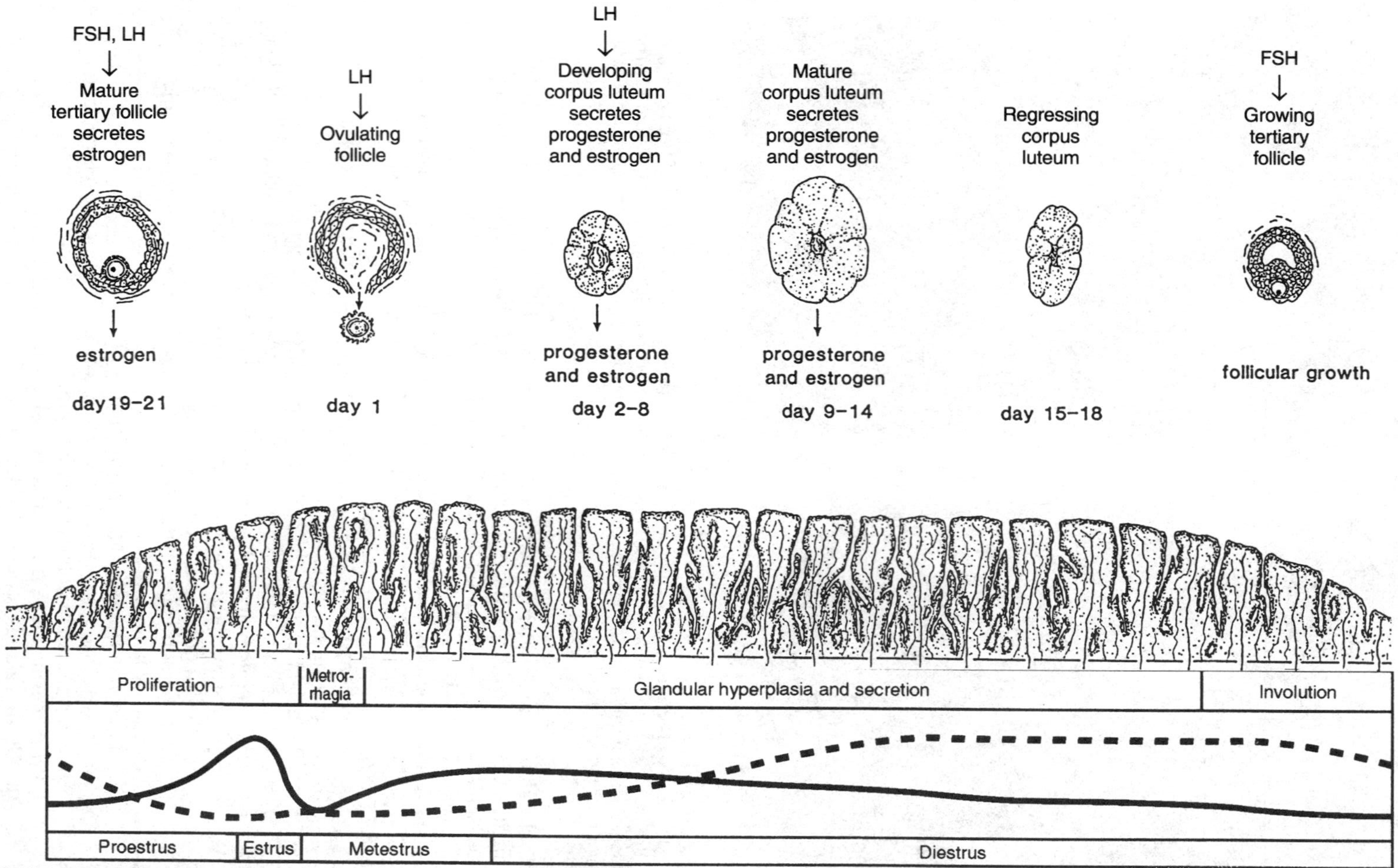

FIGURE 16-4. Schematic drawing showing the relationship of bovine ovarian and uterine changes during the estrous cycle to changes in blood levels of estrogen (*solid line*) and progesterone (dashed line). *FSH* = follicle-stimulating hormone; *LH* = luteinizing hormone. (Adapted from Dellmann H-D: *Textbook of Veterinary Histology,* 4th ed. Baltimore, Williams & Wilkins, 1993.)

(4) During **diestrus,** corpora lutea reach maturity, which causes progesterone levels to reach a maximum at about mid-diestrus.

(a) Endometrial edema and the thickness of the endometrium gradually decline, causing coiling of the uterine glands.

(b) Through mid-diestrus, the secretory activity of both the surface and glandular epithelial cells is most pronounced.

(5) In **late diestrus,** the corpus luteum regresses (unless pregnancy occurs), and further changes are associated with the decline in progesterone levels.

(a) A drastic decrease in **height of the endometrium** (i.e., involution) occurs.

(b) **Glands regress;** that is, they uncoil and become shorter, and surface and glandular epithelial cells cease secretion.

b. Cyclic changes in mares

(1) During **anestrus,** the nonedematous endometrium is lined with simple cuboidal epithelium. It contains straight uterine glands with cuboidal to low columnar epithelial cells.

(2) During **proestrus,** the endometrial epithelium is simple columnar to pseudostratified columnar. The uterine glands begin to coil.

(3) During **estrus,** the endometrium becomes edematous and thickens.

(a) The endometrial epithelium is highest during early estrus, and decreases in height in late estrus.

(b) The uterine glands proliferate and become secretory.

(c) The myometrium is contractile.

(4) **Metestrus** is not readily defined histologically.

(5) During **diestrus,** endometrial edema decreases.

(a) The endometrial lining is simple columnar.

(b) The uterine glands become increasingly coiled, and less secretory.

c. Cyclic changes in carnivores. Carnivores have only one or two estrous cycles per year.

(1) During **proestrus, metrorrhagia** occurs in bitches.

(2) Diestrus, during which corpora lutea are functional, lasts an average of 70 days in bitches and is also called **physiologic pseudopregnancy**. Endometrial changes resemble those observed during early pregnancy.

(3) **Anestrus** follows diestrus. During anestrus, the endometrium is thinnest, surface and glandular epithelia are nonsecretory, and uterine glands are straight.

d. In **species that have menstrual cycles,** the functional zone is shed at the end of diestrus and subsequently regenerates from the basal zone.

3. Histologic structure of the **cervix uteri**. The cervix is the caudalmost portion of the uterus. Its structure reflects its function as a barrier between the vagina and the body of the uterus. The mucosa of the cervical canal, through which the vagina and the uterus communicate, has species-specific characteristics (e.g., folds, interlocking cushions), but its general structure is similar in all domestic species.

a. Epithelium

(1) In **most domestic species,** the cervix is lined by simple columnar epithelium that comprises mainly **mucigenous cells,** with goblet cells and a few ciliated cells. Mucigenous cells produce mucus, most of which reaches the vagina.

(a) **During estrus,** mucus secretion increases.

(b) **During pregnancy,** the cervical canal is sealed by a mucous plug.

(2) In **bitches and sows,** however, stratified squamous epithelium lines most of the cervix.

b. Simple tubular cervical glands occur in small ruminants and the sow.

c. The **propria** is predominantly dense irregular connective tissue containing many elastic fibers. During estrus and at the time of birth, this tissue becomes edematous.

d. The **tunica muscularis** consists of irregularly arranged smooth muscle bundles with predominantly inner circular fibers and outer longitudinal fibers. The layers of the tunica muscularis are continuous with those of the uterus and vagina.

e. The **serosa** is highly vascularized, loose connective tissue.

D. Vagina

1. **Histologic structure**
   a. The **vaginal mucosa** forms low longitudinal folds and a few circular folds. The epithelium is primarily stratified squamous, but patches of simple columnar epithelium with mucigenous cells and goblet cells occur, especially between the folds.
   b. The **propria–submucosa** is loose or dense irregular connective tissue containing lymphatic nodules, which are especially numerous in the caudal vagina.
   c. The **tunica muscularis** consists of smooth muscle, usually arranged in an inner circular and an outer longitudinal layer interspersed with abundant collagen and elastic fibers.
   d. A **tunica serosa** or **tunica adventitia** is present, composed of loose connective tissue rich in blood vessels and nerves.

2. **Cyclic changes in bitches** (Figure 16-5)
   a. During **anestrus,** the stratified squamous epithelium comprises only two to three cell layers (see Figure 16-5D). Vaginal smears contain numerous unstained nonkeratinized squamous cells, a few stained larger epithelial cells with pyknotic nuclei, neutrophils, and lymphocytes.
   b. During **proestrus,** the epithelium becomes considerably thicker (up to 20 layers) and keratinizes (see Figure 16-5A). Vaginal smears contain many squamous keratinized cells and erythrocytes of uterine origin.
   c. During early **estrus,** keratinization reaches a maximum; subsequently, keratinization decreases slowly (see Figure 16-5B). Intraepithelial mucous glands are present. Vaginal smears contain squamous keratinized cells, which begin to disintegrate and become invaded by bacteria during late estrus. The number of erythrocytes decreases.
   d. During **metestrus–diestrus,** the number of epithelial cell layers decreases, as does keratinization (see Figure 16-5C). Vaginal smears are characterized by nonkera-

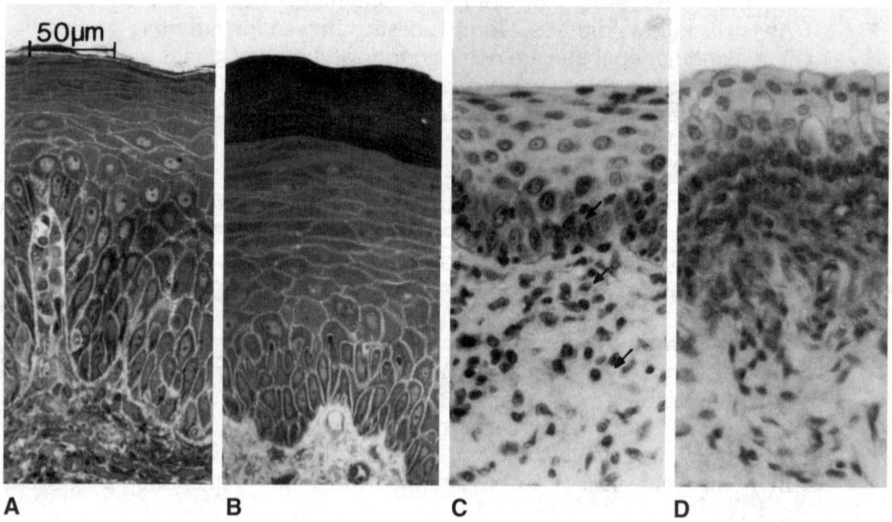

FIGURE 16-5. Cyclic epithelial changes in the canine vagina. (*A*) During proestrus, a thin, superficial, keratinized layer is present in the stratified squamous epithelium. (*B*) During estrus, several layers (darkly stained) of keratinized cells are present. (*C*) During metestrus, intraepithelial leukocytes are observed (*upper arrow*). Epithelial cells decrease in number and keratinization. (*D*) During late diestrus–early anestrus, a further reduction in the number of cell layers has occurred. (From Mosimann W, Kohler T: *Zytologie, Histologie und mikroskopische Anatomie der Haussägetiere.* Berlin–Hamburg, Paul Parey, 1990, p 246.)

tinized squamous epithelial cells; neutrophils are abundant early, and later decrease progressively in number.

E. Vestibule

1. In the vestibule, **mucosal folds** are lower than in the vagina. The lining epithelium is stratified squamous. Mucigenous cells decrease in number from cranial to caudal.
2. The **structure of the propria–submucosa** varies among different domestic species.
   a. An erectile plexus, the **bulbus vestibuli,** is present in mares and bitches.
   b. Compound glands called **major vestibular glands** are present in queens and ruminants. These glands secrete mucus to lubricate the vestibule and vagina.
   c. **Minor vestibular glands** are branched tubular mucous glands, which occur in most domestic mammals.
   d. Numerous **subepithelial lymphnodules** are present in all species.
3. The **tunica muscularis** is similar to that in the vagina. In addition to smooth muscle, circular skeletal muscle bundles (constrictor vestibuli) are present.

F. External genitalia

1. **Vulva.** The two labia are covered by skin with fine hairs and particularly numerous sebaceous glands. The dermis and hypodermis have a dense vascular plexus that becomes congested during estrus (especially in the bitch and sow). The hypodermis contains bundles of skeletal muscle (constrictor vulvae).
2. **Clitoris.** The **corpus cavernosum** of the clitoris consists of erectile tissue (endothelium-lined caverns) with numerous sensory nerve endings.

III. AVIAN FEMALE REPRODUCTIVE SYSTEM

A. Ovary. Only the left ovary develops.

1. The ovary has a **cortex** and **medulla,** but they are not as clearly defined as in the mammalian ovary.
2. **Ovarian cortex**
   a. The **main structural components** are solid, stalked ovarian **follicles** that never develop an antrum.
      (1) The oocyte is surrounded from the outside in by simple cuboidal **surface epithelium, theca externa, theca interna,** and simple columnar **granulosa** (follicular epithelium).
      (2) **Mature follicles** contain a secondary oocyte rich in yolk.
      (3) At ovulation, the oocyte and granulosa cells are released, whereas theca cells form a **transient corpus luteum**.
   b. **Additional structures.** The ovarian cortex also contains atretic and postovulatory follicles, clusters of thecal gland cells, and stromal interstitial cells.
3. The **ovarian medulla** in the mature ovary is not clearly delineated; it contains blood and lymph vessels and nerves.

B. Oviduct. While the oocyte (or zygote) is transported through the oviduct, albumin, shell membranes, and the shell are added.

1. **General structural characteristics**
   a. The height and complexity of **mucosal folds** vary among regions.
   b. The loose connective tissue of the **propria–submucosa** is rich in lymphocytes and plasma cells.

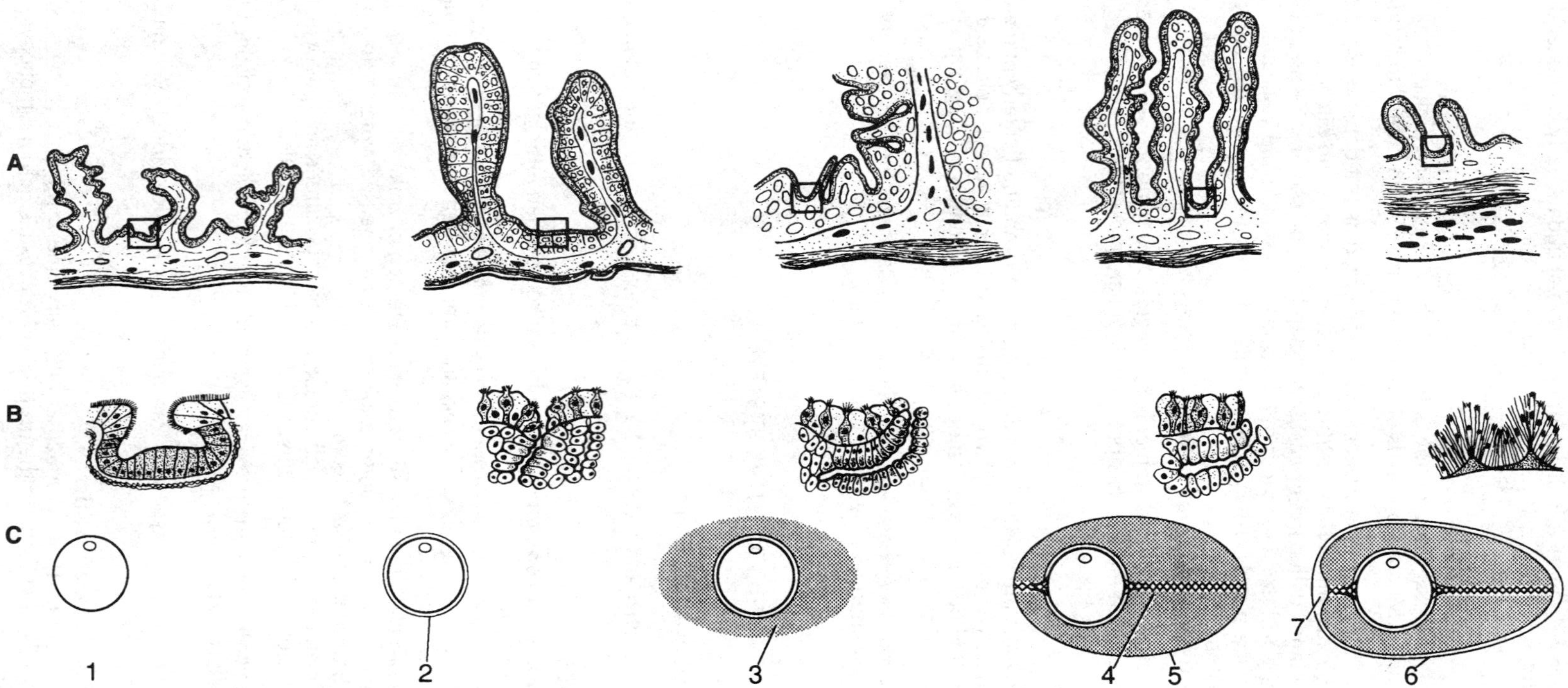

FIGURE 16-6. Schematic drawings of sections through the oviduct (*A, B*) of a laying hen and corresponding stages of egg development (*C*). *A* depicts the mucosa, muscularis, and serosa. In *B,* the surface and glandular epithelia are shown. *C* shows (*1*) blastula and yolk, (*2*) vitelline membrane, (*3*) albumin, (*4*) chalazae, (*5*) shell membrane, (*6*) shell, and (*7*) airspace at the time of entrance into the designated part of the oviduct. (Adapted from Dellmann H-D: *Textbook of Veterinary Histology,* 4th ed. Baltimore, Williams & Wilkins, 1993.)

c. The **tunica muscularis** comprises a few bundles in the infundibulum and forms two distinct layers in the remainder of the oviduct. It is thickest in the uterus, where it forms a sphincter at the uterovaginal junction, and in the vagina (where it causes expulsion of the egg).
d. The **tunica serosa** consists of a thin layer of loose connective tissue covered by mesothelium.

2. The oviduct consists of **five regions:** infundibulum, magnum, isthmus, uterus, and vagina (Figure 16-6).
   a. **Infundibulum.** The infundibulum is the site of fertilization and formation of the continuous and extravitelline membranes.
      (1) The **epithelial lining** ranges from simple columnar to pseudostratified columnar with ciliated and nonciliated cells and goblet cells.
      (2) Simple tubular glands are present in the **propria–submucosa.**
   b. **Magnum.** The magnum produces albumin for the oocyte (or zygote).
      (1) The **surface epithelium** is simple columnar with goblet cells, ciliated cells, and columnar cells that secrete ovomucin.
      (2) Branched, tubular coiled glands in the **propria–submucosa** are lined with ovalbumin- and lysozyme-secreting cells.
   c. **Isthmus**
      (1) The simple columnar **surface epithelium** comprises ciliated and nonciliated cells.
      (2) The **propria–submucosa** contains simple branched tubular glands that produce the shell membranes.
   d. **Uterus (shell gland)**
      (1) The **pseudostratified columnar lining epithelium** has ciliated cells and secretory cells that produce cuticle and shell matrix.
      (2) Simple tubular coiled glands in the **propria–submucosa** secrete the inorganic part of the egg shell.
   e. **Vagina**
      (1) The **pseudostratified columnar surface epithelium** comprises ciliated and nonciliated cells.
      (2) **Simple tubular sperm host glands,** in which spermatozoa may be stored for up to 21 days, are present at the uterovaginal junction.

STUDY QUESTIONS

DIRECTIONS: Each of the numbered items or incomplete statements in this section is followed by answers or by completions of the statement. Select the **one** numbered answer or completion that is **best** in each case.

1. Ovarian androgens that are synthesized and secreted by theca interna cells are then metabolized to estrogen by:

(1) follicular granulosa cells.
(2) theca externa cells.
(3) granulosa lutein cells.
(4) theca lutein cells.
(5) ovarian interstitial endocrine cells.

2. Early tertiary follicles are *best* described as containing:

(1) a secondary oocyte surrounded by zona pellucida and corona radiata.
(2) a primary oocyte surrounded by zona pellucida and corona radiata.
(3) an ovum surrounded by zona pellucida and corona radiata.
(4) a secondary oocyte surrounded by zona pellucida, corona radiata, and cumulus oophorus.
(5) a primary oocyte surrounded by zona pellucida, corona radiata, and cumulus oophorus.

3. Which one of the following statements *best* describes meiosis of oocytes?

(1) It is an exclusively prenatal event.
(2) It is an exclusively postnatal event.
(3) It begins prenatally and is completed postnatally.
(4) It begins and is completed immediately before ovulation.
(5) It has to be completed before fertilization can occur.

4. Follicular atresia is *best* described by which of the following statements?

(1) It is a regressive process that affects mainly tertiary follicles.
(2) It is a regressive process that affects most ovarian follicles.
(3) It does not occur until sexual maturity.
(4) It is a regressive process that affects mainly primary and secondary follicles.
(5) It is a regressive process that affects mainly primordial follicles.

5. A functional corpus luteum produces primarily progesterone and is made up of cells derived from which of the following cell types?

(1) Theca interna and ovarian interstitial cells
(2) Theca externa and ovarian interstitial cells
(3) Theca interna and theca externa
(4) Granulosa and theca interna
(5) Granulosa and theca externa

6. Which of the following statements *best* describes a secondary follicle?

(1) It contains a secondary oocyte surrounded by zona pellucida and granulosa.
(2) It contains a primary oocyte surrounded by granulosa.
(3) It contains a secondary oocyte surrounded by simple cuboidal follicular epithelium.
(4) It contains a primary oocyte surrounded by zona pellucida and stratified follicular epithelium.
(5) It contains a primary oocyte surrounded by zona pellucida, corona radiata, cumulus oophorus, and granulosa.

DIRECTIONS: Each of the numbered items or incomplete statements in this section is negatively phrased, as indicated by an italicized word such as *not, least,* or *except.* Select the **one** numbered answer or completion that is **best** in each case.

7. All of the following statements concerning the uterine tubes are correct *except:*

(1) The epithelial lining comprises ciliated and secretory cells.
(2) The zygote receives nutrients from the secretory activity of epithelial lining cells.
(3) At the time of ovulation, the infundibulum covers the entire ovarian surface.
(4) The infundibular fimbriae capture the ovulated oocyte and transport it by ciliary motion into the tubal lumen.
(5) Peristaltic contractions of the tubal musculature are primarily responsible for zygote transport toward the uterus.

8. All of the following statements concerning the uterus are correct *except:*

(1) The endometrium comprises a functional zone and a basal zone.
(2) Simple tubular branched and coiled glands are present throughout the entire endometrium in ruminants.
(3) Cyclic changes do not occur in the endometrial basal zone.
(4) Cyclic changes are prominent in the endometrial functional zone.
(5) The lining epithelium is secretory.

9. All of the following statements properly describe the bovine endometrium *except:*

(1) Endometrial congestion is maximal at metestrus.
(2) Glandular secretion is most pronounced during diestrus.
(3) Coiling of uterine glands during diestrus is primarily caused by a decrease in the height of the endometrium.
(4) Metrorrhagia occurs during endometrial involution at the end of diestrus.
(5) At proestrus, thickening, congestion, and edema of the endometrium are caused by an increase in ovarian estrogen secretion.

10. All of the following statements concerning the cervix uteri are correct *except:*

(1) Cervical mucus is mainly produced by the lining epithelial cells.
(2) Simple tubular glands are present in mares and cows.
(3) Stratified squamous epithelium lines most of the cervix in sows and bitches.
(4) The cervical connective tissue undergoes cyclic changes during the estrous cycle.
(5) Elastic fibers are prominent in the cervical propria–submucosa.

11. All of the following statements describing vaginal smears obtained from a bitch are correct *except:*

(1) Erythrocytes are present during both proestrus and estrus.
(2) Neutrophils are abundant early during metestrus–diestrus.
(3) Keratinized squamous cells and many erythrocytes are characteristic of proestrus.
(4) Keratinized squamous cells and a decreased number of erythrocytes (as compared to proestrus) are characteristic of estrus.
(5) Keratinized squamous cells but no leukocytes are present during anestrus.

12. All of the following events occur in preparation for ovulation *except:*

(1) stigma formation.
(2) loosening of the intercellular attachments between granulosa cells.
(3) rupture of the follicular wall caused by increased fluid pressure.
(4) increased follicular size.
(5) increased follicular fluid secretion.

ANSWERS AND EXPLANATIONS

1. The answer is 1 *[II A 2 d (4) (a)]*. The epithelioid cells of the theca interna synthesize and secrete androgens that are metabolized to estrogens by follicular granulosa cells. Theca externa cells are fibrocytes that do not secrete hormones. Granulosa lutein cells of the corpus luteum synthesize and secrete progesterone and relaxin. Theca lutein cells synthesize and secrete androgens. Ovarian interstitial cells synthesize and secrete androgens.

2. The answer is 5 *[II A 2 d, 3]*. Early tertiary follicles contain a primary oocyte surrounded by zona pellucida and corona radiata. The corona radiata, in turn, is surrounded by cells of the cumulus oophorus. The first meiotic division is completed shortly before ovulation (i.e., in a late tertiary follicle) in most domestic mammals, giving rise to a secondary oocyte. Only in bitches and mares does the late tertiary follicle still contain a primary oocyte; the first meiotic division is completed and a secondary oocyte is formed after ovulation in these animals. Completion of the second meiotic division requires fertilization (i.e., penetration by a spermatozoon) and gives rise to an ovum.

3. The answer is 3 *[II A 3]*. The first meiotic division of primary oocytes begins before birth. It is arrested in prophase and is resumed and completed before ovulation (in all domestic mammals except mares and bitches). In mares and bitches, the first meiotic division of primary oocytes occurs after ovulation. The second meiotic division begins immediately thereafter. It is then arrested in metaphase and completed only on penetration of a spermatozoon.

4. The answer is 2 *[II A 5 a]*. Atresia is a regressive event that affects most ovarian follicles. It involves all types of ovarian follicles both before and after sexual maturity. It results in eventual resorption and complete disappearance of the affected follicle.

5. The answer is 4 *[II A 6]*. The corpus luteum, when it is functional (i.e., during diestrus and pregnancy), produces primarily progesterone but also androgens and relaxin. Its epithelioid endocrine cells are derived mainly from the granulosa of an ovulated follicle and, to a much lesser degree, from the theca interna of the same follicle.

6. The answer is 4 *[II A 2 c]*. Secondary follicles contain a primary oocyte surrounded by zona pellucida and stratified follicular epithelium, the granulosa. The primary oocyte contained in the secondary follicle is arrested in the prophase of the first meiotic division, which is only resumed after ovulation in bitches and mares and shortly before ovulation (i.e., in a tertiary follicle) in all other domestic mammals. In tertiary (antral) follicles, the granulosa differentiates into the corona radiata and cumulus oophorus around the oocyte.

7. The answer is 3 *[II B 2 a (1), 3 a–c]*. At the time of ovulation, the infundibulum sweeps back and forth over the ovarian surface to capture the ovulated oocyte, but it does not cover the ovarian surface. The uterine tubes are lined by an epithelium that comprises both ciliated and secretory cells. The movement of the cilia is responsible for the oocyte's progression from the infundibulum into the ampulla, where further progression is achieved through the contractions of the tubal musculature. The products of the secretory cells provide initial nutrition to the zygote.

8. The answer is 2 *[II C 1 a (2), 2]*. Glandless, vascularized regions called caruncles are present in ruminants. The endometrium, the innermost layer of the uterus, is lined by an epithelium with distinct secretory activity. It comprises a subepithelial functional zone, in which drastic changes (e.g., edema) occur during the estrous cycle, and a basal zone, which does not undergo cyclic changes. Endometrial glands are simple tubular, and the degree of their branching and coiling varies within wide limits during the estrous cycle.

9. The answer is 4 *[II C 2 a; Figure 16-4]*. Metrorrhagia (i.e., endometrial hemorrhage) is a phenomenon that begins shortly before ovulation, peaks during metestrus (when endometrial congestion is maximal), and continues until mid-metestrus. Declining progesterone levels during proestrus induce a gradual rise in ovarian estrogen secretion that causes the endometrium to become congested, edematous, and thickened. During subsequent diestrus, under the influence of increasing progesterone levels, glandular and surface epithelial secretion is maximal, and the decline in endometrial thickness as a result of decreased edema causes coiling of the glands.

10. The answer is 2 *[II C 3]*. In small ruminants and sows, simple tubular glands are an additional source of mucus, but other domestic species lack cervical glands. The cervix of sows and bitches is lined mostly by a stratified squamous epithelium. The remainder of the cervix, and that of all other domestic species, is lined by a simple columnar epithelium, which has mucigenous and goblet cells that secrete mucus. The cervical connective tissue is rich in elastic fibers and becomes edematous during estrus (and at parturition).

11. The answer is 5 *[II E 2]*. During anestrus, the vaginal epithelium is not keratinized; thus, vaginal smears contain nonkeratinized squamous cells. In addition, neutrophils and lymphocytes are present. During proestrus and estrus, vaginal smears contain keratinized squamous cells. They also contain erythrocytes, but there are fewer erythrocytes present during estrus than during proestrus. During early metestrus–diestrus, neutrophils are abundant; later, the number of neutrophils declines.

12. The answer is 3 *[II A 4]*. Ovulation (i.e., the release of the oocyte from the follicle) is preceded by rupture of the follicular wall at the stigma, a spot at which the tertiary or antral follicle touches the ovarian surface. Although increased follicular fluid secretion leads to an increase in follicular size, the pressure exerted by the additional fluid is minimal and does not cause rupture of the follicular wall. Rupture of the follicular wall is induced by collagenases, prostaglandins, and histamine.

Chapter 17
Placenta

I. INTRODUCTION

A. Definition. The placenta is an organ formed during pregnancy that allows physiologic exchange between the mother and the fetus. It includes both **fetal and maternal components**.

B. Embryology

1. **Fertilization** produces the zygote.
   a. The **zygote** divides repeatedly and is transformed into a blastocyst.
   b. The **blastocyst** is a fluid-filled vesicle comprising:
      (1) An **embryonic disk,** which consists of **three primary germ layers:**
         (a) **Ectoderm,** the **outermost layer**
         (b) **Entoderm,** the **innermost layer**
         (c) **Mesoderm,** the **middle layer**
      (2) The **trophoblast,** a wall of **simple cuboidal epithelium**
         (a) In the **early blastocyst,** the **trophoblast takes up nutrients** from uterine glandular secretory products (i.e., **uterine milk**).
         (b) In the **more advanced blastocyst, membranes develop from the trophoblast** that gradually attach to the endometrium.
2. **Implantation** is the attachment of the blastocyst to the endometrium as blood vessels in the fetal membranes establish a close relationship with the maternal circulation.

II. FETAL MEMBRANES. The fetus is surrounded by or associated with four fetal membranes (Figure 17-1).

A. The **chorion** is the **outermost fetal membrane.**

1. **Origin.** The chorion is formed from the **trophoblast** and **richly vascularized mesoderm.**
2. **Characteristics**
   a. The **chorion frondosum** has **villi** or **folds,** which **establish contact with the uterine endometrium** and **enlarge the area for fetal–maternal exchange.**
   b. The **chorion laeve** is **smooth** (i.e., **nonvillous**).

B. The **amnion** is the **innermost fetal membrane.**

1. **Origin.** The amnion is formed when the **folds of the trophoblast fuse** to enclose the embryo (and later, the fetus) in a fluid-filled sac (i.e., the **amniotic cavity**).
2. **Amniochorion.** The **amniochorion** results from **fusion** of the **amnion** and **chorion.**
   a. The **amniochorion** is **present in pigs** and **ruminants.**
   b. The **amniochorion** is **absent in horses** and **carnivores.**

C. The **yolk sac** communicates with the **embryonic midgut.**

1. **Origin.** The yolk sac is formed from the **entoderm** and **mesoderm.**

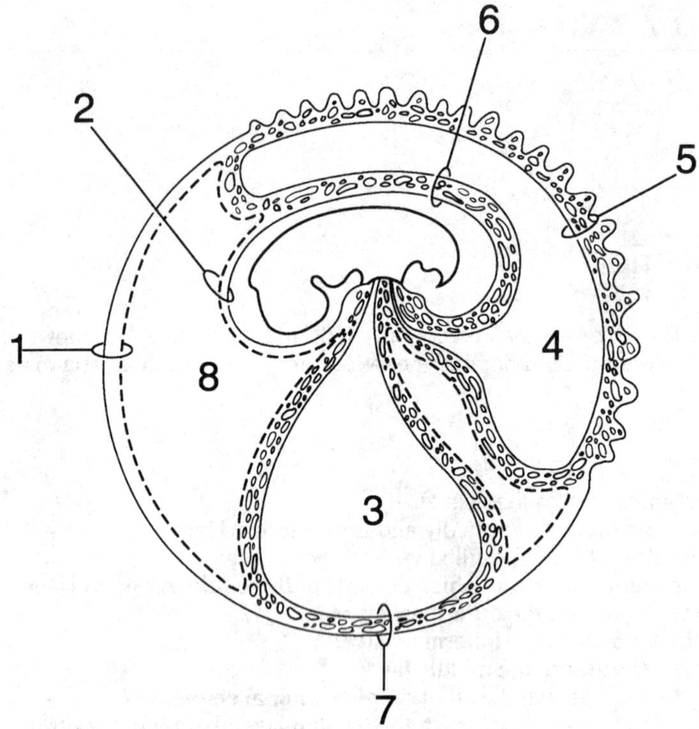

FIGURE 17-1. Schematic drawing of fetal membranes. (*1*) Chorion; (*2*) amnion, (*3*) yolk sac surrounded by yolk sac entoderm and associated vascular mesoderm; (*4*) allantois surrounded by allantoic entoderm and vascular mesoderm; (*5*) allantochorion; (*6*) allantoamnion; (*7*) choriovitelline placenta; (*8*) exocoelom. (Redrawn and modified from Dellmann H-D: *Textbook of Veterinary Histology,* 4th ed. Baltimore, Williams & Wilkins, 1993, p 256.)

2. **Characteristics. Angiogenesis** (i.e., the formation of the **first blood vessels**) and **hemopoiesis** (i.e., the development of the **first blood cells**) take place in the **mesoderm of the yolk sac wall**.

D. The **allantois** is a **diverticulum** from the **hindgut** that **gradually enlarges into the exocoelom** (i.e., the space between the amnion and chorion).

1. **Origin.** The allantois comprises **entoderm** and **mesoderm**.
2. **Allantochorion.** The allantois fuses with the chorion to form the allantochorion. The **allantoic mesoderm** is vascularized by blood vessels that connect to the embryonic vasculature. **From the vessels in the allantoic mesoderm, capillaries grow into the chorionic mesoderm** to supply the chorionic villi.
3. **Allantoamnion.** The allantois fuses with the amnion to form the allantoamnion.

III. CLASSIFICATION. There are several different methods of classifying placentae.

A. Fetal membrane contributions

1. A fetal **choriovitelline placenta** forms when the yolk sac combines with the chorion. It occurs early in gestation as a fully functional but **transitory** placenta in all domestic animals.

2. A fetal **chorioallantoic placenta** forms when the allantoic and chorionic mesoderm fuse. It is the **definitive** placenta in all domestic mammals.

B. Fate at parturition

1. **Nondeciduate placenta.** The fetal placenta **separates** from the maternal placenta (i.e., the endometrium) at parturition without damage to the uterine mucosa.
2. **Deciduate placenta.** The fetal placenta and maternal placenta are **fused** so that part of the endometrium, the **decidua,** is shed together with the fetal placenta at parturition.

C. Chorionic villi or fold distribution (Figure 17-2)

1. **Diffuse placentae. Villi** (e.g., as in **mares**) or **folds** (e.g., as in **sows**) **cover the chorionic sac**.
2. **Cotyledonary placentae** are present in **ruminants**.
   a. **Villi** are **confined to** regions of the chorion called **cotyledons,** which are attached to elevations of the endometrium called **caruncles**. The cotyledon–caruncle unit is called a **placentome**.
   b. The chorion is nonvillous between placentomes.
3. **Zonary placentae** are present in carnivores.
   a. **Villi** form a **band around the equator** of the chorionic sac.
   b. The **remainder of the chorion is nonvillous**.

D. Interhemal barriers (Figure 17-3)

1. Fetal blood may be separated from maternal blood by as many as six layers:
   a. **Fetal layers**
      (1) Allantoic capillary endothelium
      (2) Chorioallantoic mesenchyme
      (3) Chorionic (trophoblastic) epithelium
   b. **Maternal layers**
      (1) Uterine epithelium
      (2) Endometrial connective tissue
      (3) Uterine capillary endothelium
2. Although **all the fetal layers are present in all domestic mammals, some endometrial layers are lost in certain species.**
   a. In **epitheliochorial placentae,** the **endometrium remains intact**. Epitheliochorial placentae occur in ruminants, mares, and sows.
   b. In **endotheliochorial placentae,** the uterine epithelium and connective tissue are destroyed so that the **chorionic epithelium is in contact with the endothelium of the uterine capillaries**.
      (1) These placentae are **deciduate**.
      (2) Endotheliochorial placentae occur in carnivores.

IV. PLACENTAL FUNCTIONS

A. Transfer of substances

1. **Diffusion** can be **simple or facilitated**.
   a. **Diffusion barrier.** There is an **inverse relationship** between the **number of cell layers** separating the fetal and maternal blood and the **rate of diffusion**.
      (1) The rate of diffusion is lower in epitheliochorial placentae than it is in endotheliochorial placentae.
      (2) The rate of diffusion increases as gestation advances because both the **trophoblastic** and **uterine epithelial layers become thinner**.

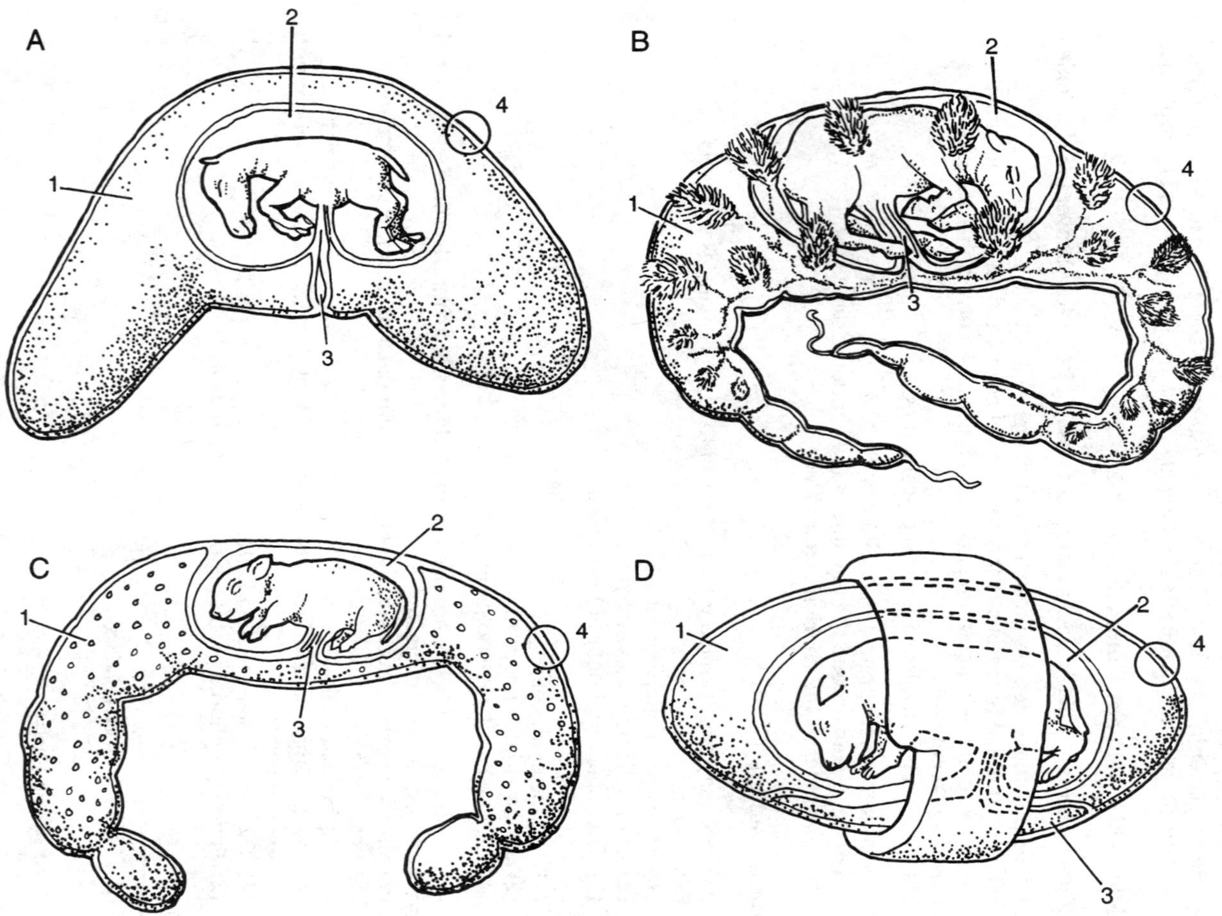

FIGURE 17-2. Three types of placentae are distinguishable macroscopically according to the distribution of the chorionic villi or folds: diffuse, cotyledonary, and zonary. (*A*) Diffuse villous placenta, as found in mares. (*B*) Cotyledonary villous placenta, as found in ruminants. (*C*) Diffuse folded placenta, as found in sows. (*D*) Labyrinthine (villous) zonary placenta, as found in carnivores. (*1*) Allantoic cavity; (*2*) amnionic cavity; (*3*) yolk sac; (*4*) allantochorion. (Redrawn and modified from Dellmann H-D: *Textbook of Veterinary Histology,* 4th ed. Baltimore, Williams & Wilkins, 1993, p 257.)

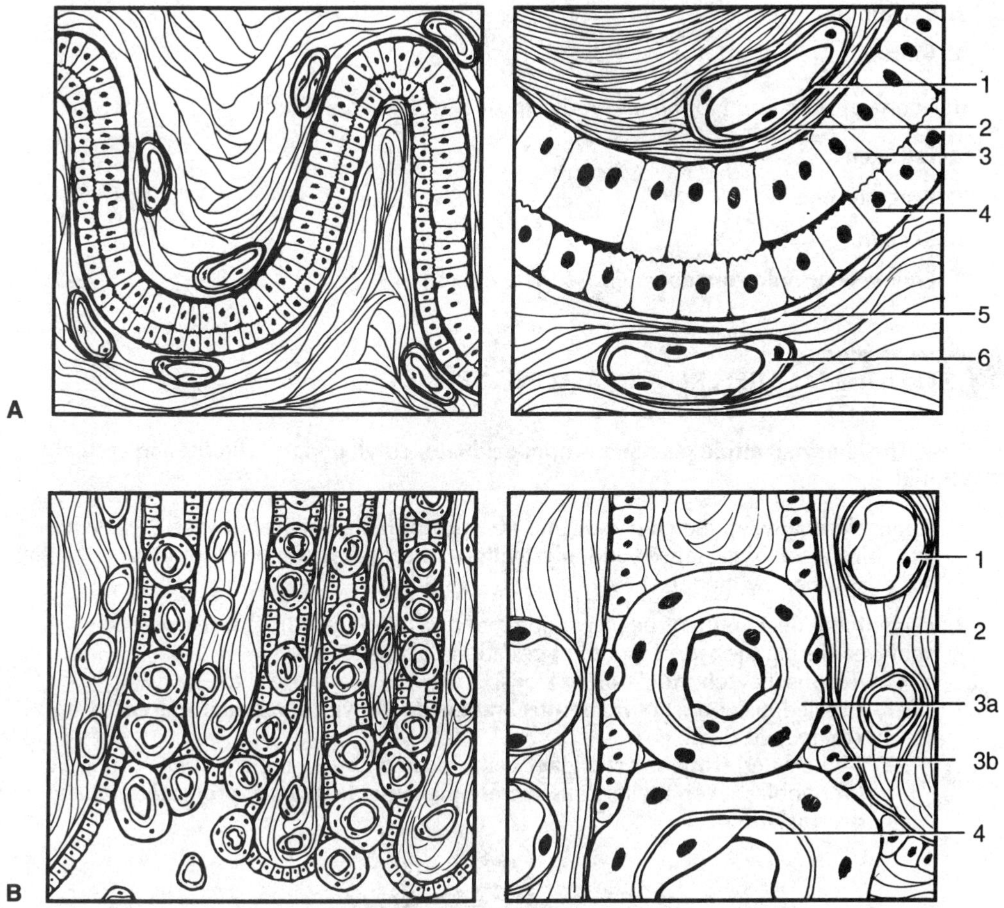

FIGURE 17-3. Schematic drawing of the two types of interhemal placental barriers. (*A*) Epitheliochorial placenta: (*1*) Allantoic capillary endothelium; (*2*) chorioallantoic mesenchyme; (*3*) chorionic (trophoblastic) epithelium; (*4*) uterine epithelium; (*5*) endometrial connective tissue; (*6*) uterine capillary endothelium. (*B*) Endotheliochorial placenta: (*1*) Allantoic capillary endothelium; (*2*) chorioallantoic mesenchyme; (*3*) chorionic (trophoblastic) epithelium, comprising (*3a*) syncytiotrophoblast and (*3b*) cytotrophoblast; (*4*) uterine capillary endothelium. Notice the loss of uterine epithelium and endometrial connective tissue in the endotheliochorial placenta. (Redrawn and modified with permission from Rüsse I, Sinowatz F: *Lehrbuch der Embryologie der Haustiere.* Berlin-Hamburg, Paul Parey, 1991, p 154.)

b. Substances transferred by diffusion include:

(1) Oxygen and **carbon dioxide** (by simple diffusion)

(2) Water and **electrolytes** (by facilitated diffusion along a concentration gradient)

(3) Iron is supplied in **erythrocytes from maternal hemorrhage** in **carnivores** [see V E 2 b (4)] and **ewes** [see V B 2 b (2)], and in **uterine milk** in **sows** (see V C 3).

(4) Sucrose

2. Active transport. Amino acids are among the substances transferred by active transport.

3. Transcytosis. Immunoglobulin transfer occurs via transcytosis, although immunoglobulin transfer is negligible in domestic mammals. Immunoglobulin G (IgG) is the only immunoglobulin that can pass the placental barrier.

B. Fetal waste removal. Substances transferred from fetal to maternal blood include:

1. Urea

2. **Creatinine**
3. **Bilirubin**

C. **Hormone production.** Hormones produced by the placenta include:

1. **Estrogen**
2. **Progesterone**
3. **Relaxin**
4. **Equine chorionic gonadotropin** [see V D 2 e (3)]

V. STRUCTURAL DIFFERENCES AMONG SPECIES

A. **Cow.** The **chorioallantoic placenta** is **nondeciduate, cotyledonary, villous,** and **epitheliochorial.**

1. **Apposition** between the **chorionic** and **uterine epithelia** begins **between the second and third week of gestation,** and **microvillous interdigitations** between these epithelia are established by the fourth week.
2. **Placentome development** begins at one month. Full placentome development is achieved during the fourth month of gestation (Figure 17-4).
   a. **Cotyledons** (i.e., chorionic protrusions)
      (1) Cotyledons consist of **numerous branched villi** with a **vascular mesenchymal connective tissue core.**
      (2) **Binucleated trophoblastic giant cells,** located among the columnar chorionic (trophoblastic) epithelial cells **secrete placental lactogens, progesterone,** and **prostaglandin.**

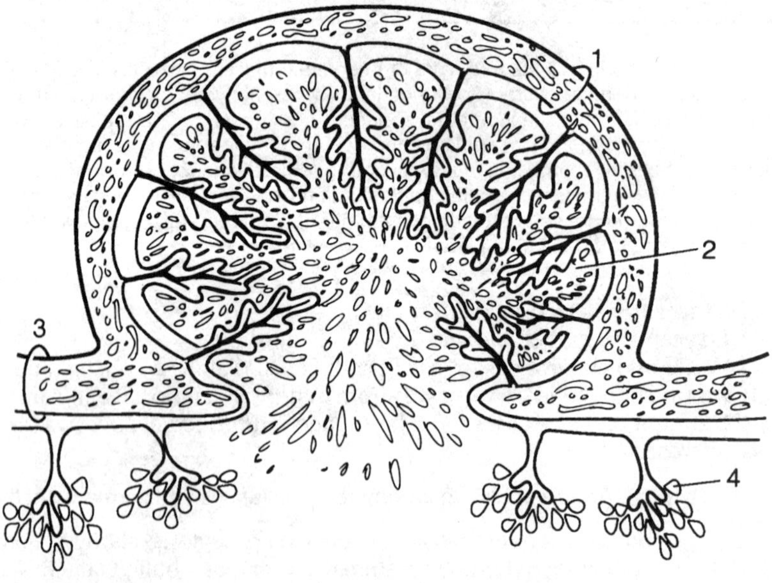

FIGURE 17-4. Schematic drawing of a bovine placentome. (*1*) Allantochorion. Note the vascularized villi, which fit into corresponding caruncular crypts. (*2*) Caruncle with crypts. The connective tissue between crypts is highly vascularized. (*3*) Nonvillous allantochorion. (*4*) Uterine glands, which are present only in the intercaruncular endometrium.

b. **Caruncles** (i.e., endometrial protrusions)
   (1) Caruncles develop **branched crypts** into which the chorionic villi grow.
   (2) **Cuboidal** or **squamous epithelium** and some **binucleated** or **trinucleated giant cells** line the caruncular crypts.

3. **Chorion laeve** adheres to the uterine epithelium between placentomes, except where **areolae** (i.e., spaces containing uterine milk) form above gland openings.

B. **Ewe.** The **chorioallantoic placenta** is **nondeciduate, cotyledonary, villous,** and **epitheliochorial.**

1. **Apposition** (i.e., contact between cell membranes of the chorionic and uterine epithelium) begins **two weeks after fertilization. Microvilli** develop a few days later.

2. **Placentome development**
   a. **Cotyledons** (similar to those in the cow) begin to develop at one month, and full development is reached before three months' gestation.
   b. **Caruncles**
      (1) The epithelium in the crypts forms large **syncytia,** within which isolated, migrated **trophoblastic giant cells** are present.
      (2) **Uterine hematomas** occur in the caruncles between chorionic and uterine epithelia. Chorionic epithelial cells phagocytose maternal erythrocytes to obtain iron for the development of fetal red blood cells.

C. **Sow.** The **chorioallantoic placenta** is **nondeciduate, diffuse, folded,** and **epitheliochorial** (Figure 17-5).

1. **Apposition** between the chorionic and uterine epithelium begins at two weeks' gestation, and **microvillous contact** develops within the next two days.

2. **Macroscopic** and **microscopic folds** develop after three weeks' gestation.

3. **Areolae** are present after one month. Figure 17-6 illustrates a porcine areola.
   a. On the **maternal side,** a smooth endometrial surface surrounds the opening of the uterine glands.
   b. On the **fetal side,** villi project into a central dome-shaped cavity where they absorb uterine milk containing **uteroferrin**. Uteroferrin is the primary source of iron for the fetus.

4. The **interhemal barrier** is reduced to four layers during **advanced gestation,** when the fetal and maternal capillaries invaginate into the chorionic and uterine epithelium, respectively.

D. **Mare**

1. A **choriovitelline placenta** is present before implantation through the first six weeks of gestation.

2. The **chorioallantoic placenta** is **nondeciduate, diffuse, villous,** and **epitheliochorial** (Figure 17-7).
   a. **Implantation.** Chorionic villi develop and **microvillous contact** between the chorionic and uterine epithelium begins at approximately 45 days of gestation.
   b. **Microplacentome development**
      (1) Microplacentomes are formed by microscopic **tufts of chorionic villi** that **fit into corresponding uterine crypts**.
      (2) Microplacentome development is complete after approximately five months' gestation.
   c. **Areolae.** Small areolae are present among the microplacentomes.
   d. **Interhemal barrier.** The interhemal barrier is reduced to five layers in advanced gestation when fetal capillaries invaginate into the chorionic epithelium.
   e. **Endometrial cups** are formed by chorionic cells.

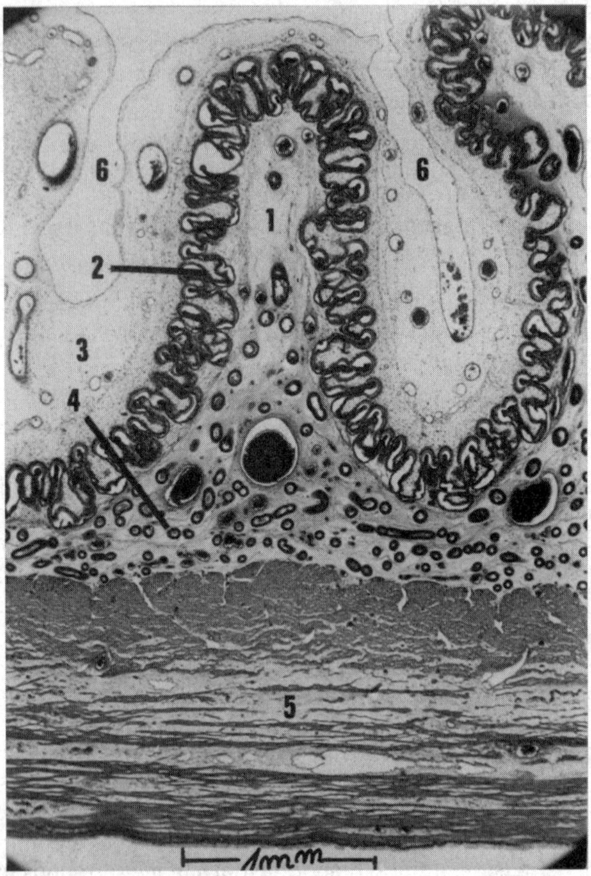

FIGURE 17-5. Section through part of the porcine placenta. (*1*) Macroscopic fold; (*2*) microscopic folds; (*3*) allantochorionic mesenchyme; (*4*) endometrium with glands; (*5*) myometrium; (*6*) allantoic cavity. (From Dellmann H-D: *Textbook of Veterinary Histology,* 4th ed. Baltimore, Williams & Wilkins, 1993, p 263.)

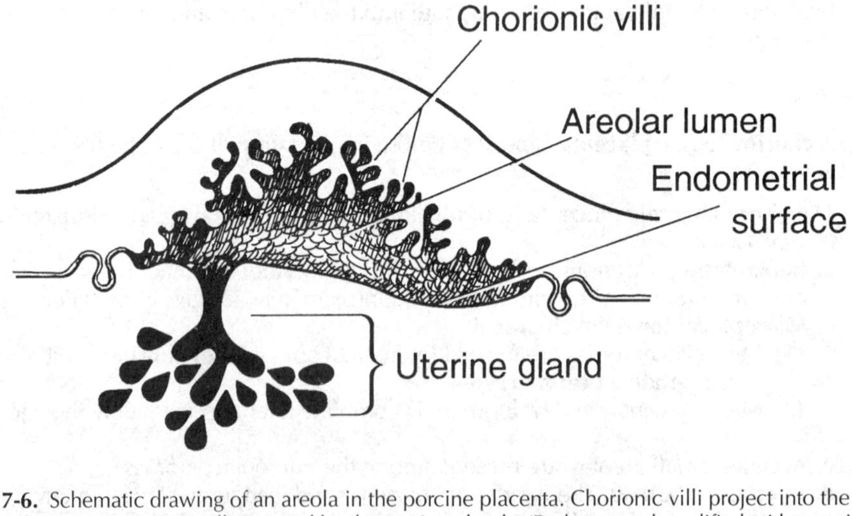

FIGURE 17-6. Schematic drawing of an areola in the porcine placenta. Chorionic villi project into the areolar lumen, which contains uterine milk secreted by the uterine glands. (Redrawn and modified with permission from Rüsse I, Sinowatz F: *Lehrbuch der Embryologie der Haustiere.* Berlin-Hamburg, Paul Parey, 1991, p 182.)

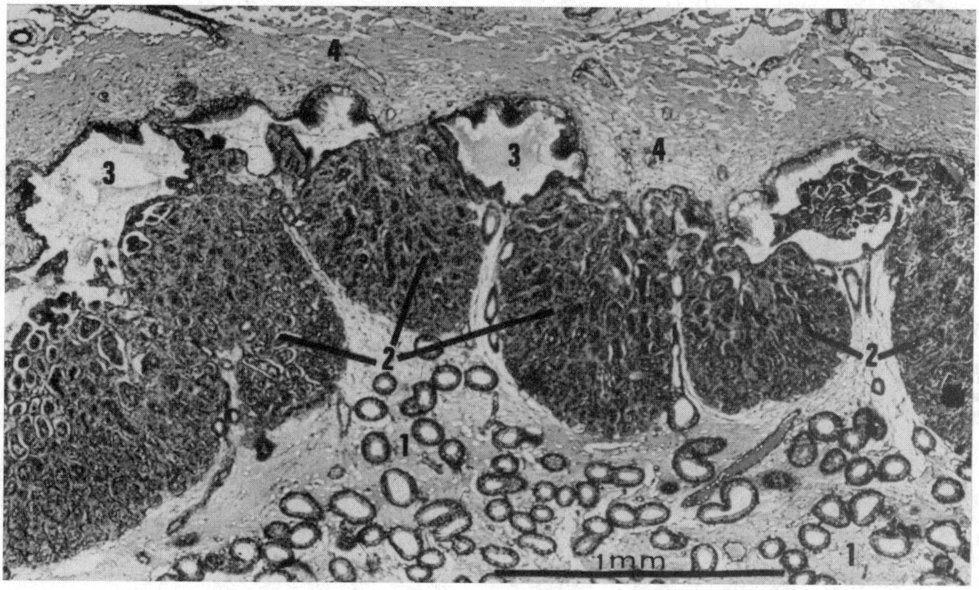

FIGURE 17-7. Section through part of the equine placenta. (*1*) Endometrium with uterine glands; (*2*) microplacentomes; (*3*) areolae (note the uterine glands that open into the areolae); (*4*) chorioallantoic mesenchyme. (From Dellmann H-D: *Textbook of Veterinary Histology,* 4th ed. Baltimore, Williams & Wilkins, 1993, p 261.)

(1) **Origin.** Chorionic cells derive from the annulate **chorionic girdle,** at the junction between the regressing yolk sac and the allantochorion.

(2) **Structure.** Chorionic cells invade the endometrial connective tissue, become hypertrophied and epithelioid, and form clusters (i.e., cups) of variable size.

(3) **Function.** The endometrial cup cells **synthesize equine chorionic gonadotropin,** a hormone that can be detected in the mare's blood between days 40 and 120 of gestation.

(4) **Degeneration.** The endometrial cups begin to degenerate after 80 days, when they detach from the uterine mucosa and are surrounded by chorionic folds to form **allantochorionic pouches**.

E. Carnivores

1. The **choriovitelline placenta** is extensive initially, but eventually disappears. The **yolk sac remains,** however, and functions as an important **hemopoietic organ** through almost two months of gestation. It is still present at parturition.

2. The **chorioallantoic placenta** is **deciduate, zonary, labyrinthine,** and **endotheliochorial** (Figure 17-8).

   a. **Implantation. Chorionic lamellae** (i.e., thin, leaf-shaped projections) penetrate the uterine mucosa before the end of the second week, forming the first contact between the chorionic and uterine epithelium.

   b. **Zone formation**

   (1) The **labyrinth** (so called because of the initial difficulty in distinguishing fetal and maternal components) is the zone of **association** between the **allantochorion** and the **uterine blood vessels**. In this region, the chorion erodes the endometrial epithelium and connective tissue.

   (a) The **fetal component** of the labyrinth is composed of **vascularized lamellae of connective tissue** and **stratified trophoblastic epithelium** [which includes discrete cells (i.e., cytotrophoblast) and fused cells (i.e., syncytiotropho-

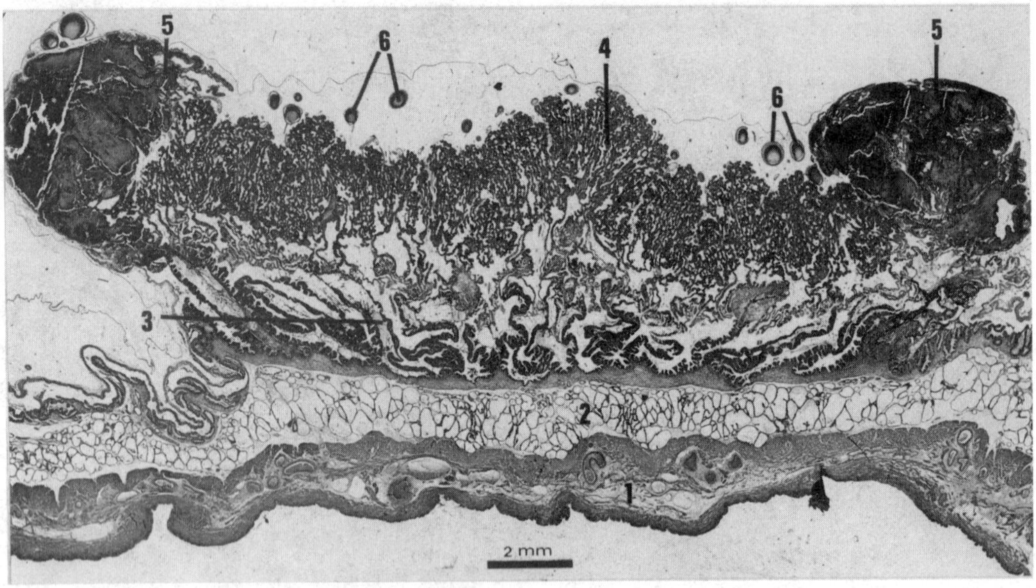

FIGURE 17-8. Cross-section through a canine zonary placenta. (*1*) Myometrium; (*2*) glandular zone; (*3*) spongy zone; (*4*) placental labyrinth; (*5*) marginal hematomas; (*6*) chorioallantoic (fetal) blood vessels. (From Dellmann H-D: *Textbook of Veterinary Histology,* 4th ed. Baltimore, Williams & Wilkins, 1993, p 260.)

blast)]. The trophoblastic epithelium forms an uninterrupted layer in direct contact with the maternal capillaries (see Figure 17-3B).

(b) The **maternal component** of the labyrinth zone is reduced to capillaries lined by cuboidal endothelium and a thick basal lamina–like amorphous layer (see Figure 17-3B).

(2) The **junctional (spongy) zone** is where separation of the placenta and endometrium occurs at parturition.

(a) **Epithelium-covered endometrial lamellae** form when uterine milk accumulates in large spaces and compresses the endometrium.

(b) **Chorionic lamellae** with absorptive trophoblast cells project into the pools of uterine milk.

(3) The **glandular zone** contains the deep portions of the uterine glands; it is separated from the junctional zone by a layer of condensed connective tissue.

(4) **Hematomas.** Hemorrhaging uterine blood vessels give rise to hematomas. **Chorionic villi** project into the hematomas, where they absorb iron for fetal hemopoiesis.

(a) In **bitches,** hematomas are **large** and **occur along the periphery** of the placental girdle; therefore, they are called **marginal hematomas**.

(b) In **queens,** hematomas are small and occur along the periphery, as well as within and outside the placental girdle (i.e., between the chorion laeve and endometrium).

STUDY QUESTIONS

DIRECTIONS: Each of the numbered items or incomplete statements in this section is followed by answers or by completions of the statement. Select the **one** numbered answer or completion that is **best** in each case.

1. Which one of the following statements concerning fetal membranes is correct?

(1) The chorion comprises the trophoblast and associated vascularized mesoderm.
(2) The amnion is a hindgut diverticulum lined by amniotic epithelium and surrounded by vascularized mesoderm.
(3) The allantois is the innermost fetal membrane that encloses the fetus in the fluid-filled allantoic cavity.
(4) The yolk sac is a typical avian feature that is lacking in mammalian embryos.
(5) The trophoblast is an outgrowth from the midgut associated with vascularized mesoderm.

2. In the cow, the definitive placenta is:

(1) choriovitelline, deciduate, cotyledonary, villous, and epitheliochorial.
(2) choriovitelline, nondeciduate, cotyledonary, villous, and epitheliochorial.
(3) chorioallantoic, nondeciduate, cotyledonary, villous, and epitheliochorial.
(4) chorioallantoic, deciduate, cotyledonary, villous, and endotheliochorial.

3. In domestic carnivores, the definitive placenta is:

(1) choriovitelline, deciduate, labyrinthine, and epitheliochorial.
(2) choriovitelline, nondeciduate, labyrinthine, and epitheliochorial.
(3) chorioallantoic, nondeciduate, zonary, labyrinthine, and endotheliochorial.
(4) chorioallantoic, deciduate, zonary, labyrinthine, and endotheliochorial.
(5) chorioallantoic, deciduate, zonary, villous, and endotheliochorial.

4. A chorioallantoic, nondeciduate, diffuse, villous, and epitheliochorial placenta is characteristic of:

(1) cows.
(2) small ruminants.
(3) sows.
(4) mares.
(5) domestic carnivores.

5. Which one of the following *best* describes a placentome?

(1) Cotyledonary villi fitting into caruncular crypts
(2) Caruncular villi fitting into cotyledonary crypts
(3) Interdigitating chorionic and uterine epithelial microvilli
(4) Chorionic villi fitting into uterine crypts
(5) Chorionic villi projecting into areolae

6. A placental labyrinth is *best* described as:

(1) interdigitating chorionic and uterine folds.
(2) chorionic villi fitting into uterine crypts.
(3) chorionic epithelium in contact with blood in marginal hematomas.
(4) chorionic epithelium in intimate contact with uterine blood vessels.
(5) caruncular crypts containing cotyledonary villi.

7. Endometrial cups are *best* described as cup-shaped:

(1) clusters of hypertrophied uterine glandular epithelial cells.
(2) clusters of hypertrophied epithelioid trophoblast cells.
(3) clusters of hypertrophied epithelioid endometrial stromal cells.
(4) clusters of hypertrophied uterine epithelioid cells.
(5) spaces between the chorion and endometrium that contain uterine milk.

ANSWERS AND EXPLANATIONS

1. The answer is 1 *[II A–D]*. The trophoblast forms at the blastocystic stage of development, forming most of the wall of the blastocyst (with the exception of the embryonic disc). When the trophoblast associates with the mesoderm, it forms the chorion. The amnion, the innermost fetal membrane, is formed when the trophoblast folds over the embryo, enclosing it in a fluid-filled cavity (i.e., the amniotic cavity). The allantois is a hindgut diverticulum; the mesenchyme surrounding the allantois fuses with that of the chorion to form the allantochorion. The yolk sac, a midgut diverticulum, is an important fetal membrane in mammalian embryos as well as avian embryos. The yolk sac plays an important role in hemopoiesis and associates with the chorion to form a transitory choriovitelline placenta in all domestic mammals.

2. The answer is 3 *[III A 2; V A]*. The definitive placenta in the cow is chorioallantoic (as it is in all domestic mammals), nondeciduate, cotyledonary, villous, and epitheliochorial. Nondeciduate placentas separate from the endometrium without loss of maternal tissue at parturition. In the cow, a line of interdigitating microvilli joins the uterine and chorionic epithelium; normally, separation occurs along this line. Retained placenta, a frequent complication in cattle, occurs when the microvilli fail to separate. The bovine placenta is characterized by large tufts of villous projections from the chorion (i.e., cotyledons) that grow into caruncular endometrial crypts. In ruminants, all six layers separating the maternal and fetal blood remain intact. Therefore, the bovine placenta is epitheliochorial because the chorionic epithelium is in contact with the endometrial epithelium.

3. The answer is 4 *[III A 2; V E]*. The definitive placenta in carnivores is chorioallantoic, deciduate, zonary, labyrinthine, and endotheliochorial. In carnivores, a part of the endometrium is lost at parturition; thus, the placenta is deciduate. Among the domestic species, only carnivores have an endotheliochorial placenta. It is endotheliochorial because endometrial epithelium and subepithelial connective tissue are eroded by histolytic action of the trophoblast. Because this erosion results in a structure in which structural details are difficult to identify at low magnification, the placenta is termed labyrinthine. In carnivores, the lamellae are located only around the equator of the chorionic sac; therefore, the placenta is classified as zonary.

4. The answer is 4 *[V D]*. The equine placenta is chorioallantoic, nondeciduate, diffuse, villous, and epitheliochorial. The placenta is chorioallantoic in all domestic mammals. It is nondeciduate in all domestic mammals except carnivores. It is diffuse in mares and sows. It is villous in all domestic mammals except sows, and epitheliochorial in all domestic mammals except carnivores.

5. The answer is 1 *[III C 2; V A 2, D 2 b]*. When the chorionic sac becomes apposed to ruminant uterine caruncles, macroscopic tufts of branched chorionic villi, called cotyledons, grow into caruncular crypts. The cotyledon–caruncle unit is called a placentome. Microscopic tufts of chorionic villi fitting into microscopic uterine crypts are present in mares and are referred to as microplacentomes. Uterine caruncles do not possess villi, and the chorionic villi that project into areolae are not designated by a special term.

6. The answer is 4 *[V E 2 b (1)]*. In the carnivore placental labyrinth, uterine blood vessels are in direct contact with the chorion (i.e., the trophoblast), which has eroded the endometrial epithelium and connective tissue. Interdigitating uterine and chorionic folds are present in sows. The association of chorionic villi and uterine crypts, which occurs in mares, is called a microplacentome. In ruminant placentomes, cotyledonary villi fit into the caruncular crypts. No special term designates the chorionic villi that project into the carnivore marginal hematomas.

7. The answer is 2 *[V D 2 e]*. Endometrial cups derive from chorionic or trophoblastic epithelial cells that have migrated into the equine endometrial stroma, where they become hypertrophied and epithelioid. They secrete equine chorionic gonadotropin. Uterine epithelial cells may hypertrophy to form giant cells (e.g., as in cows), but they do not form clusters. Neither endometrial stroma cells nor uterine glandular epithelial cells hypertrophy. Spaces between the chorion and endometrium that contain uterine milk (i.e., the secretory product of uterine glands) are referred to as areolae and commonly occur in mares (between microplacentomes) and sows, where they are particularly prominent. They are sites of uptake of uterine milk by the trophoblast.

Chapter 18

Male Reproductive System

I. INTRODUCTION

A. Components

1. The **testis** includes:
   a. Stroma and interstitial elements
   b. Convoluted seminiferous tubules
   c. Straight seminiferous tubules
   d. Rete testis
2. The **epididymis** is composed of:
   a. Ductuli efferentes
   b. Ductus epididymidis
3. The **ductus deferens**
4. The **accessory glands** include the:
   a. Vesicular gland
   b. Prostate
   c. Bulbourethral gland
   d. Glandular portion of the ductus deferens
5. The **urethra** has three portions:
   a. Prostatic
   b. Membranous
   c. Spongiose (penile)
6. The **penis** comprises the:
   a. Paired corpora cavernosa penis
   b. Corpus spongiosum penis surrounding the urethra
   c. Glans penis
7. The **prepuce**

B. Functions

1. **Spermatozoa production.** Spermatogenesis takes place in the convoluted seminiferous tubules of the testis.
2. **Transport**
   a. Spermatozoa are conveyed through the straight seminiferous tubules, the rete testis, and the ductuli efferentes to the ductus epididymidis.
   b. The ductus deferens transports spermatozoa from the tail of the epididymis to the prostatic urethra. The spermatozoa are conveyed through the urethra to the urethral opening.
3. **Hormone production.** Testicular interstitial cells synthesize and secrete **testosterone**.
4. **Spermatozoa maturation and storage.** In the head and body of the epididymis, the spermatozoa undergo maturation before their storage in the tail of the epididymis.
5. **Fluid secretion.** In the accessory glands, most of the noncellular portion of the ejaculate is produced.

6. **Copulation.** The penis is the copulatory organ, through which the ejaculate is introduced into the female reproductive system.
7. **Protection.** The prepuce provides a protective sheath for the cranial portion of the penis and the glans penis.

II. TESTIS.

TESTIS. The primary functions of the testis are the production of spermatozoa (exocrine function) and the secretion of testosterone (endocrine function).

A. Stroma and interstitial elements

1. The **tunica albuginea** is a capsule of dense irregular connective tissue that surrounds the testis. A **prominent vascular layer** is formed by branches of the testicular artery and a network of anastomosing veins (Figure 18-1).
2. **Septae (septula testis)** subdivide the testis into lobules. They are connective tissue structures that originate from the tunica albuginea.
3. The **mediastinum testis** is an area of loose connective tissue formed by converging septae. It surrounds the rete testis and large blood and lymph vessels.
4. **Myofibroblasts** are cells that form several layers around the seminiferous tubules. Myofibroblasts contract to propel the spermatozoa toward the rete testis.
5. **Epithelioid interstitial endocrine cells (Leydig cells)** form clusters between the seminiferous tubules in the testicular stroma.
   a. These cells **synthesize and secrete testosterone** and resemble other steroid hormone–producing cells.
   b. The cell clusters are abundantly vascularized by sinusoidal capillaries.

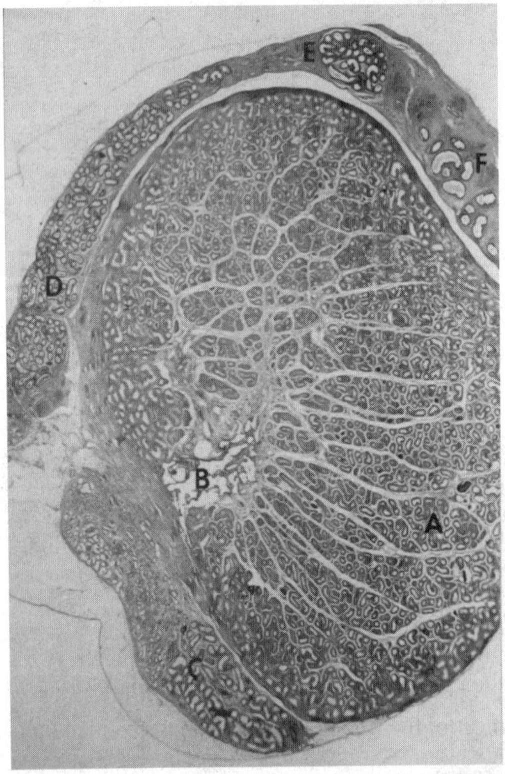

FIGURE 18-1. Low-power micrograph of a feline testis and epididymis. Testicular lobules (*A*) are separated by connective tissue septae that merge with the mediastinum testis surrounding the rete testis (*B*). In the epididymis, a head (*C*), body (*D&E*), and tail (*F*) are distinguished. (Reprinted with permission from Dellmann H-D: *Textbook of Veterinary Histology,* 4th ed. Baltimore, Williams & Wilkins, 1993, p 214.)

B. **Convoluted seminiferous tubules** form loops or begin blindly within the testicular lobules, opening through the straight seminiferous tubules into the rete testis (see Figure 18-1).

1. **Sustentacular cells (Sertoli cells)** line seminiferous tubules.
   a. **Shape.** Sustentacular cells have a broad base containing the nucleus and a highly irregular adluminal (apical) portion. Lateral processes surround spermatogenic cells.
   b. **Cytoplasmic elements.** The cytoplasm of sustentacular cells contains scattered rough endoplasmic reticulum (rER), a Golgi complex, conspicuous smooth endoplasmic reticulum (sER), microfilaments, microtubules, lysosomes, lipid inclusions, and glycogen.
   c. **Functions**
      (1) **Nutrition.** Sustentacular cells provide trophic substances for spermatogenic cells.
      (2) **Phagocytosis.** Sustentacular cells phagocytose cells that degenerate during spermatogenesis, and they phagocytose residual bodies before spermiation.
      (3) **Synthesis and secretion**
         (a) **Androgen-binding protein (ABP)** production is induced by follicle-stimulating hormone (FSH). ABP binds testosterone and maintains a high intratubular concentration of testosterone necessary for spermatogenesis.
         (b) **Inhibin** suppresses adenohypophysial FSH and hypothalamic gonadotropin-releasing hormone (GnRH) synthesis and release.
         (c) **Estrogen** may be secreted in large quantities by **Sertoli cell tumors,** which can cause feminization. Sertoli cell tumors are relatively common in dogs.

2. **Intercellular compartments** (Figure 18-2)
   a. **Spermatogenesis** (see III) occurs in compartments between adjacent sustentacular cells. These compartments contain undifferentiated to mature male germ cells (i.e., spermatogonia, primary and secondary spermatocytes, spermatids, and spermatozoa).
   b. **Tight junctions** between sustentacular cells separate the basal compartment in the tubule wall from the adluminal compartment. Passage of spermatocytes from the basal into the adluminal compartment is believed to occur through temporary zipper-like openings in the tight junctions.
      (1) The **basal compartment** extends from the basal lamina to the tight junction. It contains:
         (a) Spermatogonia
         (b) Preleptotene primary spermatocytes. (Leptotene is an early stage of meiosis.)
      (2) The **adluminal compartment** extends from the tight junction to the lumen of the tubule. It contains:
         (a) Leptotene and older primary spermatocytes
         (b) Secondary spermatocytes
         (c) Spermatids
         (d) Spermatozoa
      (3) A **blood–testis barrier,** formed by the zones of tight junctions, isolates developing spermatocytes in the adluminal microenvironment from blood-borne macromolecules.

3. The walls of the terminal segment of the convoluted seminiferous tubule contain no germ cells. Tall sustentacular cells project into and almost completely obstruct the tubular lumen, requiring spermatozoa to pass through the narrow intercellular spaces to gain access to the straight seminiferous tubules.

C. **Straight seminiferous tubules** are narrow, short tubules lined by simple squamous to columnar epithelium. They connect the convoluted seminiferous tubules to the rete testis.

D. The **rete testis** consists of a network of canals within the mediastinum testis (see Figure 18-1).

1. **Rete testis fluid** is produced by the simple squamous to columnar epithelial lining. This fluid combines with fluid produced by the seminiferous tubules to form testicular fluid.

2. **Myoid cells** surround the channels.

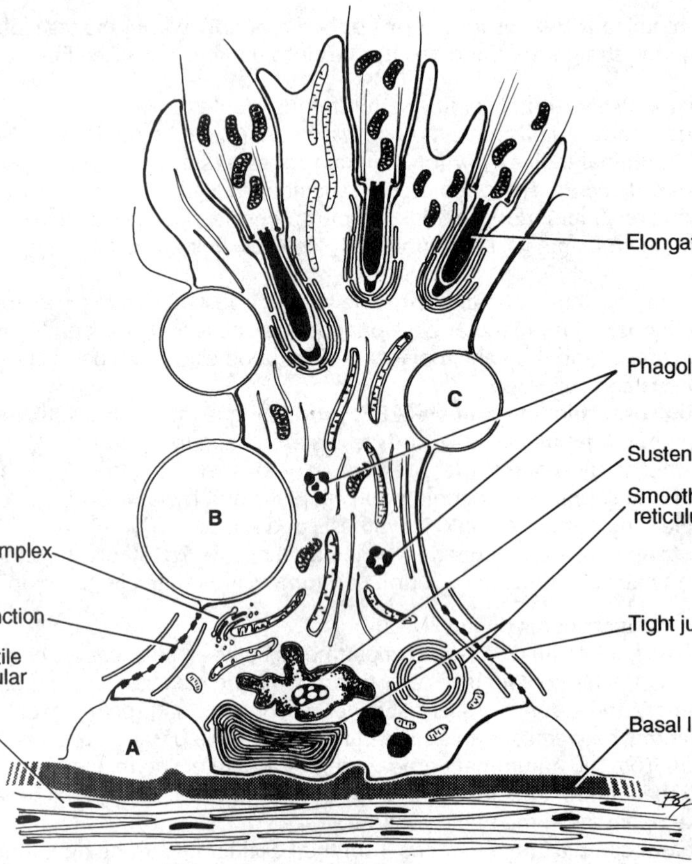

FIGURE 18-2. Diagram illustrating the relationship between a sustentacular cell and germ cells in bulls. (*A*) Space occupied by a spermatogonium. (*B*) Space occupied by a primary spermatocyte. (*C*) Space occupied by a spherical spermatid. (Redrawn with permission from Mosimann W, Kohler T: *Zytologie, Histologie und mikroskopische Anatomie der Haussäugetiere.* Berlin, Blackwell Wissenschafts-Verlag GmbH, 1990, p 210.)

E. Blood supply

1. **Arterial blood supply.** The testicular artery branches extensively within the vascular layer of the tunica albuginea. These branches supply the testicular connective tissue and parenchyma.
2. **Venous blood supply.** Veins from the testis empty into superficial veins in the tunica albuginea.
   - **a.** Together with veins from the epididymis, these veins drain into the testicular vein, which coils around the testicular artery in the spermatic cord to form the **pampiniform plexus.**
   - **b.** Cooler venous blood in the pampiniform plexus cools the arterial blood in the testicular artery to maintain the temperature of the testis below body temperature.

III. SPERMATOGENESIS

A. Spermatogenesis occurs in the convoluted seminiferous tubules of the testis. It is subdivided into **three phases:** spermatocytogenesis (production), meiosis (division), and spermiogenesis (differentiation).

1. **Spermatocytogenesis** transforms stem spermatogonia into primary spermatocytes. This process takes place in the **basal compartment** of the convoluted seminiferous tubules.
   a. **Mitosis of stem spermatogonia.** Each stem spermatogonium gives rise to one A spermatogonium and another stem spermatogonium.
   b. **Mitosis of the A spermatogonium.** Several generations of mitosis form intermediate (I) and B spermatogonia and, ultimately, preleptotene primary spermatocytes. Preleptotene primary spermatocytes undergo DNA replication, producing chromosomes consisting of two sister chromatids.
      (1) **Cytoplasmic bridges** connect all the descendants of one A spermatogonium until shortly before spermiation, permitting synchronous development of clones of cells.
      (2) **Perpetuation.** As preleptotene primary spermatocytes are being formed, stem spermatogonia are dividing and giving rise to A spermatogonia and stem spermatogonia, thus guaranteeing continuity of stem cells and spermatogenesis.

2. **Meiosis.** During meiosis, each primary spermatocyte undergoes two nuclear divisions [referred to as the first and second meiotic (maturation) divisions]. Replication of DNA does not occur before the second meiotic division, so that four haploid (i.e., containing one of each type of chromosome) spermatids result.
   a. **First meiotic division.** After DNA replication, **primary spermatocytes** pass through the tight junctions between sustentacular cells to enter the **adluminal compartment**.
      (1) **Prophase** of the first meiotic division is particularly long, as homologous chromosomes pair and participate in crossing over (i.e., the exchange of corresponding regions of the two sister chromatids of each chromosome).
      (2) **Metaphase** follows, at which time homologous chromosomes align at the equatorial plate.
      (3) **Anaphase** involves movement of the chromosomes to opposite poles of the cell.
      (4) **Telophase** gives rise to secondary spermatocytes, each containing a set of chromosomes consisting of two sister chromatids.
      (5) **Interphase** is short for secondary spermatocytes because chromosomes have already been duplicated.
   b. **Second meiotic division. Secondary spermatocytes** enter the second meiotic division, during which sister chromatids separate and are distributed to each **spermatid,** which consequently has a haploid set of chromosomes.

3. **Spermiogenesis** is the process of differentiation of spermatids into spermatozoa.
   a. Spermiogenesis comprises four phases (Figure 18-3).
      (1) **Golgi phase.** Proacrosomal granules from the Golgi complex fuse to form an acrosomal granule within an acrosomal vesicle.
      (2) **Cap phase.** The acrosomal vesicle expands to become the head cap at the anterior pole of the nucleus, and the Golgi complex becomes less extensive and moves caudad.
      (3) **Acrosomal phase.** The nucleus becomes increasingly dense and elongated.
         (a) **Acrosomal cap (acrosome).** The head cap extends further over the nucleus and becomes entirely filled by the acrosomal granule.
         (b) The cell elongates and orients itself with its head embedded in a recess of the apical cytoplasm of a sustentacular cell and its developing tail directed toward the tubular lumen.
      (4) **Maturation phase.** The middle, principal, and end pieces of the tail develop.
   b. **Spermiation.** Spermatids are released as spermatozoa into the tubular lumen, after the cytoplasmic bridges that link descendants of one proliferating spermatogonium are interrupted. Most of the excess cytoplasm is separated from the spermatozoon, forming the residual body, but some remains as the cytoplasmic droplet around the middle piece.

B. Cyclic events. The **spermatogenic cycle** is the complete sequence of cellular changes that occurs between two consecutive identical stages in a spermatogenic segment.

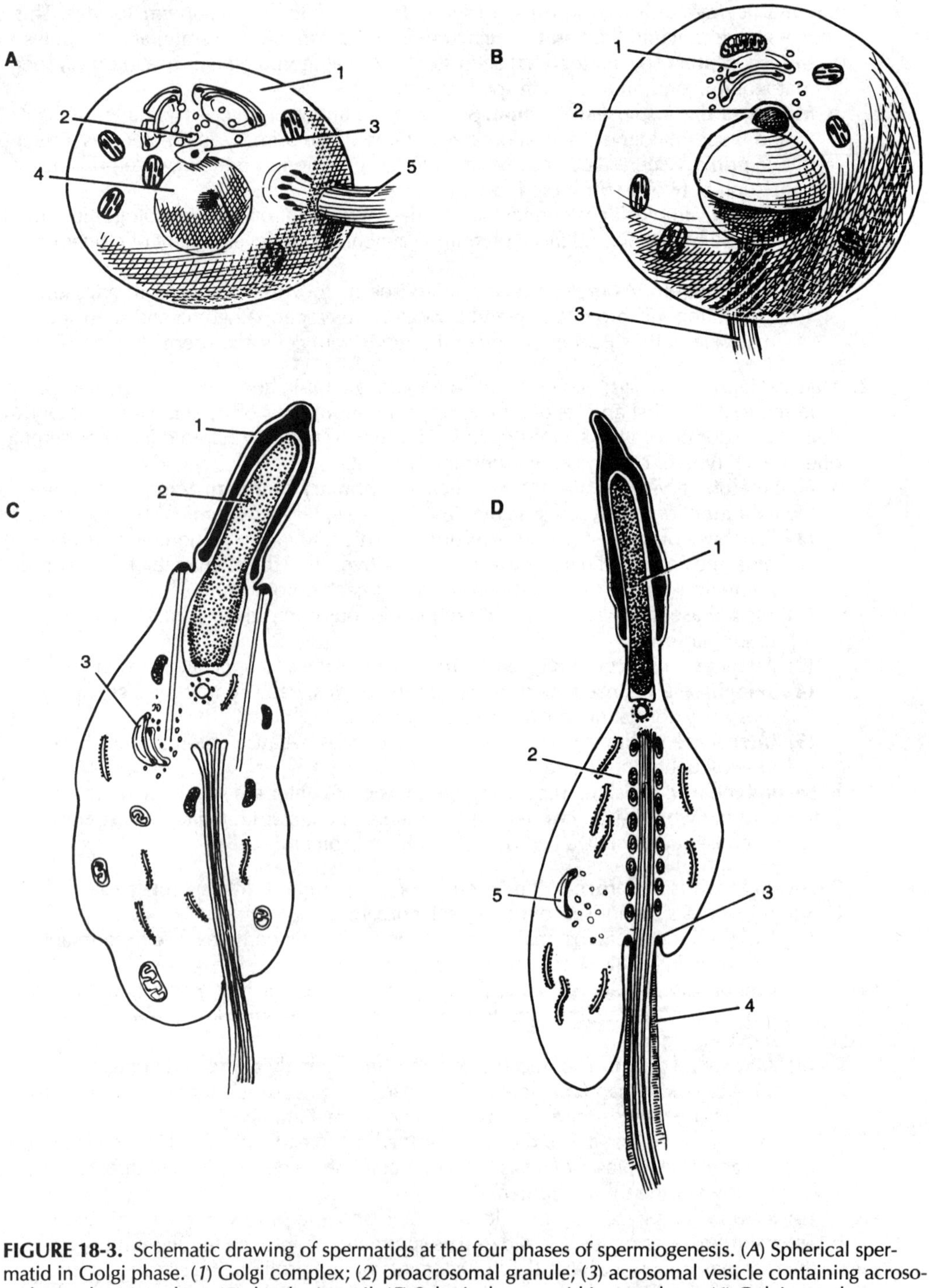

FIGURE 18-3. Schematic drawing of spermatids at the four phases of spermiogenesis. (*A*) Spherical spermatid in Golgi phase. (*1*) Golgi complex; (*2*) proacrosomal granule; (*3*) acrosomal vesicle containing acrosomal granule; (*4*) nucleus; (*5*) developing tail. (*B*) Spherical spermatid in cap phase. (*1*) Golgi complex; (*2*) head cap containing acrosome; (*3*) developing tail. (*C*) Elongated spermatid in acrosomal phase. (*1*) Acrosome; (*2*) nucleus; (*3*) Golgi complex. (*D*) Elongated spermatid in maturation phase. (*1*) Nucleus; (*2*) middle piece surrounded by mitochondria; (*3*) annulus; (*4*) principal piece; (*5*) Golgi complex. (Redrawn with permission from Mosimann W, Kohler T: *Zytologie, Histologie und mikroskopische Anatomie der Haussäugetiere.* Berlin, Blackwell Wissenschafts-Verlag GmbH, 1990, p 212.)

1. Germ cells develop synchronously within a given area of a seminiferous tubule called a **spermatogenic** segment.
2. Because several generations of germ cells develop concurrently, it is possible to observe a species-specific number of **stages** of the spermatogenic cycle within each spermatogenic segment.
3. A **spermatogenic wave** is the sequence of successive stages of the spermatogenic cycle along the length of a seminiferous tubule.

IV. STRUCTURE OF SPERMATOZOA. The spermatozoon consists of a head and a tail.

A. Head

1. The **haploid nucleus** is the major component of the head. Its shape is species dependent.
2. The **acrosomal cap** contains hydrolytic enzymes and proteases (acrosin), and it covers the nucleus.
3. The **postacrosomal sheath** surrounds the base of the nucleus. Dead spermatozoa can be identified because their postacrosomal sheaths stain with eosin or bromophenol blue.
4. **Receptor molecules** that recognize homologous oocytes are located in the postacrosomal cell membrane.

B. Tail

1. The **neck** contains a centriole and nine peripheral coarse fibers that are continuous with the outer fibers of the middle piece.
2. The **middle piece** contains two central microtubules and nine peripheral microtubule doublets surrounded by nine thick outer fibers and spirally arranged mitochondria. It terminates with a thickening of the cell membrane, the **annulus**.
3. The **principal piece** is the longest portion of the spermatozoon and is composed of the microtubular complex, the nine thick outer fibers, and a peripheral fibrous sheath.
4. The **end piece** contains only the microtubules, which lose their characteristic arrangement and terminate at various levels.

V. EPIDIDYMIS. The epididymis is composed of ductuli efferentes and the ductus epididymidis, a coiled tube that lies on the surface of the testis. It is divided into a head, body, and tail.

A. Ductuli efferentes. Several ductuli efferentes in the head of the epididymis connect the rete testis to the single ductus epididymidis.

1. The **epithelial lining** is simple columnar with ciliated and nonciliated cells.
   a. **Ciliated cells** help move testicular fluid and spermatozoa.
   b. **Nonciliated cells** resorb testicular fluid.
2. **Surrounding cells and tissues.** Ductuli efferentes are surrounded by myoid cells and loose connective tissue.

B. Ductus epididymidis. The ductus epididymidis is a long, twisted canal that makes up part of the head, and all of the body and tail of the epididymis (Figure 18-4).

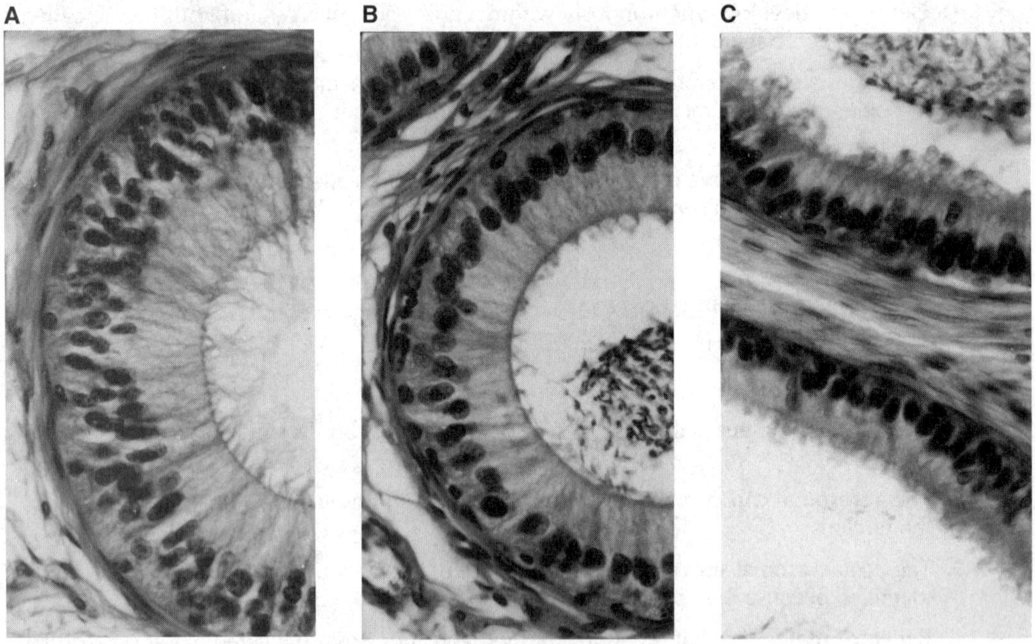

FIGURE 18-4. Micrographs illustrating sections through part of the wall of the feline ductus epididymidis in the (*A*) head, (*B*) body, and (*C*) tail of the epididymis. The pseudostratified columnar epithelium is highest in the head and lowest in the tail. The microvilli are shortest in the tail and longest in the head. Notice the increase in the thickness of the smooth muscle layer from the proximal to the distal sections. (Reprinted with permission from Dellmann H-D: *Textbook of Veterinary Histology,* 4th ed. Baltimore, Williams & Wilkins, 1993, p 222.)

1. **Histologic characteristics**
   a. The **epithelial lining** is pseudostratified columnar, comprising basal cells and columnar principal cells.
      (1) **Basal cells** are small cells of unknown significance.
      (2) **Columnar principal cells** decrease in height from the head to the tail of the epididymis.
         (a) **Resorptive activity** is indicated by apical, long, branching microvilli (stereocilia), pinocytotic vesicles, vacuoles, and multivesicular bodies.
         (b) **Secretory activity** of substances such as glycerophosphoryl choline and glycoproteins is indicated by a large supranuclear Golgi complex.
   b. **Surrounding cells and tissues**
      (1) **Smooth muscle.** The ductus epididymidis is surrounded by a layer of circular or spiral smooth muscle that increases in thickness toward the ductus deferens. Contraction of the muscle propels spermatozoa from the head to the tail of the epididymis.
      (2) **Loose connective tissue**

2. **Functions.** During their passage through the ductus epididymidis, spermatozoa acquire full **fertilization capacity**.*

---

*In some domestic species (e.g., bulls, boars, cats), changes that are necessary for fertilization of ejaculated spermatozoa take place in the female reproductive tract (i.e., **capacitation** takes place).

a. **Maturational changes** in the head and body of spermatozoa include:
   (1) Forward motility development
   (2) Surface receptor activation (necessary for homologous recognition of oocytes during fertilization)
   (3) Cell membrane stabilization
   (4) Cytoplasmic droplet loss

b. **Storage** of spermatozoa in the tail of the epididymis occurs before ejaculation.

VI. DUCTUS DEFERENS.

The ductus deferens (Figure 18-5) links the ductus epididymidis with the urethra, into which it opens at the colliculus seminalis (see VIII B 1 a).

A. The **epithelial lining** is pseudostratified columnar. It includes basal and columnar cells; the latter possess short, branched microvilli in the proximal portion of the duct.

B. The **tunica muscularis** is several layers thick.

C. **Simple branched tubuloalveolar glands** are contained in the **propria–submucosa** of the **terminal portion** in all domestic mammals. Their pseudostratified columnar glandular epithelia also line the wide glandular openings.

1. The terminal portion of the ductus deferens is dilated to form an ampulla in stallions, bulls, and dogs.
2. **Spermatozoa** are commonly present in the lumen and the glandular openings of the terminal portion.
3. **Secretory product.** The glandular portion of the ductus deferens secretes a substance rich in carbohydrates and amino acids.

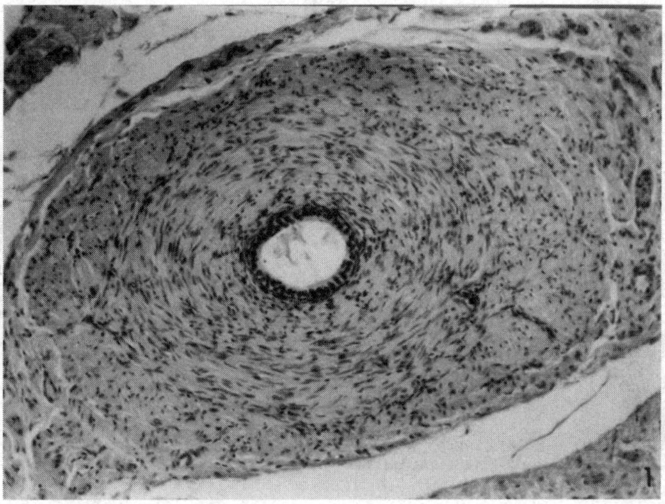

FIGURE 18-5. Cross-section through the feline ductus deferens. The relatively narrow lumen is lined by pseudostratified columnar epithelium and surrounded by several layers of smooth muscle. (Reprinted with permission from Dellmann H-D: *Textbook of Veterinary Histology,* 4th ed. Baltimore, Williams & Wilkins, 1993, p 223.)

VII. ACCESSORY GLANDS. The male accessory glands include the:

A. Glandular portion of the ductus deferens (see VI C)

B. Vesicular gland, a compound tubular or tubuloalveolar gland that is present in all domestic mammals except carnivores

1. **Histologic characteristics**
   a. **Epithelial lining**
      (1) **Gland.** The glandular epithelium is pseudostratified columnar.
      (2) **Ducts.** The ducts are lined by simple cuboidal or stratified columnar epithelium.
   b. **Surrounding tissues.** Loose connective tissue and smooth muscle surround the gland.
2. **Secretory product.** The epithelial secretion of the vesicular gland is rich in fructose, an energy source for ejaculated spermatozoa.

C. Prostate gland, a compound tubuloalveolar gland that is present in all domestic mammals

1. **Portions.** The prostate consists of a **compact external portion** and a **disseminate internal portion**.
   a. The **compact external portion** is absent in small ruminants.
   b. The **disseminate internal portion** is located in the propria–submucosa of the prostatic urethra (Figure 18-6A) in all domestic mammals except stallions.
2. **Histologic characteristics**
   a. **Epithelial lining**
      (1) **Gland.** The glandular epithelium is pseudostratified cuboidal or columnar.
      (2) **Ducts**
         (a) **Initial portions** are lined by pseudostratified cuboidal or columnar epithelium.
         (b) **Terminal portions** are lined by stratified columnar or transitional epithelium.
   b. **Surrounding tissues.** The prostate is surrounded by bundles of smooth muscle and by a capsule from which trabeculae project into the gland.

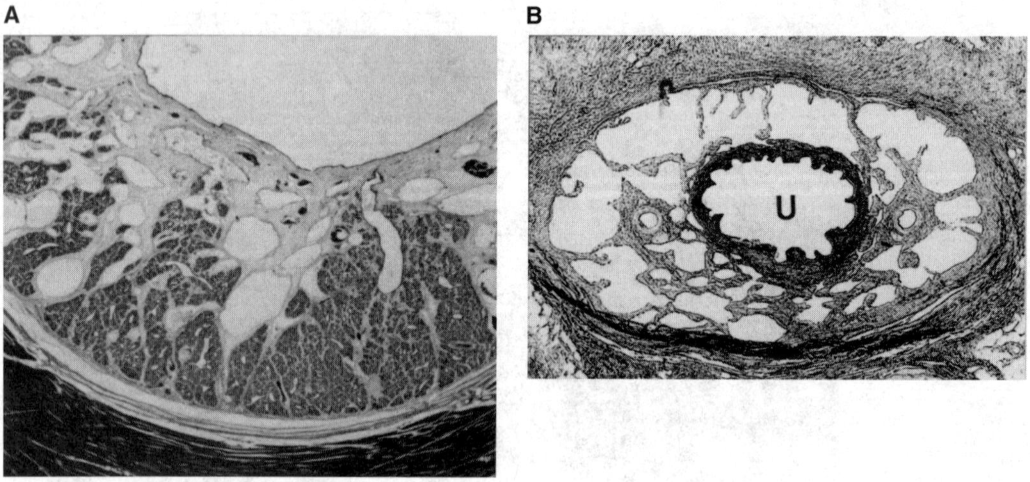

FIGURE 18-6. (*A*) Cross-section through the prostatic urethra of a bull. The propria–submucosa contains a spongiose stratum with caverns extending between the lobules of the internal portion of the prostate. The dark tissue at the bottom of the micrograph is the urethralis muscle. (*B*) Cross-section through the feline spongiose urethra (*U*), in which the propria–submucosa is occupied by the stratum spongiosum. (Reprinted with permission from Dellmann H-D: *Textbook of Veterinary Histology,* 4th ed. Baltimore, Williams & Wilkins, 1993, pp 226, 227.)

3. **Secretory product.** The prostate gland epithelium secretes proteins or mucus, which neutralize seminal plasma and initiate movement of ejaculated spermatozoa.

D. Bulbourethral gland, a compound tubular or tubuloalveolar gland that is present in all domestic mammals except dogs

1. **Histologic characteristics**
   a. **Epithelial lining**
      (1) **Gland.** The glandular epithelium is pseudostratified columnar.
      (2) **Ducts**
         (a) **Initial portions** are lined by pseudostratified cuboidal or columnar epithelium.
         (b) **Terminal portions** are lined by transitional epithelium.
   b. **Surrounding tissues.** The gland is surrounded by a dense, irregular connective tissue capsule containing skeletal muscle fibers.

2. **Secretory product.** The bulbourethral gland epithelium secretes a product that neutralizes the vaginal environment and provides lubrication. In pigs, it contributes to the formation of a postejaculatory cervical seal.

VIII. URETHRA

A. General histologic characteristics

1. The **epithelial lining** of the urethra is mostly transitional epithelium, but patches of stratified columnar or stratified cuboidal epithelium may be present. At the external urethral opening, the lining epithelium is stratified squamous.

2. The **propria–submucosa** is loose connective tissue.
   a. A **spongiose stratum (vascular stratum)** with erectile properties is formed by endothelium-lined caverns surrounded by loose connective tissue.
   b. **Lymphatic tissue.** Diffuse lymphatic tissue is frequently observed. In dogs, lymphatic nodules are present.
   c. **Urethral glands** (simple tubular mucous glands) occur in stallions and cats.

3. The **tunica muscularis** consists of smooth muscle in the vicinity of the urinary bladder and of skeletal muscle (urethralis muscle) in the remainder of the urethra.

B. Regional characteristics

1. The **prostatic urethra** begins at the urinary bladder and extends through the prostate (see Figure 18-6A).
   a. The **colliculus seminalis** is an enlargement formed by a permanent dorsomedian fold, the **urethral crest**. Structures that terminate on the colliculus seminalis are species specific and include:
      (1) Ejaculatory ducts (formed by combination of the ductus deferentes and the ducts of the vesicular glands) in ruminants and stallions
      (2) The ductus deferentes in carnivores
      (3) The ductus deferentes and the ducts of the vesicular glands in boars
   b. The **spongiose stratum** is moderately developed or absent in the prostatic urethra.
   c. The **propria–submucosa** contains the disseminate portion of the prostate in all domestic mammals except stallions.

2. **Membranous urethra.** This portion is located between the prostate and the bulb of the penis.

3. **Spongiose (penile) urethra.** This portion is the cranial continuation of the membranous urethra (see Figure 18-6B).

a. The well-developed spongiose stratum is called the **corpus spongiosum**.
b. The **urethral process** is the termination of the spongiose urethra in stallions and ruminants.

IX. PENIS

A. Corpus cavernosum penis

1. The **tunica albuginea** is a thick collagenous capsule containing many elastic fibers and smooth muscle cells. It surrounds the corpus cavernosum penis and gives rise to a **median septum** and **trabeculae**.
2. **Cavernous erectile tissue** fills the space between the trabeculae (Figure 18-7).
   a. **Caverns** are lined by endothelium and have afferent and efferent blood vessels.
      (1) **Afferent (helicine) arteries** contain longitudinal ridges or pads of smooth muscle in their tunica interna.
         (a) **Erection.** Relaxation of the muscle cells opens the arterial lumen, permitting blood to flow into the caverns.
            (i) Engorgement of these caverns causes erection of the penis.
            (ii) The venules that drain these caverns become increasingly compressed during filling of the caverns, thereby contributing to the maintenance of erection.
         (b) **Detumescence.** In the flaccid penis and during detumescence, these arterial muscle cells are contracted, thereby blocking the flow of blood into the caverns.
      (2) **Efferent venules** drain these caverns.
   b. **Pericavernous tissue** structure varies according to species.
      (1) **Stallions** have a **vascular-type penis,** in which bundles of smooth muscle interspersed with a small amount of connective tissue run parallel to the longitudinal axis of the penis.
         (a) Relaxation of the smooth muscle before urination causes the penis to protrude from the prepuce.
         (b) Relaxation of the smooth muscle and concomitant filling of the caverns with blood cause erection.
      (2) **Ruminants and boars** have a **fibrous-type penis**. Connective tissue predominates, and little or no smooth muscle is present.
      (3) **Carnivores** have an **intermediate-type penis,** in which muscle bundles are less numerous and connective tissue is more extensive than in a vascular-type penis.
3. An **os penis** (in dogs) or an **os glandis** (in cats) is continuous with the cranial corpus cavernosum.

B. Corpus spongiosum (see VIII B 3)

C. Glans penis.

Glans penis. A glans penis is an enlargement of the tip of the penis, present in dogs and stallions. Other domestic mammals lack a glans, but erectile tissue is present in the tip (cap) of the penis.

1. A **tunica albuginea,** from which trabeculae arise, surrounds the glans penis. In stallions, erectile tissue, similar to that in the corpus spongiosum, fills the spaces between trabeculae.
2. A **bulbus glandis** and a **pars longa glandis** compose the glans penis in dogs. These structures consist of large endothelium-lined caverns separated by connective tissue trabeculae rich in elastic fibers.
3. The **tip** of the penis of boars and ruminants consists of fibroblasts and abundant amorphous ground substance. An extensive subepithelial venous plexus is present.

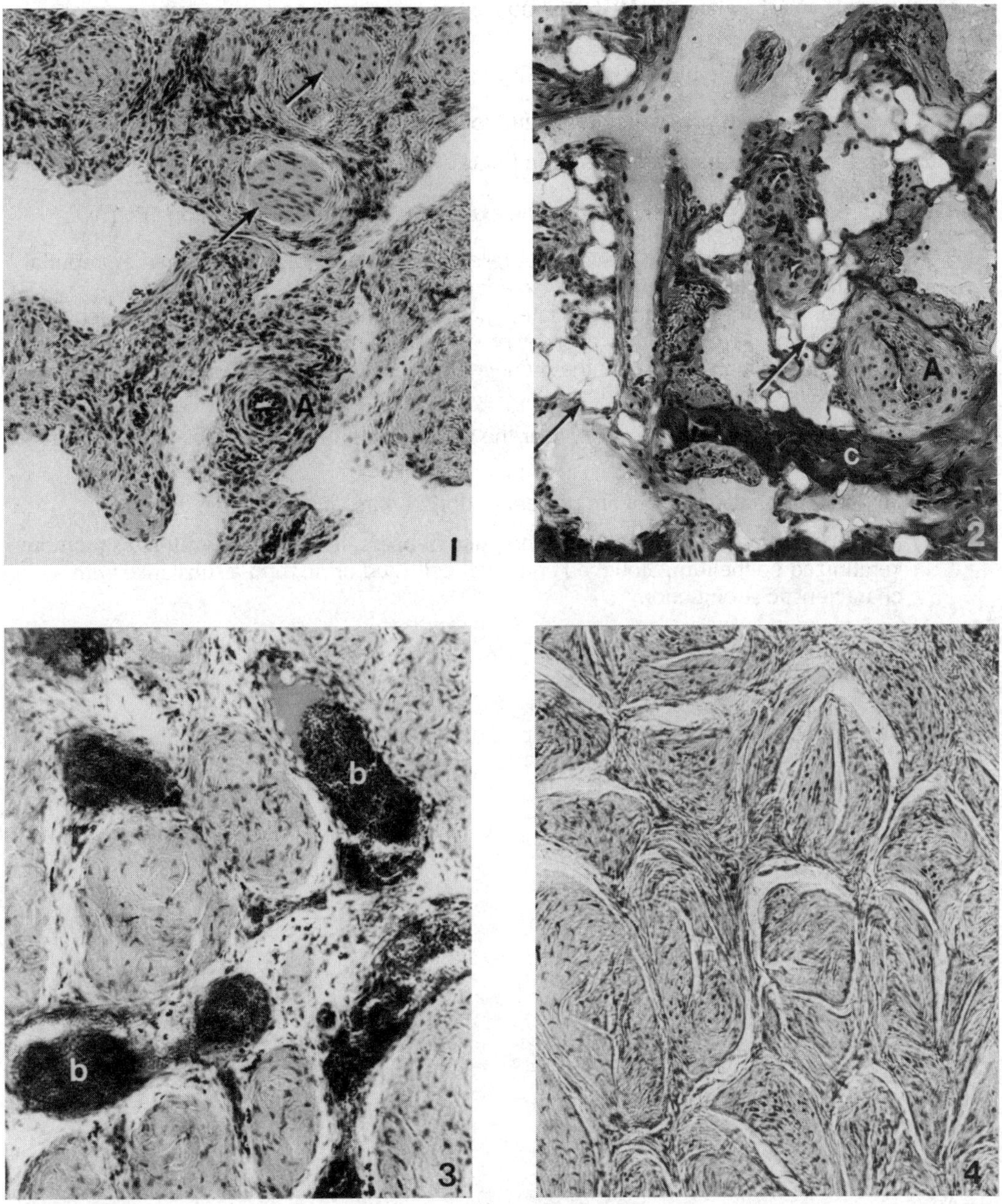

FIGURE 18-7. Corpora cavernosa of stallion, cat, boar, and bull. (*1*) Stallion. In the vascular-type penis of stallions, the pericavernous connective tissue contains bundles of smooth muscle (*arrows*). Notice the presence of a helicine artery (*A*). (*2*) Cat. In the intermediate-type penis of cats, collagen (*c*) predominates in the pericavernous tissue, and adipocytes (*arrows*) are commonly observed. Several helicine arteries (*A*) are visible. (*3*) Boar. In the fibrous-type penis of boars, the pericavernous connective tissue is abundant and virtually lacks smooth muscle. Coagulated blood (*b*) fills the caverns. (*4*) Bull. In the fibrous-type penis of bulls, notice the narrow and empty cavernous spaces and the very abundant pericavernous connective tissue. (Reprinted with permission from Dellmann H-D: *Textbook of Veterinary Histology,* 4th ed. Baltimore, Williams & Wilkins, 1993, p 229.)

X. PREPUCE.

PREPUCE. The prepuce is a tube-like fold of skin that surrounds the cranial portion of the penis and the glans penis. It is composed of an external and an internal layer.

A. The **external layer** is typical skin.

1. **Sebaceous glands** are particularly numerous at the preputial opening.
2. **Long, bristle-like hairs** are present in **boars and ruminants**.

B. The **internal layer** is a continuation of the external layer at the preputial opening.

1. **Fine hairs and associated glands** are present over varying distances from the preputial opening in all domestic mammals except cats.
   a. In stallions, the hairs and associated glands continue throughout the entire length of the internal layer and may even be present in the mucosa of the penis.
   b. **Smegma,** which collects in the prepuce in stallions, is formed when sloughed epithelial cells combine with sebum.
2. Toward the preputial fornix (i.e., near the penis), the skin gradually changes to a **cutaneous mucosa**.
3. **Solitary lymphatic nodules** are present in dogs, boars, and ruminants.
4. A **diverticulum** occurs in the dorsal prepuce of boars. It is lined by stratified squamous keratinized epithelium. Sloughed epithelial cells and urine form a substance with a very characteristic strong odor.

STUDY QUESTIONS

DIRECTIONS: Each of the numbered items or incomplete statements in this section is followed by answers or by completions of the statement. Select the **one** numbered answer or completion that is **best** in each case.

1. Testosterone synthesis takes place in:

(1) sustentacular cells in the convoluted seminiferous tubules.
(2) testicular interstitial cells.
(3) adenohypophysial gonadotropes.
(4) testicular mediastinal cells.
(5) myofibroblasts of convoluted seminiferous tubules.

2. The blood–testis barrier is formed by:

(1) the basal lamina of the convoluted seminiferous tubules and tight junctions between sustentacular cells.
(2) the basal lamina of the convoluted seminiferous tubules and surrounding myofibroblasts.
(3) myofibroblasts surrounding the convoluted seminiferous tubules.
(4) tight junctions between sustentacular cells.
(5) tight junctions between capillary endothelial cells and the capillary basal lamina.

3. Throughout the lifetime of the male, a continuous supply of spermatozoa is available because mitotic division of:

(1) a B spermatogonium gives rise to one B spermatogonium and one primary spermatocyte.
(2) a stem spermatogonium gives rise to one stem spermatogonium and one A spermatogonium.
(3) an A spermatogonium gives rise to one A spermatogonium and one I spermatogonium.
(4) an I spermatogonium gives rise to one I spermatogonium and one B spermatogonium.
(5) a primary spermatocyte gives rise to one primary spermatocyte and one secondary spermatocyte.

4. Which of the following cells are located in the basal compartment of a convoluted seminiferous tubule?

(1) Leptotene and older primary spermatocytes, secondary spermatocytes, spermatids
(2) Preleptotene and older primary spermatocytes, secondary spermatocytes, spermatids
(3) Secondary spermatocytes, spermatids
(4) Stem spermatogonia, A spermatogonia, I spermatogonia, B spermatogonia
(5) Stem spermatogonia, A spermatogonia, I spermatogonia, B spermatogonia, preleptotene primary spermatocytes

5. Which of the following events concerning spermatozoa takes place in the epididymis?

(1) Acrosome elongation
(2) Loss of residual body
(3) Formation of cell membrane receptors
(4) Loss of cytoplasmic droplet
(5) Formation of the middle piece

6. Which of the following is characteristic of the corpus spongiosum of the penis?

(1) It is surrounded by a thick tunica albuginea.
(2) Its arterial blood supply comes from helicine arteries.
(3) It consists of endothelium-lined caverns and pericavernous loose connective tissue.
(4) It contains numerous smooth muscle cells.
(5) Its erectile tissue is compartmentalized by trabeculae.

7. Spermiogenesis is *best* defined as:

(1) the sequence of mitotic divisions of spermatogonia.
(2) the entire spermatogenic cycle.
(3) the differentiation of spermatozoa from spermatids.
(4) the development of spermatids from secondary spermatocytes.
(5) the development of primary spermatocytes into secondary spermatocytes.

8. Which of the following statements *best* describes the structure of the corpus cavernosum of the penis?

(1) A sinusoidal capillary network
(2) Sinuses with afferent arterioles and efferent venules
(3) A network of dilated veins
(4) Helicine arteries supplying a capillary network that drains into endothelium-lined caverns
(5) Endothelium-lined caverns supplied by helicine arteries and drained by venules

9. Flagellar forward movement of spermatozoa:

(1) occurs during spermiation.
(2) moves spermatozoa from the convoluted seminiferous tubules to the rete testis.
(3) begins in the rete testis.
(4) is acquired in the tail of the epididymis.
(5) is acquired during capacitation.

DIRECTIONS: Each of the numbered items or incomplete statements in this section is negatively phrased, as indicated by an italicized word such as *not, least,* or *except.* Select the **one** numbered answer or completion that is **best** in each case.

10. Which of the following events does *not* take place during spermiogenesis?

(1) Formation of the acrosomal cap
(2) Development of the principal, middle, and end pieces of the spermatozoan
(3) Rearrangement of chromatin (crossing over)
(4) Reorientation of the differentiating spermatid
(5) Interruption of intercellular bridges

11. In domestic mammals, spermatogenesis takes place at temperatures slightly lower than body temperature. Which of the following does *not* participate in testicular temperature regulation?

(1) A countercurrent vascular arrangement in the spermatic cord
(2) Superficial veins in the vascular stratum of the testicular tunica albuginea
(3) Testicular location
(4) Veins draining the epididymis
(5) A countercurrent vascular arrangement in the vascular stratum of the testicular tunica albuginea

12. All of the following statements concerning sustentacular cells are correct *except:*

(1) they phagocytose degenerating spermatogenic cells.
(2) they synthesize and secrete androgen-binding protein (ABP).
(3) they synthesize and secrete inhibin.
(4) they phagocytose residual bodies.
(5) they phagocytose cytoplasmic droplets.

ANSWERS AND EXPLANATIONS

1. The answer is 2 *[II A 5 a]*. Testosterone is synthesized and secreted by testicular interstitial cells and bound to androgen-binding protein (ABP), the secretory product of sustentacular cells. Myofibroblasts around the convoluted seminiferous tubules are contractile and help move released spermatozoa toward the rete testis. The cells of the mediastinum testis are nonsecretory, and adenohypophysial gonadotropes secrete follicle-stimulating hormone (FSH) and luteinizing hormone (LH).

2. The answer is 4 *[II B 2 b (3)]*. Each sustentacular cell is linked to adjacent sustentacular cells by a zone of tight junctions that separates the adluminal compartment of the convoluted seminiferous tubules from the basal compartment, thus preventing blood-borne substances from reaching the adluminal compartment. Capillary endothelial cells, the basal laminae of capillaries and seminiferous tubules, and myofibroblasts around convoluted seminiferous tubules do not participate in the blood–testis barrier.

3. The answer is 2 *[III A 1 b 2]*. According to the prevailing opinion, the mitotic division of a stem cell spermatogonium results in one stem cell spermatogonium and one A spermatogonium. The latter undergoes a species-specific number of mitotic divisions that first yield I spermatogonia, then B spermatogonia, and finally preleptotene primary spermatocytes. At that time, the stem cell spermatogonium undergoes a mitotic division and the entire process is repeated, thus guaranteeing a never-ending supply of stem cells. According to another hypothesis, stem cells divide continuously by mitosis to give rise to other stem cells. Cyclically, certain stem cells divide by mitosis to give rise to committed spermatogonia, whose continued mitotic proliferation eventually yields preleptotene primary spermatocytes.

4. The answer is 5 *[II B 2 b (1)]*. All types of spermatogonia and preleptotene primary spermatocytes are located in the basal compartment, peripheral to the tight junctional zone between sustentacular cells. As primary spermatocytes progress through the phases of the first meiotic division, cell membrane characteristics change and, unlike spermatogonia, cells are no longer recognized as "self." Therefore, leptotene and older primary spermatocytes, secondary spermatocytes, and spermatids develop in the protected and unique microenvironment of the adluminal compartment, located above the tight junctional zone.

5. The answer is 4 *[V B 2 a (4)]*. Acrosome elongation and formation of cell membrane receptors and the middle piece are events that take place during spermiogenesis. Before spermiation, the residual body is disconnected from the spermatid and phagocytosed by the sustentacular cells. Not all of the residual cytoplasm is, however, shed before spermiation; some remains as the cytoplasmic droplet around the middle piece of the spermatozoon and is lost during passage through the epididymis.

6. The answer is 3 *[VIII A 2, B 3 a]*. The corpus spongiosum is the erectile tissue that surrounds the urethra. It is particularly well developed around the spongiose (penile) urethra. It consists of endothelium-lined caverns surrounded by loose connective tissue; however, the loose connective tissue does not contain any smooth muscle cells, is not compartmentalized by trabeculae, and is not surrounded by a tunica albuginea. Helicine arteries are characteristic of the corpus cavernosum, not the corpus spongiosum.

7. The answer is 3 *[III A 3]*. During spermiogenesis, which is the last event of spermatogenesis, spermatids differentiate into spermatozoa. Spermiogenesis is preceded by spermatocytogenesis, during which spermatogonia give rise to primary spermatocytes. Spermatocytogenesis is followed by meiosis, during which primary spermatocytes produce secondary spermatocytes (first meiotic division) and secondary spermatocytes produce spermatids (second meiotic division).

8. The answer is 5 *[IX A 2 a]*. The endothelium-lined caverns of the corpus cavernosum are supplied by helicine arteries, which open directly into the caverns, without an intervening capillary network. Caverns are drained by venules. Sinusoidal capillaries are characteristic of endocrine tissues, and blood vascular sinuses occur only in two locations: the spleen and the bone marrow.

9. The answer is 4 *[V B 2 a]*. The flagella of spermatozoa are nonmotile throughout the male reproductive system, but they acquire the capacity for forward movement while the spermatozoa are stored in the tail of the epididymis. Spermiation is the release of spermatozoa from sustentacular cells, primarily by retraction of sustentacular cell processes. The flagellum of the spermatozoon is not yet motile and does not participate in spermiation. The released spermatozoa move toward the rete testis primarily by contraction of the myofibroblasts surrounding the convoluted seminiferous tubules. Capacitation is the process during which spermatozoa acquire their fertilizing capacity in the female reproductive system.

10. The answer is 3 *[III A 2 a (1)]*. Rearrangement of chromatin (i.e., crossing over between chromatids) occurs during the prophase of the first meiotic division. Spermiogenesis, during which spermatids differentiate into spermatozoa, occurs after meiosis. The acrosomal cap (acrosome) is formed, and the differentiating spermatid reoriented, during the third phase of spermiogenesis (i.e., the acrosomal phase), and the principal, middle, and end pieces of the spermatozoon develop during the next phase, the maturation phase. Before the spermatids are released as spermatozoa into the tubular lumen, the intercellular bridges that link descendants of one spermatogonium are severed.

11. The answer is 5 *[II E]*. For spermatogenesis to proceed normally in domestic mammals, testicular temperature has to be lower than body temperature. The superficial location of the testis in the scrotum, the relaxation and contraction of the smooth muscle in the tunica dartos of the scrotum at high and low external temperatures (respectively), the extensive superficial venous plexus in the vascular layer of the testicular tunica albuginea, the veins draining the epididymis, and the venous pampiniform plexus around the testicular artery in the spermatic cord all contribute to maintaining the testicular temperature below body temperature.

12. The answer is 5 *[II B 1 c]*. Cytoplasmic droplets are residual cytoplasm that remains around the middle pieces of the spermiated (released) spermatozoa until their passage through the epididymis, where the droplets are phagocytosed by epididymal cells. Among the various functions of sustentacular cells are the phagocytosis of residual bodies that become detached from the spermatids before spermiation and phagocytosis of spermatogenic cells that degenerate during the course of their development. They also synthesize and secrete androgen-binding protein (ABP), which binds testosterone and establishes and maintains the high intratubular concentration of that hormone necessary for spermatogenesis. Sustentacular cells also synthesize and secrete inhibin, which inhibits follicle-stimulating hormone (FSH) production by adenohypophysial gonadotropes and gonadotropin-releasing hormone (GnRH) by hypothalamic neurons through a negative feedback process.

Chapter 19

Endocrine System

I. INTRODUCTION

A. Components. The endocrine system comprises **endocrine organs, groups of endocrine cells within nonendocrine organs,** and **single endocrine cells within nonendocrine organs**.

1. **Endocrine organs** include the following glands:
   a. Hypophysis
   b. Pineal gland
   c. Thyroid gland
   d. Parathyroid gland
   e. Adrenal gland
2. **Groups of endocrine cells** within nonendocrine organs comprise:
   a. Hypothalamic neurosecretory neurons
   b. Pancreatic islets
   c. Theca interna in the ovary
   d. The corpus luteum in the ovary
   e. Granulosa cells in the ovary
   f. Ovarian interstitial cells
   g. Testicular interstitial cells
   h. Atrial cardiac muscle cells
3. **Single endocrine cells** are present in the lining epithelium of the glandular stomach, intestine, and trachea (see Chapters 13 and 14).

B. Function

1. **Hormone production.** Hormones are substances that are secreted into the extracellular space; from there, they enter the vascular or lymphatic system.
   a. Effects of hormones
   (1) Most frequently, hormones exert their influence on distant cells or on specific tissues or organs (**target organs**).
   (2) Hormones may also act locally, in a **paracrine** manner.
   b. Types of hormones
   (1) Proteins or glycoproteins (e.g., adenohypophysial hormones, thyroxine)
   (2) Steroids (e.g., testosterone, progesterone)
   (3) Biogenic amines (e.g., epinephrine, serotonin)
   (4) Peptides [antidiuretic hormone (ADH), cholecystokinin (CCK)]
2. The endocrine and the nervous systems often work closely together—many of their functions are linked, coordinated, and, occasionally, integrated.

II. ENDOCRINE ORGANS

A. Hypophysis. The hypophysis has two embryologically and morphologically distinct portions, the adenohypophysis and the neurohypophysis (Figure 19-1).

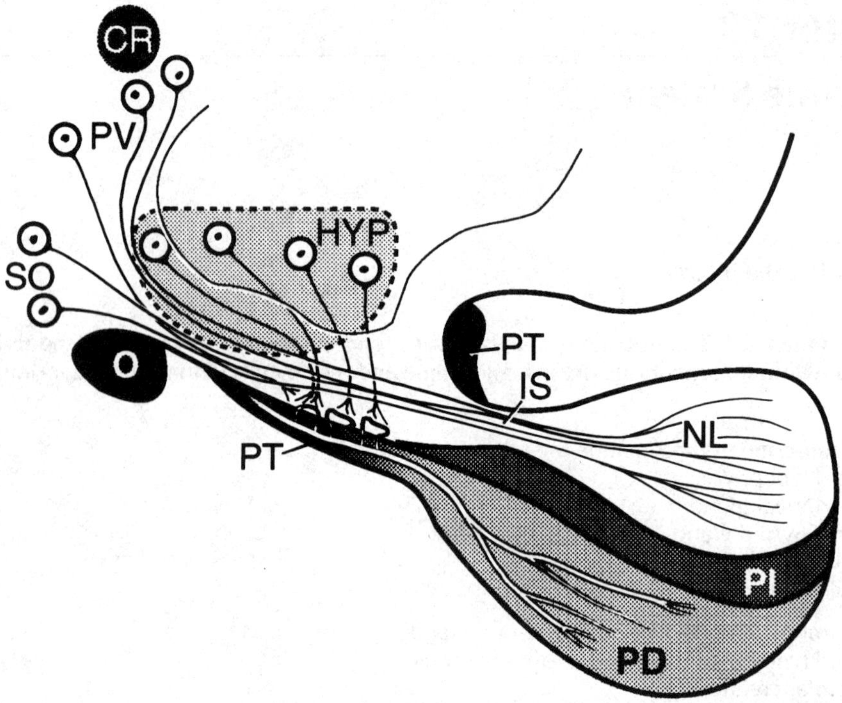

FIGURE 19-1. Schematic drawing of a midline sagittal section through the basal hypothalamus and hypophysis. The *dotted line* delineates the hypophysiotropic area of the hypothalamus (*HYP*). Axons from the neurons in this area terminate at the primary capillaries of the hypophysial portal system in the external zone of the median eminence. Releasing or inhibiting hormones are released into these capillaries and reach the secondary capillaries in the pars distalis (*PD*) of the adenohypophysis through portal venules that traverse the pars tuberalis (*PT*) of the adenohypophysis. Oxytocin and antidiuretic hormone (ADH) are synthesized in the hypothalamic supraoptic (*SO*) and paraventricular (*PV*) nuclei and transported by way of axons through the infundibular stalk (*IS*) to their site of release from axon terminals in the neural lobe (*NL*). *CR* = rostral commissure; *O* = optic chiasm; *PI* = pars intermedia. (Redrawn with permission from Dellmann H-D: *Textbook of Veterinary Histology,* 4th ed. Baltimore, Williams & Wilkins, 1993, p 271.)

1. **Adenohypophysis.** The adenohypophysis is derived from the epithelium of the pharynx.
   a. **Structure.** The adenohypophysis comprises three parts: the pars distalis (anterior lobe), the pars intermedia (intermediate lobe), and the pars tuberalis (tuberal lobe).
      (1) **Pars distalis.** The anterior lobe is the largest lobe, consisting of clusters and cords of cells: acidophils, basophils, and chromophobes (Figure 19-2). The cells are surrounded by delicate connective tissue and vascularized by a dense network of sinusoidal capillaries.
         (a) **Acidophils** contain eosinophilic granules. Two cell types may be distinguished using immunohistochemical staining methods.
            (i) **Somatotropes** give a positive staining reaction for somatotropin, a protein hormone.
            (ii) **Lactotropes** give a positive staining reaction for prolactin, a protein hormone.
         (b) **Basophils** secrete glycoprotein hormones and, therefore, give a strong periodic acid-Schiff (PAS) reaction. There are three types of basophils.
            (i) **Gonadotropes** give a positive immune reaction for follicle-stimulating hormone (FSH) and luteinizing hormone (LH).
            (ii) **Thyrotropes** give a positive immune reaction for thyroid-stimulating hormone (TSH).

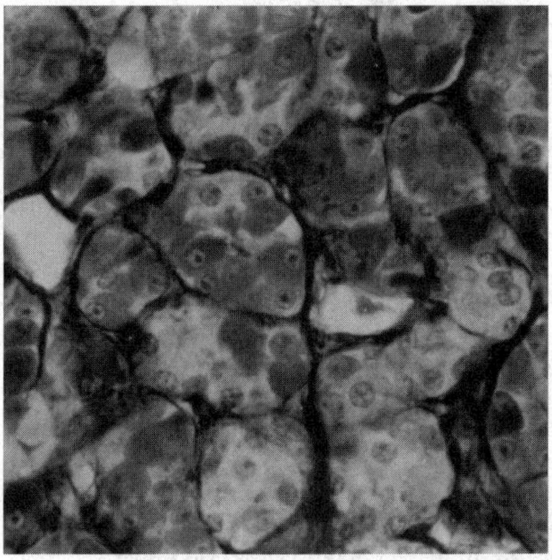

FIGURE 19-2. In this micrograph of the pars distalis of the bovine adenohypophysis, both basophils (*dark-staining cells*) and acidophils (*light-staining cells*) are present in most cell clusters. (Reprinted with permission from Dellmann H-D: *Textbook of Veterinary Histology,* 4th ed. Baltimore, Williams & Wilkins, 1993, p 272.)

(iii) **Corticotropes** give a positive immune reaction for adrenocorticotropic hormone (ACTH) and β-lipoprotein (β-LPH).

(c) **Chromophobes** comprise three cell types.

(i) The most numerous chromophobic cells are considered to be a **resting, degranulated form of all chromophilic cells**.

(ii) **Follicular cells** line follicles of unknown significance.

(iii) **Stellate cells** are also of unknown significance and are scattered among the other cells of the pars distalis.

(2) **Pars intermedia.** The intermediate lobe is located adjacent to the neural lobe of the neurohypophysis. In most domestic mammals, the pars intermedia is separated from the pars distalis by the **hypophysial cleft**. The pars intermedia is poorly vascularized. Its cells frequently form small, colloid-filled follicles.

(a) **Melanotropes,** the principal cell type of the pars intermedia, give a positive immune reaction for melanocyte-stimulating hormone (MSH) and, in some species, for lipotropin (LPH).

(b) **Other cell types** are subject to great variation among species and include:

(i) Typical cells of the pars distalis

(ii) Follicular cells

(iii) Stellate cells

(iv) Cells lining the hypophysial cleft

(3) **Pars tuberalis.** The tuberal lobe completely surrounds the median eminence of the neurohypophysis and consists of clusters of epithelial cells and numerous hypophysial portal venules.

(a) **Typical pars tuberalis cells** contain **secretory granules** of unknown significance.

(b) A few **gonadotropes** and **thyrotropes** commonly occur in the pars tuberalis.

b. **Hypothalamo-adenohypophysial system.** The hypothalamo-adenohypophysial system is a functional unit formed by the adenohypophysis and the hypophysiotropic region of the hypothalamus.

(1) **Components of the hypothalamo-adenohypophysial system**

(a) **Neuronal component** (i.e., the hypophysiotropic region of the hypothalamus and the median eminence)

(i) **Neurosecretory cells** are located in the hypophysiotropic area of the hypothalamus.

(ii) The **neuronal perikarya** synthesize **releasing and inhibiting hormones and factors** that control the release of specific adenohypophysial hormones [see II A 1 b (2) (b)].

(iii) These substances are transported intraaxonally to **pericapillary axon terminals** in the external zone of the median eminence, where they are released and enter the primary capillaries of the hypophysial portal system.

(b) **Vascular component.** The **hypophysial portal system** is the link between the pericapillary axon terminals in the median eminence and the pars distalis. It has three components.

(i) **Primary capillaries** form loops in the external zone of the median eminence. These loops are supplied by branches of the arterial circle of the brain.

(ii) **Portal venules** pass through the pars tuberalis from the primary capillaries to the pars distalis.

(iii) **Secondary capillaries** form a plexus that permeates the pars distalis.

(c) **Glandular component.** The **pars distalis** and **pars intermedia** of the adenohypophysis form the glandular component of the hypothalamo-adenohypophysial system.

(2) **Functions**

(a) **Adenohypophysial hormones**

(i) **Somatotropin** promotes postnatal growth. Hyposecretion causes dwarfism, and hypersecretion induces gigantism in young animals and acromegaly (enlargement of the extremities and head) in adults.

(ii) **Prolactin** stimulates development of the mammary gland before lactation and causes milk secretion in the lactating animal.

(iii) **FSH** stimulates spermatocytogenesis and meiosis in the male and growth of ovarian follicles in the female.

(iv) **LH** is required for spermiogenesis and synthesis and release of testosterone in the male. It is required for maturation of ovarian follicles, estrogen secretion, ovulation (together with FSH), corpus luteum development, and progesterone secretion in the female.

(v) **TSH** induces synthesis and release of the thyroid hormones thyroxine [tetraiodothyronine (T_4)] and triiodothyronine (T_3).

(vi) **ACTH** regulates the secretion of glucocorticoids in the zona fasciculata and zona reticularis of the adrenal cortex.

(vii) **MSH** provokes melanosome dispersion in amphibians. In mammals, there is evidence that it causes pigmentation of hair and that it plays a role in fetal growth, learning, and memory.

(b) **Control of adenohypophysial hormone release.** The following hormones and factors released by the hypothalamus control the release of adenohypophysial hormones:

(i) Somatotropin-releasing hormone (SRH)
(ii) Somatostatin (SST) [inhibitory]
(iii) Prolactin-releasing factor (PRF)
(iv) Prolactin-inhibiting factor (PIF)
(v) Thyrotropin-releasing hormone (TRH)
(vi) Gonadotropin-releasing hormone (GnRH)
(vii) Corticotropin-releasing hormone (CRH)
(viii) Melanotropin-inhibiting factor

2. **Neurohypophysis.** The neurohypophysis is derived from the basal hypothalamus, to which it remains intimately connected, both morphologically and functionally, in the hypothalamo-neurohypophysial system.

a. **Components of the hypothalamo-neurohypophysial system**

(1) **Hypothalamic component**

(a) **Magnocellular secretory neurons** in the hypothalamic paraventricular and supraoptic magnocellular nuclei synthesize and secrete a variety of biologically active substances. These nuclei are the major sites of synthesis of the polypeptide hormones:

(i) **Oxytocin**
(ii) **Antidiuretic hormone (ADH),** also called **vasopressin** (Figure 19-3)

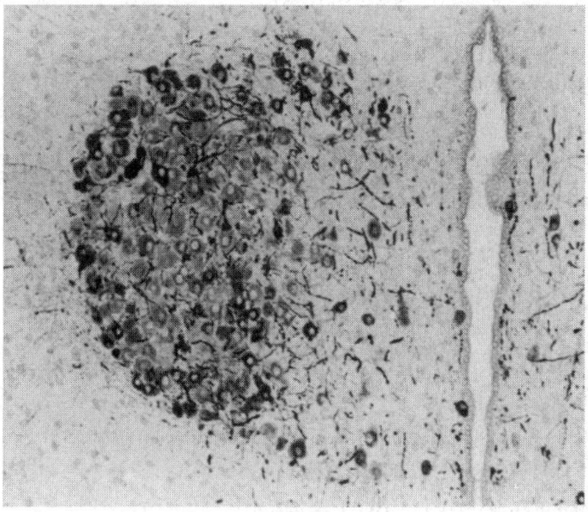

FIGURE 19-3. These cells in the hypothalamic paraventricular nucleus of the rat show a positive immune reaction for antidiuretic hormone (ADH). (Reprinted with permission from Dellmann H-D: *Textbook of Veterinary Histology,* 4th ed. Baltimore, Williams & Wilkins, 1993, p 276.)

(b) **Neurosecretory granules** contain these hormones, which are synthesized within separate neuronal perikarya.

(c) **Axons** convey the neurosecretory granules through the hypothalamo-neurohypophysial tract to their site of release in the neural lobe.

(2) **Neurohypophysial component.** The neurohypophysial portion has three parts—the median eminence, the infundibular stalk, and the neural lobe—each of which is composed of axons and pituicytes (supporting glial cells).

(a) **Median eminence and infundibular stalk.** The hypothalamo-neurohypophysial tract traverses the internal zone of the median eminence, passing through the infundibular stalk on its way to the neural lobe. The median eminence and infundibular stalk are primarily sites of axon passage.

(b) **Neural lobe.** The neurosecretory axons branch repeatedly in the neural lobe. Their pericapillary terminals (at sinusoidal capillaries) are sites of storage and release of neurosecretory granules.

b. Neurohypophysial hormones

(1) ADH

(a) **Function.** ADH renders the distal convoluted tubules and collecting ducts in the kidney permeable to water, increasing **water conservation**. Lack of ADH causes **diabetes insipidus,** which is characterized by increased urine output, decreased urine osmolarity, and increased water consumption.

(b) **ADH release** is triggered by a variety of stimuli related to body fluid balance (e.g., hypovolemia, decreased blood pressure, and increased plasma osmolarity).

(2) Oxytocin

(a) **Functions**

(i) Oxytocin induces **milk ejection** (milk let-down) by causing contraction of myoepithelial cells in the mammary gland.

(ii) During parturition, oxytocin causes **uterine muscular contractions**.

(b) **Oxytocin release** is caused by mechanical stimulation of the teat or the uterine cervix.

(3) A number of substances [e.g., acetylcholine (ACh), enkephalin, dynorphin, galanin, and other peptides] coexist with ADH or oxytocin and appear to modulate the release of these hormones.

B. Pineal gland.

B. Pineal gland. The mammalian pineal gland is derived from the dorsal diencephalon, to which it is attached by a stalk.

1. Structure

a. Connective tissue. The pineal gland is surrounded by pial connective tissue, which penetrates the gland to form trabeculae and septa that incompletely subdivide the parenchyma into lobules.

b. **Cells**
   (1) **Pinealocytes,** epithelioid secretory cells with numerous processes, are derived from glial cells. They frequently establish perivascular contacts with sinusoidal capillaries.
   (2) **Astrocytes** surround individual pinealocytes or groups of pinealocytes.

c. **Corpora arenacea** (i.e., intercellular calcium deposits) are frequently observed. Their significance is unknown.

2. **Function. Melatonin** is the main secretory product of the pinealocytes.
   a. **Melatonin secretion.** Melatonin synthesis and release are stimulated by the **dark phase of the photoperiod**.
      (1) The hypothalamic suprachiasmatic nuclei relay information about light from the retina to the cranial cervical ganglia.
      (2) Postganglionic fibers from the ganglia convey stimulatory impulses to the pinealocytes through synaptic contact.
   b. **Functions of melatonin.** In a variety of laboratory animals, melatonin is known to participate in **circadian** and **photoperiod-induced rhythms, sexual behavior, reproduction,** and **thermoregulation**. Its action in domestic mammals is still unclear.

C. Thyroid gland

1. **Structure.** The thyroid gland is surrounded by a connective tissue capsule from which thin septa or trabeculae subdivide the gland into irregular lobules. Within the lobules, **follicles** and **parafollicular cells** are well vascularized by sinusoidal capillaries.
   a. **Thyroid follicles** are complete spheres lined by simple epithelium, which consists of follicular epithelial cells (Figure 19-4). The follicles contain colloid.
      (1) **Thyroid follicular cells** vary in height, depending on physiological conditions.
         (a) **Resting.** Follicular epithelial cells are simple squamous or low cuboidal when at rest.
         (b) **Stimulated.** Follicular epithelial cells become high cuboidal to columnar and possess a distinct structural polarity when stimulated by TSH.
            (i) The spherical nucleus in the cell base is surrounded by abundant rough endoplasmic reticulum (rER) and numerous mitochondria.
            (ii) A large Golgi complex lies between the nucleus and the apical cell surface.
            (iii) Abundant secretory vesicles are located in the apical cytoplasm, containing:
               Thyroglobulin, a glycoprotein
               Endocytic, colloid-containing vesicles

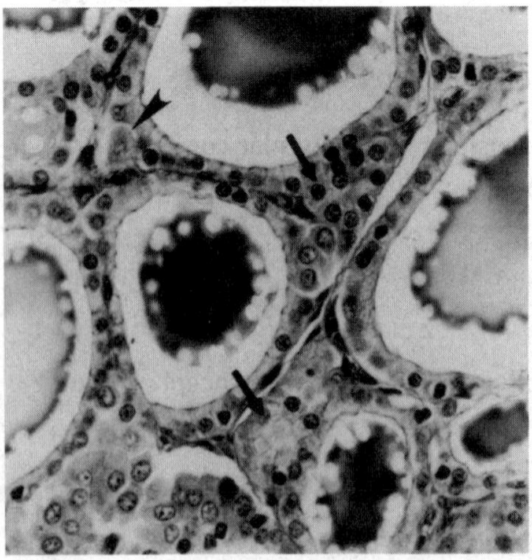

FIGURE 19-4. These thyroid follicles, lined with simple cuboidal to columnar epithelium, contain colloid. The space between follicular epithelium and colloid is an artifact, and the vacuoles in the colloid are considered to be indicative of colloid uptake. The *arrows* point to two groups of parafollicular cells; each *arrowhead* specifically points to a single parafollicular cell. (Reprinted with permission from Dellmann H-D: *Textbook of Veterinary Histology,* 4th ed. Baltimore, Williams & Wilkins, 1993, p 278.)

Lysosomes
Phagolysosomes

(iv) Apical junctional complexes join adjacent cells.

(2) **Thyroid colloid** is a suspension of iodinated thyroglobulin.

(a) Thyroglobulin is the **storage form** of the thyroid hormones T_4 and T_3.

(b) Thyroglobulin is **amphoteric** (i.e., it stains with either acid or basic dyes, depending on the pH).

b. **Parafollicular cells,** also called **C cells,** are derived from the neural crest.

(1) Parafollicular cells occur singly or in groups between follicular epithelial cells and the surrounding basal lamina; they also occur as isolated groups between follicles, surrounded by their own basal lamina (see Figure 19-4).

(2) Parafollicular cells contain many mitochondria, a well-developed rER, an extensive Golgi complex, and numerous secretory vesicles that contain **calcitonin (thyrocalcitonin)**.

2. Functions

a. **Thyroid hormone synthesis and release** are controlled by TSH. Thyroid hormones increase metabolic activities in almost all organs and tissues.

(1) **Thyroid hormone synthesis**

(a) **Thyroglobulin** is synthesized in the rER and Golgi complex of the thyroid follicular cells and secreted into the follicular lumen.

(b) **Thyroperoxidase** is also synthesized and secreted into the follicular lumen.

(c) **Iodide** is taken up through the basal cell membrane, transported through the cell, and released into the follicular lumen.

(d) **Oxidation of iodide** and **iodination of thyroglobulin** are mediated by thyroperoxidase in the follicular lumen. Iodinated thyroglobulin is stored in the follicular lumen.

(2) **Thyroid hormone release**

(a) TSH induces the formation of **pseudopods (microfolds)** at the luminal surface of follicular epithelial cells.

(b) Colloid, containing iodinated thyroglobulin, is taken up by **endocytosis** into vesicles.

(c) Colloid-containing vesicles fuse with lysosomes to form **phagolysosomes**. Inside the phagolysosomes, proteolysis splits the iodinated thyroglobulin to yield thyroxine (T_4) and triiodothyronine (T_3).

(d) T_3 and T_4 reach the pericapillary extracellular space through **diffusion**.

b. **Calcitonin release.** Calcitonin regulates the level of calcium in the blood. High levels of blood calcium induce the secretion of calcitonin, which then lowers blood calcium levels by suppressing resorption of bone.

D. Parathyroid glands

1. Structure

a. A **thin connective tissue capsule** surrounds the parathyroid glands.

b. **Parenchymal cells** occur in clusters, strands, or cords. They are highly vascularized by sinusoidal capillaries.

(1) **Principal (chief) cells** (Figure 19-5)

(a) **Active (dark) principal cells** contain abundant rER, an extensive Golgi complex, numerous mitochondria, and numerous secretory granules.

(b) **Inactive (light) principal cells** usually predominate. They contain few organelles, few secretory granules, and glycogen in some species, especially cats.

(2) **Oxyphil cells** are large acidophilic cells.

(a) Oxyphil cells occur singly or in clusters in horses and ruminants but are rare in other domestic mammals.

(b) They contain inconspicuous rER, an inconspicuous Golgi complex, sparse secretory granules, and numerous mitochondria.

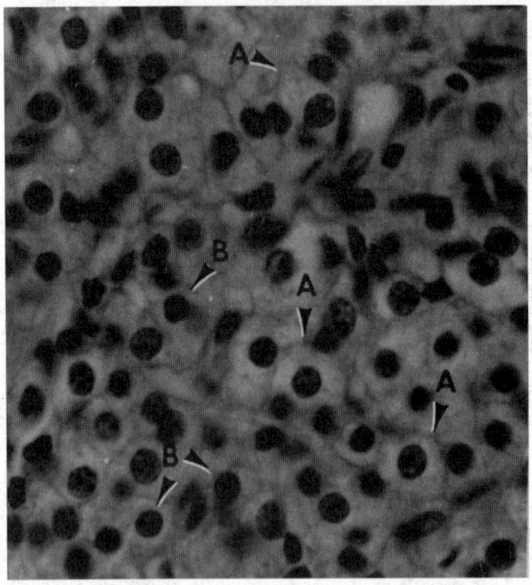

FIGURE 19-5. In this parathyroid gland, inactive (light) principal cells predominate (*A*) and are readily distinguished from active (dark) principal cells (*B*). (Reprinted with permission from Dellmann H-D: *Textbook of Veterinary Histology,* 4th ed. Baltimore, Williams & Wilkins, 1993, p 279.)

2. **Functions.** The principal cells of the parathyroid gland secrete **parathormone** in response to low blood calcium levels. Parathormone raises blood calcium levels by:
   a. **Increasing calcium absorption from bone.** Parathormone stimulates **osteocytes** to release calcium from bone. If parathormone remains chronically elevated, it stimulates **osteolysis** by **osteoclasts**.
   b. **Decreasing renal calcium excretion.**
   c. **Increasing calcium absorption from the diet.** Parathormone affects the synthesis of a vitamin D metabolite, **1,25-dihydroxycholecalciferol,** that increases intestinal absorption of dietary calcium.

E. Adrenal gland

1. **Structure.** The adrenal gland is surrounded by a thin connective tissue capsule, and its parenchymal cells are arranged in clusters or cords. The adrenal gland is subdivided into an outer **cortex** of mesodermal origin and an inner **medulla** of neuroectodermal origin (Figure 19-6).
   a. **Adrenal cortex.**The adrenal cortex is subdivided into zones, based on cell characteristics, arrangement of cells, and function.
      (1) The **zona glomerulosa (zona arcuata)** is the **outermost zone**.
         (a) The cells in this zone are arranged in clusters in ruminants and in arcs in all other domestic mammals (Figure 19-7).
         (b) The cuboidal to columnar cells have all the characteristics of steroid hormone–producing cells, including extensive smooth endoplasmic reticulum (sER) and numerous lipid droplets.
         (c) Only the cells of this zone contain the enzymes required for the final stages of **aldosterone synthesis**.
      (2) The **zona intermedia** is inconspicuous, except in horses, dogs, and cats, where its location between the zona glomerulosa and zona fasciculata is readily identifiable. The zona intermedia consists of apparently undifferentiated cells that are thought to give rise to the cells of the zona fasciculata.
      (3) The **zona fasciculata** contains cells arranged in radial cords or fascicles that are usually one cell layer thick (Figure 19-8A).
         (a) The cells are cuboidal to columnar and have all the characteristics of steroid hormone–producing cells.
         (b) The cells contain abundant lipid droplets that appear as vacuoles in routine histologic preparations; therefore, they are frequently called **spongiocytes**.

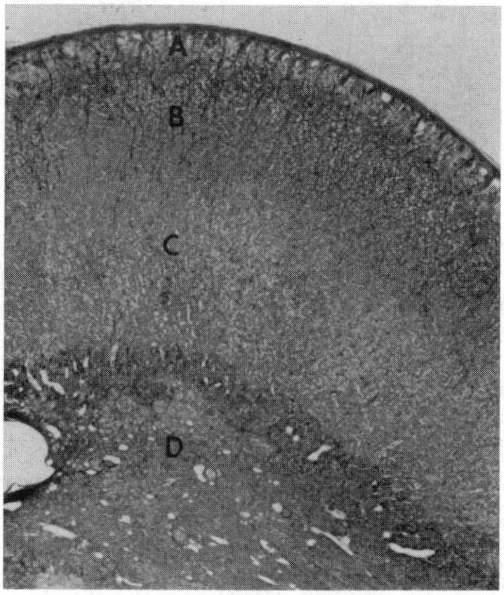

FIGURE 19-6. In this section through the equine adrenal gland, the cortex (*A,B,C*) is clearly distinguished from the medulla (*D*). The subdivision of the cortex into zona glomerulosa (*A*), zona fasciculata (*B*), and zona reticularis (*C*) is evident. (Reprinted with permission from Dellmann H-D: *Textbook of Veterinary Histology,* 4th ed. Baltimore, Williams & Wilkins, 1993, p 279.)

(4) The **zona reticularis** is the innermost cortical zone, in which the cells form irregularly anastomosing cords (Figure 19-8B).

(a) The cells are usually polyhedral and are smaller than those in the zona fasciculata.

(b) The cells also possess the structural characteristics of steroid hormone–producing cells, but lipid droplets are scant and lipofuscin is more abundant.

b. Adrenal medulla. The adrenal medulla is composed of irregular cords and clusters of **monoamine-secreting cells,** which are modified postganglionic sympathetic neurons. Monoamine-secreting cells are also called **chromaffin cells** because they stain dark brown when fixed with fixatives containing dichromate ions.

(1) Epinephrine and **norepinephrine** are the principal monoamines produced by the adrenal medulla.

A

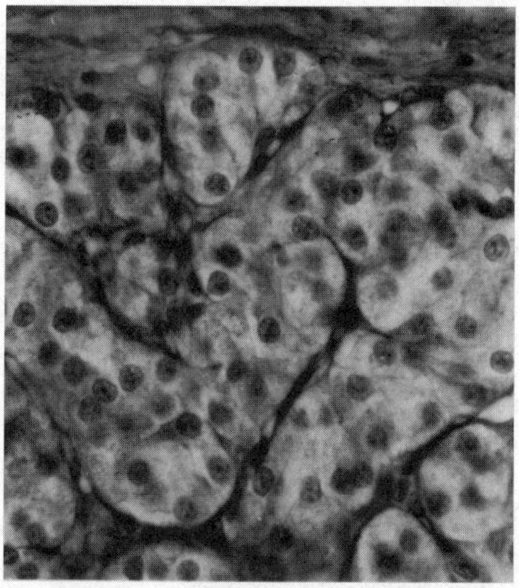

B

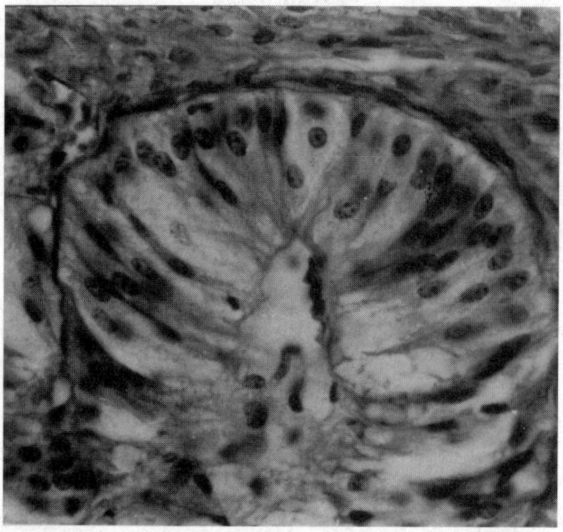

FIGURE 19-7. In the outermost zone of the adrenal cortex (zona glomerulosa or zona arcuata), cells may be arranged in clusters called glomeruli (*A*) or in arcades (*B*), depending on the species. (Reprinted with permission from Dellmann H-D: *Textbook of Veterinary Histology,* 4th ed. Baltimore, Williams & Wilkins, 1993, p 280.)

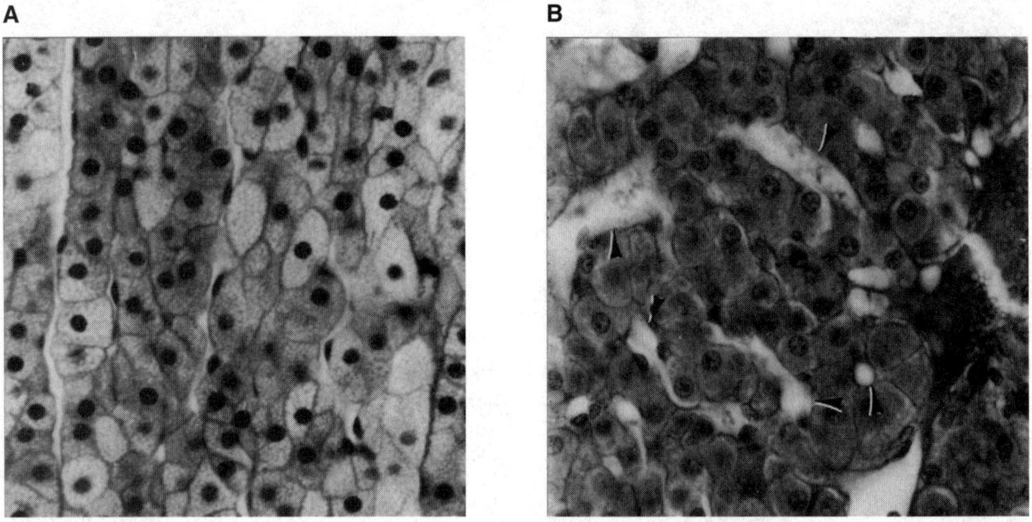

FIGURE 19-8. (*A*) In the zona fasciculata of the adrenal cortex, cells are organized into fascicles. Notice the spongy appearance of the cytoplasm, which results from the dissolution of lipid droplets. (*B*) In the zona reticularis of the adrenal cortex, cells are arranged in anastomosing cords. Each cell is in contact with a sinusoidal capillary (*arrowheads*). (Reprinted with permission from Dellmann H-D: *Textbook of Veterinary Histology,* 4th ed. Baltimore, Williams & Wilkins, 1993, pp 280, 281.)

(a) In horses, cows, sheep, and pigs, **epinephrine** is produced by large columnar cells located around the **periphery** of the medulla, and **norepinephrine** is produced by small polyhedral cells in the **center**.

(b) In other domestic mammals, zones are lacking.

(2) **Monoamine-secreting cells** contain numerous mitochondria, moderately abundant rER, a Golgi complex, and secretory granules.

2. **Vascularity and nerve supply**

a. **Sinusoidal capillaries** in a dense network supply the adrenal cortex and medulla.

(1) Cortical capillaries receive blood from arterioles located superficially in the cortex and drain into venules located between the cortex and the medulla (i.e., at the corticomedullary junction).

(2) The medullary capillary network is supplied by arterioles that traverse the cortex without giving off branches before reaching the medulla, and it drains into medullary venules.

(3) A large central vein drains the cortical and medullary venules.

b. **Sympathetic preganglionic axons** innervate mainly the adrenal medulla, where they make synaptic contacts with the monoamine-producing cells.

3. **Functions**

a. **Adrenal cortex.** The adrenal cortex produces mineralocorticoids and glucocorticoids.

(1) **Mineralocorticoids.** Cholesterol precursors in the **zona glomerulosa** produce the principal mineralocorticoid, **aldosterone**.

(a) The **renin–angiotensin system** (see Chapter 15 II C 2) regulates aldosterone synthesis.

(b) Aldosterone controls sodium retention (and, indirectly, water retention) by the renal distal convoluted tubule and collecting ducts.

(2) **Glucocorticoids.** The **zonae fasciculata and reticularis** synthesize **cortisol** and **corticosterone**.

(a) **Glucocorticoid secretion** is controlled by hypothalamic CRH and adenohypophysial ACTH.

(i) CRH (and consequently, ACTH) secretion is regulated through negative feedback from glucocorticoids and a wide range of external and internal factors, such as stress.

(ii) Hypophysectomy causes atrophy and decreased secretory activity of the cells of the zonae fasciculata and reticularis.

(b) Glucocorticoids have **numerous functions,** including facilitation of gluconeogenesis, release of fatty acids from adipocytes, and inhibition of cellular and fibrous proliferation (antiinflammatory effect).

b. Adrenal medulla. The adrenal medulla secretes epinephrine and norepinephrine. This process is under direct synaptic control by preganglionic cholinergic sympathetic neurons.

(1) **Epinephrine** has predominantly **metabolic effects,** including:

(a) **Liver glycogenolysis** accompanied by glucose liberation

(b) **Lipolysis** (i.e., mobilization of triglycerides from adipocytes)

(c) **Muscle glycogenolysis** accompanied by release of lactic acid

(2) **Norepinephrine** has primarily **cardiovascular effects,** including **vasoconstriction** (which, in turn, increases peripheral resistance and blood pressure).

III. GROUPS OF ENDOCRINE CELLS

A. Pancreatic islets

1. **Structure.** Pancreatic islets are generally spherical or ovoid clusters of irregularly anastomosing cords of several types of endocrine cells (Figure 19-9). Pancreatic islets are well vascularized by sinusoidal capillaries.

   a. **A cells** (5%–30% of islet cells) secrete **glucagon**. They characteristically contain large, electron-dense, membrane-bounded granules.

   b. **B cells** (60%–80% of islet cells) secrete **insulin**. They are structurally similar to A cells, but their secretory granules are crystalloid (except in horses).

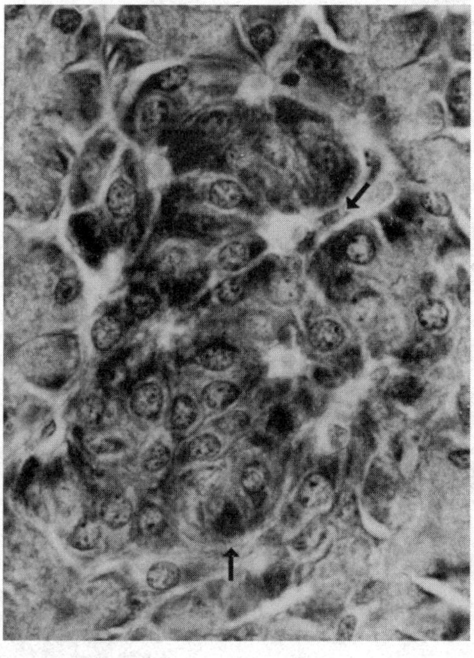

FIGURE 19-9. In this pancreatic islet, the many dark-staining cells (*arrows*) are B cells. With the histologic staining method used, the light-staining cells cannot be identified specifically. (Reprinted with permission from Dellmann H-D: *Textbook of Veterinary Histology,* 4th ed. Baltimore, Williams & Wilkins, 1993, p 283.)

c. **C cells** have few (if any) secretory granules and are considered to be immature **precursors** of other islet cells.
d. **D cells,** which secrete **somatostatin,** are relatively rare. They contain granules of medium electron density.
e. **F cells,** which contain **pancreatic polypeptide,** have been reported in dogs.
f. **Other cells** synthesize **gastroenteropancreatic hormones,** such as vasoactive intestinal polypeptide (VIP) or CCK.

2. **Functions.** Pancreatic functions are independent of adenohypophysial influences.
a. **Insulin** stimulates the synthesis and storage of glycogen in liver and muscle and the conversion of glucose into fat for storage in adipocytes. Insufficient insulin secretion causes diabetes mellitus, which is characterized by varying degrees of hyperglycemia and glucosuria.
b. **Glucagon** counteracts the effects of insulin. It stimulates glycogen breakdown and glucose synthesis in the liver and causes an increase in glucose in the blood.
c. **Somatostatin** acts on nearby cells in a paracrine manner. It inhibits the secretion of insulin and glucagon.
d. **Other hormones** produced by cells in the pancreatic islets have functions that are covered with the enteroendocrine cells (see Chapter 13 II D 3 b).

B. Other groups of endocrine cells

1. Hypothalamic neurosecretory neurons are discussed under II A 2.

2. Other groups of endocrine cells in the heart, ovary, and testis are discussed in Chapters 11, 16, and 18, respectively.

IV. SINGLE ENDOCRINE CELLS

A. Single endocrine cells **in the digestive system** are discussed in Chapter 13.

B. Single endocrine cells **in the respiratory system** are discussed in Chapter 14.

C. **APUD cells,** which are found throughout the body, are characterized by **a**mine **p**recursor **u**ptake and **d**ecarboxylation, which occur during synthesis of amines or peptide hormones. All APUD cells have similar fine structural morphology.

1. APUD cells include:
a. Enteroendocrine cells
b. Endocrine cells in the mucosa of the respiratory system
c. Juxtaglomerular cells
d. Epinephrine- and norepinephrine-producing cells in the adrenal medulla
e. Pancreatic islet cells
f. Thyroid parafollicular cells
g. Chemoreceptor cells in the carotid body
h. Corticotropes and melanotropes in the adenohypophysis

2. Some APUD cells (e.g., the cells of the adrenal medulla, the parafollicular cells, and the cells in the respiratory system) are of neural crest origin, and are therefore members of the **diffuse neuroendocrine system**.

STUDY QUESTIONS

DIRECTIONS: Each of the numbered items or incomplete statements in this section is followed by answers or by completions of the statement. Select the **one** numbered answer or completion that is **best** in each case.

1. Which of the following cell types is commonly observed in the pars tuberalis of the adenohypophysis?

(1) Corticotrope
(2) Lactotrope
(3) Somatotrope
(4) Gonadotrope
(5) Chromophobe

2. A releasing factor and inhibitory factor both exist for which of the following hormones?

(1) Thyrotropin
(2) Gonadotropin
(3) Somatotropin
(4) Corticotropin
(5) Melanotropin

3. Antidiuretic hormone (ADH) and oxytocin are synthesized in hypothalamic neuronal perikarya and released from perivascular axon terminals in the:

(1) hypothalamus.
(2) internal zone of the median eminence.
(3) neural lobe.
(4) external zone of the median eminence.
(5) infundibular stalk.

4. Which one of the following stimuli triggers release of antidiuretic hormone (ADH)?

(1) Hypervolemia
(2) Decreased plasma osmolarity
(3) Increased blood pressure
(4) Hypovolemia
(5) Excessive water consumption

5. All endocrine organs have which one of the following?

(1) Lymphatic capillaries
(2) Sinusoids
(3) Epithelioid cells
(4) Sinusoidal capillaries
(5) Porous capillaries

6. Which of the following is a component of thyroid follicular cells that is not observed in any other endocrine organ?

(1) Lysosomes
(2) Autophagolysosomes
(3) Phagolysosomes
(4) Smooth endoplasmic reticulum (sER)
(5) Exocytotic vesicles

7. An outstanding characteristic of the cells of the zona fasciculata is the presence of:

(1) numerous ribosomes.
(2) large Golgi complexes.
(3) extensive rough endoplasmic reticulum (rER).
(4) many lipid droplets.
(5) abundant glycogen.

8. Which of the following endocrine organs, parts of endocrine organs, or endocrine cell groups is affected by hypophysectomy?

(1) Adrenal zona glomerulosa
(2) Adrenal medulla
(3) Pancreatic A cells
(4) Pinealocytes
(5) Ovarian corpus luteum

9. The cells of the adrenal medulla are:

(1) of mesodermal origin.
(2) modified parasympathetic neurons.
(3) modified glial cells.
(4) modified sympathetic neurons.
(5) of entodermal origin.

DIRECTIONS: Each of the numbered items or incomplete statements in this section is negatively phrased, as indicated by an italicized word such as *not, least,* or *except.* Select the **one** numbered answer or completion that is **best** in each case.

10. All of the following are characteristic of adrenal medullary cells *except:*

(1) numerous mitochondria.
(2) rough endoplasmic reticulum (rER).
(3) abundant smooth endoplasmic reticulum (sER).
(4) secretory granules.
(5) a Golgi complex.

11. Which of the following is *not* part of the adenohypophysis?

(1) Pars distalis
(2) Pars tuberalis
(3) Anterior lobe
(4) Posterior lobe
(5) Intermediate lobe

12. Which of the following is *not* a cell type of the pars distalis?

(1) Corticotrope
(2) Gonadotrope
(3) Somatotrope
(4) Thyrotrope
(5) Melanotrope

ANSWERS AND EXPLANATIONS

1. The answer is 4 *[II A 1 a (3) (b)]*. In addition to cells that are characteristic of the pars tuberalis, whose function is unknown, gonadotropes and thyrotropes are present in the pars tuberalis. After hypophysectomy in which the pars tuberalis is spared, female rats occasionally continue to have estrous cycles, and spermatogenesis proceeds normally in the male. Corticotropes, lactotropes, somatotropes, and chromophobes are found in the pars distalis.

2. The answer is 3 *[II A 1 b (2) (b)]*. Somatotropin-releasing factor (somatotropin-releasing hormone) stimulates, and somatostatin inhibits, the release of somatotropin. Thyrotropin, gonadotropin, and corticotropin are released under the influence of stimulating factors or hormones, and an inhibitory factor regulates the release of melanocyte-stimulating hormone (MSH, melanotropin).

3. The answer is 3 *[II A 2 a]*. The axons of the magnocellular hypothalamic neurons that synthesize antidiuretic hormone (ADH) and oxytocin traverse the hypothalamus, the internal zone of the median eminence, and the infundibular stalk. They terminate at the sinusoidal capillaries of the neural lobe. It is from these axon terminals that the hormones are released. Axons of neurons in the hypothalamic hypophysiotropic area that synthesize releasing and inhibitory factors and hormones terminate in the external zone of the median eminence.

4. The answer is 4 *[II A 2 b (1) (b)]*. In hypovolemia, there is an urgent need for water preservation, which is accomplished by antidiuretic hormone (ADH) release and an increase in water consumption. Hypervolemia, an increase in blood pressure, a decrease in plasma osmolarity, and high water consumption all inhibit ADH secretion.

5. The answer is 4 *[II A 1 a (1), 2 a (2) (b), B 1 b (1), C 1, D 1 b, E 2 a]*. Sinusoidal capillaries are fenestrated capillaries whose shape is adapted to the surrounding cells. They are present in all endocrine organs and in endocrine cell groups. Lymphatic capillaries are present in all endocrine organs except in the neural lobe and the pineal gland, which are part of the central nervous system (CNS), which lacks lymphatics. Sinusoids are unique to the liver. Epithelioid cells are present in all endocrine organs except the neural lobe. Porous capillaries are found in renal glomeruli.

6. The answer is 3 *[II C 1 a (1) (b) (iii), 2 a (2) (c)]*. Phagolysosomes are a unique feature of thyroid follicular cells. They are important in thyroid hormone secretion because iodinated thyroglobulin that has been taken up from the follicular lumen by endocytosis is enzymatically split into thyroxine (T_4) and triiodothyronine (T_3), which then diffuse out of the cell. Lysosomes and autophagolysosomes are observed in almost all cells of the organism and especially in secretory cells. Exocytotic vesicles are commonly observed in most secretory cells. Smooth endoplasmic reticulum (sER) occurs in virtually all cells, but it is particularly abundant in steroid hormone–synthesizing cells and liver cells.

7. The answer is 4 *[II E 1 a (3) (b)]*. The cells of the zona fasciculata synthesize steroid hormones (deoxycorticosterone and aldosterone) and thus possess the fine structural characteristics of steroid hormone–synthesizing cells, including abundant smooth endoplasmic reticulum (sER), mitochondria of the tubular type, and many lipid droplets. Numerous free ribosomes are characteristic of cells that synthesize proteins for use by the cell. Cells that synthesize secretory proteins have extensive rough endoplasmic reticulum (rER) and large Golgi complexes. Glycogen (a storage form of glucose) occurs in many cells and is especially abundant in hepatocytes and skeletal muscle cells.

8. The answer is 5 *[II A 1 b (2) (a) (iv)]*. Progesterone secretion by the corpus luteum is under the influence of adenohypophysial luteinizing hormone (LH). Hypophysectomized animals do not normally have estrous cycles (exceptions may occur if the pars tuberalis, which is usually not removed during hypophysectomy, contains numerous gonadotropes); therefore, a corpus luteum would not even develop. The secretory activities of the adrenal zona glomerulosa, the adrenal medulla, pancreatic A cells, and pinealocytes are not under adenohypophysial control.

9. The answer is 4 *[II E 1 b]*. The monoamine-secreting cells of the adrenal medulla are of ectodermal origin. They are sympathetic neurons that are modified to secrete epinephrine or norepinephrine on synaptic stimulation by preganglionic sympathetic neurons.

10. The answer is 3 *[II E 1 b (2)]*. Adrenal medullary cells secrete monoamines and, therefore, have numerous mitochondria, rough endoplasmic reticulum (rER), a Golgi complex, and many secretory granules. A small amount of smooth endoplasmic reticulum (sER) is present, as it is in all cells; but it is not abundant as it is, for example, in the steroid hormone–synthesizing cells of the adrenal cortex.

11. The answer is 4 *[II A 1 a]*. The posterior lobe, which is also called the neural lobe, is part of the neurohypophysis, not the adenohypophysis. The adenohypophysis is composed of three lobes: the pars distalis (anterior lobe), the pars tuberalis (tuberal lobe), and the pars intermedia (intermediate lobe).

12. The answer is 5 *[II A 1 a]*. Melanotropes are the principal and predominant cells of the pars intermedia and do not occur in the pars distalis. The pars distalis of the adenohypophysis contains somatotropes, lactotropes, gonadotropes, thyrotropes, corticotropes, and chromophobes.

Chapter 20

Integument

I. INTRODUCTION

A. Components. The integument comprises the **skin** and **its appendages** and **special epidermal structures** (Figure 20-1).

1. **Skin.** The skin (cutis) consists of two layers, the **epidermis** and the **dermis**. The **hypodermis** (subcutis), which is not part of the skin, anchors the skin to the underlying fascia, skeletal muscle, or bone.
   a. The **epidermis** is the **outermost layer** of the skin. It consists of **keratinized stratified squamous epithelium** comprising keratinocytes and other specialized cells.
      (1) Its thickness varies with the species and body region according to friction and pressure. Therefore, the epidermis is thickest on palmar and plantar surfaces and thinnest under the hair coat. The heavier the protective hair coat, the thinner the epidermis.
      (2) The epidermis has ridges in some locations.

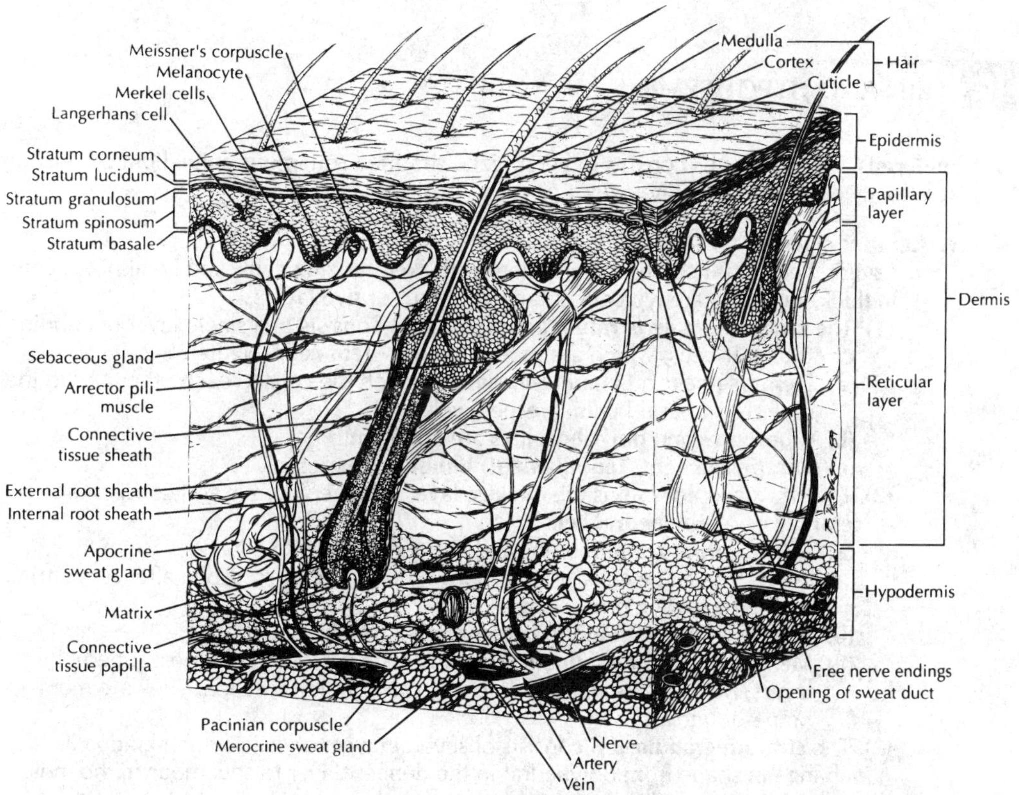

FIGURE 20-1. Schematic drawing of the mammalian skin and underlying hypodermis. (Reprinted with permission from Monteiro-Riviere NA: Comparative anatomy, physiology and biochemistry of mammalian skin. In *Dermal and Ocular Toxicology: Fundamentals and Methods.* Edited by DW Hobson, Boca Raton, FL, CRC Press, 1991, p 5.)

b. The **dermis,** which comprises **dense irregular connective tissue,** is usually the thickest layer of the skin.
c. The **hypodermis** is a layer of **loose connective tissue**.

2. **Special epidermal structures** include **hooves, claws, horns, mammary glands,** and **feathers**.

B. Functions

1. **Environmental (diffusion) barrier**
2. **Mechanical protection**
3. **Body temperature regulation** through hairs or feathers, sweat glands, and dermal blood flow
4. **Sensory reception** by specialized epithelial cells and free and encapsulated nerve endings
5. **Immune responses** through intradermal antigen-presenting cells
6. **Secretion** of sweat, sebum, and milk
7. **Individual recognition** and **adornment** through hair coat or feather color or horns and through odoriferous substances secreted by apocrine sweat glands
8. **Locomotion** through hooves or feathers
9. **Capture of prey** through claws

II. SKIN AND HYPODERMIS

A. Epidermis.

The epidermis consists of keratinized stratified squamous epithelium comprising keratinocytes and nonkeratinocytes.

1. **Keratinocytes**
   a. **Layers.** The keratinocytes include stem cells, keratinizing cells, and keratinized cells. In thick skin, they are typically arranged in four or five layers.
      (1) The **stratum basale (stratum germinativum)** consists of a single layer of cuboidal or columnar cells, which are predominantly **stem cells** (Figure 20-2).
         (a) **Desmosomes** and **hemidesmosomes** attach the cells to each other and to the underlying basal lamina, respectively.
         (b) **Ribosomes** and **polyribosomes** are abundant.
         (c) **Keratin filament (tonofilament) bundles** are present.
      (2) The **stratum spinosum** is the thickest layer of the epidermis and consists of several layers of **polyhedral cells.**
         (a) **Desmosomes** are numerous and connect adjacent cells. Because of these connections, the cells appear "spiny" under the microscope after they shrink during histologic processing.
         (b) **Keratin filament bundles** are prominent (see Figure 20-2).
         (c) **Membrane-coating (lamellar) granules** are present in the most superficial layers, but they are not visible under the light microscope. They are membrane-bounded.
      (3) The **stratum granulosum** consists of several layers of cells, which gradually change in shape from polyhedral in the deepest layer to squamous in the most superficial layer (Figure 20-3).
         (a) **Keratohyalin granules,** which are not membrane-bounded, are prominent under the light microscope.
         (b) **Membrane-coating granules** become more numerous and larger in the upper layers and are released from the uppermost cells.

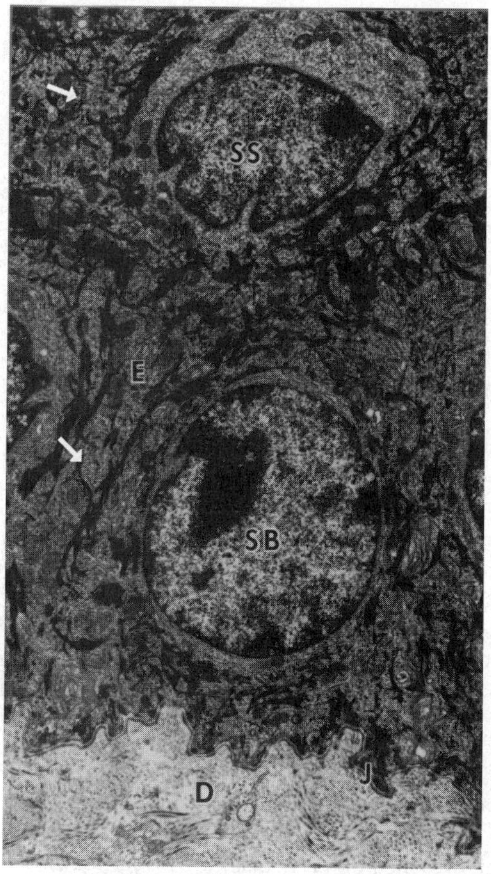

FIGURE 20-2. In this electron micrograph, a cell of the stratum basale (*SB*) in the epidermis (*E*) is seen interdigitating with the connective tissue of the underlying dermis (*D*). This cell and, to a larger extent, the keratinocyte in the stratum spinosum (*SS*) contain bundles of keratin filaments (*arrows*). The junction (*J*) of the epidermis and dermis is clearly visible. (Reprinted with permission from Dellmann H-D: *Textbook of Veterinary Histology,* 4th ed. Baltimore, Williams & Wilkins, 1993, p 288.)

(4) A brightly stained **stratum lucidum,** consisting of several layers of squamous keratinized cells, is present in most thick and hairless epidermis.

(a) Organelles and **nuclei** are absent.

(b) Keratin filaments are prominent.

(5) The **stratum corneum** consists of several (3–50, depending on location) layers of keratinized squamous cells.

(a) The **stratum disjunctum** is the uppermost layer, which is constantly shed.

(b) A **bidirectional barrier** effectively blocks passage of fluids and other substances. It is formed by released **lamellar granules,** which completely fill the intercellular space, and **keratinized cells**.

(i) The keratinized cells are filled with a dense, amorphous **keratohyalin matrix,** into which keratin filaments are embedded. The keratinized cells lack both organelles and nuclei.

(ii) A thick **subplasmalemmal layer** reinforces the cell membrane and provides protection against microorganisms and environmental agents.

b. Keratinization is the process by which keratin is formed, but this term is commonly used to designate the process of **cornification** (i.e., the **differentiation of epidermal keratinocytes**). Keratinization results in a protective layer of differentiated cells and relatively impermeable intercellular substance. This layer is continuously shed at the surface and replaced by differentiating cells in the deeper epidermal strata.

(1) As keratinocytes migrate upward in the epidermis, keratin filaments, keratohyalin granules, and lamellar granules are formed. Nuclei and organelles progressively disintegrate.

(2) Membrane-coating granules are released into and completely fill the intercellular space.

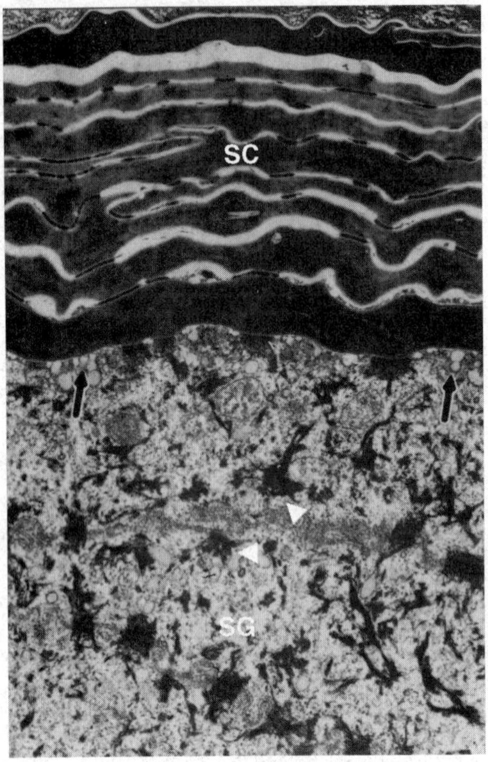

FIGURE 20-3. This electron micrograph depicts cells of the upper stratum granulosum (*SG*) with membrane-coating granules in the process of exocytosis (*arrows*). Keratohyalin granules and associated keratin filaments can also be seen (*arrowheads*). The cells of the stratum corneum (*SC*) lack organelles. The dark intercellular lines are the thickened dense intercellular component of desmosomes. (Reprinted with permission from Dellmann H-D: *Textbook of Veterinary Histology,* 4th ed. Baltimore, Williams & Wilkins, 1993, p 288.)

(3) The cell membrane is reinforced by a subplasmalemmal layer.

c. Types of keratin

(1) Hard keratin is characterized by the presence of many disulfide bridges between the polypeptide chains that make up keratin filaments. It is found in hooves, claws, horns, the cortex and cuticle of hairs, and feathers.

(2) Soft keratin has fewer disulfide bonds and is contained in nonspecialized epidermis.

2. Nonkeratinocytes

a. Melanocytes

(1) Origin. They are derived from the neural crest.

(2) Location. Most melanocytes lie near or in the stratum basale, but they also occur in the external root sheath of hairs and among the cells lining the ducts of sweat and sebaceous glands.

(3) Structure

(a) Melanocytes synthesize **melanin,** which is packaged in **melanosomes** (membrane-bounded, elliptical granules).

(b) Long processes from melanocytes usually penetrate between adjacent keratinocytes. Melanosomes move into the cell processes, the ends of which are phagocytosed by keratinocytes. Within the keratinocytes, melanosomes are often concentrated above the nucleus.

(4) Function. Melanosomes **confer color** to skin, hair, and other specialized epidermal structures (e.g., hooves, feathers).

b. Merkel cells

(1) Location. Merkel cells are located in the stratum basale of hairless and hairy skin. They are particularly numerous in the:

(a) Planum rostrale of pigs

(b) Planum nasale of carnivores

(c) External root sheath of tactile hairs

(2) **Structure**
(a) Merkel cells are **flat**.
(b) **Dense-core vesicles** are found in the light-staining, vacuolated cytoplasm.
(c) **Desmosomes** are common.
(3) **Function. Tactile discs,** which function as **mechanoreceptors,** are Merkel cells and the neurites that terminate as flat menisci on the basal aspect of these cells.

c. **Langerhans cells**
(1) **Origin.** Langerhans cells are derived from bone marrow.
(2) **Location.**
(a) Pigs are the only domestic mammals in which these cells have been observed.
(b) Langerhans cells are most common in the **upper stratum spinosum** and extend long, branched processes into the **stratum granulosum**.
(3) **Structure.** Langerhans cells contain characteristic rod- or racket-shaped granules.
(4) **Function.** Langerhans cells are **antigen-presenting cells**.

B. Dermis.
Dermis. The dermis is usually the thickest layer of the skin. It has a superficial and a deep layer.

1. The **superficial (papillary) layer** forms a continuous subepidermal layer that also surrounds hairs and glands. Protrusions of the superficial layer into the epidermis are called **dermal papillae**.
a. The superficial layer comprises **loose connective tissue** consisting of thin collagen fibers, many elastic fibers, and numerous fibrocytes, histiocytes, mast cells, and plasma cells.
b. It contains a network of **subepithelial capillaries** and many **nerve fibers**.
c. The **papillary body** of the integument comprises all papillae that are formed by the superficial layer.
(1) Papillae are low or nonexistent in hairy skin.
(2) Papillae are high in hairless skin and the skin of pigs (which has sparse hairs).
(3) In hooves and claws, the papillary body is composed of long papillae, laminae, and ridges (see IV B 1 a (3), 3 a).

2. The **deep (reticular) layer,** the thickest layer of the dermis, is composed of **dense irregular connective tissue,** which contains thick collagen fibers, some elastic fibers, and relatively few fibrocytes.
a. **Few blood vessels** are contained in the deep layer.
b. **Arrectores pilorum** muscles are present in hairy skin [see III A 1 c (3)].
c. **Smooth muscle fibers** that are not associated with hairs are present in the tunica dartos of the scrotum and may occur in the dermis of the penis and teat.
d. **Cutaneous skeletal muscle fibers** that are anchored in the deep layer permit voluntary movements of the skin.

C. Hypodermis

1. Highly flexible **loose connective tissue** predominates in the hypodermis, permitting displacement or movement of the skin.
a. It is most flexible in carnivores and sheep.
b. It is less flexible in horses, large ruminants, and goats.
c. It is least flexible in pigs, where it contains large masses of metabolic adipose tissue.

2. Less flexible **structural adipose tissue,** reinforced by bundles of collagen fibers, predominates in the shock-absorbing digital, carpal, and metacarpal pads.

3. **Certain regions** (e.g., the wall and sole of hooves and claws, horns, teats, and eyelids) **lack a hypodermis**.

III. SKIN APPENDAGES.

The skin appendages comprise hairs, hair follicles, and their associated glands (Figure 20-4).

A. Hair and hair follicles

1. Structure

a. Hairs are flexible epidermal structures that provide mechanical protection and function in temperature regulation and sensory perception.

(1) The **hair shaft** protrudes above the surface of the skin.

(2) The **hair root** is located within the hair follicle and terminates with a thickened **hair bulb** above the **dermal hair papilla.**

(3) The shaft and root are composed of **three layers.**

(a) The **cuticle** is the outermost layer.

(i) It comprises squamous keratinized cells that overlap in a shingle-like manner with their free edges directed toward the distal end of the hair.

(ii) The shape and size of the cells and the configuration of their free border are species-specific.

(b) The **cortex** comprises several concentric layers of squamous keratinized cells held together by desmosomes.

(c) The **medulla,** which may be absent in secondary hairs (see III A 2 b), consists of loosely packed cells. The thickness of both the cortex and the medulla varies by region and hair type and is species-specific.

b. The **hair follicle** is an invagination of the epidermis into the dermis and sometimes into the hypodermis. It surrounds the hair root and bulb.

(1) The **external root sheath** corresponds to the strata basale and spinosum of the epidermis, with which it is continuous.

(2) **Internal root sheath**

(a) The internal root sheath comprises **three layers.**

(i) The **outer pale epithelial layer** (Henle's layer) is adjacent to the internal root sheath and usually consists of one layer of keratinized cells.

(ii) The **inner granular epithelial layer** (Huxley's layer) consists of one to three layers of cuboidal epithelial cells. These cells contain many trichohyalin granules (keratohyalin granules of hair), which become fewer proximodistally.

(iii) The **cuticle** of the internal root sheath is formed by keratinized squamous cells, which overlap in a manner similar to that of the cuticle of the hair but with the free edges oriented toward the hair bulb. This arrangement provides firm attachment for the hair.

(b) The growing hair and the internal root sheath advance at the same rate in a proximodistal direction. Immediately below the opening of the sebaceous gland into the hair follicle, the internal root sheath disintegrates and mixes with the secretory product of the sebaceous gland.

(3) **Hair matrix cells** cover the dermal hair papilla [see III A 1 c (2)] and make up most of the hair bulb.

(a) **Hard keratin** is synthesized by nondesquamating keratinocytes, which arise from hair matrix cells.

(b) Hair matrix cells are characterized by **mitotic activity** and quiescent periods in alternating **hair cycles** (see III A 3).

c. A **dermal sheath,** which is continuous with the superficial layer of the dermis, surrounds the hair follicle. It is a delicate network of collagen and elastic fibers.

(1) **Glassy membrane.** This thick basal lamina separates the follicle from the dermal sheath.

(2) **Dermal hair papilla.** Formed by the dermal sheath at the level of the hair bulb, the dermal hair papilla provides nutrition for the hair matrix cells of the growing hair.

(a) The papilla contains many fibrocytes and at least one capillary.

(b) It undergoes morphologic changes during the hair cycle (see III A 3).

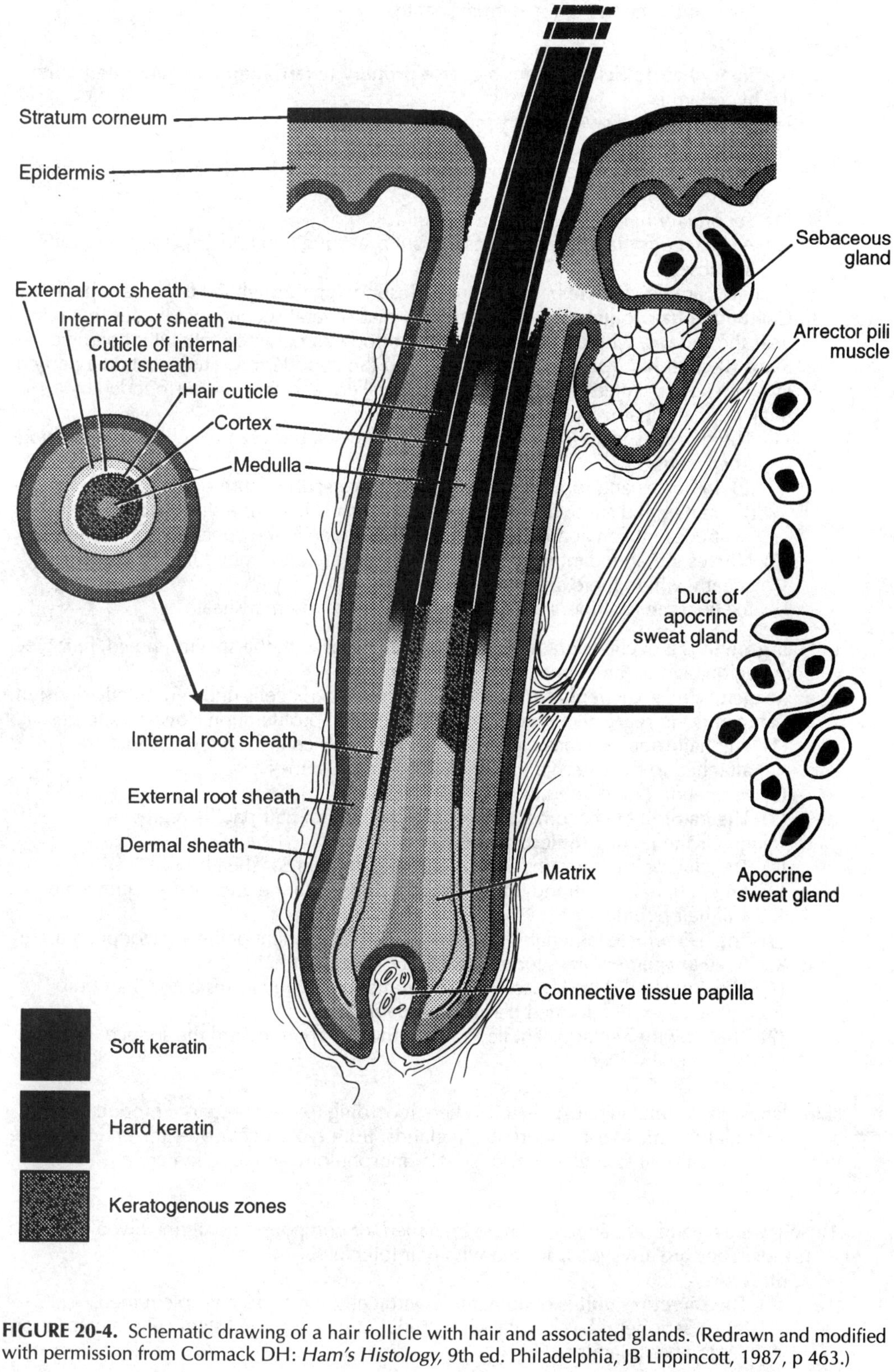

FIGURE 20-4. Schematic drawing of a hair follicle with hair and associated glands. (Redrawn and modified with permission from Cormack DH: *Ham's Histology,* 9th ed. Philadelphia, JB Lippincott, 1987, p 463.)

(3) **Arrector pili muscle.** This smooth muscle originates from the superficial dermal layer and attaches to the dermal sheath.

2. **Types**
   a. A **primary hair follicle** contains a coarse **primary (guard) hair** and may extend into the hypodermis.
      (1) Sebaceous and sweat glands open into the follicle.
      (2) An arrector pili muscle is present.
   b. A **secondary hair follicle** contains a **secondary hair (underhair)** and is usually confined to the dermis.
      (1) Secondary hairs usually lack a medulla.
      (2) A sebaceous gland may be present, but a sweat gland and arrector pili muscle are absent.
   c. A **single (simple) follicle** has only one hair surfacing through the follicular opening.
   d. **Compound hair follicles** have one primary and several secondary follicles that join near the surface, where their hairs emerge through a common follicular opening.
   e. **Sinus (tactile) hair follicles** extend deep into the hypodermis. They contain a particularly thick hair, called a **tactile hair** (e.g., whisker), and they are surrounded by a thick dermal sheath.
      (1) The dermal sheath forms inner and outer layers, between which there is a **blood-filled sinus.**
         (a) In horses and ruminants, trabeculae traverse the entire sinus.
         (b) In pigs and carnivores, the inner dermal sheath forms a sinus pad that protrudes into an annular sinus free of trabeculae in the upper portion of the sinus.
      (2) **Nerves** are abundant in the inner dermal sheath and extend into the outer root sheath, where there are many tactile discs.
      (3) **Skeletal muscle fibers** are attached to the outer dermal sheath.

3. **Hair growth** is a cyclic event (Figure 20-5) that varies with the species, breed, hair type, body region, age of the animal, and the season.
   a. **Anagen** is the **growth phase,** during which hair matrix cells undergo mitotic division.
   b. **Catagen** is the **regressive phase,** during which cell proliferation slowly decreases.
      (1) The hair root becomes club-shaped. The club's cells form rootlets that are attached to the external root sheath via desmosomes.
      (2) Formation of the internal root sheath ceases.
      (3) The hair follicle becomes shorter and the dermal hair papilla regresses.
   c. **Telogen** is the **resting (quiescent) phase.**
      (1) The club hair is surrounded only by the external root sheath.
      (2) An epithelial cell strand connects the follicle with the area of the regressed dermal hair papilla.
      (3) The hair follicle terminates near the level of attachment of the arrector pili muscle.
   d. **Renewed anagen** involves formation of a replacement hair.
      (1) The epithelial strand becomes thicker and eventually forms a new hair bulb above a newly reformed dermal hair papilla.
      (2) The growing replacement hair pushes the club hair toward the surface, where it is eventually shed.

B. Skin glands. Skin glands are usually classified according to their secretory product into sebaceous glands and sweat (sudoriferous) glands. Both types occur over the entire surface of the skin. Additional skin glands with special morphology and function are present in other locations.

1. **Sebaceous glands** are simple, simple branched, or compound holocrine alveolar glands. They are always associated with hair follicles.
   a. **Structure**
      (1) The **secretory unit** is entirely filled with cells and lacks a visible lumen.
         (a) A peripheral layer of flat or cuboidal undifferentiated stem cells is present on the basal lamina.

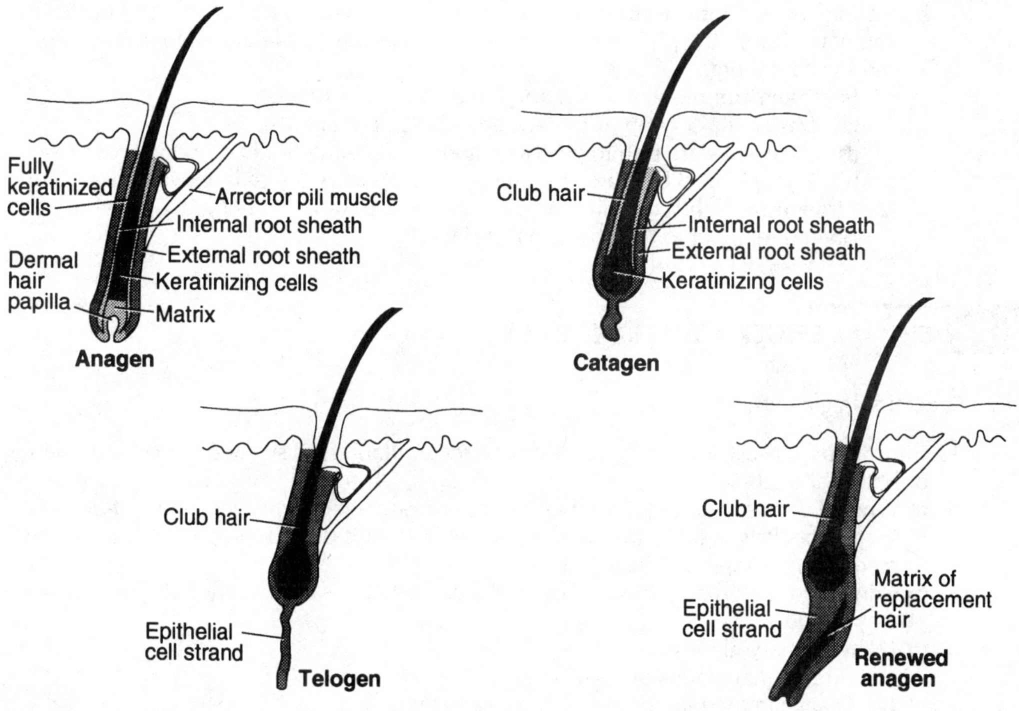

FIGURE 20-5. The hair cycle. (Redrawn with permission from Mosimann W, Kohler T: *Zytologie, Histologie und mikroskopische Anatomie der Haussäugetiere*. Berlin, Blackwell Wissenschafts-Verlag GmbH, 1990, p 289.)

(b) Mitotic divisions give rise to cells that move away from the basal lamina, enlarge, and accumulate lipid droplets. Their nuclei become pyknotic and eventually disappear. The cells disintegrate, forming the sebaceous secretory product.

(2) **Short ducts** are lined by stratified squamous epithelium. They open into the hair follicles below the opening of apocrine sweat glands (see III B 2 a).

b. Location

(1) Sebaceous glands are particularly well developed at **transition sites between skin and mucosae,** such as the **lip, nose, anus, prepuce,** and **vulva**.

(2) Sebaceous glands are not found in the bovine planum nasolabiale, the planum nasale of small ruminants and carnivores, the planum rostrale of pigs, the teat of cows, footpads, digital organs, and horns.

2. Sweat glands are simple or simple branched tubular glands.

a. Apocrine sweat glands predominate in domestic mammals. They are usually associated with hair follicles.

(1) **Secretory tubules** are coiled and have a wide lumen.

(a) The secretory tubules are lined with cuboidal to columnar secretory cells with protruding apices.

(b) **Myoepithelial cells** are located between the secretory cells and the surrounding basal lamina.

(2) A **straight duct** is lined with stratified cuboidal epithelium and opens into a hair follicle above the opening of the sebaceous gland.

(3) **Sweat** is a viscous secretory product containing 95%–98% water.

(a) It is produced in significant amounts only in horses. In horses and large ruminants, sweat functions in thermoregulation.

(b) In other domestic mammals, it is scant and viscous, and it functions in communication among individuals.

b. **Merocrine (eccrine) sweat glands** occur in the footpads of carnivores and horses (the frog of the hoof), the planum nasolabiale, the planum nasale and planum rostrale, and the carpal organ of pigs.
   (1) **Secretory tubules** are coiled and have a narrow lumen.
      (a) **Dark cells** contain numerous apical mucin granules.
      (b) **Clear cells** are rich in glycogen and produce the fluid component of sweat.
      (c) **Myoepithelial cells** are present between the secretory cells and the basal lamina.
   (2) **Straight** or **slightly coiled ducts** are lined with stratified cuboidal epithelium and open directly onto the epidermal surface.

IV. SPECIAL EPIDERMAL STRUCTURES

A. Special skin glands

1. **Introduction.** Most special skin glands are accumulations of sweat or sebaceous glands or both (Table 20-1).
   a. Whenever these glands are well-delineated or associated with special skin structures, such as pockets or folds, they are referred to as organs or have proper names (e.g., submental organ, inguinal sinus).
   b. Skin glands may be so specialized that their cutaneous origin is not obvious. Examples include:
      (1) Mammary glands
      (2) Circumanal glands of carnivores
      (3) Glands in the planum nasolabiale of cattle
      (4) Glands in the planum nasale of small ruminants

2. **Mammary gland.** This is a compound tubuloalveolar gland, which is divided into lobules by interlobular connective tissue. In animals that produce copious amounts of milk, such as cows and goats, the tubular secretory portions of the gland have virtually disappeared and are reduced to mere connections between adjacent alveoli.
   a. **Active (lactating) gland**
      (1) **Secretory alveoli.** Several secretory alveoli open into a large collecting space, or collecting alveolus (Figure 20-6).
         (a) **Secretory cells.** Alveoli are lined by simple cuboidal to columnar epithelium, depending on the stage of secretory activity.
            (i) **Lipid droplets** form in the cell base and become larger in the cell apex. They cause protrusion of the apical surface and are released surrounded by a small amount of cytoplasm and part of the cell membrane (apocrine secretion).
            (ii) **Protein micelles** are released by exocytosis (merocrine secretion).
         (b) **Myoepithelial cells,** which are responsible for milk let-down, lie between the secretory cells and the surrounding basal lamina.
      (2) **Ducts**
         (a) **Interlobular ducts** continue into **lactiferous ducts,** which open into the **lactiferous sinus**. The lactiferous sinus is continuous with the **teat sinus,** which opens onto the teat surface via the **papillary duct**.
         (b) **Duct linings**
            (i) The simple cuboidal lining epithelium of the smallest ducts may be secretory in lactating mammary glands.
            (ii) Larger ducts and sinuses are lined by bistratified cuboidal to columnar epithelium.
            (iii) The papillary duct is lined by keratinized stratified squamous epithelium.
            (iv) Myoepithelial cells are abundant in the ducts.
      (3) **Interstitial connective tissue**
         (a) **Interalveolar tissue** is relatively **sparse**. It is **well vascularized** and **plasma cells** are abundant.

TABLE 20-1. Special Skin Glands of Domestic Mammals

Gland	Location	Species	Characteristics
Nasolabial glands	Planum nasolabiale	Cattle	Compound tubuloacinar merocrine glands
Planum nasale glands	Planum nasale	Sheep, goat	Compound tubular merocrine glands
Planum rostrale glands	Planum rostrale	Pig	Compound tubular merocrine glands
Tarsal glands	Eyelid	All domestic mammals	Multilobar sebaceous glands
Ceruminous glands	External ear canal	All domestic mammals	Apocrine sweat glands and sebaceous glands
Infraorbital sinus glands	Infraorbital sinus	Sheep	Predominantly sebaceous glands and a few apocrine sweat glands
Mental glands	Mental organ	Pig	Apocrine sweat glands and sebaceous glands
Submental glands	Submental organ	Cat	Predominantly sebaceous glands and a few apocrine sweat glands
Postcornual glands	Base of horn	Buck	Sebaceous glands and apocrine sweat glands
Supracaudal glands	Supracaudal organ	Dog, cat	Predominantly sebaceous glands and a few apocrine sweat glands
Ventral caudal glands	Subcaudal organ	Goat	Sebaceous glands
Infracaudal glands	Infracaudal organ	Sheep	Sebaceous glands and apocrine sweat glands
Anal sac glands	Anal sacs	Dog, cat	Apocrine sweat glands (dog, cat) and sebaceous glands (cat)
Circumanal glands	Perianal region, prepuce	Dog, cat	Sebaceous glands and hepatoid glands
Perineal glands	Perineum	Horse	Sebaceous glands and apocrine sweat glands
Inguinal glands	Inguinal sinus	Sheep	Sebaceous glands and apocrine sweat glands
Carpal glands	Carpal organ	Pig	Merocrine sweat glands
Interdigital sinus glands	Interdigital sinus	Sheep	Sebaceous glands and apocrine sweat glands

(b) **Interlobular septa** are formed by dense irregular connective tissue. **Elastic fibers** are abundant.

b. **Inactive (involuting) gland.** Sudden arrest of milking or suckling leads to intraalveolar accumulation of milk and an intracellular increase in the number and confluence of lipid droplets.

(1) **Granulocytes** and **macrophages** invade the interalveolar connective tissue. Macrophages phagocytose the accumulated milk.

(2) The **alveoli collapse,** and alveolar epithelial cells are phagocytosed by macrophages.

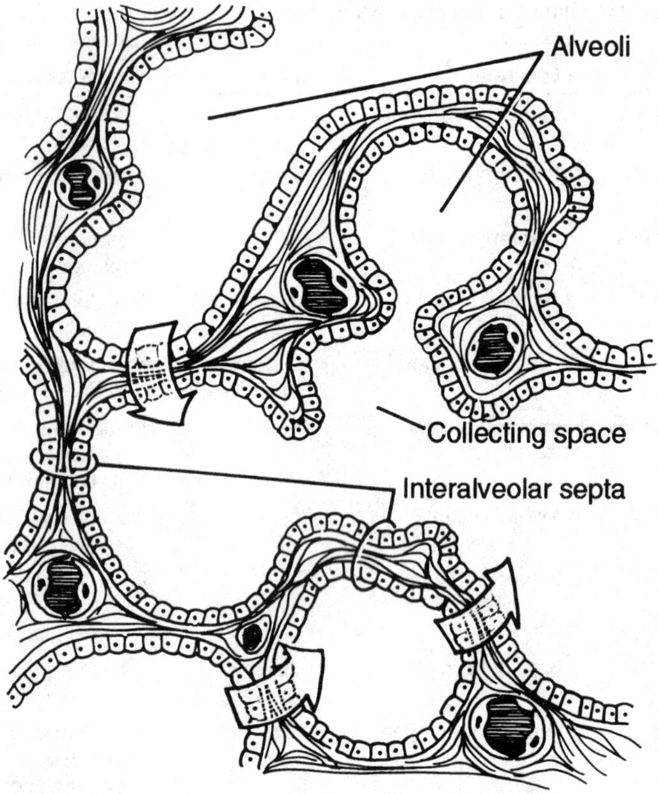

FIGURE 20-6. Schematic drawing of a section taken from a lactating mammary gland, illustrating a group of alveoli, a collecting space, and interalveolar septa. The *arrows* indicate areas where interalveolar communications are present above or below the plane of sectioning. (Redrawn with permission from Mosimann W, Kohler T: *Zytologie, Histologie und mikroskopische Anatomie der Haussäugetiere.* Berlin, Blackwell Wissenschafts-Verlag GmbH, 1990, p 289.)

(3) A few small **new alveoli** lined by nonsecretory cells are formed.
(4) **Interalveolar loose connective tissue** and **adipose tissue** become abundant.
(5) **Corpora amylacea** are concentrically layered concretions formed by casein and degenerated cells in the alveoli, ducts, and interstitium.

c. Teat

(1) The **mucosa** merges imperceptibly with the skin, which is hairless and glandless in cows and sows.
  (a) The mucosa is lined by stratified cuboidal epithelium.
  (b) It is surrounded by a thick layer of dense irregular connective tissue containing smooth muscle bundles and numerous veins that have a thick muscular media.
(2) **Alveoli** are present in the subepithelial connective tissue.
(3) The **papillary duct** is tightly closed by smooth muscle bundles oriented both circularly and longitudinally.

B. Digital organs and horns. In the digital organs and horns, the epidermis and dermis (also called **corium**) are highly modified, whereas the hypodermis is either absent or considerably thickened (e.g., in the digital pads). These structures are supported by bones.

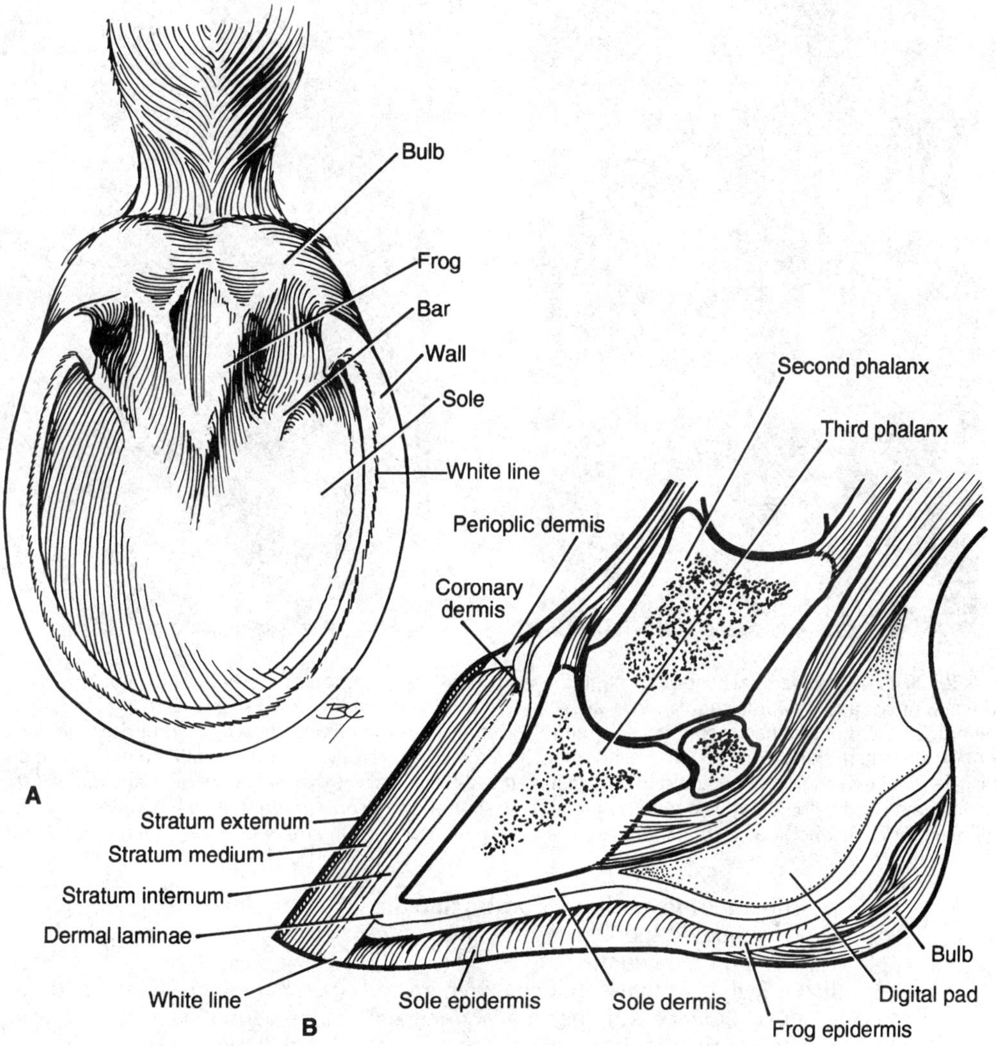

FIGURE 20-7. (*A*) Longitudinal section through the equine hoof. (*B*) Ventral view of the hoof. (Modified and redrawn with permission from Nickel R, Schummer A, Seiterle E: *Lehrbuch der Anatomie der Haustiere,* 3rd ed. Berlin/Hamburg, Paul Parey, 1984, pp 498, 499.)

1. **Equine hoof.** The hoof consists of the **wall,** which extends from the coronary band to the ground; the **sole,** which fills the space between the wall and the bars on the ventral surface; and the **frog,** a wedge-shaped mass between the bars and the sole (Figure 20-7A).
   - **a.** The **wall** comprises three layers (Figure 20-7B).
     - **(1) Stratum externum (tectorium)**
       - **(a)** The stratum externum is a thin layer of **soft tubular and intertubular horn** that arises from the stratum basale above and between the relatively thin and short papillae of the perioplic dermis.
       - **(b)** The bulbs of the hoof are formed toward the palmar/plantar (heel) surface of the foot, where the perioplic dermis and epidermis widen.
     - **(2) Stratum medium** (Figure 20-8A)
       - **(a)** This thickest layer of the wall consists of hard tubular and intertubular horn.
         - **(i) Tubular horn** consists of **solid rods** with a medulla and cortex. They arise from the stratum basale above the long papillae of the coronary dermis.

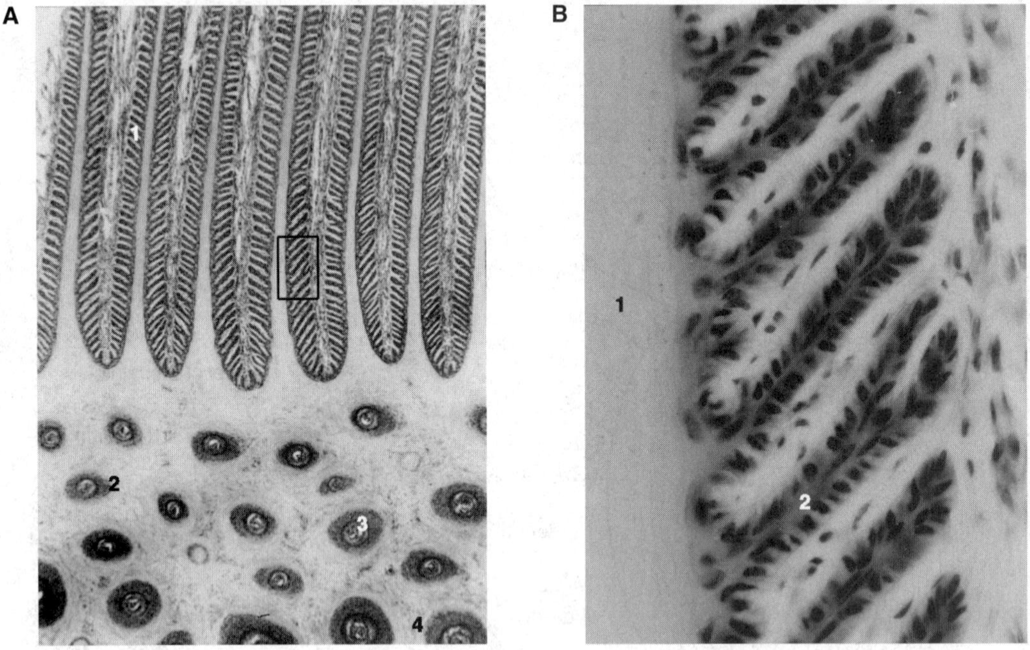

FIGURE 20-8. (*A*) Horizontal section through the wall of the equine hoof. In the stratum lamellatum (*1*), primary and secondary epidermal laminae are seen to interdigitate with corresponding dermal laminae. The primary dermal laminae merge imperceptibly with the stratum medium (*2*), which comprises tubular horn (*3*) and intertubular horn (*4*). (*B*) Higher magnification of an area similar to that outlined in (*A*). The primary dermal lamina (*1*) consists entirely of keratinized cells. The cells of the secondary dermal laminae (*2*) are nucleated and belong to the stratum basale and the stratum spinosum. (Reprinted with permission from Dellmann H-D: *Textbook of Veterinary Histology,* 4th ed. Baltimore, Williams & Wilkins, 1993, pp 308, 309.)

- **(ii) Intertubular horn** is **unstructured** and fills the space between the tubules. It originates from the stratum basale above the interpapillary coronary dermis.

(b) Growth in both the stratum externum and stratum medium is proximodistal, in accordance with the vertical orientation of the dermal papillae. The wall grows proximodistally at an average rate of 6.4 millimeters per month.

(3) Stratum internum (lamellatum)

(a) The stratum internum consists of vertical primary and secondary **epidermal laminae,** which are fused with the stratum medium (see Figure 20-8A&B).

- **(i) Primary epidermal laminae** are composed of hard keratin. They originate between the proximal ends of dermal laminae at the inner (deep) edge of the coronary dermis and grow in a proximodistal direction.
- **(ii) Secondary epidermal laminae** comprise only the stratum basale, which lies on the secondary dermal laminae, and the stratum spinosum, which forms the core of the epidermal laminae.

(b) The **dermis (corium)** underneath the stratum internum consists of **primary** and **secondary laminae,** which interdigitate with those of the epidermis, and a deeper layer that merges imperceptibly with the periosteum of the third phalanx.

- **(i)** The dermis is **well vascularized** and **innervated dense irregular connective tissue**.
- **(ii) Laminitis** is an extremely painful condition in which engorgement of the vascular bed compresses sensory nerve endings between the bone and the rigid hoof wall.

(c) The **white line** comprises an inner layer of unpigmented horn of the stratum medium and the nonpigmented epidermal laminae of the stratum internum that interdigitate with the pigmented tubular and intertubular horn of the sole.

b. The **sole** is composed of **tubular** and **intertubular horn,** which arise from the stratum basale above and among **dermal papillae.**

c. The **frog** is also composed of **tubular** and **intertubular horn,** which is softer than in any other part of the hoof.

(1) The papillated dermis rests upon a **thick hypodermis** that is rich in adipose cell clusters among strands of collagen and elastic fibers.

(2) Merocrine sweat glands are present.

2. **Ruminant and porcine claws** differ in a few respects from hooves of horses.

a. Only **primary epidermal laminae** are found on the stratum internum of the wall and the corresponding dermis.

b. The **sole** is very narrow.

c. The **bulb,** which comprises soft tubular and intertubular horn, occupies most of the ventral surface.

3. **Carnivore claws**

a. **Wall (claw plate).** The wall consists of densely packed flat keratinocytes. The keratinocytes originate above the proximodistally oriented **papillae of the coronary dermis.**

(1) Little growth occurs over the ridges of the wall dermis, over which the plate glides proximodistally. Ridges merely anchor the claw plate.

(2) The **dorsal ridge** is the region above the dorsal surface of the third phalanx. Both the claw plate and the underlying dermis are particularly thick in this region.

b. **Sole.** The sole epidermis consists of soft, thick keratinized stratified squamous epithelium, which arises from the stratum basale above the papillae of the underlying dermis.

c. The **claw fold** covers the claw plate proximally.

(1) The claw fold is typical skin on its outer aspect and hairless skin on its inner aspect.

(2) The epidermis of the inner surface of the claw fold produces a thin layer of keratinocytes that covers the claw plate proximally, similar to the stratum externum of the equine hoof.

4. **Digital pads** contact the ground.

a. **Epidermis.** The digital pads are covered by **thick keratinized stratified squamous epithelium.** The epithelial surface is **smooth in cats** and **papillated in dogs.**

b. **Dermis. Papillae** are prominent on the dermis.

c. **Hypodermis**

(1) The **digital cushion** is formed by the hypodermis. It consists of clusters of adipocytes separated and enclosed by septa of collagen and elastic fibers.

(2) Merocrine sweat glands are present in the digital cushion.

5. **Chestnuts and ergots** are areas of equine epidermis that consist of tubular and intertubular horn arising above long dermal papillae.

6. The **horn** of ruminants arises above the papillated dermis, which covers the cornual process of the frontal bone.

a. It consists of **hard tubular** and **intertubular horn.**

b. The **epikeras** is a thin layer of soft horn, similar to the stratum externum of the hoof. It extends a short distance distally from the base of the horn.

V. AVIAN INTEGUMENT

A. The **epidermis** comprises four layers:

1. **Stratum basale**

2. **Stratum intermedium** (corresponding to the mammalian stratum spinosum)
3. **Stratum transitivum** (corresponding to the mammalian stratum granulosum)
4. **Stratum corneum**

B. The **dermis** comprises three main layers.

1. The **superficial layer** is comparable to that of mammalian skin.
2. The **deep layer** includes a:
   a. **Stratum compactum** of dense irregular connective tissue
   b. **Stratum laxum,** a deeper layer of loose connective tissue into which feather follicles and their associated muscles extend
3. **Deep elastic stratum**

C. The **hypodermis** is rich in adipose tissue.

D. **Skin appendages**

1. **Uropygial (preen) gland.** This bilobed gland is the only gland in avian skin.
   a. **Tubular secretory units** are similar to mammalian sebaceous glands.
   b. **Secretory tubules** open into a common **primary cavity,** which continues into the relatively narrow **excretory duct**. This duct is lined with keratinized stratified squamous epithelium and opens onto the epidermal surface on the tip of a large papilla.
2. **Feathers** are epidermal structures of diverse morphology. Only contour feathers, down feathers, and filoplumes are described here.
   a. **Contour feathers** are the predominant feather type. They comprise a shaft and a vane.
      (1) The **shaft (quill)** comprises a tubular **calamus,** implanted in the feather follicle, and a solid **rachis,** projecting above the epidermis.
      (2) On each side of the rachis is a **vane,** composed of parallel **barbs** (i.e., lateral oblique projections from the rachis).
         (a) Each barb has proximal and distal branches, called **barbules**.
         (b) Barbules of adjacent barbs interlock (i.e., hooklets on the distal barbules of a given barb attach to indentations between tooth-like projections on the proximal barbules of the following barb). This creates a tightly knit vane.
   b. **Downs** of adult birds often have a short rachis, long barbs, and thin, long barbules that are not tightly interlocking. Entrapped air has a highly insulating effect.
   c. **Filoplumes** are the hair-like feathers that remain after a bird has been plucked. They have barbs only at the tip of the rachis, and their barbules are similar to those of downs.
3. **Scales** on avian feet consist of keratinized stratified squamous epithelium with a thick multilayered stratum corneum. The overlapping scales are separated by grooves (sulci) in which the keratin is of the soft variety.

STUDY QUESTIONS

DIRECTIONS: Each of the numbered items or incomplete statements in this section is followed by answers or by completions of the statement. Select the **one** numbered answer or completion that is **best** in each case.

1. Which one of the following layers is only present in thick and hairless epidermis?

(1) Stratum corneum
(2) Stratum spinosum
(3) Stratum basale
(4) Stratum lucidum
(5) Stratum granulosum

2. Which one of the following statements is true concerning the stratum spinosum?

(1) Membrane-coating granules are present in keratinocytes of the most superficial layers.
(2) Stem cells divide mitotically in the deeper layers.
(3) Tonofibrils link adjacent cells.
(4) Keratohyalin granules are present in the uppermost layers.
(5) Hemidesmosomes are abundant.

3. Which one of the following statements regarding melanosomes is true?

(1) Melanosomes are melanin-containing lysosomes.
(2) Melanosomes are melanocyte-derived secretory granules in the intercellular space between keratinocytes.
(3) Melanosomes are the ribosomes responsible for melanin synthesis.
(4) Melanosomes are melanin-containing phagosomes in melanocytes.
(5) Melanosomes are melanin-containing phagosomes in keratinocytes.

4. Which one of the following best describes the sweat glands of the hairy skin of domestic mammals?

(1) Merocrine
(2) Both apocrine and merocrine
(3) Apocrine
(4) Holocrine
(5) Both apocrine and holocrine

5. Which one of the following statements concerning merocrine sweat glands in domestic mammals is correct?

(1) They lack myoepithelial cells.
(2) They are associated with hairs and open into hair follicles.
(3) They function in thermoregulation.
(4) They are straight tubular glands.
(5) They are present in hairless regions.

6. Which of the following statements best describes mammary gland alveolar epithelial cells?

(1) They are cuboidal when at the height of their secretory activity.
(2) They secrete according to a holocrine mode of secretion.
(3) They secrete lipids according to a merocrine mode of secretion.
(4) They secrete proteins according to an apocrine mode of secretion.
(5) They are underlaid by myoepithelial cells.

7. Which one of the following best describes the stratum externum of the equine hoof?

(1) It is a thin layer of stratified squamous epithelium.
(2) It consists of primary horny laminae.
(3) It consists of primary and secondary horny laminae.
(4) It is hard tubular and intertubular horn.
(5) It is soft tubular and intertubular horn.

DIRECTIONS: Each of the numbered items or incomplete statements in this section is negatively phrased, as indicated by an italicized word such as *not, least,* or *except.* Select the **one** numbered answer or completion that is **best** in each case.

8. All of the following statements concerning the dermis are correct *except:*

(1) It is composed of both loose and dense connective tissue.
(2) Collagen fibers predominate.
(3) It has a rich superficial capillary bed.
(4) It is poorly innervated.
(5) Its deep layer contains few blood vessels.

9. All of the following statements concerning the dermal sheath of the hair follicle are correct *except:*

(1) It is a continuation of the superficial layer of the dermis.
(2) It is dense irregular connective tissue.
(3) It includes the hair papilla.
(4) The arrector pili muscle attaches to it.
(5) It is separated from the external root sheath by the glassy membrane.

10. All of the following statements concerning the characteristics of a tactile hair follicle are correct *except:*

(1) The outer root sheath contains many tactile discs.
(2) The dermal sheath is richly innervated.
(3) The dermal sheath comprises an inner and an outer layer.
(4) The hair papilla contains a blood-filled sinus.
(5) Voluntary movements are possible through skeletal muscle fibers.

11. All of the following statements concerning the mammary gland are correct *except:*

(1) Milk may be secreted by the lining epithelium of small ducts.
(2) The interstitial connective tissue contains numerous elastic fibers.
(3) Plasma cells commonly occur among the alveolar epithelial cells.
(4) Both alveoli and ducts contain myoepithelial cells.
(5) The larger ducts are lined with bistratified cuboidal epithelium.

ANSWERS AND EXPLANATIONS

1. The answer is 4 *[II A 1 a]*. The stratum lucidum is usually present in thick and hairless epidermis but usually not in thin and hairy epidermis. The stratum corneum, stratum spinosum, stratum basale, and stratum granulosum may be present in both hairy and hairless epidermis.

2. The answer is 1 *[II A 1 a (2)]*. The keratinocytes of the most superficial layers of the stratum spinosum contain membrane-coating granules, also called lamellar granules, which are released into the stratum granulosum. Stem cells divide in the stratum basale but not in the stratum spinosum. Tonofibrils are bundles of keratin filaments, or tonofilaments, that are confined to individual cells and do not cross the intercellular space. Keratohyalin granules are evident only in the stratum granulosum. Hemidesmosomes are characteristic of those keratinocytes in the stratum basale that are adjacent to the basal lamina.

3. The answer is 5 *[II A 2 a (3) (a)–(b)]*. Melanosomes are membrane-bounded melanin granules. They are synthesized in melanocytes, but they are present in keratinocytes as well. Melanosomes are not secreted by exocytosis; consequently, they are never present in the intercellular space. From the melanocyte cell body they move into the cell processes and are subsequently transferred to keratinocytes by phagocytosis of melanocyte processes.

4. The answer is 3 *[III B 2 a]*. The sweat glands of the hairy skin of domestic mammals are exclusively apocrine glands. Apocrine sweat glands are also present in many of the special skin glands. Merocrine sweat glands are restricted to a few hairless areas (e.g., the digital pad of carnivores). In the skin, only sebaceous glands are holocrine.

5. The answer is 5 *[III B 2 b]*. In the integument of domestic mammals, merocrine sweat glands are present in a few restricted hairless regions, such as the foot pads of carnivores and the planum nasale. They are coiled tubular glands with an epithelium that includes myoepithelial cells. In humans, merocrine sweat glands are present in both the hairy and the hairless skin and play an important role in body temperature regulation. The functional significance of merocrine sweat glands in domestic mammals remains largely obscure. In the digital pads, secretion is believed to improve traction.

6. The correct answer is 5. *[IV A 2 a (1)]*. Myoepithelial cells are prominent and play an important role in the emptying of alveoli (milk let-down). When at maximum secretory activity, mammary gland alveolar epithelial cells are columnar in shape; when at rest, they assume a low cuboidal shape. Secretory products are released by both apocrine (for lipids) and merocrine (for protein) secretion.

7. The answer is 5 *[IV B 1 a (1)]*. The stratum externum of the equine hoof is a thin layer of soft tubular and intertubular horn that has a tendency to wear off. Hard tubular and intertubular horn are present in the stratum medium. The stratum internum comprises primary and secondary horny laminae.

8. The answer is 4 *[II B]*. The dermis has a rich sensory nerve supply, particularly in the subepithelial loose connective tissue, which also contains a dense capillary plexus. Dense irregular connective tissue forms the bulk of the dermis (i.e., the deep layer) into which intradermal injections are made. Injected substances are resorbed very slowly because of the density of the tissue and the relatively poor blood supply. There are elastic fibers in the dermis, but they are outnumbered by collagen fibers.

9. The answer is 2 *[III A 1 c]*. The dermal sheath of the hair follicle is loose connective tissue. It is continuous with the superficial layer of the dermis and is separated from the epithelial external root sheath by a glassy membrane (i.e., a thickened basal lamina). It includes the hair papilla and serves as an attachment site for the arrector pili muscle. In the deep layer of the dermis, dense irregular connective tissue is present; but that layer is not part of the dermal sheath.

10. The answer is 4 *[III A 2 e]*. The hair papilla of a tactile hair does not contain a blood-filled sinus and does not differ structurally from the papilla of a nontactile hair. A blood-filled sinus is present between the outer and inner layers of the dermal sheath, both of which are abundantly supplied with nerves, some of which continue into the outer root sheath to terminate in tactile discs

(Merkel cells). Tactile hairs can voluntarily be moved by contraction of the skeletal muscle fibers that attach to the outer dermal sheath.

11. The answer is 3 *[IV A 2 a]*. Plasma cells are numerous in the mammary gland, but they lie within the interstitial connective tissue rather than among the alveolar epithelial cells. The lining epithelium is simple cuboidal to columnar in alveoli and small ducts, and it is secretory in both. It is bistratified in the larger ducts and not secretory. The interstitial connective tissue, especially where it is abundant (e.g., in interlobular septa), is rich in elastic fibers. Myoepithelial cells lie between secretory cells and the surrounding basal lamina in the alveoli and ducts.

Chapter 21

The Eye and Its Accessory Organs

I. INTRODUCTION

A. Structure of the eye (Figure 21-1)

1. **Tunics**
   a. **Fibrous tunic.** This outer tunic comprises the **sclera** and **cornea**.
   b. **Vascular tunic.** This middle tunic includes the **choroid, ciliary body,** and **iris**.
   c. **Neuroepithelial tunic.** This inner tunic is the **retina**.

2. **Compartments**
   a. **Anterior compartment**
      (1) This compartment is located **between the cornea and the vitreous body**.
      (2) It is divided into **two chambers**.
         (a) The **anterior chamber** is located between the cornea and iris.
         (b) The **posterior chamber** is located between the iris and vitreous body, and it contains the **lens**.
      (3) **Aqueous humor** fills the anterior compartment.

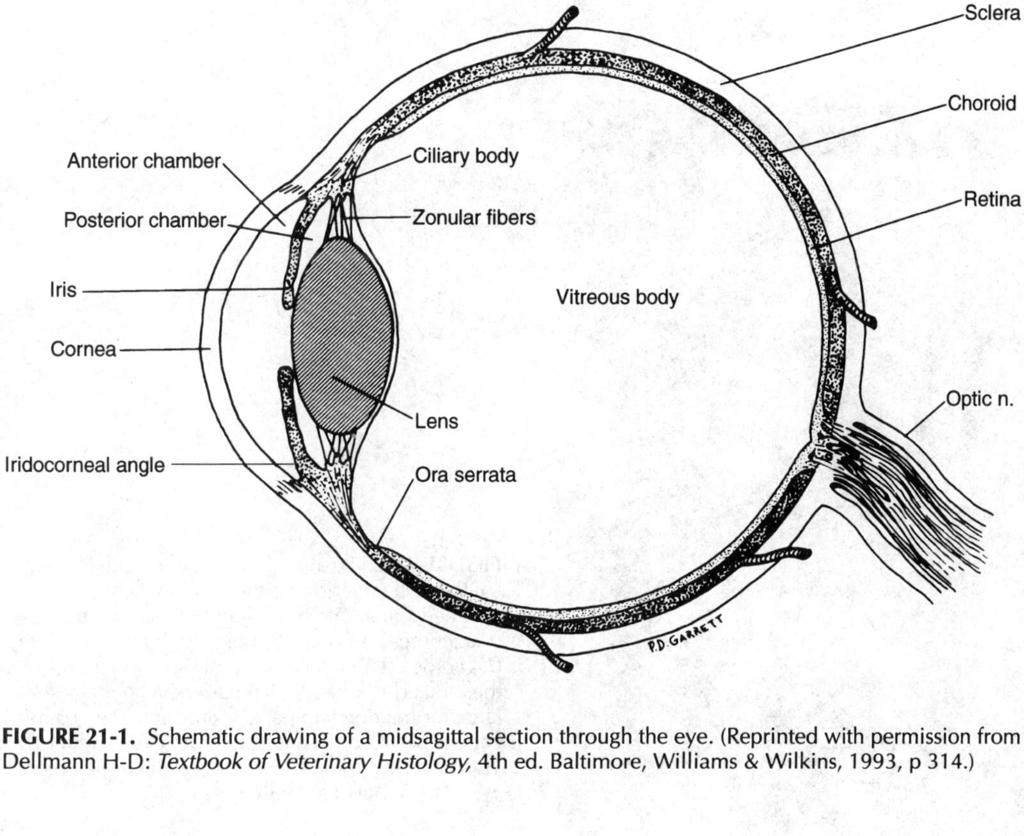

FIGURE 21-1. Schematic drawing of a midsagittal section through the eye. (Reprinted with permission from Dellmann H-D: *Textbook of Veterinary Histology,* 4th ed. Baltimore, Williams & Wilkins, 1993, p 314.)

b. Posterior compartment

(1) This compartment is located **between the lens and the retina**.

(2) The **vitreous body** fills the posterior compartment.

B. **Accessory organs** include the eyelids, the third eyelid (nictitating membrane), the conjunctiva, and the lacrimal apparatus.

C. **Functions.** The eye transforms light into electrical impulses that are transmitted to the brain, where they form images and influence circadian rhythms.

II. TUNICS

A. Fibrous tunic

1. The **sclera** is a poorly vascularized, tough protective layer that maintains the shape of the eye and serves as an attachment site for the extrinsic eye muscles.
   - **a.** It is composed of **dense irregular connective tissue** in which bundles of collagen fibers and a few elastic fibers are arranged parallel to the surface of the globe (eyeball).
   - **b.** Melanocytes may be present, subject to species-dependent and individual variations.
2. The **cornea** is an avascular, richly innervated, transparent convex and concave lens that plays an important role in image formation. It is composed of five layers (Figure 21-2).
   - **a. Corneal epithelium (anterior epithelium)** covers the anterior surface of the cornea.
     - **(1)** It is **nonkeratinized stratified squamous epithelium** with many free nerve endings.
     - **(2)** **Mitosis** and **cell migration** ensure **fast healing** of injured epithelium.

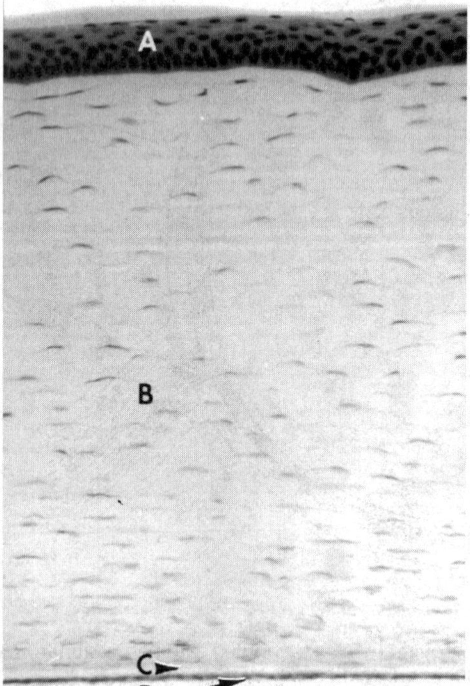

FIGURE 21-2. Section through the canine cornea. (*A*) Corneal (anterior) epithelium (nonkeratinized stratified squamous epithelium); (*B*) substantia propria (corneal stroma); (*C*) posterior limiting lamina; (*D*) corneal endothelium (simple squamous epithelium). The subepithelial basement membrane (anterior limiting lamina) is visible at higher magnifications between (*A*) and (*B*). (From Dellmann H-D: *Textbook of Veterinary Histology,* 4th ed. Baltimore, Williams & Wilkins, 1993, p 314.)

b. The **subepithelial basement membrane (anterior limiting lamina)** consists of a **basal lamina** and a **reticular layer**.

c. The **substantia propria (corneal stroma)** is the thickest layer of the cornea.

(1) It consists of **layers of collagen fibers** and **fibrocytes** arranged parallel to the corneal surface and oriented at right angles in adjacent layers.

(2) **Amorphous ground substance** is abundant.

(a) It is **rich in sulfated glycosaminoglycans** (i.e., chondroitin sulfate and keratan sulfate).

(b) **Adequate hydration** of the amorphous ground substance is **necessary for corneal transparency**.

d. The **posterior limiting lamina (Descemet's membrane)** is a thick refractile layer of **atypical collagen fibrils in hexagonal arrays**.

e. **Posterior epithelium (corneal endothelium)** is composed of **simple squamous epithelium**. Integrity of the corneal endothelium is important for maintaining corneal transparency.

3. **Corneoscleral junction (limbus).** The sclera overlaps the cornea at the corneoscleral junction (see Figure 21-1).

a. The posterior epithelium gradually changes into conjunctival epithelium (see IV C 1). The subepithelial basement membrane terminates at the limbus.

b. The collagen fibers of the substantia propria gradually become irregularly arranged and merge with those of the sclera.

c. The posterior limiting lamina divides to continue into the trabecular meshwork [see II B 4 a (2)].

d. The posterior epithelium continues into the mesothelium covering the trabecular meshwork.

e. Nutrients reach the cornea via diffusion from blood vessels at the corneoscleral junction and from the aqueous humor.

B. Vascular tunic

1. The **choroid** is a thick and richly vascularized coat between the sclera and retina. It is subdivided into five layers (Figure 21-3).

a. The **suprachoroid layer** is adjacent to the sclera. It is composed of collagen fibers, elastic fibers, fibroblasts, and numerous melanocytes.

b. The **vascular layer** contains a network of arteries and veins that is connected to capillaries of the choriocapillary layer (see II B 1 d).

c. The **tapetum lucidum** lies between the vascular layer and the choriocapillary layer, primarily in the dorsal half of the fundus of the eye. Depending on the species, collagen fibers or intracellular rods reflect and diffract incoming light, possibly improving low-light vision.

(1) In carnivores, the tapetum lucidum consists of several layers of flat polygonal cells packed with parallel crystalline rods rich in zinc.

(2) In herbivores, it consists of parallel collagen fibers and fibrocytes.

d. The **choriocapillary layer** is composed of a dense capillary network adjacent to the pigmented epithelium of the retina. Retinal pigmented epithelial cells and receptor cells receive nutrients via these capillaries.

(1) Where capillaries face the pigmented epithelium, the endothelium is fenestrated.

(2) The basal laminae of capillaries and pigmented epithelium are often fused.

e. The **basal complex (Bruch's membrane)** separates the choroid and retina.

(1) It usually consists of collagen fibers, elastic fibers, fibrocytes, and the basal laminae of the choriocapillary layer and pigmented retinal epithelium.

(2) In many areas, it comprises only the fused basal laminae of capillaries and pigmented epithelium.

2. The **ciliary body** is a rostral continuation of the choroid that **extends from the ora serrata to the iris** (see Figure 21-1).

a. **Ciliary processes** are rostral projections of the ciliary body. They form the **ciliary crown (pars plicata)** as they project into the posterior chamber.

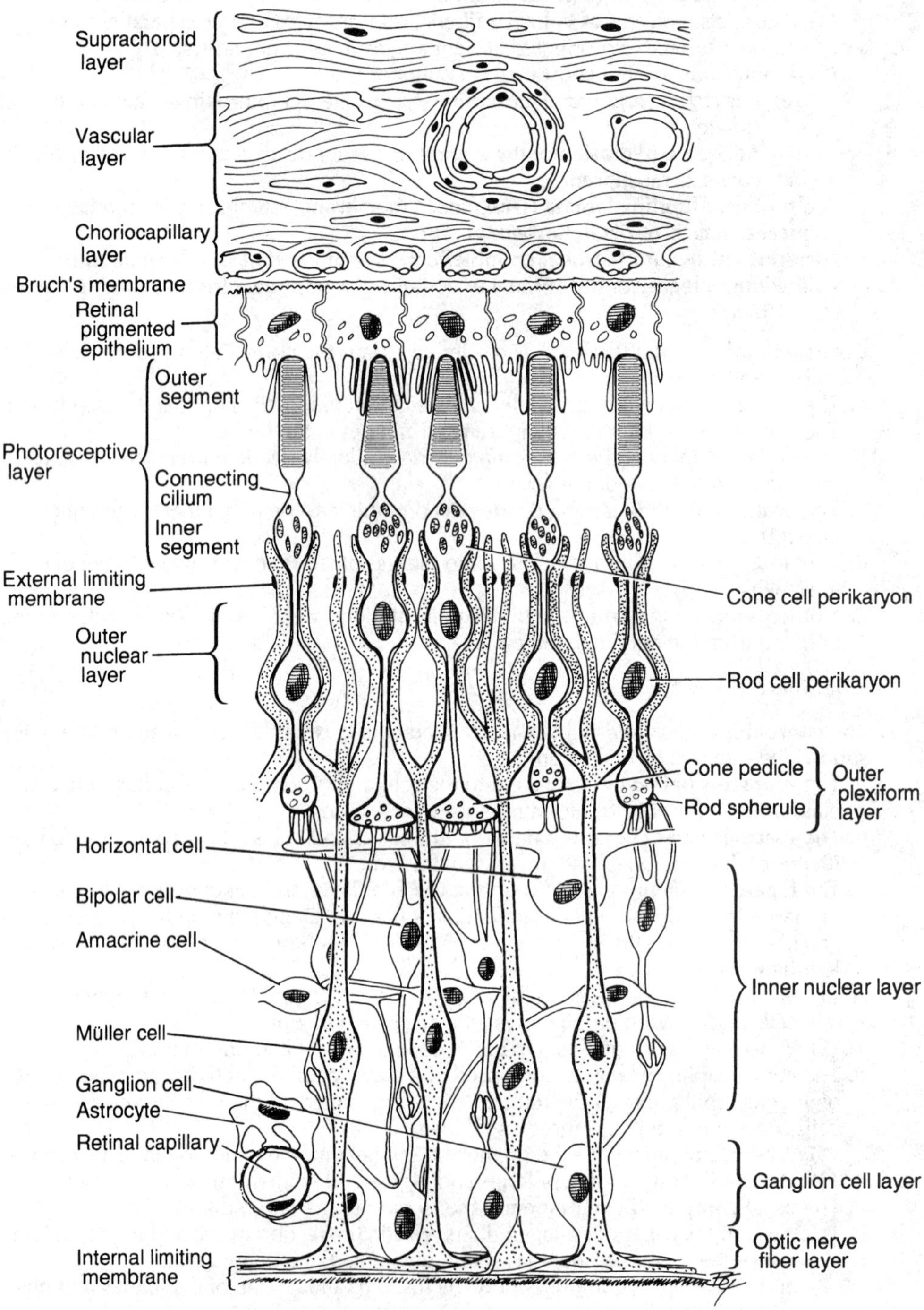

FIGURE 21-3. Schematic drawing of the retina and adjacent choroid. (Redrawn and modified from Mosimann W, Kohler T: *Zytologie, Histologie und mikroskopische Anatomie der Haussäugetiere.* Berlin, Blackwell Wissenschafts-Verlag GmbH, 1990, p 312.)

b. The **pars plana** is the flat, caudal portion of the ciliary body.

c. Ciliary muscle. This smooth muscle is located within the loose connective tissue of the ciliary body. Its fibers are arranged predominantly meridionally.

(1) Contraction of the ciliary muscle fibers reduces tension of the zonular fibers of the lens. Consequently, the elastic lens becomes more convex and thus accommodates (i.e., focuses on nearby objects).

(2) Relaxation of the ciliary muscle fibers has the opposite effect.

d. Epithelium. The two layers of epithelium that cover the ciliary body (i.e., the pars ciliaris retinae) are of retinal origin.

(1) The **outer pigmented epithelial layer** is simple cuboidal epithelium that is continuous with the pigmented epithelium of the retina. Microvillous apical projections interdigitate with similar projections from the adjacent nonpigmented epithelium.

(2) The **inner nonpigmented epithelial layer** is simple cuboidal or columnar epithelium resting on a basal lamina that faces the posterior chamber.

e. Aqueous humor, a watery fluid that nourishes the lens and cornea, is elaborated by the ciliary epithelium, capillaries of the ciliary processes, and fibrocytes. It is continuously renewed and flows through the pupil into the anterior chamber, from which it is drained via the iridocorneal angle (see II B 4).

3. The **iris** is the most anterior part of the choroid. It is located rostral to the lens, between the anterior and posterior chambers, which communicate through the centrally located **pupil**. It comprises stroma, two muscles, and two layers of epithelium.

a. The **stroma** of the iris occupies the most anterior part of the iris.

(1) Its **anterior lining** is **discontinuous flattened mesothelium.**

(2) It is **richly vascularized connective tissue** with many **collagen fiber bundles**.

(3) Melanocytes, together with the posterior pigmented epithelium, determine the color of the iris.

b. Muscles. Two muscles of neuroepithelial origin regulate the aperture of the pupil.

(1) The **sphincter muscle (m. sphincter pupillae)** is composed of circularly arranged muscle cells at the pupillary margin.

(2) The **dilator muscle (m. dilator pupillae)** consists of radially arranged contractile cells that have differentiated from the deep (anterior) pigmented epithelial cell layer of the iris epithelium.

c. Epithelium. Iris epithelium (i.e., pars iridica retinae) is continuous with ciliary epithelium.

(1) The **deep (anterior) layer** forms the dilator muscle.

(2) The **superficial (posterior) layer** is pigmented.

(3) Granula iridica are found in ungulates. They are localized proliferations of the two epithelial layers that project into the anterior chamber of the eye at the dorsal and ventral pupillary margins.

4. The **iridocorneal angle (iris or drainage angle)** is located at the periphery of the anterior chamber, where the corneoscleral junction, iris, and ciliary body meet.

a. Structure

(1) The **pectinate ligament** is formed by connective tissue strands covered by flattened mesothelial cells.

(2) The **trabecular meshwork** is deeper tissue, continuous with the pectinate ligament. Fluid-filled spaces (**spaces of Fontana**) are present among the trabeculae.

(3) Trabecular veins within the trabecular meshwork drain into a **scleral venous plexus** (the **canal of Schlemm** of primates).

b. Function. Drainage of aqueous humor occurs through the spaces of the pectinate ligament and trabecular meshwork into trabecular veins. Inadequate drainage results in increased intraocular pressure (glaucoma).

C. **Neuroepithelial tunic.** The **retina** is the light-sensitive layer of the eye.

1. **Layers.** Ten layers of orderly arranged cells can be identified (see Figure 21-3).
   a. **Retinal pigment epithelium,** the outermost layer, is **simple cuboidal epithelium.**
      (1) **Histologic appearance**
         (a) The **bases** of the epithelial cells have many membrane infoldings associated with mitochondria.
         (b) Cell **apices** are joined by **tight junctions.**
         (c) **Apical microvillous or leaf-like processes** surround the outer segments of rods and cones, respectively.
         (d) **Melanin granules** are numerous, except in the region of the tapetum lucidum.
      (2) **Functions**
         (a) **Light absorption**
         (b) **Transport of nutrients** to photoreceptor cells (i.e., rods and cones)
         (c) **Phagocytosis and degradation** of discarded membranous disks of the outer segments of photoreceptor cells [see II C 1 b (1) (a) (ii)]
   b. **Photoreceptive layer.** This layer of **rods and cones** contains the photoreceptive portion of the first neuron of the visual pathway.
      (1) **Histologic appearance.** Both rods and cones consist of:
         (a) An **outer segment** containing **stacked membranous disks**
            (i) **Visual pigment (rhodopsin)** is contained within disk membranes. This pigment absorbs light rays.
            (ii) Disks are continuously replaced. Old disks are shed distally while new disks form proximally at the base of the outer segment through plasma membrane invagination.
         (b) A **cilium,** which connects the outer and inner segments
         (c) An **inner segment** containing numerous mitochondria and the basal body of the cilium
      (2) **Functions**
         (a) **Low-light vision. Rod cells** are stimulated by dim light.
         (b) **Color vision. Cone cells** are stimulated by bright light and are responsible for color vision.
   c. The **external limiting membrane** is formed by zonulae adherentes between processes of **radial glial (Müller) cells** and rod and cone cells.
   d. The **outer nuclear layer** contains the perikarya of the rod and cone cells.
   e. In the **outer plexiform layer,** rod and cone axon terminals (i.e., rod spherules and cone pedicles) synapse with dendrites of bipolar cells and processes of horizontal cells.
   f. In the **inner nuclear layer, bipolar cells,** the second neurons in the visual neuronal chain, predominate. **Horizontal cells, amacrine cells,** and **radial glial cells** are also present.
   g. In the **inner plexiform layer,** synaptic contact between bipolar cells and ganglion cells and between amacrine cells and ganglion cells occurs.
   h. The **ganglion cell layer** contains the large perikarya of the **ganglion cells,** the third neurons of the visual pathway.
   i. The **optic nerve fiber layer** contains the axons of the ganglion cells, some astrocytes, and microglial cells. Converging axons form the **optic nerve** as they exit the retina at the optic disk.
   j. The **internal limiting membrane** consists of a layer of flattened radial glial cell processes [resembling the glia limitans in the central nervous system (CNS)] and a basal lamina.

2. The **area centralis** is the region of most acute vision. Compared with the rest of the retina, it has more cone cells and ganglion cells, a thicker inner plexiform layer, a thinner optic nerve fiber layer, and no large blood vessels.

III. REFRACTIVE MEDIA. The cornea, aqueous humor in the anterior and posterior chambers, lens, and vitreous body contribute to light refraction.

A. Lens. The lens is a biconvex, transparent structure, suspended by zonular fibers between the iris and the vitreous body. Its diameter is controlled by contraction or relaxation of the ciliary muscle.

1. **Lens structure.** The lens consists of a lens capsule, lens epithelium, and lens fibers.
   - a. **Lens capsule.** Several layers of collagen fibrils embedded into basal lamina material form the lens capsule.
   - b. **Lens epithelium** is simple cuboidal epithelium that covers the anterior surface of the lens.
   - c. **Lens fibers** are long, prism-shaped, interdigitating fibers without nucleus and organelles. Through continuous differentiation and addition of fibers, the lens grows throughout life.
     - (1) Lens fibers are formed by elongation and differentiation of lens epithelial cells at the equator of the lens.
     - (2) They are interconnected by gap junctions and desmosomes.
     - (3) In aged individuals, the lens fibers decrease in elasticity and plasticity.
2. **Zonular fibers** are bundles of collagen fibrils that arise from the basal lamina of the ciliary body epithelium and attach to the outer layers of the lens capsule at the equator.

B. The **vitreous body** is a gel that occupies the posterior compartment between the lens and the retina.

1. It contains **99% water** and is **rich in hyaluronic acid**.
2. The **hyaloid membrane** is formed by collagen fibrils and fibrocytes (hyalocytes) concentrated in the periphery of the vitreous body.

IV. ACCESSORY ORGANS

A. Eyelids. The rostral surface of the eyelid is typical skin, and the inner surface is covered by conjunctiva.

1. **Eyelashes** are present at the free margins of the eyelids in most domestic species. They are more numerous on the upper eyelid than on the lower one. Tactile hairs may also be present.
2. **Tarsal (Meibomian) glands** are large multilobar sebaceous glands. Their secretory product helps prevent lacrimal (tear) overflow over the margin of the eyelid.
3. The **tarsus** is a plate of collagen and elastic fibers attached to the periosteum at the base of the eyelid. It makes the eyelid rigid.

B. The **third eyelid** is a conjunctival fold.

1. A **cartilaginous plate** confers rigidity.
2. Both the **superficial gland** and the **deep (Harderian) gland** of the third eyelid resemble the lacrimal gland structurally (see IV D 1).

C. Conjunctiva. The bulbar and palpebral conjunctivae link the globe and eyelids.

1. **Conjunctival epithelium** is stratified cuboidal to columnar epithelium with goblet cells. It varies widely among species.

2. The **lamina propria** is highly vascular loose connective tissue that contains lymphocytes, plasma cells, and solitary (and, occasionally, aggregated) lymphatic nodules.

D. Lacrimal apparatus

1. The **lacrimal gland** is a compound tubuloalveolar or tubuloacinar serous or seromucous gland, drained by several main ducts.
2. The **lacrimal lake** is an accumulation of lacrimal fluid. It is formed by a medial widening of the conjunctiva.
3. **Lacrimal canaliculi** and the **lacrimal sac** convey lacrimal fluid to the **nasolacrimal duct**. These structures are lined with conjunctival epithelium.

STUDY QUESTIONS

DIRECTIONS: Each of the numbered items or incomplete statements in this section is followed by answers or by completions of the statement. Select the **one** numbered answer or completion that is **best** in each case.

1. Which one of the following statements concerning the cornea is correct?

(1) The stroma consists of several layers of collagen and elastic fibers.
(2) The stroma contains abundant amorphous ground substance.
(3) The posterior limiting lamina (Descemet's membrane) is a thick layer of elastic fibers.
(4) The corneal endothelium is simple cuboidal.
(5) The cornea receives its nutrients from a rich peripheral capillary plexus.

2. Which one of the following statements concerning the ciliary body is correct?

(1) Contraction of the ciliary muscle causes the lens to become less convex.
(2) Zonular fibers are elastic fibers originating from the basal lamina of the nonpigmented epithelial layer.
(3) The ciliary epithelium participates in the production of aqueous humor.
(4) Ciliary processes are projections of the ciliary crown into the anterior chamber of the eye.
(5) The pigmented epithelium is modified to form the dilator muscle of the pupil.

3. Which one of the following statements concerning the retina is correct?

(1) The pigment epithelium reflects light onto the rods and cones.
(2) Rods and cones are light-sensitive dendrites of nerve cells in the outer nuclear layer.
(3) Axons of rod and cone cells form the optic nerve fiber layer.
(4) Ganglion cells are the second neurons in the visual pathway.
(5) Glial cells are absent.

4. Which one of the following statements concerning the lens is correct?

(1) Elastic zonular fibers originating from the equator attach the lens to the ciliary body.
(2) The lens receives nutrients via capillaries that enter the lens at the equator.
(3) Lens fibers are differentiated lens epithelial cells.
(4) The lens is surrounded by a thin capsule of elastic fibers and amorphous ground substance.
(5) Lens epithelium surrounds the lens underneath the capsule.

DIRECTIONS: Each of the numbered items or incomplete statements in this section is negatively phrased, as indicated by an italicized word such as *not, least,* or *except.* Select the **one** numbered answer or completion that is **best** in each case.

5. Which one of the following statements is *not* correct regarding the anterior epithelium of the cornea?

(1) It is stratified squamous keratinized epithelium.
(2) It is rich in free nerve endings.
(3) It responds to injury with mitosis.
(4) It responds to injury with cell migration.
(5) It rests on a basement membrane.

6. All of the following statements correctly describe a characteristic of the choroid *except:*

(1) A dense network of capillaries is present adjacent to the retinal pigmented epithelium.
(2) Retinal pigmented epithelium and capillaries are separated by Bruch's membrane (basal complex).
(3) A prominent vascular layer contains large blood vessels that supply and drain the choriocapillary layer.
(4) The light-reflecting tapetum lucidum consists of several layers of parallel elastic fibers and fibrocytes.
(5) Numerous melanocytes confer a dark color to the choroid.

ANSWERS AND EXPLANATIONS

1. The answer is 2 *[II A 2 c (2)]*. The corneal stroma consists of several layers of parallel collagen fibers between which abundant amorphous ground substance (mainly keratan sulfate and chondroitin sulfate) is present. Elastic fibers are absent in the cornea. The corneal endothelium (posterior epithelium) is simple squamous epithelium through which nutrients diffuse from the aqueous humor into the cornea. Blood-borne nutrients diffuse into the cornea from blood vessels in the corneoscleral junction; the cornea itself does normally not contain any blood vessels.

2. The answer is 3 *[II B 2 e]*. Aqueous humor is produced by the ciliary body; both the inner and outer epithelium as well as capillaries in the underlying connective tissue and the fibroblasts of the connective tissue are involved in its elaboration. Contraction of the predominantly meridional fibers of the ciliary muscle causes relaxation of the collagen zonular fibers; by virtue of its elasticity, the lens becomes more convex. The zonular fibers are attached to the basal lamina of the inner nonpigmented ciliary epithelium; however, they are not elastic. The ciliary crown is the most rostral portion of the ciliary body and projects with numerous processes into the posterior chamber of the eye (located between the iris and the vitreous body), not into the anterior chamber (located between the iris and the cornea). The pigmented epithelium of the ciliary body is a continuation of the pigmented epithelium of the retina and has virtually the same structural characteristics. It is the pigmented epithelium of the iris that is contractile and forms the dilator muscle of the pupil.

3. The answer is 2 *[II C 1 b]*. Rod cells and cone cells are the first neurons of the visual pathway. Their perikarya are located in the outer nuclear layer. Their dendrites consist of an outer and an inner segment and a connecting cilium. The actual light-sensitive structures, flattened disks with membranes that contain visual pigment, are in the outer segments. The pigment epithelium is the outermost layer of the retina; it absorbs light and does not reflect it. The light-reflecting layer of the eye is the tapetum lucidum, which is part of the choroid. Light is able to reach the tapetum lucidum because the pigmented epithelium of the retina lacks pigment where it overlies the tapetum lucidum. Axons of the retinal ganglion cells, the third neurons of the visual pathway, form the optic nerve fiber layer of the retina. The retina contains glial cells. Radial glial cells that span the entire thickness of the retina are the most numerous (and probably most important) glial cells. Astrocytes and the less numerous microglial cells are mainly present in the optic nerve fiber layer.

4. The answer is 3 *[III A 1 c]*. Lens fibers originate from lens epithelial cells throughout the life of the animal. When, through displacement by mitotic divisions, lens epithelial cells arrive at the equator, they elongate and gradually lose their organelles, including the nucleus, and are interconnected through numerous interdigitations. On its anterior surface, the lens is covered by simple cuboidal lens epithelium, but it has no epithelium on its posterior surface. It is, however, completely surrounded by a capsule in which layers of collagen fibers alternate with basal lamina material. At the equator, collagen fibrils that make up the zonular fibers, which originate primarily from between the ciliary processes of the ciliary body, attach to the lens equator. The nutrient supply of the lens is derived from the aqueous humor; the lens is avascular.

5. The answer is 1 *[II A 2 a]*. The anterior epithelium of the cornea is nonkeratinized stratified squamous epithelium. If it were keratinized, perception of foreign objects on the cornea would be difficult and damage repair would be much less efficient. Damaged epithelium is repaired through mitosis and cell migration. The anterior epithelium of the cornea is rich in free nerve endings. It rests on the subepithelial basement membrane.

6. The answer is 4 *[II B 1 c]*. The tapetum lucidum is one of the five layers of the choroid. In herbivores, the tapetum is made up of collagen fibers and fibrocytes; in carnivores it consists of several layers of flat cells that contain parallel rods rich in zinc. Both collagen fibers and cells reflect and diffract light.

Chapter 22
The Ear

I. INTRODUCTION

A. Components (Figure 22-1)

1. The **external ear** comprises the **auricle (pinna)** and the **external auditory canal**.
2. The **middle ear** is separated from the external ear by the tympanic membrane and is connected to the nasopharynx via the auditory tube. It contains three **auditory ossicles**.
3. The **internal ear** is composed of the **osseous labyrinth,** a system of bony canals and cavities within the petrous part of the temporal bone, and the **membranous labyrinth,** which fits into the osseous labyrinth (see Figure 22-1). The membranous labyrinth is composed of the **vestibular apparatus** and the **cochlear duct**.

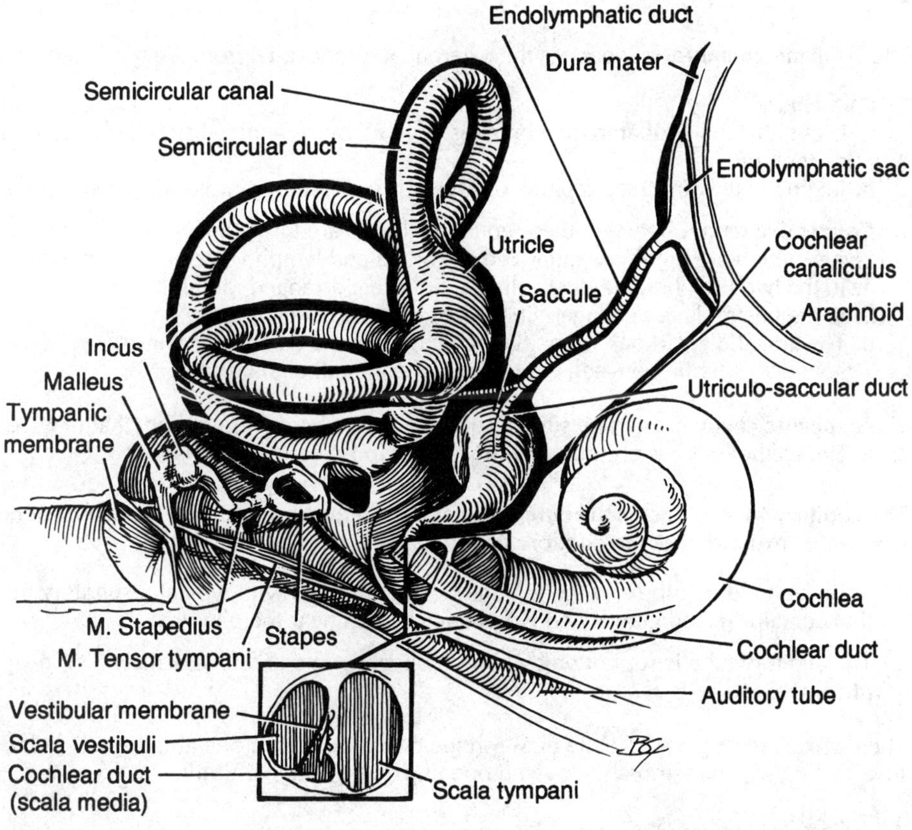

FIGURE 22-1. Schematic drawing of the middle and inner ear.

B. Functions

1. **Hearing.** Sound vibrations are transduced into electrical impulses in the spiral organ of the cochlear duct.
2. **Position awareness.** Linear and rotary acceleration induce electrical impulses via receptors in the vestibular apparatus.

II. EXTERNAL EAR

A. The **auricle** consists of an elastic cartilaginous plate covered on both sides by typical skin.

B. The **external auditory canal** is mostly surrounded by elastic cartilage. It is lined with skin containing small hair follicles, associated sebaceous glands, and ceruminous glands (apocrine sweat glands). Cerumen, a waxy substance found in the external auditory canal, repels insects and other vermin. It is a combination of the secretions of ceruminous glands, sebum, and sloughed epithelial cells.

III. MIDDLE EAR

A. The **tympanic membrane** separates the external auditory canal from the tympanic cavity.

1. **Epithelium**
   a. Externally, the tympanic membrane is covered by keratinized stratified squamous epithelium.
   b. Internally (toward the tympanic cavity), it is covered by simple squamous epithelium.
2. **Connective tissue.** Between these epithelial layers are three thin connective tissue layers, which are highly vascularized (by blood and lymph vessels) and innervated.
   a. In the two peripheral layers, collagen fibers are arranged radially.
   b. In the central layer, collagen fibers are arranged concentrically.
   c. The dorsal, flaccid part of the tympanic membrane contains a single layer of loose connective tissue between the two peripheral epithelial layers.

B. The **tympanic cavity** is lined by simple squamous or cuboidal epithelium that may be ciliated. The epithelium lies on top of a thin layer of loose connective tissue.

C. The **auditory tube** connects the tympanic cavity and the nasopharynx. The **guttural pouch** is a ventral expansion of the auditory tube in horses.

1. Both the auditory tube and the guttural pouch are lined with typical respiratory mucosa that contains mixed glands and lymphatic nodules near the pharynx.
2. The auditory tube is supported by bone proximally and cartilage distally (i.e., near the pharynx).

D. The **ossicles** (see Figure 22-1) lie between the tympanic membrane and the vestibular (oval) window, the membrane-covered opening of the scala vestibuli.

1. The ossicles comprise:
   a. The **malleus,** which inserts into the connective tissue of the tympanic membrane
   b. The **incus,** which connects the malleus and stapes
   c. The **stapes,** which attaches to the membrane that covers the vestibular window

2. The ossicles are joined by synovial articulations and held in place by ligaments. Their movements are modulated by the **tensor tympani** and **stapedius muscles**.

3. The ossicles transmit vibrations of the tympanic membrane to the **perilymph** of the inner ear.

IV. INTERNAL EAR

A. The **osseous labyrinth** comprises three major portions.

1. **Vestibule.** This centrally located space communicates with the tympanic cavity via the vestibular window.

2. **Semicircular canals.** The **anterior, posterior,** and **lateral canals** originate from and terminate at the vestibule. They lie at right angles to each other, and each has a dilated end (**ampulla ossea**).

3. **Cochlea**
   a. **Modiolus.** The cochlea, a cone-shaped structure, contains a central osseous column, the modiolus.
      (1) The modiolus is hollow, and the opening at its base forms the **internal acoustic meatus.**
      (2) The modiolus contains the cochlear division of the **eighth cranial nerve,** including its nerve cells, which form the **spiral ganglion.**
   b. **Cochlear canal.** The modiolus is surrounded by the cochlear canal, a spiral-shaped perilymphatic structure divided into dorsal and ventral compartments by the **spiral lamina,** a bony projection, and by the **basilar membrane,** a connective tissue membrane.
      (1) The **scala vestibuli,** the **dorsal compartment,** extends from the vestibular window to the **cupula,** the apex of the cochlea.
      (2) The **scala tympani,** the **ventral compartment,** extends from the cochlear window to the cupula.
      (3) The **helicotrema** is a small opening at the cupula through which the scala vestibuli and scala tympani communicate.

B. The **membranous labyrinth** is a series of membranous ducts and sacs contained within the osseous labyrinth.

1. **General structural characteristics**
   a. The membranous labyrinth is lined by simple squamous epithelium and filled with **endolymph.**
   b. It is surrounded by the perilymphatic space and held in place by a fine trabecular meshwork of connective tissue filled with perilymph.
   c. The **cochlear canaliculus** connects the perilymphatic space with the subarachnoid space.

2. **Subdivisions**
   a. The **vestibular apparatus** consists of the **utricle, saccule,** and **semicircular ducts** (see Figure 22-1). The utricle and saccule are joined by the utriculosaccular duct, which in turn communicates with the subarachnoid endolymphatic sac via the endolymphatic duct.
      (1) **Macula utriculi** and **macula sacculi** are sensory areas within the utricle and saccule that detect linear acceleration and changes in head position, enabling control of posture, gait, and equilibrium.

(a) Maculae consist of **supporting cells** and **two types of receptor (hair) cells** (Figure 22-2). Receptor cells are in contact with afferent and efferent nerve fibers.

(b) Maculae are covered by the **statoconial (otolithic) membrane,** a gelatinous mass containing **statoconia** (calcium carbonate crystals). **Stereocilia** (long, apical microvilli) and cilia of the hair cells penetrate this mass.

(2) **Cristae ampullares** (Figure 22-3) are ridge-shaped sensory receptor areas within membranous ampullae in the semicircular ducts.

(a) **Supporting cells** and **two types of epithelial receptor cells** are present in the cristae. Apical stereocilia and cilia of the sensory cells project into the cupula.

(b) The **cupula** is a gelatinous crest that extends to the opposite wall of the ampulla. Motion of the cupula permits detection of changes in the speed of rotation.

b. The **cochlear duct (scala media)** is an endolymphatic compartment located between the perilymphatic scala vestibuli dorsally and the scala tympani ventrally (see Figures 22-1 and 22-4).

(1) The cochlear duct is separated from the scala vestibuli by the vestibular (Reissner's) membrane and from the scala tympani by the basilar membrane. It is connected to the saccule via the ductus reuniens.

(2) The **stria vascularis** is the outer wall of the cochlear duct.

(a) The stria vascularis consists of stratified cuboidal epithelium, penetrated by numerous capillaries.

(b) It participates in the production of endolymph and maintains the high potassium and low sodium levels of the endolymph.

(3) The **spiral organ (organ of Corti)** is contained within the cochlear duct. It is the **receptor organ for sound** and contains sensory and supporting cells.

(a) **Supporting cells** provide the supporting framework of the spiral organ (see Figure 22-4).

(i) **Inner border cells** are the innermost supporting cells.

(ii) **External supporting cells (cells of Claudius)** are the outermost supporting cells.

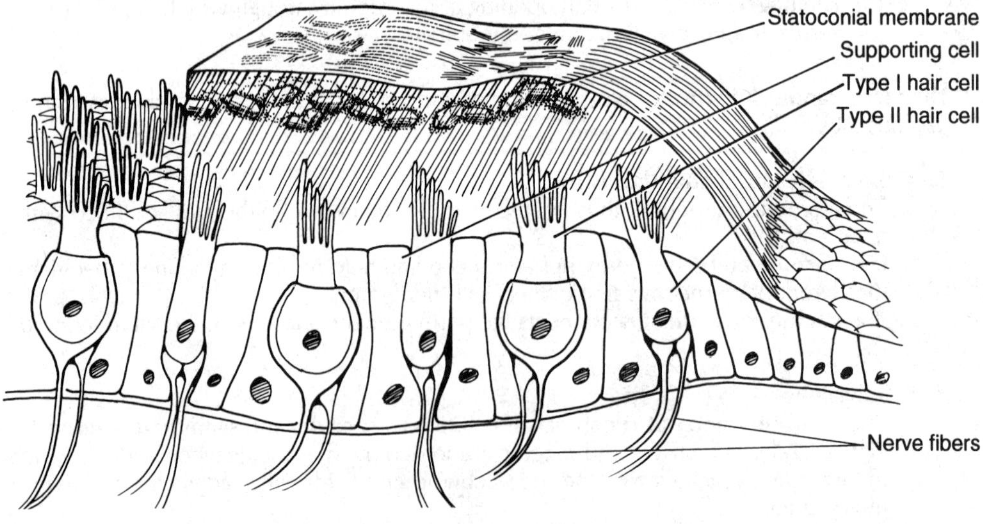

FIGURE 22-2. Schematic drawing of the macula sacculi, showing the statoconial membrane with statoconia (calcium carbonate crystals) embedded into its surface. The underlying supporting and sensory epithelial cells are identical to those present in the cristae ampullares. (Modified and redrawn from Dellmann H-D: *Textbook of Veterinary Histology,* 4th ed. Baltimore, Williams & Wilkins, 1993, p 329.)

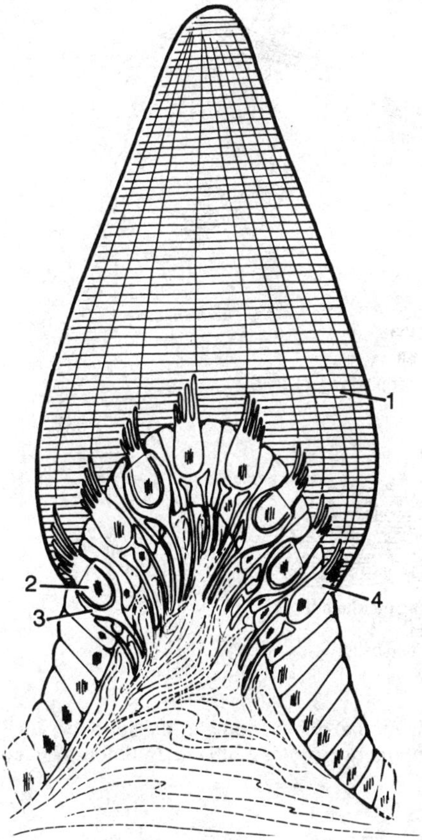

FIGURE 22-3. Schematic drawing of a crista ampullaris. The crest-like connective tissue core is covered by supporting cells and, at the level of the gelatinous cupula (*1*), sensory cells. (*2*) Type 1 sensory cell, which is flask-shaped; (*3*) afferent nerve terminal, which almost completely surrounds the type I cell and is itself contacted by an efferent terminal; (*4*) type II sensory cell, which is cylindric; (*5*) afferent and efferent terminals, which are both in direct contact with the type II cell. (Modified and redrawn from Dellmann H-D: *Textbook of Veterinary Histology,* 4th ed. Baltimore, Williams & Wilkins, 1993, p 329.)

- **(iii)** **Outer** and **inner phalangeal cells** are cup-shaped and provide support for the sensory cells.

(b) Spaces between the supporting cells form **three canals:** the outer, middle, and inner tunnels (see Figure 22-4).
- **(i)** **Outer limiting cells (cells of Hensen)** line the outer tunnel externally.
- **(ii)** **Outer phalangial cells** line the outer tunnel internally.
- **(iii)** **Pillar cells** line the inner tunnel.

(c) **Sensory cells** are called **inner** and **outer hair cells**.
- **(i)** Hair cells are almost entirely enveloped by phalangeal cells.
- **(ii)** The apex of each hair cell is studded with stereocilia arranged in a "W" pattern.
- **(iii)** Inner and outer hair cells are in synaptic contact with afferent nerve fibers. Outer hair cells are also contacted by efferent nerve fibers.

(d) The **tectorial membrane** is a gelatinous structure that lies over the spiral organ.
- **(i)** It is produced by epithelial cells, called **interdental cells**.
- **(ii)** The tips of most stereocilia of the sensory cells are attached to the tectorial membrane.

V. MECHANISM OF HEARING

A. Sound-induced vibrations of the tympanic membrane are transmitted to the ossicles and, via the footplate of the stapes, to the perilymph of the scala vestibuli.

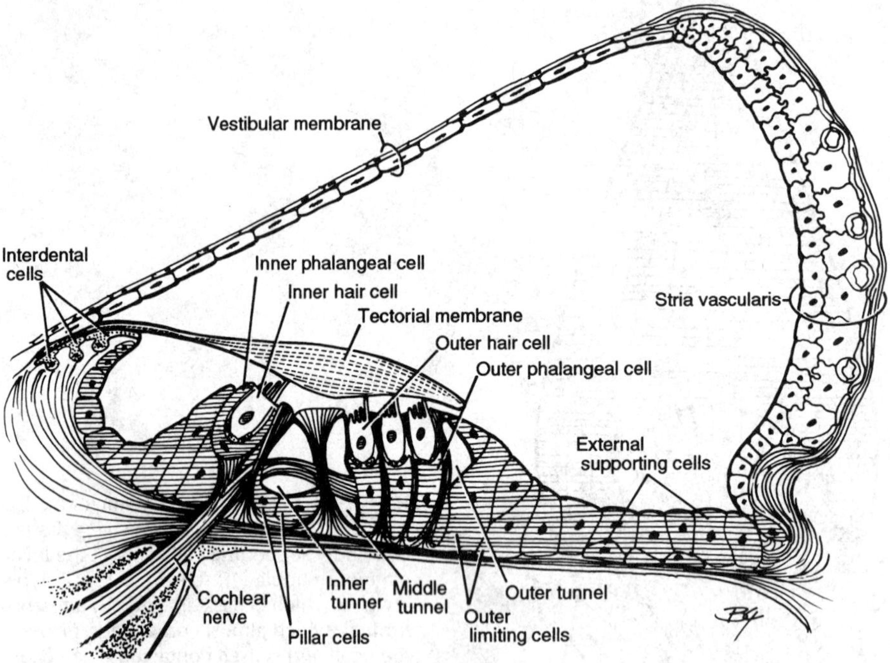

FIGURE 22-4. Schematic drawing of the cochlear duct (scala media), which contains the spiral organ. (Modified and redrawn from Dellmann H-D: *Textbook of Veterinary Histology,* 4th ed. Baltimore, Williams & Wilkins, 1993, p 332.)

B. Pressure change in the perilymph causes displacement of the basilar membrane. The basilar membrane is narrowest at the base of the cochlea and increases steadily in width toward the apex of the cochlea. This change in width allows tonotopic localization of various frequencies along the length of the basilar membrane.

1. High-frequency sounds cause deflection of the narrower (basal) part of the basilar membrane.
2. Low-frequency sounds cause deflection of the wider (apical) part of the basilar membrane.

C. Displacement of the basilar membrane causes displacement of the sensory cell stereocilia, which are embedded into the fixed tectorial membrane. Movement of the stereocilia prompts opening of ion channels in the cell membrane and subsequent transmitter release at the afferent synapse.

STUDY QUESTIONS

DIRECTIONS: Each of the numbered items or incomplete statements in this section is followed by answers or by completions of the statement. Select the **one** numbered answer or completion that is **best** in each case.

1. Which one of the following statements concerning the auditory tube is correct?

(1) It is lined with stratified squamous epithelium.
(2) It is lined with simple squamous or simple cuboidal epithelium.
(3) It is lined with respiratory mucosa.
(4) It contains no glands.
(5) It contains fine hairs.

2. Which one of the following statements concerning the tympanic membrane is correct?

(1) The central connective tissue layer has an elastic component.
(2) The footplate of the stapes inserts into the connective tissue layer.
(3) It is poorly vascularized and lacks lymph capillaries.
(4) It has a rich nerve supply.
(5) Externally, it is covered by stratified squamous nonkeratinized epithelium.

3. Which one of the following statements concerning the cochlear duct is correct?

(1) It is also referred to as the scala vestibuli.
(2) It is separated from the scala tympani by the tympanic membrane.
(3) It is connected to the sacculus via the cochlear canaliculus.
(4) It contains perilymph.
(5) Its outer wall is the stria vascularis.

4. Which one of the following statements is correct concerning the spiral organ?

(1) The dendrites of the bipolar nerve cells of the spiral ganglion are in contact with the tectorial membrane.
(2) Receptor cells have stereocilia that are moved by movements of the tectorial membrane.
(3) Sound-induced vibrations of the perilymph cause displacement of the tectorial membrane.
(4) The basilar membrane is displaced by sound-induced pressure changes in the perilymph.
(5) Receptor cells are the first neuron in a chain of three neurons that are required for sound perception.

ANSWERS AND EXPLANATIONS

1. The answer is 3 *[III C 1]*. The auditory tube is lined with typical respiratory mucosa (i.e., ciliated pseudostratified columnar epithelium with goblet cells); glands are present in the propria–submucosa; hairs are absent. Stratified squamous epithelium lines the external auditory canal. Simple squamous or simple cuboidal epithelium is the lining of the tympanic cavity, from which the auditory tube originates (to terminate in the nasopharynx).

2. The answer is 4 *[III A]*. The tympanic membrane is richly innervated, and it also is densely vascularized by blood and lymph capillaries. A central connective tissue layer is located between two peripheral epithelial layers: an external keratinized stratified squamous epithelium that faces the external auditory canal, and an internal simple squamous epithelium that faces the tympanic cavity. The orderly arrangement of collagen fibers in this central connective tissue layer confers a certain rigidity to the tympanic membrane. Sound waves are transmitted from the tympanic membrane to the perilymph of the inner ear via the ossicles. It is the malleus, not the stapes, that inserts into the connective tissue layer of the tympanic membrane. The footplate of the stapes is firmly attached to the membrane that covers the vestibular window.

3. The answer is 5 *[IV B 2 b]*. The stria vascularis is a prominent stratified cuboidal epithelial layer that lines the outer wall of the cochlear duct; the adjective "vascularis" refers to the many capillaries that deeply penetrate that epithelium. The cochlear duct is also called the scala media, because it lies between the scala vestibuli dorsally and the scala tympani ventrally. The scala tympani is separated from the cochlear duct by the basilar membrane; the scala vestibuli is separated from the cochlear duct by the vestibular membrane. The tympanic membrane separates the external auditory canal from the middle ear. The cochlear duct contains endolymph, whereas the scalae vestibuli and tympani contain perilymph. The cochlear canaliculus is the connection between the perilymphatic and subarachnoid spaces; the connection between the cochlear duct and sacculus is the ductus reuniens.

4. The answer is 4 *[IV B 2 b (3); V]*. Sound-induced movements of the tympanic membrane are transmitted via the ossicles to the perilymphatic compartment, causing deflection of the basilar membrane. The apices of the stereocilia of the receptor cells, which are epithelial cells and not neurons, are embedded in the tectorial membrane. Because that membrane is fixed, movements of the basilar membrane deflect the stereocilia, causing subsequent transmitter release at the afferent nerve terminal (from the bipolar spiral ganglion cells). Unlike the visual pathway, in which three neurons are involved, the auditory pathway consists of only one neuron.

COMPREHENSIVE EXAM

QUESTIONS

Directions: Each of the numbered items or incomplete statements in this section is followed by answers or by completions of the statement. Select the **one** numbered answer or completion that is **best** in each case.

1. Which one of the following is a function of centrioles?

(1) Organization of the basal bodies of cilia
(2) Disassembly of the mitotic apparatus after cell division occurs
(3) Movement of chromosomes to the center of the cell in preparation for cell division
(4) Formation of a new nuclear envelope after cell division occurs
(5) Organization of the Golgi complex

2. In which one of the following ways does endochondral osteogenesis differ from intramembranous osteogenesis?

(1) Collagen and ground substance are the first substances secreted by osteoblasts.
(2) Cartilage is destroyed before bone is formed.
(3) Osteoblasts are surrounded by bone before becoming osteocytes.
(4) Appositional growth is responsible for enlarging the original bony spicules.
(5) Osteoblasts secrete alkaline phosphatase.

3. Which one of the following statements best describes the ground substance of connective tissue?

(1) Its two main constituents are glycosaminoglycans and structural glycoproteins.
(2) It is basophilic.
(3) It is highly structured.
(4) Its constituents are remarkably uniform throughout the body.
(5) It contains a large amount of free water.

4. Olfactory epithelium typically comprises:

(1) olfactory cells, columnar ciliated cells, and basal cells.
(2) olfactory cells, columnar ciliated cells, goblet cells, basal cells, and sustentacular cells.
(3) olfactory cells, basal cells, and sustentacular cells.
(4) olfactory cells, sustentacular cells, basal cells, and goblet cells.
(5) olfactory cells, basal cells, sustentacular cells, and columnar ciliated cells.

5. A unique characteristic of epithelia is:

(1) the presence of type IV collagen in the extracellular matrix.
(2) the presence of gap junctions.
(3) merocrine secretion.
(4) rich vascularity.
(5) the presence of keratin intermediate filaments.

6. Pinocytosis is best described as:

(1) a regulated endocytic process.
(2) the nonselective uptake of extracellular fluids.
(3) the selective uptake of extracellular fluids.
(4) a continuous process.
(5) the process cells use to transport materials across the cytoplasm.

7. The definitive type of placenta in all domestic mammals is:

(1) deciduate.
(2) nondeciduate.
(3) choriovitelline.
(4) chorioallantoic.
(5) chorioamniotic.

8. Heparin and histamine are present in the specific granules of:

(1) lymphocytes.
(2) monocytes.
(3) neutrophils.
(4) eosinophils.
(5) basophils.

9. Which one of the following statements concerning epidermal strata is correct?

(1) In the stratum basale, keratin filaments are absent.
(2) In the stratum spinosum, eleidin granules are contained in the uppermost layers.
(3) In the stratum granulosum, keratohyalin granules are released.
(4) In the stratum lucidum, lamellar granules are released.
(5) In the stratum corneum, keratohyalin forms an amorphous matrix containing keratin filaments.

10. Lipofuscin granules are best described as:

(1) residual bodies containing yellow-brown pigment.
(2) characteristic of active phagocytes.
(3) most numerous in short-lived cells with a high turnover rate.
(4) autophagic vesicles.
(5) heterophagosomes.

11. Which one of the following statements is true concerning contractile filaments?

(1) Thick filaments are composed of myosin and tropomyosin.
(2) One of the troponin subunits of thin filaments has adenosine triphosphatase (ATPase) activity.
(3) Thick filaments contain desmin.
(4) Thin filaments are attached to α-actinin.
(5) Thick filaments are attached to the cell membrane.

12. Which of the following organs lacks endocrine cells?

(1) Ovary
(2) Skeletal muscle
(3) Pancreas
(4) Testis
(5) Hypothalamus

13. Which one of the following statements regarding chondrocytes is true?

(1) They communicate through gap junctions.
(2) They secrete chondromucoproteins.
(3) They are nourished by nearby capillaries.
(4) They are incapable of division.
(5) They destroy cartilage.

14. Which of the following is a complete list of cell types occurring in the intestinal epithelium?

(1) Columnar absorptive cells, columnar mucus-secreting cells, goblet cells, enteroendocrine cells, undifferentiated cells
(2) Columnar absorptive cells, goblet cells, enteroendocrine cells, undifferentiated cells, parietal cells
(3) Columnar absorptive cells, goblet cells, undifferentiated cells, chief cells
(4) Columnar absorptive cells, goblet cells, undifferentiated cells, enteroendocrine cells
(5) Columnar absorptive cells, columnar mucus-secreting cells, enteroendocrine cells, undifferentiated cells

15. Progesterone and relaxin are synthesized and secreted by:

(1) granulosa lutein cells.
(2) theca externa cells.
(3) theca interna cells.
(4) ovarian interstitial cells.
(5) follicular granulosa cells.

16. Which one of the following statements correctly describes a difference between humoral and cellular immune responses?

(1) Microorganisms that live outside the cells of the host are more likely to initiate a humoral response, and those that enter the host's cells are more likely to initiate a cellular response.
(2) Macrophages are involved only in cellular responses.
(3) Humoral responses do not necessarily involve an antigen.
(4) No cellular changes are produced in humoral immune responses.
(5) Memory cells are produced only in cellular responses.

17. Which one of the following statements correctly describes the function of a cytoplasmic inclusion?

(1) Lipid droplets are storage depots for unmetabolized byproducts of metabolism.
(2) Hemoglobin is a breakdown product of red blood cells.
(3) Mitochondria produce chemical energy from products of digestion.
(4) Hemosiderin is secreted in the bile, where it aids in digestion and absorption.
(5) Melanin helps to protect some animals from predators.

18. Which one of the following statements concerning maculae is correct?

(1) They are located in the utricle, saccule, and semicircular ducts.
(2) They are covered by a gelatinous mass called the cupula.
(3) Their receptor cells are ciliated.
(4) Their epithelium comprises nerve cells and supporting cells.
(5) They detect movements of the endolymph caused by rotation.

19. The Golgi complex can best be described as:

(1) receiving newly formed proteins from the rough endoplasmic reticulum (rER) for further processing and packaging.
(2) present only in secretory cells.
(3) a system of ribosome-studded and smooth-surfaced membranes.
(4) staining strongly with basophilic dyes.
(5) undetectable with the light microscope because of its small size.

20. The most common storage place of spermatozoa prior to ejaculation is the:

(1) head of the epididymis.
(2) rete testis.
(3) tail of the epididymis.
(4) vesicular gland.
(5) ampulla of the ductus deferens.

21. Which one of the following structures is *not* part of the membranous labyrinth?

(1) Utricle
(2) Saccule
(3) Semicircular ducts
(4) Cochlear canal
(5) Cochlear duct

22. What is a motor unit?

(1) A sarcomere
(2) A skeletal muscle cell
(3) A motor neuron
(4) An axon and all the muscle cells it innervates
(5) A spray-like arborization of an axon terminal on a muscle cell

23. The juxtaglomerular apparatus is best described as:

(1) afferent arteriolar endothelial cells, juxtaglomerular cells, and macula densa cells.
(2) efferent arteriolar endothelial cells, juxtaglomerular cells, and macula densa cells.
(3) juxtaglomerular cells, extraglomerular mesangial cells, and macula densa cells.
(4) juxtaglomerular cells, glomerular mesangial cells, and macula densa cells.
(5) epithelioid smooth muscle cells, glomerular mesangial cells, and macula densa cells.

24. Brush borders are best described as:

(1) especially well developed in the upper airways.
(2) typically covered by a layer of mucus.
(3) appearing as a layer of striations parallel to the free surface in light microscopic preparations.
(4) detectable only with the electron microscope.
(5) characteristic of a surface that is specialized for absorption.

25. Which one of the following statements is true of body fluids?

(1) Interstitial fluid is confined between the cell membrane and the subcellular organelles.
(2) Body fluids are separated into three compartments.
(3) Lymph is carried in a one-way vascular system.
(4) Erythrocytes, platelets, and macromolecules are confined within the cardiovascular system.
(5) Lymph has the same composition as amorphous ground substance.

26. The omasum is characterized by:

(1) laminae of variable length that lack papillae.
(2) two muscle layers derived from the tunica muscularis in the center of the laminae.
(3) the lack of a lamina muscularis.
(4) laminae of variable length studded with prominent papillae.
(5) a lining of simple columnar epithelium that has absorptive capacities.

27. Which of the following statements best describes the basement membrane?

(1) It is a layer that separates epithelial cells from each other.
(2) It is an amorphous layer that underlies almost all epithelia.
(3) It is a well-developed feature in malignant tumors.
(4) It is a layer containing fibrillar type IV collagen.
(5) It is a product of the connective tissue underlying an epithelium.

28. Meiosis is the process during which:

(1) spermatids differentiate into spermatozoa.
(2) secondary spermatocytes differentiate into spermatids.
(3) primary spermatocytes give rise to spermatids.
(4) spermatogonia become primary spermatocytes.
(5) primary spermatocytes differentiate into secondary spermatocytes.

29. Neurosensory olfactory cells are present in which one of the following structures?

(1) Larynx
(2) Nasopharynx
(3) Nasal vestibule
(4) Vomeronasal organ
(5) Paranasal sinuses

30. Which one of the following statements is true regarding the conducting system of the heart?

(1) The atrioventricular node is richly innervated by the autonomic nervous system.
(2) The first part of the ventricular myocardium to receive the action potential is adjacent to the atrioventricular septum.
(3) Specialized conductive cells transmit the action potential from the sinoatrial node to the ventricular myocardium.
(4) Contractile cells of the atrial myocardium form the connection between the sinoatrial and atrioventricular nodes.
(5) Conductive cells spread through the subepicardium to reach all parts of the ventricular myocardium.

31. Which statement best describes platelets?

(1) They become sticky in the presence of connective tissue fibers.
(2) They contain no specific granules.
(3) They synthesize the vasoconstrictor serotonin.
(4) They are able to phagocytose bacteria.
(5) They release heparin.

32. Which one of the following statements best describes cytoplasmic filaments in skeletal muscle cells?

(1) Thick, intermediate, and thin filaments are the contractile elements.
(2) No intermediate filaments are present.
(3) Most microfilaments are located just under the cell membrane.
(4) Thin filaments are composed of overlapping molecules of myosin, and thick filaments are polymers of globular actin molecules (G-actin).
(5) Thick filaments are composed of overlapping molecules of myosin, and thin filaments contain polymers of G-actin.

33. Which of the following is a component of the ground substance of blood?

(1) Hyaluronic acid
(2) Chondroitin sulfate
(3) Hemoglobin
(4) Immunoglobulin
(5) Platelets

34. An endotheliochorial placenta is present in:

(1) domestic carnivores.
(2) sows.
(3) mares.
(4) small ruminants.
(5) cows.

35. Which of the following is the primary germ layer that gives rise to most connective tissue, most muscle, and some epithelium?

(1) Mesoderm
(2) Mesothelium
(3) Entoderm
(4) Endothelium
(5) Ectoderm

36. The development of T lymphocytes in the thymus involves:

(1) gradual movement of developing T lymphocytes from the medulla to the cortex.
(2) clonal expansion of T lymphocytes in the medulla and differentiation to effector cells in the cortex.
(3) an environment in which developing T lymphocytes are protected from the effects of cytokines.
(4) death of approximately 90% of the developing T lymphocytes.
(5) replacement of surface receptors for "self" markers with receptors for "nonself" markers.

37. Which one of the following statements concerning the iris is correct?

(1) The stroma is poorly vascularized connective tissue.
(2) Its anterior and posterior surfaces are covered by mesothelium.
(3) The color of the iris is determined by the number of melanosomes.
(4) Radially arranged muscle fibers in the stroma make up the dilator muscle of the pupil.
(5) Granula iridica are focal proliferations of the iris stroma that project into the anterior chamber.

38. In which way does the amorphous ground substance of cartilage differ from that of loose connective tissue?

(1) It contains sulfated glycosaminoglycans.
(2) Its proteoglycans bind with hyaluronic acid.
(3) Its proteoglycans bind with collagen.
(4) It does not contain bound water.
(5) It does not contain hyaluronic acid.

39. Which of the following best describes macrophages?

(1) They have a characteristic appearance that varies little with their functional state.
(2) They are the body's first line of defense against bacteria.
(3) They are important in stimulating the healing process.
(4) They die within a few days after entering the tissue.
(5) They secrete all the extracellular elements of connective tissue.

40. Which one of the following statements describes the second meiotic division of oocytes?

(1) It begins and is completed in secondary follicles.
(2) It begins and is completed in tertiary follicles.
(3) It begins in secondary follicles and is completed in tertiary follicles.
(4) It begins in early tertiary follicles and is completed in late (i.e., preovulatory) tertiary follicles.
(5) It begins in tertiary follicles and is completed after fertilization (i.e., penetration of the oocyte by the spermium).

41. Which one of the following statements is true regarding the organization of cardiac muscle?

(1) Fasciae adherentes (attachment plaques) join large areas of the lateral cell membranes.
(2) Cells are joined end to end by gap junctions.
(3) No basal laminae are present between cardiac muscle cells.
(4) Desmosomes join adjacent lateral cell membranes.
(5) Interweaving chains of cells anastomose and run in different directions.

42. Cells in connective tissue include those that:

(1) have entered the tissue from the blood.
(2) produce only elastic fibers.
(3) are specialized for contraction.
(4) line the peritoneal, pleural, and pericardial cavities.
(5) secrete hormones.

43. Which one of the following statements is true regarding the general organization of blood vessels?

(1) Smooth muscle is present only in the tunica media.
(2) Smooth muscle may be present in any of the three tunics.
(3) The external elastic membrane, if present, is the outermost layer of the tunica interna.
(4) The outer surface is covered by mesothelium.
(5) Vasomotor nerves terminate in the subendothelial layer.

44. Which one of the following statements regarding marginated leukocytes is true?

(1) Marginated cells immediately move into the connective tissue by diapedesis.
(2) Most marginated cells are monocytes and neutrophils reentering the blood from the connective tissue.
(3) Marginated cells are no longer functional.
(4) Marginated cells form a reserve pool of cells that can be severalfold larger than the number of circulating cells.
(5) The marginal pool is the only place leukocytes can be stored.

45. In which one of the following ways do B lymphocytes differ from T lymphocytes?

(1) B lymphocytes have antibodies on the surface of their cell membranes.
(2) B lymphocytes are stimulated by antigens.
(3) B lymphocytes have a subcategory of regulatory cells.
(4) B lymphocytes recognize malignant cells.
(5) B lymphocytes are the most abundant type of lymphocytes in the circulating blood.

46. Which one of the following statements best describes the formation of microtubules?

(1) Polymerization is regulated by the amount of tubulin present in the cytoplasm.
(2) A cell's full complement of microtubules is formed by the time the mitotic apparatus disappears at the end of cell division.
(3) Microtubules form and dissolve in response to cellular regulatory signals.
(4) Polymerization is enhanced in the presence of the drugs colchicine and vincristine.

47. Movement of spermatozoa through the ductus epididymidis is accomplished by:

(1) beating of cilia on columnar epithelial lining cells.
(2) flagellar movement of spermatozoa.
(3) contraction of the smooth muscle cells of the ductus epididymidis.
(4) continued flow of testicular fluid.
(5) the pressure of continued production of spermatozoa in the testis.

48. In which one of the following ways do most central nervous system (CNS) capillaries differ from capillaries in most other tissues?

(1) They are usually fenestrated.
(2) The endothelial cells are joined only by adhering junctions.
(3) They have a relatively well-developed layer of reticular fibers surrounding the basal lamina.
(4) They have few or no transcytotic vesicles.
(5) They are continuous capillaries.

49. Basophils most resemble what other cell type?

(1) Mast cells
(2) Neutrophils
(3) Eosinophils
(4) Plasma cells
(5) Pericytes

50. The structure of the axoneme (i.e., the motile apparatus in the shaft of a cilium) is *best* described as:

(1) containing microfilaments.
(2) having a core composed of 20 microtubules.
(3) resembling an elongated centriole with two additional central microtubules.
(4) surrounded by mitochondria.
(5) containing tonofilaments.

51. Which one of the following lingual papillae is gustatory papillae?

(1) Filiform papillae
(2) Conical papillae
(3) Lenticular papillae
(4) Marginal papillae
(5) Fungiform papillae

52. Viewing smooth muscle through an electron microscope reveals that:

(1) bundles of thick and thin filaments run obliquely in many directions through the cells.
(2) intermediate filaments are absent.
(3) the T tubule system is well developed.
(4) the cells contain no sarcoplasmic reticulum.
(5) each cell is totally isolated by a continuous basal lamina.

53. Classification of cartilage is based on:

(1) whether it is immature or mature.
(2) whether it is derived from mesenchyme or other types of connective tissue.
(3) the types of fibers in the matrix.
(4) whether or not it is attached to bone.
(5) its shape.

54. Which of the following is an example of an immigrant cell of connective tissue?

(1) Mast cell
(2) Neutrophil (microcyte)
(3) Macrophage (histiocyte)
(4) Mesenchymal cell
(5) Pericyte

55. Which one of the following structures is classified as a cytoskeletal element?

(1) Microvillus
(2) Microtubule
(3) Nuclear envelope
(4) Endoplasmic cytosol
(5) Smooth endoplasmic reticulum (sER)

56. Which one of the following statements is true of bone cells?

(1) Osteoclasts are derived by fusion of osteocytes.
(2) Osteoclasts are joined to the surrounding cells by gap junctions.
(3) Osteocytes are functionally active cells that work in a coordinated manner.
(4) Osteoclasts are the only cells that can break down bone matrix.
(5) Osteocytes are capable of phagocytosing their surrounding matrix.

57. When part of the endometrium is shed together with the fetal placenta at parturition, the placenta is referred to as:

(1) diffuse.
(2) villous.
(3) deciduate.
(4) epitheliochorial.
(5) cotyledonary.

58. Iodinated thyroglobulin is stored in:

(1) thyroid follicles, extracellularly.
(2) secretory granules.
(3) endocytotic vesicles.
(4) phagolysosomes.
(5) Golgi saccules.

59. Reticular fibers differ from collagen fibers in that they:

(1) are more acidophilic.
(2) are more densely packed.
(3) tend to form bundles instead of networks.
(4) are produced only by connective tissue cells.
(5) have a carbohydrate-rich surface coating.

60. Members of the mononuclear phagocyte system (MPS) include:

(1) cells that present antigenic fragments to lymphocytes to initiate the immune response.
(2) cells that can be recognized in a wide variety of tissues by their common morphological features.
(3) cells that are called microphages when they are active in the tissue.
(4) all the granulocytes.
(5) all cells with receptor-mediated phagocytosis.

61. Gap junctions are best described as:

(1) junctions that permit attached cells to act independently.
(2) attachment sites where the apposing cell membranes are widely separated.
(3) junctions that characterize mature tissues and fully functional organs.
(4) junctions that allow efficient transfer of large molecules between adjacent cells.
(5) sites where both metabolic and electrical coupling can occur.

62. Which one of the following characteristics differentiates bone from cartilage?

(1) Bone is in contact with dense connective tissue.
(2) Cells on the bone surface are capable of initiating appositional growth.
(3) Nutrients and wastes are able to diffuse to and from bone cells through the rigid matrix.
(4) Bone cells are supplied by a system of nutrient capillaries.
(5) The bone matrix appears homogeneous under the light microscope.

Directions: Each of the numbered items or incomplete statements in this section is negatively phrased, as indicated by an italicized word such as *not, least,* or *except.* Select the **one** numbered answer or completion that is **best** in each case.

63. All of the following statements concerning sebaceous glands are correct *except:*

(1) They are alveolar glands.
(2) Lipids are released by apocrine secretion.
(3) Undifferentiated stem cells continuously give rise to secretory cells.
(4) Their secretory product is emptied into the hair follicle.
(5) Their ducts are lined with stratified squamous epithelium.

64. All of the following are part of the sole plate of a neuromuscular synapse *except:*

(1) mitochondria.
(2) myofibrils.
(3) rough endoplasmic reticulum (rER).
(4) glycogen.
(5) nuclei.

65. Repair and renewal of epithelium is believed to involve all of the following *except:*

(1) migration of epithelial cells through the basement membrane in wounded areas.
(2) division of stem cells to produce one stem cell and one cell that will give rise to differentiated epithelial cells.
(3) renewal rates that range from a few days to several years in different epithelia.
(4) ameboid movement of epithelial cells to cover a wounded area.

66. All of the following are functions of monocytes *except:*

(1) secretion of growth factors.
(2) initiation of the inflammation response.
(3) phagocytosis of bacteria, viruses, and other particles in the circulating blood.
(4) nonselective phagocytosis of dust particles.
(5) secretion of tumor necrosis factor α (TNFα).

67. All of the following statements concerning hairs are correct *except:*

(1) The shaft comprises three layers: cuticle, cortex, and medulla.
(2) The root comprises four layers: cuticle, cortex, medulla, and internal root sheath.
(3) The medulla may be absent in secondary hairs.
(4) The morphology of the cells of the cuticle is species-specific.
(5) The hair bulb is the terminal (proximal) portion of the hair root.

68. All of the following statements are true of lymph capillaries *except:*

(1) They are more permeable than capillaries or postcapillary venules.
(2) They are held open by attachments between endothelial cells and surrounding tissue elements.
(3) They are present only in the lymphatic organs.
(4) They have a discontinuous basal lamina.
(5) Their contents appear milky in the intestine.

69. Which of the following are *not* affected by hypophysectomy?

(1) Thyroid follicular cells
(2) Adrenal zona reticularis
(3) Adrenal zona fasciculata
(4) Pancreatic B cells
(5) Testicular interstitial cells

70. The proximal tubule has all of the following characteristics *except:*

(1) It extends from the cortex into the outer medulla.
(2) It is a component of the cortical labyrinth and the loop of the nephron.
(3) It forms the macula densa.
(4) It is lined by cuboidal epithelial cells with an extensive apical microvillous border.
(5) It has convoluted and straight segments.

71. All of the following statements concerning the hypodermis are correct *except:*

(1) It is composed of both metabolic and structural adipose tissue.
(2) It is a highly flexible layer.
(3) It is richly vascularized.
(4) It is absent in certain specialized regions of the integument.
(5) Elastic fibers predominate.

72. All of the following are functions of the complement system *except:*

(1) lysing foreign cells and microorganisms.
(2) inducing degranulation of mast cells and basophils.
(3) attracting neutrophils.
(4) activating T lymphocytes.
(5) enhancing phagocytosis.

73. All of the following are characteristics of brown adipose tissue *except:*

(1) it is multilocular.
(2) it is able to elevate body temperature.
(3) it is widespread in the body.
(4) its mitochondria are responsible for its brown hue.
(5) its mitochondria oxidize lipids.

74. All of the following are myeloid elements *except:*

(1) erythrocytes.
(2) granulocytes.
(3) platelets.
(4) lymphocytes.
(5) monocytes.

75. A presynaptic element contains all of the following *except:*

(1) synaptic vesicles.
(2) endocytosed membranes of synaptic vesicles.
(3) mitochondria.
(4) lysosomes.
(5) microtubules and neurofilaments.

76. Which of the following organs does *not* contain endocrine cells in the lining epithelium?

(1) Glandular stomach
(2) Trachea
(3) Duodenum
(4) Esophagus
(5) Cecum

77. Which one of the following is *not* a characteristic of epithelial bronchioles?

(1) Simple cuboidal or columnar epithelial lining
(2) Absence of glands in the propria–submucosa
(3) Absence of cartilage
(4) Clara cells
(5) Goblet cells

78. Which of the following is *not* a zone of the adrenal cortex?

(1) Zona fasciculata
(2) Zona pellucida
(3) Zona glomerulosa
(4) Zona reticularis
(5) Zona arcuata

79. Which of the following statements does *not* correctly describe a function of neuroglial cell types?

(1) Astrocytes form the glia limitans.
(2) Ependymal cells may participate in the formation of the glia limitans.
(3) Microglial cells are potentially phagocytic.
(4) Oligodendrocytes form myelin sheaths in white matter but are absent from gray matter.
(5) Schwann cells are myelin-forming cells in the peripheral nervous system (PNS).

80. All of the following statements regarding centrioles are true *except:*

(1) Centrioles usually lie in the cytocentrum.
(2) Centrioles replicate before cell division occurs.
(3) Centrioles are essential for cell division.
(4) Centrioles are involved in intracellular movement systems.
(5) Centrioles cannot be detected light microscopically.

81. Which one of the following statements concerning the external auditory canal is *incorrect*?

(1) It is lined with skin.
(2) It contains hairs.
(3) Apocrine sweat glands are present.
(4) It contains sebaceous glands.
(5) Cerumen is the secretory product of the apocrine glands.

82. All of the following cells are found in gastric fundic glands *except:*

(1) Mucous neck cells
(2) Parietal cells
(3) Enteroendocrine cells
(4) Undifferentiated cells
(5) Goblet cells

83. All of the following statements concerning the conjunctiva are correct *except:*

(1) It is continuous with the corneal epithelium and the epithelium covering the free surface of the eyelid.
(2) It forms a fold, the third eyelid.
(3) Its epithelium contains many goblet cells.
(4) Its subepithelial connective tissue is poorly vascularized.
(5) Lymphatic nodules are present in the lamina propria.

84. Which of the following statements concerning neuroglial cells is *incorrect*?

(1) In craniospinal and autonomic ganglia, Schwann cells surround ganglion cells and are called satellite cells.
(2) In gray matter, astrocytes ensheathe synapses.
(3) In gray matter, oligodendrocytes surround neurons and are called satellite oligodendrocytes.
(4) In white matter, astrocytes react to injury by becoming phagocytic.

Directions: Each group of items in this section consists of numbered options followed by a set of numbered items. For each item, select the **one** numbered option that is most closely associated with it. Each numbered option may be selected once, more than once, or not at all.

Questions 85–90

Match each descriptive phrase with the associated structure.

(1) Multivesicular body
(2) Peroxisome (microbody)
(3) Lysosome
(4) Mitochondrion
(5) Residual body
(6) Smooth endoplasmic reticulum (sER)
(7) Rough endoplasmic reticulum (rER)

85. Responsible for cellular respiration

86. Involved in both disease processes and defense

87. Able to divide, fuse, move about the cell, and change shape

88. Gives rise to smooth endoplasmic reticulum (sER)

89. Essential for lysosome production

90. Vesicle-containing structure related to the lysosomal system

Questions 91–92

For each leukocyte, select the most appropriate function.

(1) Phagocytoses products of other leukocytes
(2) Initiates immune responses
(3) Phagocytoses and destroys pathogenic bacteria
(4) Helps initiate inflammation response
(5) Promotes healing

91. Eosinophil

92. Basophil

Questions 93–96

Match each description with the appropriate numbered structure in the micrograph.

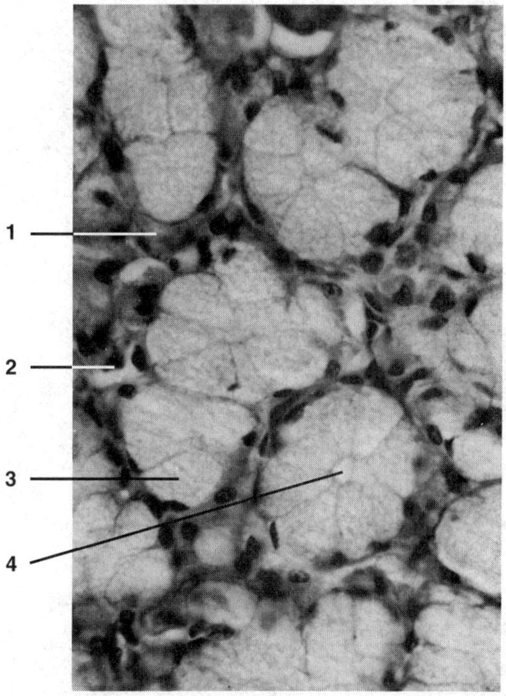

93. Its secretory product combines with water to form mucus.

94. It produces a watery secretory product that is rich in proteins.

95. It is called a demilune.

96. It produces a secretory product that is rich in acidic glycoproteins.

Questions 97–98

Match each function with the type of vessel that performs it.

(1) Arterioles
(2) Metarterioles
(3) Elastic arteries
(4) Muscular arteries
(5) Capillaries

97. Regulates blood flow to specific organs

98. Major regulator of blood pressure

Questions 99–103

Match each descriptive phrase with the associated lymphatic organ.

(1) Thymus
(2) Hemal node
(3) Spleen
(4) Peyer's patch
(5) Cloacal bursa

99. Contains blood-filled subcapsular sinuses

100. Contains epithelial cells, some of which present antigens and some of which take up antibodies

101. Site of mast cell differentiation from progenitor cells

102. Among the domestic species, are numerous only in ruminants

103. Site of prenatal erythropoiesis

ANSWERS AND EXPLANATIONS

1. The answer is 1 *[Chapter 3 I C 2 b (2) (b)]*. Not only do centrioles organize the formation of basal bodies of cilia and flagella, a centriole can itself act as a basal body. The basic structure of basal bodies is the same as that of centrioles. Centrioles organize the formation of the mitotic apparatus in preparation for cell division. They then act as poles for the movement of chromosomes away from the center of the cell to form the nuclei of two daughter cells. The endoplasmic reticulum (ER) forms a new nuclear envelope after cell division occurs. Although the centrioles are usually located near the Golgi complex, they are not believed to play a role in its organization.

2. The answer is 2 *[Chapter 7 III E 2]*. Because endochondral osteogenesis replaces a temporary cartilaginous skeleton, the cartilage must be removed to make space for the bone to form. Collagen and ground substance are the first secretions of all osteoblasts. Osteoblasts become osteocytes when they are surrounded by bone in all osteogenic processes. Bony spicules in endochondral osteogenesis have a core of calcified cartilage; but their growth, like that of spicules formed by intramembranous osteogenesis, is by appositional growth. All osteoblasts secrete alkaline phosphatase, which promotes mineralization of the organic matrix.

3. The answer is 1 *[Chapter 6 II A 1]*. The two main constituents of the ground substance of connective tissue are glycosaminoglycans and structural glycoproteins. Ground substance is poorly stained, and areas it occupies appear empty in histologic sections. Although its components are attached to each other at many points, its fibrous elements are randomly arranged in a loose network. The relative proportions of its components vary widely in different parts of the body, contributing to the differences in viscosity and firmness in different regions. Most of the water is bound in hydration layers around macromolecules of the ground substance.

4. The answer is 3 *[Chapter 14 II A 1 c; Figure 14-2]*. Only three cell types—olfactory cells, basal cells, and sustentacular cells—make up typical olfactory epithelium. Goblet cells and ciliated columnar cells are the major cell types of nonolfactory respiratory epithelium in the larger conducting airways.

5. The answer is 5 *[Chapter 5 II D]*. Intermediate filaments in epithelia are composed of the family of proteins called keratins, found only in epithelia. Moreover, each type of epithelium has a characteristic type or mixture of types of keratin. Type IV collagen is present in basal laminae. Gap junctions are common between cells of several tissue types. Merocrine secretion is the type of exocytosis practiced by all cell types except certain epithelial cells. Epithelia are avascular.

6. The answer is 4 *[Chapter 4 III A 2]*. Pinocytosis, which can involve either selective or nonselective uptake of extracellular fluids, is continuous and unregulated (i.e., it is a constitutive process). Uptake and transport of material across the cell to be released into a different extracellular compartment is called transcytosis. Pinocytosis is involved with the uptake segment of this process, but has nothing to do with the transport of materials across the cell.

7. The answer is 4 *[Chapter 17 III A 2]*. A chorioallantoic placenta is the definitive placenta in all domestic mammals. The highly vascularized allantois fuses with the nonvascular chorion to form the allantochorion, which becomes closely apposed to the endometrium, forming the chorioallantoic placenta. The fusion between yolk sac and chorion forms a choriovitelline placenta. This type of placenta occurs early during fetal development in all domestic mammals, but it is transitory in nature. In ruminants and pigs, the amnion merges with the chorion to form an amniochorion. A nondeciduate placenta, in which the endometrium remains intact at parturition, occurs in all domestic mammals except carnivores. Carnivores have a deciduate placenta (i.e., part of the endometrium is lost at parturition).

8. The answer is 5 *[Chapter 8 II B 6 a (2) (b)]*. Granules of basophils (like those of mast cells) contain heparin, which is an anticoagulant, and histamine, which increases the permeability of small blood vessels and constricts the small airways. The granules also contain other highly potent substances that promote the inflammation response. Widespread degranulation of basophils, mast cells, or both can cause anaphylactic shock.

9. The answer is 5 *[Chapter 20 II A 1 a (5)].* In the keratinocytes of the stratum corneum, the keratin filaments are embedded in the amorphous matrix formed by keratohyalin. Keratohyalin granules are synthesized in the stratum granulosum; they are not membrane-bounded. As the cells move up in the epidermis, the granules become amorphous and closely associated with keratin filaments. These filaments are already prominent in the stratum basale. The stratum spinosum does not contain eleidin granules, which are characteristic of the stratum lucidum of thick skin. Keratohyalin granules are never released from the keratinocytes, but lamellar granules are released in the stratum granulosum.

10. The answer is 1 *[Chapter 2 I F 3].* Residual bodies, which are former lysosomes that contain undigestible remnants, may accumulate the yellow-brown lipid called lipofuscin, or "wear and tear pigment." When large enough to see with the light microscope, such structures are called lipofuscin granules. They are most numerous in long-lived cells (such as muscle, liver, and nerve cells). Autophagic vesicles and heterophagosomes are active lysosomes that may evolve into lipofuscin granules if they are unable to digest all their contents.

11. The answer is 4 *[Chapter 10 II B 1 a–b, 2 a (2)].* α-Actinin attaches one end of the thin filaments to the Z line or to the cell membrane. Tropomyosin is a component of thin filaments, not thick filaments. The heads of the myosin molecules of thick filaments have adenosine triphosphatase (ATPase) activity. Desmin is an intermediate filament, not a component of thick filaments. Thin filaments, not thick filaments, are attached to the cell membrane.

12. The answer is 2 *[Chapter 19 I A 2].* Skeletal muscle cells do not have any known endocrine activity. In the ovary, interstitial cells secrete estrogens, cells of the theca interna secrete androgens, cells of the granulosa convert androgens to estrogens, and the corpus luteum secretes progesterone and relaxin. Testicular interstitial cells secrete testosterone. The pancreatic islets secrete a variety of hormones, most importantly insulin and glucagon. Neurons in the hypothalamus secrete hypophysiotropic hormones, antidiuretic hormone (ADH), and oxytocin.

13. The answer is 2 *[Chapter 7 II A 1 a (2), D 1 a (2) (a)].* Chondrocytes secrete glycosaminoglycans and proteins that form the chondromucoproteins of the cartilage matrix. They have no intercellular junctions; each cell is isolated in the matrix. Their nourishment must diffuse through the chondromatrix from capillaries outside the cartilage because the cartilage is avascular. They can divide in young cartilage, producing isogenous groups. They form and maintain cartilage; they do not destroy it.

14. The answer is 4 *[Chapter 13 II E 1 a].* It is possible to find columnar absorptive cells, goblet cells, undifferentiated cells, and enteroendocrine cells throughout the intestinal epithelium. Columnar mucus-secreting cells do not occur in the intestine; they are the characteristic lining epithelial cells of the glandular stomach. Chief cells and parietal cells do not occur in the intestine; they are characteristic of the fundic glands of the stomach.

15. The answer is 1 *[Chapter 16 II A 6 c (2)].* Granulosa lutein cells synthesize and secrete both progesterone and relaxin. The cells of the theca externa do not secrete any hormones; those of the theca interna synthesize and secrete androgens. Ovarian interstitial cells are the source of androgens. In follicular granulosa cells, androgens that are synthesized and secreted by the cells of the theca interna are metabolized to estrogens.

16. The answer is 1 *[Chapter 12 I C 3].* Humoral responses are initiated by bacteria that live outside cells of the host and their toxins; cellular immunity is stimulated by microorganisms that enter the host's cells or their products. Humoral responses require B cell activation, which usually requires interaction with a T cell and a macrophage (the macrophage activates the T cell, which then activates the B cell). All humoral responses are initiated by antigens. In a humoral immune response, clones of B cells are changed to antibody-producing plasma cells. Memory cells are produced in both humoral and cellular responses.

17. The answer is 5 *[Chapter 3 II B 3].* Melanin is a pigment that is present in skin and hair, where its distribution can camouflage the animal. Lipid droplets store fats that provide energy between feedings; unmetabolizable materials are stored in residual bodies. Hemoglobin is the oxygen- and carbon dioxide-carrying pigment in healthy red blood cells. The breakdown products of hemoglobin are hemosiderin, which is reused to make hemoglobin in new red blood cells, and bilirubin, which is secreted in the bile to emulsify fats in the intestine.

18. The answer is 3 *[Chapter 22 IV B 2 a (1) (b)].* Receptor cells in the maculae of the utricle and saccule, and also those of the cristae ampullares in the semicircular ducts, possess one cilium and many stereocilia that are embedded in the statoconial membrane. The statoconial membrane is a gelatinous mass containing calcium carbonate crystals (statoconia). The cupula is the crest-shaped gelatinous mass without statoconia in the cristae ampullares. The epithelium of the maculae is composed of supporting cells and sensory receptor cells, not nerve cells (which are present in olfactory epithelium). The maculae detect linear, not rotary, acceleration.

19. The answer is 1 *[Chapter 1 II D 2 a].* Newly formed proteins carried from the rough endoplasmic reticulum (rER) in transfer vesicles are further processed in the Golgi complex—for example, by removing parts of the molecules or complexing the proteins with fats or polysaccharides. They are also packaged in membranes of the appropriate type, depending on whether the proteins are lysosomal enzymes or secretory products. Nonsecretory cells need a Golgi complex to perform such essential functions as production of lysosomal enzymes. The size of the Golgi complex is well within the resolving power of the light microscope. It can be demonstrated with special stains or detected as an unstained region (called a negative image) in cells that contain large amounts of rER or numerous granules in their cytoplasm; however, it is not seen using most routine preparations because no ribosomes are attached to any part of the Golgi complex, and its smooth-surfaced membranes have no particular staining affinity.

20. The answer is 3 *[Chapter 18 V B 2 b].* Spermatozoa traverse the rete testis to enter the head of the epididymis through the efferent ductules. In the head and body of the epididymis, they undergo maturational changes, and then they are stored in the tail prior to ejaculation. The vesicular glands (also called seminal vesicles) do not store spermatozoa, but they contribute to the seminal fluid, as does the ampulla of the ductus deferens. In bulls, the ampulla of the ductus deferens has been reported to store large quantities of spermatozoa (sufficient for one normal ejaculate following castration or vasectomy).

21. The answer is 4 *[Chapter 22 IV A 3 b, B].* The cochlear canal is the osseous canal that winds in two to three turns around the central modiolus of the cochlea. The utricle, saccule, and semicircular ducts make up the vestibular apparatus. The cochlear duct, also referred to as the scala media, is located within the cochlear canal between the scala vestibuli dorsally and the scala tympani ventrally.

22. The answer is 4 *[Chapter 10 II C 2 a].* A motor unit comprises a nerve fiber (i.e., the axon of a motor neuron) and all the muscle cells it innervates. A sarcomere is the structural and functional unit of a skeletal or cardiac muscle cell. The arborization of an axon terminal on a muscle cell is called a motor endplate.

23. The answer is 3 *[Chapter 15 II C].* The juxtaglomerular apparatus consists of epithelioid secretory (renin) smooth muscle cells (referred to as juxtaglomerular cells and located most frequently in the afferent arteriole of the glomerulus), extraglomerular mesangial cells, and the cells of the macula densa in the distal tubule. Neither endothelial cells in the afferent or efferent arteriole nor glomerular mesangial cells are part of the juxtaglomerular apparatus.

24. The answer is 5 *[Chapter 4 II C 2].* The hundreds of finger-like microvilli comprising a brush border function to significantly increase the surface area available for absorption. Cilia, not microvilli, are characteristic of the upper airways and are often covered by a layer of mucus. Brush borders were so named by light microscopists to describe an easily seen, intensely stained layer with striations that are perpendicular, not parallel, to the surface. Microvilli, which are responsible for the striated pattern, were later discovered using the electron microscope.

25. The answer is 3 *[Chapter 11 V].* Lymph returns substances that have escaped from the blood into the interstitial fluid back to the venous system via one-way lymphatic vessels. Lymph comprises macromolecules and fluids that have escaped from the blood and mixed with the interstitial fluid. Molecules in the amorphous ground substance have many cross-linkages that form tissue-wide networks; therefore, these molecules do not enter the lymph vessels. Interstitial fluid, also called extracellular fluid, is located between cells; cellular fluid is contained within the cell membrane; and cytosol is located between the cell membrane and organelles. There are four body fluid compartments: cellular fluid, interstitial fluid, blood, and lymph. Erythrocytes and platelets do not leave the intact cardiovascular system, but macromolecules escape from exchange vessels (e.g., capillaries).

26. The answer is 4 *[Chapter 2 II C 3 a].* The omasum of the ruminant forestomach is characterized by laminae of variable length that are studded with prominent papillae. Papillae on omasal laminae are essential for the grinding function of that organ. This function is mediated by two peripheral layers of muscle derived from the lamina muscularis and one central muscle layer derived from the tunica muscularis. The two outer layers parallel the lamina muscularis; the central layer is perpendicular to it. The lining epithelium of the omasum is stratified squamous, as in the rumen and reticulum. Only the abomasum is lined with simple columnar epithelium.

27. The answer is 2 *[Chapter 5 II C 2].* The basement membrane, a continuous amorphous layer, lies beneath all epithelia, except in some small capillaries and lymphatic capillaries. It separates the epithelial layer from the underlying connective tissue but does not extend between epithelial cells. Loss of a continuous basement membrane is characteristic of invasive tumors, and its disruption is considered clinical evidence of metastasis. Type IV collagen forms highly cross-linked elastic networks rather than fibrils. The connective tissue may produce a reticular lamina composed of fibrillar collagen, but the portion of the basement membrane that is always present, the basal lamina, is produced by epithelia.

28. The answer is 3 *[Chapter 18 III A 2].* Following a number of mitotic divisions during which stem cell spermatogonia give rise to primary spermatocytes (a process referred to as spermatocytogenesis), each primary spermatocyte undergoes two meiotic divisions. The first meiotic division results in two secondary spermatocytes, and the second meiotic division produces four spermatids. This is not a process of differentiation. Differentiation occurs in a subsequent step called spermiogenesis, in which spermatids differentiate into spermatozoa.

29. The answer is 4 *[Chapter 14 II A 1 c, 3].* Neurosensory receptor cells are present only in the olfactory mucosa and the vomeronasal organ. Volatile substances from the mouth cavity are sucked into the blind-ending vomeronasal organ through the incisive duct. The suction is created by contraction of the blood vessels in the propria–submucosa of the vomeronasal organ. The substances are expelled when the vessels dilate. The vomeronasal organ is thought to play a role in male and female sexual behavior and in maternal behavior.

30. The answer is 4 *[Chapter 11 II B 2 c (2)].* Waves of depolarization that begin in the sinoatrial node are spread through the atrial myocardium to the atrioventricular node. The sinoatrial node (not the atrioventricular node) is innervated by the autonomic nervous system. The action potential is transmitted to the ventricular myocardium by specialized conductive cells that reach the apex of the heart first. The system then delivers the impulse closer and closer to the atrioventricular septum, creating a wave of contraction that squeezes the blood from the apex toward the pulmonary artery and aorta. The conductive cells from the atrioventricular node form the atrioventricular bundle, which passes through the subendocardial layer (not the subepicardium) of the ventricles until it branches into the myocardium.

31. The answer is 1 *[Chapter 8 II C 2 b (1)].* In the presence of basal lamina, collagen fibers, or elastic fibers (any of which could be exposed in a blood vessel with a damaged endothelium), platelets become sticky. This causes them to adhere to the fibrous material and to agglutinate with each other, forming a platelet plug. Their specific granules (alpha granules) contain clotting factors and growth factors. They take up the vasoconstrictor serotonin from the blood and store it in dense bodies, which are extruded through exocytosis during degranulation. The vasoconstrictor activity of serotonin helps prevent blood loss in damaged vessels. Platelets are not phagocytic, but they promote leukocytic phagocytosis of bacteria by sticking to the surface of the bacteria. Because one of the main functions of platelets is to promote clotting, they release anti-heparin. Heparin is an anti-clotting agent released by mast cells and basophils.

32. The answer is 5 *[Chapter 10 II B 1].* Myosin molecules are elongated dimeric (two-part) proteins that combine in a staggered overlapping pattern to form thick filaments. Thin filaments comprise polymers of globular actin (G-actin) and associated proteins. Only thick and thin filaments are contractile; the intermediate filaments in skeletal muscle cells support the arrays of contractile filaments and help to attach the thin filaments to the plasma membrane. Most microfilaments, which are components of thin filaments in skeletal muscle, are arranged in highly ordered arrays with thick filaments in the center of the muscle cell. In other cell types, microfilaments tend to be abundant near the cell membrane.

33. The answer is 4 *[Chapter 8 I A 1].* Immunoglobulins and other plasma proteins are components of blood plasma, the ground substance of blood. Hyaluronic acid is present in the ground substance of formed connective tissues and is especially abundant in soft tissues, such as loose connective tissue. Chondroitin sulfate is present primarily in cartilage matrix. Hemoglobin is confined within erythrocytes. Platelets are considered part of the cellular components of blood.

34. The answer is 1 *[Chapter 17 III D 2 b (2), V E 2].* Among the domestic mammals, only carnivores have an endotheliochorial placenta. In all other domestic mammals, the placenta is epitheliochorial. Fetal blood may be separated from maternal blood by as many as six layers: allantoic endothelium, chorioallantoic mesenchyme, chorionic (trophoblastic) capillary endothelium, uterine epithelium, endometrial connective tissue, and uterine capillary endothelium. In endotheliochorial placentae, the uterine epithelium and endometrial connective tissue are destroyed so that the chorionic epithelium is in direct contact with the uterine capillary endothelium.

35. The answer is 1 *[Chapter 5 I C].* Mesoderm, the middle of the three primary germ layers, gives rise to most connective tissue and most muscle. It also gives rise to two adult types of epithelium; namely, endothelium, which lines the cardiovascular system, and mesothelium, which lines the closed body cavities. In addition to mesoderm, the primary germ layers include ectoderm, the outermost layer, and entoderm, the innermost layer.

36. The answer is 4 *[Chapter 12 III B 3 a (5)].* Over 90% of developing T lymphocytes die and are phagocytosed by the many macrophages in the thymic cortex. During development, T lymphocytes undergoing clonal expansion in the cortex are pushed toward the medulla by incoming T progenitor cells, which enter the peripheral cortex. Eventually, the successful T lymphocytes enter postcapillary venules near the corticomedullary junction. Development is stimulated by cytokines [e.g., interleukin 1 (IL-1) from macrophages and thymosins from reticular epithelial cells]. Development of T cells includes acquisition of surface receptors for both "self" and "nonself" antigens.

37. The answer is 3 *[Chapter 21 II B 3 a (3)].* The color of the iris is dependent on the number of melanosomes. When many pigmented melanocytes are present, the iris appears brown. When only a few melanocytes are present together with a pigmented epithelium, the iris is blue. Lack of pigmentation in the stroma and epithelium makes the iris appear red in albinos. The stroma of loose connective tissue with many collagen bundles is well-vascularized. The stroma is covered anteriorly by a discontinuous mesothelial layer, but its posterior surface is covered by two layers of epithelial cells (the continuation of the epithelium covering the ciliary body). Unlike the epithelium on the ciliary processes, both epithelial layers on the iris are pigmented. The dilator muscle of the pupil is not located within the stroma of the iris because it differentiates from the anterior epithelial layer. The smooth muscle bundles of the sphincter muscle lie in the stroma near the pupillary margin. Granula iridica occur in ungulates and can be seen with the naked eye; they look like granules of varying sizes, representing focal proliferations of the epithelial layers of the iris.

38. The answer is 2 *[Chapter 7 II D 1 b (1) (b); Figure 7-2].* Cartilage has many cross-links between its proteoglycans (called chondromucoproteins) and hyaluronic acid, but proteo glycans in loose connective tissue do not bind to hyaluronic acid. In cartilage, a single filamentous hyaluronic acid polymer can anchor the protein cores of up to 200 proteoglycans. Because the other ends of the proteoglycans are bound electrostatically to collagen and to many layers of water molecules, the overall structure is rigid. Sulfated glycosaminoglycans are present in proteoglycans of both cartilage and loose connective tissue, and in both tissues their net negative charge is responsible for the binding of the proteoglycans with collagen and with solvation water.

39. The answer is 3 *[Chapter 6 II C 1 g (4) (b)]*. Macrophages secrete substances involved in healing, including several growth factors. Their appearance varies widely, depending on their functional state and the nature of any material they have phagocytosed. They phagocytose and destroy bacteria, but are not as specialized for bactericidal action as are neutrophils. They are considered resident cells of the connective tissue because they live in the tissues for several months (after only about 40 hours in the blood). However, they do not secrete extracellular matrix and fibers.

40. The answer is 5 *[Chapter 16 II A 3 d]*. The second meiotic division is an event that begins immediately after completion of the first meiotic division, around the time of ovulation. The second meiotic division is then arrested in metaphase; it resumes and is completed after penetration of the oocyte by the spermium. The oocyte is then called an ovum. When the two nuclei, also called pronuclei, merge, the cell is called a zygote.

41. The answer is 5 *[Chapter 10 III A 3 a]*. Cardiac cells bifurcate longitudinally, allowing anastomoses between chains of cells, which run in all directions. The tightly interwoven mass formed by this arrangement permits the atria and ventricles to squeeze the blood out of their lumens effectively. Fasciae adherentes and desmosomes, both of which are attachment types of intercellular junctions, are characteristic of the transverse portions of the intercalated disks that join the ends of cardiac muscle cells. Gap junctions are common between lateral cell membranes and lateral segments of intercalated disks. Each cardiac muscle cell is surrounded by basal lamina except where these junctions occur.

42. The answer is 1 *[Chapter 6 II C 1]*. Connective tissue cells include immigrants from the blood as well as cells derived from local mesenchymal cells. Connective tissue cells that produce elastic fibers also produce collagen fibers and often reticular fibers. Muscle cells (and myoepithelial cells) are specialized for contraction. Epithelial cells line the closed body cavities and secrete hormones.

43. The answer is 2 *[Chapter 11 III A]*. Smooth muscle is most abundant in the tunica media in most blood vessels but may also be present in the tunica interna and tunica externa. The internal elastic membrane is the outermost layer of the tunica interna; the outermost elastic lamina of the tunica media is called the external elastic membrane. Blood vessels are embedded in connective tissue and have no outer free surface; therefore, their outermost layer is a tunica externa that blends into the surrounding connective tissue. Vasomotor nerves terminate in or near the tunica media; they do not penetrate to the tunica interna.

44. The answer is 4 *[Chapter 8 II B 1 b (1)]*. The number of marginated neutrophils and monocytes can equal or surpass by severalfold the number of circulating cells, forming an important ready reserve of defense cells. Most cells are marginated only temporarily; some are attracted into the tissue, and some reenter the circulation. Once they have left the blood vessels, monocytes and neutrophils do not reenter the circulation. Marginated cells have their functional life ahead of them. In addition to the marginal pool, the bone marrow is a storage site for many leukocytes.

45. The answer is 1 *[Chapter 12 II A 2, B 2]*. B lymphocytes have antibodies on their cell membranes; T lymphocytes have antigen receptors on their surface. Both T and B lymphocytes are stimulated by antigens, although they may not respond to the same antigens. T lymphocytes, not B lymphocytes, have subcategories of regulatory cells and recognize malignant cells. T lymphocytes are the most abundant circulating lymphocytes, normally accounting for 60%–90% of the lymphocytes in the blood.

46. The answer is 3 *[Chapter 3 I C 1 b (1) (b)]*. Microtubules, other than those found in centrioles, cilia, and flagella, are labile structures that form and dissolve readily as needed in response to regulatory signals in the cytoplasm. However, microtubule formation is initiated only at microtubule-organizing centers, which may be present throughout the cytoplasm. The drugs colchicine and vincristine cause net depolymerization of microtubules, thereby inhibiting functions that require microtubules.

47. The answer is 3 *[Chapter 18 V B 1 b].* The ductus epididymidis has a muscle layer that increases in thickness from the proximal to distal end (i.e., from the head to the tail). Contraction of the muscle layer moves the spermatozoa into the tail, where they are stored prior to ejaculation. The columnar cells of the lining epithelium do not have motile cilia; they have long microvilli (stereocilia) that participate in resorptive activity of these cells. Testicular fluid is resorbed in the efferent ductules and ductus epididymidis and does not contribute to the movement of spermatozoa through the ductus epididymidis, and neither does the continued production of spermatozoa. Flagellar forward movement of spermatozoa is acquired in the tail of the epididymis, but actual movements do not occur prior to ejaculation.

48. The answer is 4 *[Chapter 11 IV C 2 b (1) (b) (i)].* Capillaries in most of the central nervous system (CNS) constitute a blood–brain barrier, which is possible because of a paucity or absence of transcytotic vesicles and the relatively impermeable tight junctions between endothelial cells. Except in a few specialized regions, capillaries in the CNS are continuous (not fenestrated) capillaries, the most common type of capillaries in the body. Capillaries in the CNS, unlike other capillaries, are not surrounded by reticular fibers.

49. The answer is 1 *[Chapter 6 II C 2 a (1)].* The contents of the specific granules of basophils and mast cells are very similar (in some species they are identical), and their functions are also the same. For many years it was suspected that mast cells were basophils that had entered the connective tissue, but it is now known that they arise from different stem cells. Neutrophils and eosinophils are also white blood cells, but their morphology and functions are totally different from those of basophils. Plasma cells are derived from white blood cells but are structurally and functionally different from basophils. Pericytes are not blood cells.

50. The answer is 2 *[Chapter 4 II B 1 a].* The microtubules that form the core of cilia are arranged in 9 peripheral doublets and 2 central singlets, for a total of 20. Centrioles differ in structure from the shafts of cilia because they have 9 peripheral triplets and no central microtubules. Microfilaments are found in the cores of microvilli, not axonemes. Cilia are about two and one-half times larger in diameter than microvilli, and they are much longer than most microvilli.

51. The answer is 5 *[Chapter 13 II A 3 a (1) (b) (i)].* Fungiform papillae contain taste buds in their surface epithelium and are therefore classified as gustatory papillae. Filiform papillae, conical papillae, lenticular papillae, and marginal papillae are mechanical papillae. Filiform papillae assist in the prehension of food in large ruminants, the uptake of fluids in carnivores, and grooming in cats. Conical papillae and lenticular papillae help move food toward the pharynx. Marginal papillae are present in newborn carnivores and swine; they contribute to a tight seal around the teat during suckling.

52. The answer is 1 *[Chapter 10 IV B 1].* Bundles of thick and thin filaments run in many directions through smooth muscle cells. Many intermediate filaments are present. Intermediate filaments provide support for the contractile filaments and transmit the forces they generate to the stroma and, hence, to the rest of the tissue. There is no T tubule system, but the cells do contain sarcoplasmic reticulum. A basal lamina surrounds the cells but not completely; it is absent in the areas of intercellular junctions, which are common in many smooth muscle tissues.

53. The answer is 3 *[Chapter 7 II D].* Cartilage is classified as hyaline, elastic, or fibrocartilage on the basis of the types of fibers present. Immature cartilage is simply an early stage of mature cartilage, not a different type. Cartilage that arises in mesenchyme is no different from that formed in other tissues. Both hyaline cartilage and fibrocartilage may be attached to bone, and the shape of cartilage is not a basis for classification.

54. The answer is 2 *[Chapter 6 II C 2 b].* Immigrant cells are white blood cells that normally enter the connective tissue only during an inflammation reaction. Neutrophils, also called microphages, are immigrant cells that are attracted in large numbers by substances released in an inflamed area. Mast cells resemble white blood cells in that they are derived from bone marrow precursors, but they are normal occupants of the connective tissue. Macrophages (histiocytes) arise from white blood cells (monocytes), but they are considered resident connective tissue cells because they are normally present. Mesenchymal cells are embryonic connective tissue cells and pericytes are multipotential cells of the connective tissue; both are resident cells.

55. The answer is 2 *[Chapter 3 I]*. Microtubules, along with microfilaments and intermediate filaments, are classified as cytoskeletal elements. Microvilli are finger-like projections of the cell surface that contain a core of microfilaments. The nuclear envelope and smooth endoplasmic reticulum (sER) are membranous organelles that are derived from the rough endoplasmic reticulum (rER). The endoplasmic cytosol is the fluid cytoplasmic matrix that surrounds organelles and other cytoplasmic structures.

56. The answer is 3 *[Chapter 7 III B 1 b; Chapter 19 II D 2 a]*. Osteocytes remain functionally important after they are surrounded by matrix. They are essential for maintaining the bone matrix, which disintegrates if the cells are killed, and they help maintain the appropriate levels of blood calcium and other ions. Because they are joined by gap junctions, their activities are coordinated. Osteoclasts form by fusion of blood-derived monocytes. They are not joined to the other types of bone cells. Although osteoclasts are capable of the most massive breakdown of bone matrix, osteocytes are also able to destroy the matrix. They do this by releasing proteases (including collagenase) and organic acids, not by phagocytosis. Osteocytic osteolysis affects only a very small amount of matrix surrounding each lacuna, but its cumulative effect is significant in maintaining calcium homeostasis.

57. The answer is 3 *[Chapter 17 III B 2]*. When part of the endometrium is shed together with the fetal placenta at parturition, the placenta is referred to as "deciduate." In domestic carnivores, part of the uterus, called the decidua (derived from the Latin term *deciduus,* which means "fallen off"), is lost at parturition. "Villous" refers to the presence of villi, projections from the chorion that increase the area of fetal–maternal association. The term "diffuse" describes the distribution of villi or folds on the chorionic sac. "Epitheliochorial" describes the apposition of the endometrial and chorionic epithelia, and "cotyledonary" refers to the presence of cotyledons (i.e., tufts of chorionic villi).

58. The answer is 1 *[Chapter 19 II C 2 a (1) (d)]*. Intrafollicular thyroid colloid is mainly iodinated thyroglobulin, a glycoprotein and the storage form of thyroid hormone. The hormone becomes activated by proteolytic processing of the iodinated thyroglobulin in phagolysosomes into active thyroxine (T_4) and triiodothyronine (T_3). Secretory granules originating from the Golgi complex (in which no storage occurs) contain the noniodinated thyroglobulin. Endocytotic vesicles take up iodinated thyroglobulin from the follicular lumen and merge with lysosomes to become phagolysosomes, but they do not store iodinated thyroglobulin.

59. The answer is 5 *[Chapter 6 II B 2 a]*. Reticular fibers are composed primarily of collagen; but unlike collagen fibers, they have a surface coating of glycoproteins and proteoglycans. They are not acidophilic; in fact, they are not stained by routine methods. However, they are periodic acid–Schiff (PAS) positive and can be stained with silver stains. Reticular fibers are composed of loosely packed fibrils, as opposed to the denser arrangement of fibrils in collagen. They form networks (hence the term "reticular"), not bundles. In smooth muscle, where they are abundant, reticular fibers are produced by the smooth muscle cells.

60. The answer is 1 *[Chapter 6 II C 1 g (3); Chapter 8 II B 3 c (1)]*. The mononuclear phagocyte system (MPS) comprises macrophages throughout the body. Members of the MPS present antigenic fragments to lymphocytes to initiate the immune response. MPS cells appear quite different in different tissue, ranging from small cells called microglia in the central nervous system (CNS) to large, multinucleated osteoclasts in bone. They are called macrophages when they are active in the tissue. They are derived from monocytes, which are a type of agranulocyte. Microphages, which arise from neutrophils, are *not* members of the MPS. Neutrophils and eosinophils also exhibit receptor-mediated phagocytosis.

61. The answer is 5 *[Chapter 4 II A 3 b]*. Metabolic coupling refers to the spread of nutrients, ions, and regulatory molecules through groups of cells, and electrical coupling occurs when waves of depolarization are passed directly from one conductive cell to another. Both processes are accomplished by gap junctions, which allow the attached cells to act as a unit, rather than independently. Gap junctions are named for the very narrow gap that separates the lipid bilayers of adjacent cells. Initially, these junctions appeared to be fused, but when viewed with an electron microscope at high magnification and with good resolution, the gap became apparent. Gap junctions are especially abundant between embryonic cells, where they are believed to be important routes for communicating developmental instructions during morphogenesis. Membrane proteins are aligned in adjacent membranes to form channels whose lumens join the cytoplasm of the two cells, but only ions and small molecules are able to pass.

62. The answer is 4 *[Chapter 7 II A 3, III B 3].* Bone is richly vascularized with nutrient capillaries. In fact, compact bone is organized around its capillary supply. Both bone and cartilage (except for articular cartilage) are in contact with dense connective tissue. The deep (cambium) layer of both perichondrium and periosteum contains osteoprogenitor cells. Whether they differentiate into chondroblasts or osteoblasts is determined by the concentration of oxygen in the tissue. If oxygen tension is low, chondroblasts are favored; if it is high, osteoblasts develop. The lamellae and cement lines of bone matrix are visible under the light microscope.

63. The answer is 2 *[Chapter 20 III B 1].* The mode of secretion in sebaceous glands is holocrine (i.e., following synthesis of the secretory product, the entire cell is secreted). This process necessitates continuous replacement of cells by stem cells, which are located in the periphery of the secretory alveoli. Sebaceous glands are connected to hair follicles via a short duct lined with stratified squamous epithelium. They empty their secretory product into this duct, where it mixes with the cells of the disintegrating inner root sheath to form sebum.

64. The answer is 2 *[Chapter 9 III B 1 b (2) (a) (iii)].* The sole plate is an oval area of sarcoplasm, subjacent to the motor end-plate, from which myofibrils are conspicuously lacking. It contains numerous nuclei, rough endoplasmic reticulum (rER), free ribosomes, mitochondria, and glycogen.

65. The answer is 1 *[Chapter 5 II C 2 c (2) (c); V].* Migration of epithelial cells through the basement membrane is characteristic of malignant neoplasms, not normal wound healing. Although normally nonmotile, epithelial cells may exhibit ameboid movement to cover surface wounds. Renewal rates vary from a few days in some epithelia to years in others. Division of stem cells to produce one stem cell and one cell that gives rise to differentiated epithelial cells ensures ongoing cell renewal.

66. The answer is 2 *[Figure 6-2; Chapter 8 II B 3 b].* Macrophages, which are derived from monocytes, do not initiate the inflammatory response; however, they contribute to inflammation responses that have been initiated by other cells. Macrophages are also important in promotion of the healing process, in that they secrete growth factors and antigenic factors. They phagocytose bacteria, viruses, and other particles in the circulating blood, as well as in formed tissues. Alveolar macrophages of the lung also exhibit nonselective phagocytosis of dust particles. Macrophages secrete tumor necrosis factor α (TNFα).

67. The answer is 2 *[Chapter 20 III A 1 a (3)].* Both the root and the shaft of a hair have three layers: the outermost cuticle of the hair, the cortex, and the medulla. The internal root sheath is part of the hair follicle, which surrounds the hair root. In secondary hairs or underhairs, the medulla may indeed be absent. The cells of the cuticle of the hair have species-specific characteristics that are of importance in forensic medicine. The hair bulb is the thick terminal or proximal portion of the hair root; it is located above the dermal papilla and is predominantly made up of hair matrix cells.

68. The answer is 3 *[Chapter 11 V B 1].* Lymph capillaries exist throughout the body, except the central nervous system (CNS), parts of the eye, bone, and cartilage. They are present in some, but not all, lymphatic organs. Lymph capillaries are more permeable than capillaries and postcapillary venules. Their basal lamina is discontinuous, and they are held open by attachments between endothelial cells and surrounding tissue elements. In the intestine, they are called lacteals because of the milky appearance of their contents.

69. The answer is 4 *[Chapter 19 II A 1 b (2); III A 2]*. Insulin secretion by pancreatic B cells is regulated by blood glucose level and is independent of adenohypophysial hormones. Following hypophysectomy, the secretions of thyroid follicular cells, the cells of the adrenal zonae reticularis and fasciculata, and testicular interstitial cells decrease and eventually cease because of the lack of adenohypophysial stimulating factors or hormones. Morphologic changes (cellular atrophy, reduction of cellular organelles involved in secretion) parallel the functional changes.

70. The answer is 3 *[Chapter 15 II B 1 d]*. The macula densa is formed by the distal, not proximal, tubule. The proximal convoluted tubule is located in the cortical labyrinth. Its continuation is the proximal straight tubule in a medullary ray, where it descends as the thick descending limb of the loop of the nephron into the outer medulla and continues as the thin tubule into the inner medulla. The ascending limb of the loop of the nephron comprises the ascending thin tubule and the distal straight tubule. A dense microvillous apical border is characteristic of the proximal tubule, but it is more extensive in the convoluted portion. Water is reabsorbed in the proximal tubule; it passively follows the active transport of sodium through the tubular epithelial cells.

71. The answer is 5 *[Chapter 20 II C]*. The hypodermis is a flexible layer of loose connective tissue, which enables the skin to readily shift over hard or rough bony surfaces without being damaged. Like all loose connective tissue, it has a rich blood supply and it contains packets of adipose cells that are both structural (e.g., footpads) and metabolic (e.g., back fat of pigs). In certain regions of the integument (e.g., hoof, horn), the hypodermis is lacking.

72. The answer is 4 *[Chapter 12 I B 3 b, II B 3 a]*. T lymphocytes are activated by interaction with a macrophage or an antigen-presenting cell, not by the complement system. Primary functions of the complement system include lysing foreign cells and bacteria, inducing degranulation of mast cells and basophils, attracting neutrophils, and enhancing phagocytosis, all activities that generally result in inflammation.

73. The answer is 3 *[Chapter 6 III F 2 a]*. Brown adipose tissue is limited to certain localized deposits in the body, primarily the axilla, interscapular region, mediastinum, mesenteries, and around the kidneys. It is multilocular and its many mitochondria, which oxidize lipids to produce heat, impart a brown hue.

74. The answer is 4 *[Chapter 8 III A 1 b]*. Myeloid elements are those that develop in the red bone marrow (i.e., erythrocytes, granulocytes, platelets, monocytes, and lymphocytic stem cells). Lymphocyte progenitor cells arise in the bone marrow, but they migrate to lymphatic organs to produce lymphocytes.

75. The answer is 4 *[Chapter 9 III A 1 c–d]*. Presynaptic terminals normally do not contain lysosomes; worn-out organelles are transported in a retrograde manner to the perikaryon for disposal. Synaptic vesicles are prominent organelles in a presynaptic element, as are empty synaptic vesicles (i.e., synaptic vesicular membranes that have undergone endocytosis after transmitter release). Both microtubules and neurofilaments are present in presynaptic elements. Mitochondria supply energy for the presynaptic element.

76. The answer is 4 *[Chapter 19 I A 3]*. Single endocrine cells are present in the lining of the gastrointestinal and respiratory systems, which are lined with simple columnar or pseudostratified columnar epithelium, respectively, but not in those portions of the digestive system lined with stratified squamous epithelium.

77. The answer is 5 *[Chapter 14 II E 1 b (1)]*. Bronchioles are lined by simple cuboidal or columnar epithelium that includes ciliated and Clara cells (bronchiolar exocrine cells), but not goblet cells. Both glands and cartilage are lacking in bronchioles, but both are present in the propria–submucosa of bronchi. Glands are sometimes present in the early bronchioles of certain species.

78. The answer is 2 *[Chapter 19 II E 1 a]*. The zona pellucida is a homogeneous amorphous glycoprotein layer surrounding primary oocytes in secondary and older ovarian follicles.

79. The answer is 4 *[Chapter 9 IV B 2 a]*. Oligodendrocytes are the myelin-forming cells in white matter, but they are also present in gray matter, where they are called satellite oligodendrocytes because they are closely associated with neuronal perikarya. In most of the central nervous system (CNS), the glia limitans is formed by astrocytes, and both types of astrocytes participate in its formation. There are, however, locations in the CNS, such as the ventral hypothalamus (floor of the third ventricle) and circumventricular organs (e.g., subfornical organ) where long basal processes of ependymal cells (tanycytes) project to the brain surface and participate in the formation of the glia limitans. Microglial cells are dormant phagocytes that become activated by appropriate stimuli. Myelin sheaths in the peripheral nervous system (PNS) are formed by Schwann cells.

80. The answer is 5 *[Chapter 3 I C 4 b]*. Centrioles can be seen in good light microscopic preparations, especially if the tissue is stained with iron hematoxylin. They appear as minute rods surrounded by a small, clear area, the cytocentrum. Replication of centrioles is the first event that precedes cell division. Centrioles organize the mitotic apparatus and act as poles toward which chromosomes move during cell division; therefore, they are essential for cell division.

81. The answer is 5 *[Chapter 22 II B]*. The secretory product of the apocrine ceruminous glands is sweat, which combines with sebum produced by the sebaceous glands and with sloughed squamous epithelial cells from the stratum corneum of the epithelium to form cerumen.

82. The answer is 5 *[Chapter 13 II D 2 a (2); Figure 13-7]*. Goblet cells are present neither in fundic glands nor in the gastric lining epithelium, but they occur throughout the entire intestine. Mucous neck cells, parietal cells, chief cells, enteroendocrine cells, and undifferentiated cells are all found in the gastric fundic glands.

83. The answer is 4 *[Chapter 21 IV C 2]*. The lamina propria is a highly vascularized loose connective tissue that contains many lymphatic nodules. The vascularity and lymphatic nodules are visible grossly, especially when conjunctivitis occurs. The third eyelid is a conjunctival fold. Conjunctival epithelium is continuous with the corneal epithelium and the epithelium covering the free surface of the eyelid. The epithelium contains many goblet cells.

84. The answer is 4 *[Chapter 9 IV B 1 b (4)]*. Astrocytes do not become phagocytic in reaction to injury (e.g., stab wound, abscess). Instead, they proliferate and form a multilayered scar, analogous to the glia limitans, that reestablishes the protected environment of the central nervous system (CNS). In both craniospinal and autonomic ganglia, satellite cells (a form of Schwann cell) are intimately associated with ganglion cells. In the CNS, satellite cells are likewise present; they are oligodendrocytes associated with neurons. Synapses in white matter are ensheathed by astrocytes and are thus isolated from the surrounding neuropil.

85–90. The answers are: 85-4 *[Chapter 2 IV C 1]*, **86-3** *[Chapter 2 I D 3 a, E]*, **87-4** *[Chapter 2 IV A 1]*, **88-7** *[Chapter 2 III A 1]*, **89-7** *[Chapter 1 II C 2]*, **90-1** *[Chapter 2 I A 2]*. Mitochondria are the organelles of cellular respiration. They use oxygen from the air to oxidize the products of digestion, converting the energy from food to adenosine triphosphate (ATP), a high-energy compound that can be used to power other cellular reactions.

Lysosomes have roles in both defense and disease. They are important elements in the defense system because they contain enzymes that can kill or break down most foreign material that may threaten the cell. However, the release of lysosomal enzymes from wounded tissue or dead cells of the defense system contributes to tissue damage in inflamed areas. When phagocytic cells encounter foreign substances that the lysosomes cannot digest, particle diseases may result. Because lysosomes fuse with phagosomes, they are especially vulnerable to the effects of exogenous substances. A congenital lack of certain lysosomal enzymes causes storage diseases or the inability to fight some types of infection. Because lysosomes are not immediately essential for cell survival, lysosomes are more likely than other organelles to have genetic deficiencies.

Mitochondria, which are believed to be derived from bacteria, fuse with each other, change shape, and move about the cell. They also divide, which is how they reproduce.

Smooth endoplasmic reticulum (sER) is formed by rough endoplasmic reticulum (rER). The ribosomes of rER are necessary to synthesize the protein components of the sER membrane.

Rough endoplasmic reticulum (rER) is essential for lysosome production because it is the site where the lysosomal contents, which are primarily proteins, are synthesized and compartmentalized. Lysosomes undergo final processing in the Golgi complex.

Multivesicular bodies are vesicles that contain smaller vesicles and function as lysosomes.

91–92. The answers are: 91-1 *[Chapter 8 II B 5 b (3)]*, **92-4** *[Chapter 8 II B 6 b (1)]*. Eosinophils phagocytose antigen–antibody complexes (antibodies are produced by lymphocytes) and granules released by basophils and mast cells. Their numbers increase in the blood during allergic reactions and also during inflammation responses and parasitic infections. Although many specific facts have been determined about eosinophils, their functions are not yet well understood.

Receptor-mediated degranulation of basophils and mast cells, which closely resemble each other in many ways, initiates the inflammation response.

93–96. The answers are: 93-3 *[Chapter 5 IV C 4 a; Figure 5-7]*, **94-1** *[Chapter 5 IV C 4 b; Figure 5-7]*, **95-1** *[Chapter 5 IV C 4 c; Figure 5-7]*, **96-3** *[Chapter 5 IV C 4 a; Figure 5-7]*. Mucous cells release mucin, which combines with water to form mucus after it is released from the cell. The mucous cells are very lightly stained except for their heterochromatic flattened basal nuclei. Most of the cytoplasm is filled with unstained secretory granules, which gives it a foamy appearance.

Serous cells produce a watery protein-rich secretory product. Both mucous and serous cells are present in this figure, but the serous cells are more darkly stained and their nuclei are round or oval. The serous cells that have been pushed to the periphery of the secretory unit form more darkly stained crescents, called demilunes, around the more lightly stained mucous cells.

Mucus, the secretory product of mucous cells, is rich in acidic glycoproteins.

97–98. The answers are: 97-4 *[Chapter 11 III B 2 a]*, **98-1** *[Chapter 11 IV A 1 b]*. Muscular arteries are relatively well innervated and are also responsive to local chemical signals, enabling them to regulate the rate of blood flow to specific organs and organ systems. Arterioles and metarterioles are within organs; therefore, the domains they control are much smaller. Elastic arteries are conducting arteries that are not equipped to divert blood flow between regions.

Arterioles, which are responsible for half of the total resistance in the circulatory system, are the major regulators of blood pressure. Capillaries have no muscle in their walls to affect the blood pressure. When blood enters the capillaries, it is already close to the pressure of the surrounding tissue. Elastic arteries and muscular arteries are important in maintaining the blood pressure, but less so than arterioles.

99–103. The answers are: 99-2 *[Chapter 12 IV E 2 a]*, **100-4** *[Chapter 12 I C 3 a (3), IV B 2 b, 3 b (2)]*, **101-1** *[Chapter 12 III B 3 b]*, **102-2** *[Chapter 12 IV E 1]*, **103-3** *[Chapter 8 III A 1 b; Chapter 12 IV D 2 b (4)]*. The structure of hemal nodes is similar to that of lymph nodes except that their wide sinuses, including the subcapsular sinus, are filled with blood.

M cells in Peyer's patches are attenuated epithelial cells that take up antigens in the lumen of the ileum and present them to underlying lymphocytes. Adjacent absorptive cells take up immunoglobulin A (IgA) dimers produced by plasma cells in the Peyer's patches. These cells synthesize transport proteins that attach to the IgA dimers, and they secrete the resulting complexes into the intestinal lumen, where they can inactivate antigens before they have a chance to enter the tissue.

The medulla of the thymus is believed to be the site where mast cells differentiate from marrow-derived progenitor cells.

Among the domestic species, hemal nodes are present primarily in ruminants.

The spleen is an erythropoietic organ in fetal life and can resume that activity in adult animals if necessary.

Index

Note: Page numbers in italics denote illustrations, those followed by *t* denote tables, those followed by Q denote questions, and those followed by E denote explanations.

D

E

F

G

M

N

R

S